HANDBOOK OF

Carcinogens and Hazardous Substances

HANDBOOK OF

Carcinogens and Hazardous Substances

Chemical and Trace Analysis

Edited by MALCOLM C. BOWMAN
Division of Chemistry
National Center for Toxicological Research
U.S. Food and Drug Administration
Jefferson, Arkansas

MARCEL DEKKER, INC. New York and Basel

This volume was edited by Malcolm C. Bowman in his private capacity. No official support or endorsement by the U.S. Food and Drug Administration is intended or should be inferred.

Library of Congress Cataloging in Publication Data
Main entry under title:

Handbook of carcinogens and hazardous substances.

Includes bibliographies and index.
Contents: An overview of chemical carcinogens Thomas J. Haley -- Alkylating agents Alexej B. Borkovec and Charles W. Woods -- Aromatic amines and azo compounds Charles R. Nony -- [etc.]
1. Carcinogens--Analysis. I. Bowman, Malcolm C., [date].
RC268.6.H35 1982 616.99'4071 82-9779
ISBN O-8247-1683-3 AACR2

MARCEL DEKKER, INC.
270 Madison Avenue, New York, New York 10016

Current printing (last digit):
10 9 8 7 6 5 4 3 2 1

PRINTED IN THE UNITED STATES OF AMERICA

Preface

Within the last decade, chemical toxicology has been highlighted by the accumulation of considerable quantities of new analytical data, such as the isolation and identification of chemicals, metabolites, reaction products, and adducts of body constituents, as well as by the development of new and improved analytical equipment and techniques.

One will find a wealth of information related to toxicology, and particularly to the use of analytical chemistry in this field in the ten chapters of this volume. This series of subjects may be read for pleasure by the specialist or for profit by the student and junior investigator. The book will be helpful to research workers who wish to obtain an up-to-date picture outside the purview of their own specialty. This is especially important because of the plethora of regulations dealing with carcinogens.

These chapters are written by experts in their particular field of endeavor. They present their topics in a stimulating and interesting manner without the detractions of obfuscating minutiae.

Malcolm C. Bowman

Contributors

WILLIAM M. BLAKEMORE Research Chemist, Division of Chemistry, National Center for Toxicological Research, U.S. Food and Drug Administration, Jefferson, Arkansas

ALEXEJ B. BORKOVEC Chief, Insect Reproduction Laboratory, Agricultural Research Center, U.S. Department of Agriculture, Beltsville, Maryland

DAVID H. FINE Director of Research, New England Institute for Life Sciences, Waltham, Massachusetts

LAWRENCE FISHBEIN Acting Deputy Director, Office of Scientific Intelligence, National Center for Toxicological Research, U.S. Food and Drug Administration, Jefferson, Arkansas

THOMAS J. HALEY Science Advisor to the Director, Office of Scientific Intelligence, National Center for Toxicological Research, U.S. Food and Drug Administration, Jefferson, Arkansas

EDWARD D. HELTON* Senior Research Chemist, Molecular Biology, National Center for Toxicological Research, U.S. Food and Drug Administration, Jefferson, Arkansas

PETER W. JONES† Electric Power Research Institute, Palo Alto, California

Present affiliations:

*Chief, Division of Biochemical Toxicology, Associate Professor of Chemistry and Biology, Primate Research Institute, New Mexico State University, Holloman Air Force Base, New Mexico
†President, Peter Jones & Associates, Morgan Hill, California

IRA S. KRULL* Senior Scientist, New England Institute for Life Sciences, Waltham, Massachusetts

MILTON A. LUKE Supervisory Chemist, Executive Director of Regional Operations, U.S. Food and Drug Administration, Los Angeles, California

HERBERT T. MASUMOTO Pesticide Specialist, Executive Director of Regional Operations, U.S. Food and Drug Administration, Los Angeles, California

CHARLES R. NONY Research Chemist, Division of Chemistry, National Center for Toxicological Research, U.S. Food and Drug Administration, Jefferson, Arkansas

ALBERT E. POHLAND Bureau of Foods, U.S. Food and Drug Administration, Washington, D.C.

ROBERT H. PURDY Foundation Scientist, Organic and Biological Chemistry, Southwest Foundation for Research and Education, San Antonio, Texas

CHARLES W. THORPE Bureau of Foods, U.S. Food and Drug Administration, Washington, D.C.

MARY C. WILLIAMS Associate Foundation Scientist, Department of Clinical Sciences and Reproductive Biology, Southwest Foundation for Research and Education, San Antonio, Texas

CHARLES W. WOODS Research Chemist, Agricultural Research Service, U.S. Department of Agriculture, Beltsville, Maryland

Present affiliation:

*Senior Scientist, Institute of Chemical Analysis, Applications, and Forensic Science, Northeastern University, Boston, Massachusetts

Contents

HANDBOOK OF

Carcinogens and Hazardous Substances

1

An Overview of Chemical Carcinogens

THOMAS J. HALEY National Center for Toxicological Research, U.S. Food and Drug Administration, Jefferson, Arkansas

I. INTRODUCTION

From a historical point of view, the association of scrotal cancer with soot and the lack of bathing by chimney sweeps noted by Sir Percivall Pott represents the beginning of the field of chemical carcinogenesis. His precise description follows:

> Everybody is acquainted with the disorders to which painters, plummers, glaziers, and the workers in white lead are liable; but there is a disease as peculiar to a certain set of people which has not, at least to my knowledge, been publicly noticed; I mean the chimney sweepers' cancer. . . .
>
> The disease seems to derive its origin from a lodgment of soot in the rugae of the scrotum, and at first not to be a disease of the habit. In other cases of a cancerous nature, in which the habit is too frequently concerned, we have not often so fair a prospect of success by the removal of the distempered part; and are obliged to be content with means, which I wish I could say were truly palliative. But here the subjects are young, in general good health (at least at first), the disease brought on them by their occupation, and in all probability local; which last circumstance may, I think, be fairly presumed from its always seizing the same part: all this makes it (at first) a very different case from cancer which appears in an elderly man, whose fluids are become acrimonius from time, as well as in other cases [1].

Pott's reference to occupationally induced cancer refers to Hill's description of "polypusses" of the nasal cavity resulting from excessive use of snuff. Hill wrote:

> Whether or not polypusses, which attend Snuff-takers, are absolutely caused by that custom: or whether the principles of the disorder were there before, and Snuff only irritated the parts, and hastened the mischief, I shall not pretend to determine: but even supposing the latter to be the case, the damage is certainly more than the indulgence is worth: for who is able to say, that the Snuff is not the absolute cause, or that he has not the seeds of such a disorder which Snuff will bring into action. With respect to cancers of the nose, they are as dreadful and as fatal as any others. . . .
>
> It is evident therefore that no man should venture upon Snuff, who is not sure that he is not far liable to a cancer: and no man can be sure of that. [2]

Apparently, there exists a lack of appreciation regarding the role that occupation plays in cancer induction. Two hundred and four years after Pott's report, some coke oven workers are still dying of lung cancer caused by the same chemicals [3]. A similar situation exists with regard to lung cancer induced by radon daughter products in uranium miners, where the cause was enunciated in 1879 and proven in 1944 [4, 5]. Arsenic-induced lung and lymphatic cancer are other examples that clearly show what results from poor industrial hygienic controls of a known hazard [6-10]. Bladder cancer caused by exposure to aromatic amines was first reported in 1895 and is still a major cause of death in American workers [11-13]. Asbestos workers and their families are still being subjected to lung fibrosis and cancer, even though these pathological findings were described as long ago as 1907 [14-17]. As if to prove that our occupationally induced problems are never ending, vinyl chloride was shown to be a potent inducer of angiosarcoma of the liver in workers in the polymer industry [18]. Lately, benzene, in addition to being a producer of aplastic anemia, has been shown to induce leukemia in workers [19]. Ethylenethiourea, a neoprene rubber accelerator and curing agent for polyacrylate rubber, has caused thyroid and liver cancer in mice and may well do the same in humans [20]. Another curing agent of concern is 4,4'-methylene-bis(2-chloroaniline), which causes cancer in animals and skin lesions in humans [21]. Last, but not least, are the polychlorinated biphenyls (PCBs). Malignant melanoma and liver cancer have been associated with industrial exposure to these compounds [22,23].

One of the reasons that detection of carcinogenic chemicals takes so long is the inability of the investigator to find an animal model that duplicates the cancer observed in humans. This is illustrated by the fact that Pott [1] found scrotal cancer in 1775, but it was not until

1914-1915 that Japanese workers produced cancer of the skin of the rabbit ear following prolonged painting with coal tar [24]. Although latency is probably involved, not all species respond to a given carcinogen in the same target organ. Another reason is that, in the past, it was not possible to separate complex mixtures into their component parts and then identify the active chemicals. Extensive work on coal tar, including the production of synthetic coal tar, resulted in the identification in 1932 of a fluorescent fraction that contained 1,2:5,6-dibenzanthracene and 3,4-benzpyrene [25-30]. Further work led to the discovery of methylcholanthrene [31,32]. The isolation and synthesis of these chemical carcinogens were aided by the development of analytical procedures which allowed the investigators to follow each step during the isolation and synthesis in the processes.

This volume has been written with the idea of bringing up to date the various analytical methods used in the identification, separation, and quantitation of both new and old carcinogens, thereby enabling the investigator to obtain valid results. Throughout this discussion of chemical carcinogens we will be speaking of target organs first defined by Ehrlich, who stated:

> I have made extensive experiments with many hundreds of different compounds, and in all of these I have discovered only one substance to which I am inclined to ascribe substituting action on protoplasm. This substance, vinylamine, discovered by Gabriel and described by him in a masterly manner, is formed by abstracting bromine from bromoethylamine by means of potassium thus bromoethylamine forms vinylamine. Since then, however, Marckwald has shown convincingly (1900-1901) that this substance cannot, as was supposed, contain a double bond (ethylene linkage), for it does not reduce permanganate at ordinary temperature nor take up bromine. It can therefore only possess the constitution of a dimethyleneimine. [33]

II. ALKYLATING AGENTS

It has been shown that alkylating agents induce cancer by interacting with sensitive groups in DNA [34]. The therapeutic use of alkylating agents has resulted in cancer in patients; 245 workers, exposed occupationally and followed for 20 years, were shown to have developed malignant tumors, especially bronchial carcinoma, bladder carcinoma, and leukemia [35]. These compounds, because of their N, S, Cl, or P atoms, can readily be determined by gas chromatography using the appropriate detector. 1-Phenyl-3,3-dimethyltriazene, phenylmonomethyltriazene, and 1-(pyridyl-3)-3,3-dimethyltriazene and its N-oxide have all been shown to be potent alkylating agents which induce a variety of tumors in experimental animals [36]. Data from preclinical investigations of a comprehensive list of alkylating agents in cancer chemotherapy were

Table 1 Naturally Occurring Alkylating Agents and Their Toxicities to Male Rats

Alkaloid	LD_{50} in male rats (mg/kg)
Heliosupine	60
Lasiocarpine	72
Seneciphylline	77
Senecionine	85
Latifoline	125
Heleurine	140
Monocrotaline	175
Echimidine	200
Spectabiline	220
Cynaustine	260
7-Angelylheliotridine	260
Heliotrine	300
Echinatine	350
Supinine	450
Rinderine	550
Europine	>1000
Intermediate + lycopsamine	>1000
Heliotridine	1200
Heliotrine N-oxide	5000

Source: Ref. 38.

reported by Goldin and Wood [37]. Naturally occurring alkylating agents such as the pyrrolizidine alkaloids have also been extensively investigated; some of these compounds, together with their toxicities to rats, are listed in Table 1 [38]. Their alkylating activity appears to be related to the cleavage of the alkyl oxygen of the allylic ester group. Members of the cycad family of plants produce cycasin, β-D-glucosyloxyazoxymethane, which is degraded to its aglycone, methylazoxymethanol, a very potent alkylating agent which has caused sickness and death in humans who consumed unprepared or poorly prepared cycad seed ground into flour [39]. The insect chemosterilants (derivatives of aziridine) Tepa, Metepa, Tretamine, and Apholate have been widely used and, as a result, have contributed substantially to environmental pollution. Although their mode of action is poorly understood, they are potent alkylating agents [40]. Other alkylating agents in current use include the methanesulfonates, epoxides, and ethyleneimines. The use of ethylene oxide and propylene oxide as sterilizing agents gives rise to persistent toxic chlorohydrins, which are potent carcinogens. Another sterilizant, β-propionolactone (widely used), is

Table 2 Common Azo Dyes and Pigments and Their Color Index Number

Dye or pigment	Color Index number	Dye or pigment	Color Index number
	Benzidine-based		
Mordant Yellow 36	14135	Direct Blue 6	22610
Pigment Red 39	21080	Direct Brown 1	30045
Direct Red 28	22120	Direct Brown 1A	30110
Direct Orange 8	22130	Direct Brown 154	30120
Direct Red 10	22145	Direct Brown 6	30140
Direct Red 13	22155	Direct Brown 95	30145
Direct Red 37	22240	Direct Black 38	30235
Direct Red 1	22310	Direct Black 4	30245
Direct Brown 2	22311	Direct Green 1	30280
Direct Orange 1	22370	Direct Green 6	30295
	22375	Direct Green 8	30315
	22430	Direct Brown 31	35660
Direct Violet 1	22570	Direct Brown 74	36300
Direct Blue 2	22590		
	3,3'-Dimethoxybenzidine-based		
Pigment Orange 16	21160	Direct Blue 1	24410
Direct Blue 15	24400	Direct Blue 8	24140
Direct Blue 76	24411	Direct Blue 98	23155
	3,3'-Dichlorobenzidine-based		
Pigment Yellow 12	21090	Pigment Yellow 14	21095
Pigment Yellow 17	21105	Pigment Orange 13	21110
Pigment Orange 34	21115	Pigment Red 38	21120
	3,3'-Dimethylbenzidine-based		
Direct Red 2	28500	Direct Red 39	23630
Acid Red 114	23635	Direct Blue 25	23790
Direct Blue 14	23850	Direct Blue 26	31930
Azoic coupling component 5	37610		

Source: Ref. 43.

is considered to be a potent carcinogen [41]. Details concerning the alkylating agents are presented in Chapter 2.

III. AROMATIC AMINES

Aromatic amines have been indicted as carcinogenic chemicals ever since Rehn [11] discussed "aniline tumors" in 1895. It was later shown that the actual carcinogens involved were benzidine and 2-naphthylamine. Aromatic amines that have produced cancer in animals and humans include 2-naphthylamine, 4-aminobiphenyl, and benzidine [42]. Benzidine congeners are widely used in industry. These compounds, reported by Lurie [43], include nitrobenzidine, dinitrobenzidine, ethoxybenzidine, benzidine disulfonic acids, benzidine sulfones, toluidine disulfonic acids, benzidine dicarboxylic acids, and a wide variety of azo dyes and pigments. The principal difficulty with analysis of these compounds is the fact that they are not the ultimate carcinogens but must be metabolized and conjugated in the liver to compounds that can penetrate the target organ(s). Aromatic amines and amides are metabolically converted and activated to precarcinogens. Present evidence indicates that N hydroxylation produces the precarcinogen, but the activation step appears to be esterification. The carcinogenically active forms in vivo may be the conjugates of the aromatic amine noted above [44]. These active forms react with DNA, resulting in alteration, deletions, or rearrangements of the nucleotide sequence, which, in turn, causes cancer [45]. Such theoretical considerations become very important when the carcinogenic potential of various benzidine, dimethylbenzidine, dimethoxybenzidine, and dichlorobenzidine dyes is evaluated. Some of the common azo dyes and pigments are listed in Table 2 [43]. It should be noted that each dye has a Color Index number to identify its color but not its chemical purity. The dyes also contain diluents, unreacted amine and acid, and various other constituents from side reactions. Moreover, the azo linkage is weak; and enzymes, both microbial and those in the liver, can split the dye into its original components. Chapter 3 deals with the chemistry and analysis of the aromatic amines.

IV. ESTROGENS

It has long been known that the injudicious use of estrogens can cause cancer, and this fact was reinforced when it was discovered that some of the offspring of women treated with diethylstilbestrol to prevent abortion developed cancer 20 years later [47-49]. Dienestrol and hexestrol have also been implicated as producers of both cervical and vaginal adenocarcinoma in young girls [50]. A list of some of the more important estrogenic hormones is presented in the *Handbook of Chemistry and Physics* [51]. The widespread use of oral contraceptives since their introduction in 1960 led to some speculation that such drugs might induce cancer of the cervix but as yet this has apparently not occurred [52]. However, prolonged use of estrogen may be associated with an increased risk of endometrial hyperplasia followed by atypical adenomatous hyperplasia leading to well-differentiated adenocarcinoma of the endometrium [53]. Contraceptive steroids have been associated with an increased number of hepatic adenomas and related lesions in women [54]. Details pertaining to the chemistry and analysis of estrogens are presented in Chapter 4.

V. MYCOTOXINS

The aflatoxins are a group of potent, naturally occurring carcinogens formed when various *Aspergillus* species grow on edible nuts, oil seeds, grains, and figs [55]. Wogan [56] has summarized the evidence for the carcinogenicity of aflatoxins in rainbow trout, salmon, guppy, duck, rat, mouse, ferret, monkey, marmoset, and tree shrew. Evidence of liver tumors in humans is somewhat contradictory because the usual time interval between exposure and occurrence of tumor in humans covers a period of up to 20 years. The carcinogenic effect of aflatoxin B_1 in the rat and hamster has been correlated with binding to liver nucleic acids and protein [57]. Trichothecenes are another group of fungal metabolites produced by species of *Fusarium, Myrothecium, Trichoderma, Cephalosporium, Verticimonosporium,* and *Stachybotrys* which have been associated with fatal toxicosis from consumption of contaminated grains. An excellent overview of the role of mycotoxins in human and animal health was presented by Ueno [58]. Zearalenone and its derivatives are phytoestrogens produced by *Fusarium* species on moldy maize [59]. They produce a high incidence of symptoms of hyperestrogenicity in swine, including tumefaction of the vulva, prolapse of the vagina, and hypertrophy of the mammae, resulting in infertility in swine herds [60]. There are numerous other mycotoxins, but these are discussed in Chapter 5.

VI. NITROSO COMPOUNDS

The nitroso compounds comprise a group of very potent carcinogens [46]. The dialkylnitrosamines are enzymatically dealkylated to diazoalkane, diazotate, or alkyldiazonium, followed by decomposition which yields the alkylating carcinogen. Druckrey et al. [61] have observed more than 200 cases of carcinoma of the esophagus induced by nonsymmetrical dialkylnitrosamines. The acylalkylnitrosamides are also very potent carcinogens, as are the 1,2-dialkylhydrazines, azo- or azozyalkanes, and 1-aryl-3,3-dialkyltriazenes. Some of the nitroso

Table 3 Acute Oral Toxicities of Nitroso Compounds in Rats

Compound	LD_{50} (mg/kg)
N-Nitrosodimethylamine	27-41
N-Nitrosodiethylamine	216
N-Nitrosodi-n-butylamine	1200
N-Nitroso-n-butylmethylamine	130
N-Nitroso-tert-butylmethylamine	700
N-Nitroso-n-amylamine	1750
N-Nitrosomethylphenylamine	200
N-Nitrosobenzylmethylamine	18
N-Nitrosoethylisopropylamine	1100
N-Nitroso-n-butylethylamine	380
N-Nitroso-tert-butylethylamine	1600
N-Nitrosoethylvinylamine	88
N-Nitrosoethyl-2-hydroxyethylamine	>7500
N-Nitroso-di-2-hydroxyethylamine	>5000
N-Nitrosobutyl-4-hydroxybutylamine	1800
N-Nitrosomorpholine	282
N-Nitrososarcosine	>4000
N-Nitrososarcosine ethyl ester	>5000
N,N'-Dinitroso-N,N'dimethylethylenediamine	150
N-Methyl-N-nitrosourea	180
N-Methyl-N-nitrosourethane	240
N-Nitrosotrimethylurea	250
Azoxyethane	530
Diazoethylacetate	400

Source: Ref. 63.

compounds occur in the environment as a result of interaction between secondary amines and nitrite [62]. The nitrosourea compounds constitute another group of potent carcinogens. Table 3 lists the acute oral LD_{50} values in rats for a series of nitroso compounds. It can be seen that, in general, these chemicals have a relatively low toxicity. However, there is no correlation between acute toxicity and carcinogenicity. Moreover, very low doses of nitroso compounds administered for long intervals produce cancer in most species tested. There are exceptions to this rule in that some nitroso compounds induce cancer after a single dose of a rapidly eliminated chemical. This indicates a rapid interaction between the nitroso compound and/or its decomposition product(s) with some cell component shortly after administration [63]. Such rapid events make analysis of tissue components for the nitroso compound and/or its decomposition product(s) extremely difficult. The chemistry and analytical methods for determining nitrosamines are discussed in Chapter 6.

VII. PESTICIDES

When one considers the pesticide field, it is easy to understand the confusion that exists even among professionals because of the number of chemical groupings involved and the great diversity of chemical structures reported [64]. When DDT began to lose its effectiveness and pest resistance became a problem, many other organochlorine compounds, such as lindane, aldrin, dieldrin, chlordane, heptachlor, and mirex, were synthesized. With the discovery of the bioaccumulation and possible carcinogenic effects of the organochlorine pesticides, biodegradable and shorter-acting chemicals were synthesized. The "newer" pesticide classes and some representative chemicals of each class are: carbamates (carbaryl, propoxur, promecarb, and terbutol); phosphonates (tetraethyl pyrophosphate, trichlorfon, mevinphos, dichlorvos, naled, and dicrotophos); phosphonothioates (parathion, methyl parathion, EPN, fenitrothion, dicapthon, and leptophos); and phophorodithioates (malathion, dimethoate, phenkapton, and phosmet), This list is by no means complete; see Ref. 64 for most of the compounds in current use. The pesticidal compounds can produce teratogenic, mutagenic, and carcinogenic effects in animals, but their potency is extremely variable. Recently, it has been suggested that naturally occurring nitrate, or that derived from fertilizers, can interact with the carbamate pesticides to produce carcinogenic nitrosamines [65]. Pesticides are discussed in detail in Chapter 7.

VIII. POLYCYCLIC AROMATIC HYDROCARBONS

We now return to the components of coal tar and soot, the polycyclic aromatic hydrocarbons originally involved in the first occupationally encountered cancer [1,3,24-32]. A comprehensive survey of some of the chemicals in this group was reported by McCaustland et al. [66]. Many derivatives of these chemicals have been synthesized, some of which are not carcinogenic because they cannot be activated to the ultimate carcinogen. Potential reaction mechanisms resulting in ultimate carcinogens are discussed in Refs. 67 to 75. McCaustland et al. [66] also illustrated the K-region of polycyclic aromatic hydrocarbons, where oxides are formed enzymatically in vivo which, in turn, react with both nuclear DNA and polydeoxy nucleotides to form covalent adducts [76]. Under the right circumstances these products lead to carcinogenesis [77]. Similar reactions involving the induction of a nucleophilic attack on diol epoxides, Bay-region and non-Bay-region tetrahydro epoxides, and K-region and non-K-region arene oxides have been suggested as structural features required in the induction of carcinogenesis [78]. Such chemical derivatives are extremely difficult to isolate and determine analytically. Moreover, the monitoring of polycyclic aromatic hydrocarbons in the environment, where they are in such low concentrations, requires analytical methods of high specificity and sensitivity which, in most cases, are not available and must be developed. Furthermore, comparable data from different laboratories do not exist. Further complicating the situation are the variability in samples with time, and the concentrations, which occur below the level of detection [79]. Details concerning the chemistry and analysis of polycyclic aromatic hydrocarbons are presented in Chapter 8.

IX. METALS

Many metals have proven to be carcinogenic in animals, including compounds containing arsenic, beryllium, cadmium, chromium, iron, lead, and nickel.

Exposure to arsenic increases the incidence of epidermoid carcinoma of the skin and lungs and precancerous dermal keratoses in humans [80-84]. However, there is little evidence that arsenic is carcinogenic in animals [85,86].

Beryllium produces lung cancer in workers, especially those with bronchitis and pneumonitis [87]. Chronic pulmonary berylliosis has been reported to develop cancer in the respiratory tract [88]; however, this has been denied in other studies [89]. Inhalation of beryllium aerosols by rats and monkeys resulted in pulmonary carcinomas [90-93].

Cancer of the lung and prostate induced by cadmium has been reported [94-96]; but when the tenuous evidence was reviewed, there did not appear to be a relationship between occupational exposure to cadmium and prostatic cancer [97,98]. Parenteral administration of cadmium compounds to rats produces acute testicular necrosis followed by Leydig cell tumors [90,100].

Workers in chromium refineries have a predilection for development of cancer of the lung, nose, pharynx, and sinuses [101,102]. It has been suggested that pulmonary neoplasia is caused by hexavalent chromium compounds and not by any other valance state [103]. Intrabronchial implantation of pellets of calcium chromate in rats resulted in induction of squamous cell carcinomas and adenocarcinomas in the lungs of rats [104,105]. Mice developed alveolar adenomas and adenocarcinomas from chronic inhalation of calcium chromate [106].

It has been suggested that hematite miners have an increased risk of developing occupationally induced pulmonary carcinoma [107]. Patients have developed sarcomas from injections of iron-dextran complexes, and similar results have been obtained in animals [108-110].

There is no evidence that lead poisoning causes cancer induction in humans, but lead phosphate has produced renal carcinomas in rats, and feeding lead acetate has induced Leydigiomas in this species [111-113].

Nickel is one of the best known inducers of cancer of the lung and nasal cavities [114-118]. Inhalation of nickel carbonyl or nickel dust by animals induces pulmonary carcinomas and sarcomas in various organs [119].

Hopefully, this introduction to chemical carcinogenesis will set the stage for my colleagues to describe the various analytical methods available for quantitative determination of the diverse chemicals and metals involved in the carcinogenesis process.

REFERENCES

1. P. Pott, Cancer scroti. In *Chirurgical Observations.* Hawes, Clarke and Collins, London, 1775, pp. 63-68.
2. J. Hill, *Cautions Against the Immoderate Use of Snuff.* London, 1759.
3. J.W. Lloyd. Long term mortality study of steel workers: V. Respiratory cancer in coke plant workers. J. Occup. Med. *13*, 53-68 (1971).
4. F. H. Hartung and W. Hesse. Der Lungenkrebs die Bergkrankheit in den Schneebergen Gruben. Vrtl. Jhrssch. Gerichtl. Med. *30*, 296-301; *31*, 102-132, 313-337 (1879).
5. E. Lorenz. Radioactivity and lung cancer: critical review of lung cancer in miners of Schneeberg and Joachimstahl. J. Natl. Cancer Inst. 5, 1-15 (1944).
6. J. A. Paris. *Pharmacologia*, 3rd ed. W. Phillips, London, 1820, p. 282.
7. National Institute for Occupational Safety and Health. *Occupational Exposure to Inorganic Arsenic*, Vol. 16. Stock No. 1733-00030. U.S. Government Printing Office, Washington, D.C. 1973.
8. A. M Lee and J. F. Fraumeni. Arsenic and respiratory cancer in man—an occupational study. J. Natl. Cancer Inst. *42*, 1045-1052 (1969).
9. S. Milham and T. Strong. Human arsenic exposure in relation to a copper smelter. Environ. Res. 7, 176-182 (1974).
10. M. G. Oh, B. B. Holder, and H. L. Gordon. Respiratory cancer and occupational exposure to arsenicals. Arch. Environ. Health *29*, 250-255 (1974).
11. L. Rehn. Blasengeschwulste bei Anilinarbeitern. Arch. Klin. Chir. *50*, 588-600 (1895).
12. M. R. Zavon, U. Hoegg, and E. Bingham. Benzidine exposure as a cause of bladder tumors. Arch. Environ. Health *27*, 1-7 (1973).

13. T. J. Haley. Benzidine revisited. Clin. Toxicol. *8,* 13-42 (1975).
14. H. M. Murray. *Report of the Department Committee on Compensation for Industrial Disease.* H.M. Stationery Office, London, 1907.
15. M. L. Newhouse and H. Thompson. Mesothelioma of pleura and peritoneum following exposure to asbestos in the London area. Br. J. Ind. Med. *22,* 261-269 (1965).
16. J. Lieben and H. Pistawka. Mesothelioma and asbestos exposure. Arch. Environ. Health *14*, 559-563 (1967).
17. T. J. Haley, Asbestosis: a reassessment of the overall problem. J. Pharm. Sci. *64*, 1435-1449 (1975).
18. T. J. Haley. Vinyl chloride: how many unknown problems? J. Toxicol. Environ. Health *1*, 47-43 (1975).
19. T. J. Haley. An evaluation of the health effects of benzene inhalation. Clin. Toxicol. *11*, 531-548 (1977).
20. *IARC Monographs on the Evaluation of Carcinogenic Risk,* Vol. 7. International Agency for Research on Cancer, Lyon, France, 1974.
21. S. R. Cowles. Cancer in the workplace–Percivall Pott to the present. Mil. Med. *143*, 395-400 (1978).
22. A. K. Bahn, I. Rosenwaike, N. Herrmann, P. Grover, J. Stellman, and K. O'Leary. Melanoma after exposure to PCB's. N. Engl. J. Med. *295*, 450 (1976).
23. M. Kuratsune, T. Yoshimura, J. Matsuzaka, and A. Yamaguchi. Epidemiologic study on yusho, a poisoning caused by ingestion of rice oil contaminated with a commercial brand of polychorinated biphenyls. Environ. Health Perspect. *1*, 119-128 (1972).
24. K. Yamagiwa and K. Ichikawa. Experimental study of the pathogenesis of carcinoma. J. Cancer Res. *3*, 1-29 (1918).
25. J. W. Cook, I. Hieger, E. L. Kennaway, and W. V. Mayneord. The production of cancer by pure hydrocarbons, Part I, Proc. R. Soc. Lond. B, *111*, 455-484 (1932).
26. J. W. Cook. The production of cancer by pure hydrocarbons, Part II. Proc. R. Soc. Lond. B, *111*, 485-496 (1932).
27. G. Barry, J. W. Cook, G. A. D. Haslewood, C. L. Hewett, I. Hieger, and E. L. Kennaway. The production of cancer by pure hydrocarbons, Part III. Proc. R. Soc. Lond. B, *117,* 318-351 (1935).
28. W. E. Bachmann, J. W. Cook, A. Dansi, G. M. de Norms, G. A. D. Haslewood, C. L. Hewett, and A. M. Robinson. The production of cancer by pure hydrocarbons, Part IV. Proc. R. Soc. Lond. B, *123*, 343-368 (1937).
29. G. M. Badger, J. W. Cook, C. L. Hewett, E. L. Kennaway, N. M. Kennaway, R. H. Martin, and A. M. Robinson. The production of cancer by pure hydrocarbons, Part V. Proc. R. Soc. Lond. B, *129*, 439-467 (1940).

30. G. M. Badger, J. W. Cook, C. L. Hewett, E. L. Kennaway, N. M. Kennaway, and R. H. Martin. The production of cancer by pure hydrocarbons, Part VI. Proc. R. Soc. Lond. B, *131*, 170-182 (1942).
31. H. Wieland and H. Dane. The constitution of the bile acids: LII. The place of attachment of the side chain. Z. Physiol. Chem. *219*, 240-244 (1933).
32. J. W. Cook and G. A. D. Haslewood. Conversion of a bile acid into a hydrocarbon derived for 1,2-benzoanthracene. Chem. Ind. *38*, 758-759 (1933).
33. P. Ehrlich. In *The Collected Papers of Paul Ehrlich*, Vol. 1. Pergamon Press, Oxford, 1956, p. 596.
34. P. Brooks. Chemical carcinogenesis. Ann. Clin. Biochem. *13*, 471 (1976).
35. A. Weiss and B. Weiss. Karzinogenese durch Lost-Exposition beim Menschen, ein wichtiger Hinweis fuer die Alkylantien-Therapie. Dtsch. Med. Wschr. *100*, 919-923 (1975).
36. R. Preussmann, H. Druckrey, S. Ivankovic, and A. V. Hodenberg. Chemical structure and carcinogeicity of aliphatic hydrazo, azo, and azoxy compounds and of triazenes, potential in vivo alkylating agents. Ann. N. Y. Acad. Sci. *163*, 697-714 (1969).
37. A. Goldin and H. B. Wood, Jr. Preclinical investigation of alkylating agents in cancer chemotherapy. Ann. N.Y. Acad. Sci. *163*, 954-1005 (1969).
38. C. C. J. Culvenor, D. T. Downing, and J. A. Edgar. Pyrrolizidine alkaloids as alkylating and antimitotic agents. Ann. N.Y. Acad. Sci. *163*, 837-847 (1969).
39. M. Spatz. Toxic and carcinogenic alkylating agents from cycads. Ann. N.Y. Acad. Sci. *163*, 837-847 (1969).
40. A. B. Borkovec. Alkylating agents as insect chemosterilants. Ann. N.Y. Acad. Sci. *163*, 860-868 (1969).
41. L. Fishbein. Degradation and residues of alkylating agents. Ann. N.Y. Acad. Sci. *163*, 869-894 (1969).
42. M. C. Bowman. Trace analysis: a requirement for toxicological research with carcinogens and hazardous substances. J. Assoc. Off. Anal. Chem. *61*, 1253-1262 (1978).
43. A. P. Lurie. Benzidine and related diaminobiphenyls. In *Kirk-Othmer Encyclopedia of Chemical Technology*, 2nd ed., Vol. 3 (R. E. Kirk and D. F. Othmer, Eds.). Interscience, New York, 1964, pp. 408-420.
44. J. A.Miller and E. C. Miller. The metabolic activation of carcinogenic aromatic amines and amides. Prog. Exp. Tumor Res. *11*, 273-301 (1969).
45. J. A. Miller and E. C. Miller. Chemical carcinogenesis: mechanisms and approaches to its control. (Guest Editorial). J. Natl. Cancer Inst. *47*, v-xiv (1971).

46. *IARC Monographs on the Evaluation of Carcinogenic Risk of Chemicals to Man*, Vol. 4; *Some Aromatic Amines, Hydrazine and Related Substances, N-Nitroso Compounds and Miscellaneous Alkylating Agents*. International Agency for Research on Cancer, Lyon, France, 1974.

47. A. L. Herbst, H. Ulfelder, and D. C. Poskanzer. Adenocarcinoma of the vagina. Association of maternal stilbestrol therapy with tumor appearance in young women. N. Engl. J. Med. *184*, 878-881 (1971).

48. A. L. Herbst, S. J. Robboy, R. E. Scully, and D. C. Poskanzer. Clear cell adenocarcinoma of the vagina and cervix in girls. Analysis of 170 Registry cases. Am. J. Obstet. Gynecol. *119*, 713-724 (1974).

49. S. J. Robboy, R. E. Scully, W. I. Welch, and A. L. Herbst. Intrauterine diethylstilbestrol exposure and its consequences. Pathologic characteristics of vaginal adenosis, clear cell adenocarcinomas and related lesions. Arch. Pathol. Lab. Med. *101*, 1-5 (1977).

50. A. L. Herbst. Summary of the changes in the human female genital tract as a consequence of maternal diethylstilbestrol therapy. J. Toxicol. Environ. Health *1*, 13-20 (1976).

51. R. C. Weast (Ed). *Handbook of Chemistry and Physics*, 57th ed. CRC Press, Cleveland, 1976-1977, pp. C760-C766.

52. V. A. Drill. History of the first oral contraceptive. J. Toxicol. Environ. Health *3*, 133-138 (1977).

53. K. S. Moghissi. Oral contraceptives and endometrial and cervical cancer. J. Toxicol. Environ. Health *3*, 243-265 (1977).

54. C.-R. Garcia, J. Gordon, and V. A. Drill. Contraceptive steroids and liver lesions. J. Toxicol. Environ. Health *3*, 197-206 (1977).

55. L. Stoloff. Aflatoxins–an overview. In *Mycotoxins in Human and Animal Health* (J. V. Rodricks, C. W. Hesseltine, and M. A. Mehlman, Eds.). Pathotox Publishers, Park Forest South, Ill., 1977, pp. 7-28.

56. G. N. Wogan. Aflatoxin carcinogenesis. In *Methods in Cancer Research* (H. Busch, Ed.), Vol. 7. Academic Press, New York, 1973, pp. 309-344.

57. R. C. Garner and C. M. Wright. Binding of [^{14}C]aflatoxin B_1 to cellular macromolecules in the rat and hamster. Chem.-Biol. Interact. *11*, 123-131 (1975).

58. Y. Ueno. Trichothecenes: overview address. In *Mycotoxins in Human and Animal Health* (J. V. Rodricks, C. W. Hesseltine, and M. A.Mehlman, Eds.). Pathotox Publishers, Park Forest South, Ill., 1977, pp. 189-207.

59. C. J. Mirocha, S. V. Pathre, and C. M. Christensen. In *Mycotoxins in Human and Animal Health* (J. V. Rodricks, C. W. Hesseltine, and M. A. Mehlman, Eds.). Pathotox Publishers, Park Forest South, Ill., 1977, pp. 345-364.

60. M. Stob, R. S. Baldwin, J. Tuite, F. N. Andrews, and K. G. Gillette. Isolation of an anabolic, uterotropic compound from corn infected with *Gibberella zeae*. Nature (Lond.) *196*, 1318 (1962).
61. H. Druckrey, R. Preussmann, and S. Ivankovic. N-Nitroso compounds in organotropic and transplacental carcinogenesis. Ann. N.Y. Acad. Sci. *163*, 676-695 (1969).
62. P. N. Magee. In vivo reactions of nitroso compounds. Ann. N.Y. Acad. Sci. *163*, 717-729 (1969).
63. P. N. Magee and J. M. Barnes. Carcinogenic nitroso compounds. Adv. Cancer Res. *10*, 163-246 (1967).
64. K. Packer. *Nanogen Index: A Dictionary of Pesticides and Chemical Pollutants*. Nanogen International, Freedom, Calif., 1975, p. 256.
65. L. Fishbein. Teratogenic, mutagenic and carcinogenic effects of insecticides. In *Insecticide Biochemistry and Physiology* (C. F. Wilkinson, Ed.). Plenum, New York, 1976, pp. 555-603.
66. D. J. McCaustland, D. L. Fisher, K. C. Kolwyck, W. P. Duncan, J. C. Wiley, Jr., C. S. Menon, J. F. Engel, J. K. Selkirk, and P. P. Roller. Polycyclic aromatic hydrocarbon derivatives: synthesis and physiochemical characterization. In *Carcinogenesis—A Comprehensive Survey*, Vol. 1 (R. I. Freudenthal and P. Jones, Eds.). Raven Press, New York, 1976, pp. 349-411.
67. P. O. P. Ts'o, W. J. Caspary, B. I. Cohen, J. C. Leavitt, S. A. Lesko, R. J. Lorentzen, and L. M. Schechtman. Basic mechanisms in polycyclic hydrocarbon carcinogenesis. In *Chemical Carcinogenesis*, Part A (P. O. P. Ts'o and J. A. DiPaolo, Eds.). Marcel Dekker, New York, 1974, pp. 113-147.
68. C. Nagata, Y. Tagashira, and M. Kodama. Metabolic activation of benzo[a]pyrene: significance of free radical. In *Chemical Carcinogenesis*, Part A (P. O. P. Ts'o and J.A. DiPaolo, Eds.). Marcel Dekker, New York, 1974, pp. 87-111.
69. A. Dipple, P. D. Lawley, and P. Brookes. Theory of tumor initiation by chemical carcinogens: dependence of activity on structure of ultimate carcinogen. Eur. J. Cancer *4*, 493-506 (1968).
70. J. Fried. One-electron oxidation of polycyclic aromatics as a model for the metabolic activation of carcinogenic hydrocarbons. In. *Chemical Carcinogenesis*, Part A (P. O. P. Ts'o and J. A. DiPaolo, Eds.). Marcel Dekker, New York, 1974, pp. 197-215.
71. E. Cavaliere and R. Auerbach. Reactions between activated benzo[a]pyrene and nucleophilic compounds, with possible implications on the mechanism of tumor initiation. J. Natl. Cancer. Inst. *53*, 393-397 (1974).
72. J. W. Flesher and K. L. Sydnor. Possible role of 6-hydroxymethylbenzo[a]pyrene as a proximate carcinogen of benzo[a]-pyrene and 6-methylbenzo[a]pyrene. Int. J. Cancer *11*, 433-437 (1973).

73. N. H. Sloane and T. K. Davis. Hydroxymethylation of the benzene ring. Microsomal hydroxymethylation of benzo[a]pyrene to 6-hydroxymethylbenzo[a]pyrene. Arch. Biochem. Biophys. *163*, 46-52 (1974).
74. M. S. Newman and D. R. Olson. A new hypothesis concerning the reactive species in carcinogenesis by 7,12-dimethylbenz[a]-anthracene. The 5-hydroxy, 7,12-dimethylbenz[a]antrhacen-5 (6H)-one equilibrium. J. Am. Chem. Soc. *96*, 6207-6208 (1974).
75. D. M. Jerina and J. W. Daly. Arene oxides: a new aspect of drug metabolism. Science *185*, 537-582 (1974).
76. W. M. Baird and L. Diamond. The nature of benzo[a]pyrene-DNA adducts formed in hamster embryo cells depends on the length of time of exposure to benzo[a]pyrene. Biochem. Biophys. Res. Commun. *77*, 162-167 (1977).
77. S. K. Yang, H. V. Gelboin, B. F. Trump, H. Astrup, and C. C. Harris. Metabolic activation of benzo[a]pyrene and binding to DNA in cultured human bronchus. Cancer Res. *37*, 1210-1215 (1977).
78. A. R. Becker, J. M. Janusz, D. Z. Rogers, and T. C. Bruice. Structural features which determine the carcinogenesis, mutagenesis, and rates of acid- and water-mediated solvolysis of a nucleophilic attack upon diol epoxides, Bay-region and non-Bay region tetrahydro epoxides, and K-region and non-K region arene oxides. J. Am. Chem. Soc. *100*, 3244-3246 (1978).
79. R. Preussmann. Chemical carcinogens in the human environment. Problems and quantitative aspects. Oncology *33*, 51-57 (1976).
80. G. Ehlers. Klinische und histologische Untersuchungen zur Frage arzneimittelbedingter Arsen-tumoren. Z. Haut. Geschlechstkr. *43*, 763-774 (1974).
81. E. G. Friedrich, Jr. Vulvar carcinoma in situ in identical twins-an occupational hazard. Obstet. Gynocol. *39*, 837-841 (1972).
82. A. L. Goldman. Lung cancer in Bowen's disease. Am. Rev. Respir. Dis. *108*, 1205-1207 (1973).
83. A. M. Lee and J. F. Fraumeni, Jr. Arsenic and respiratory cancer in man: an occupational study. J. Natl. Cancer Inst. *42*, 1045-1052 (1969).
84. M. Oh, B. B. Holder, and H. L. Gordon. Respiratory cancer and occupational exposure to arsenicals. Arch. Environ. Health *29*, 250-255 (1974).
85. D. V. Frost. Arsenicals in biology–retrospect and prospect. Fed. Proc. *26*, 194-208 (1967).
86. C. Baroni, G. J. vanEsch, and U. Saffiotti. Carcinogenesis tests of two inorganic arsenicals. Arch. Environ. Health *7*, 668-674 (1963).
87. T. F. Mancuso. Relation of duration of employment and prior respiratory illness to respiratory cancer among beryllium workers. Environ. Res. *3*, 251-275 (1970).

88. F. M. Hasan and H. Kazemi. Chronic beryllium disease: a continuing epidemiologic hazard. Chest *65*, 289-293 (1974).
89. D. Bayliss. Expected and observed deaths by selected causes occurring to beryllium workers. In National Institute of Occupational Health and Safety, *Criteria for a Recommended Standard: Occupational Exposure to Beryllium.* U.S. Dept. of Health, Education and Welfare, Washington, D.C., 1972, pp. IV-23.
90. G. W. H. Scheppers. Biological action of beryllium, reaction of the monkey to inhaled aerosols. Ind. Med. Surg. *33*, 1-16 (1964).
91. A. J. Vorwald and A. L. Reeves. Pathological changes induced by beryllium compounds. Arch. Ind. Health *19*, 190-199 (1959).
92. A. L. Reeves, D. Deitch, and A. J. Vorwald. Beryllium carcinogenesis: I. Inhalation exposure of rats to beryllium sulfate aerosol. Cancer Res. *27*, 439-445 (1967).
93. A. L. Reeves and A. J. Vorwald. Beryllium carcinogenesis: II. Pulmonary deposition and clearance of inhaled beryllium sulfate in the rat. Cancer Res. *27*, 446-451 (1967).
94. C. L. Potts. Cadmium proteinuria. The health of battery workers exposed to cadmium oxide dust. Ann. Occup. Hyg. *8*, 55-61 (1965).
95. M. D. Kipling and J. A. H. Waterhouse. Cadmium and prostatic cancer. Lancet *1*, 730-731 (1967).
96. H. Holden. Cadmium toxicology. Lancet *2*, 57 (1969).
97. W. Winkelstein and S. Kantor. Prostatic cancer: relationship to suspended particulate air polution. Am. J. Public Health *59*, 1134-1138 (1969).
98. D. Malcolm. Potential carcinogenic effect of cadmium in animals and man. Ann. Occup. Hyg. *15*, 33-36 (1972).
99. O. J. Lucis, R. Lucis, and K. Aterman. Tumorigenesis by cadmium. Oncology *26*, 53-57 (1972).
100. J. Reddy, D. Svoboda, D. Azarnoff, and R. Dawes. Cadmium-induced Leydig cell tumors of rat testis: morphologic and cytochemical study. J. Natl. Cancer Inst. *51*, 891-903 (1973).
101. A. M. Baetjer. Pulmonary carcinoma in chromate workers: I. Review of the literature and report of cases. Arch. Ind. Hyg. Occup. Med. *2*, 487-504 (1950).
102. P. E. Enterline. Respiratory cancer among chromate workers. J. Occup. Med. *16*, 523-526 (1974).
103. A. M. Baetjer, D. J. Birmingham, P. E. Enterline, W. Mertz, and J. V. Pierce II. *Chromium.* National Academy of Sciences, Washington, D.C., 1974.
104. S. Laskin, M. Kuschner, and R. T. Drew. Studies in pulmonary carcinogenesis. In *Inhalation Carcinogenesis* (M. G. Hanna, Jr., P. Nettesheim, and J. R. Gilbert, Eds.). U.S. Atomic Energy Commission, Washington, D.C., 1970, pp. 321-351.

105. M. Kuschner and S. Laskin. Experimental models in environmental carcinogenesis. Am. J. Pathol. *64*, 183-191 (1971).
106. P. Nettesheim, M. G. Hanna, Jr., D. G. Dohertz, R. F. Newell, and A. Hellman. Effect of calcium chromate dust, influenza virus and 100 R whole-body x-radiation on lung tumor incidence in mice. J. Natl. Cancer Inst. *47*, 1129-1144 (1971).
107. J. T. Boyd, R. Dall, J. S. Faulds, and J. Leiper. Cancer of the lung in iron ore (hematite) miners. Br. J. Ind. Med. *27*, 97-105 (1970).
108. A. E. MacKinnon and J. Bancewicz. Sarcoma after injection of intramuscular iron. Br. Med. J. *2*, 277-279 (1973).
109. E. Myhre. Sarkom etter intramuskulaer injeksjon ar jern. Tidsskr. Nor. Laegeforen. *93*, 2500-2501 (1973).
110. A. Haddow and E. S. Horning. On the carcinogenicity of an iron-dextran complex. J. Natl. Cancer Inst. *24*, 109-147 (1960).
111. I. Dingwall-Fordyce and R. E. Lane. A follow-up study of lead workers. Br. J. Ind. Med. *20*, 313-315 (1963).
112. H. U. Zollinger. Druch chronische Bleivergiftung erzeugte Nierenadenoma und -carcinome bei Ratten und ihre Beziehungen zu den entsprechenden Neubildungen des Menschen. Virchows Arch. Pathol. Anat. *323*, 694-710 (1953).
113. B. Zawirska and K. Medras. Tumors and disorders of porphyrin metabolism in rats with chronic experimental lead poisoning. Zentralbe Allg. Pathol. *111*, 1-12 (1968).
114. R. Doll, L. G. Morgan, and F. E. Speizer. Cancers of the lung and nasal sinuses in nickel workers. Br. J. Cancer *24*, 623-632 (1970).
115. E. Pederson, A. C. Hogetveit, and A. Canderson. Cancer of respiratory organs among workers at a nickel refinery in Norway. Int. J. Cancer *12*, 32-41 (1973).
116. A. V. Saknyn and N. K. Shabynina. Epidemology of malignant neoplasms in nickel plants. Gig. Tr. Prof. Zabol. *17*, 25-28 (1973).
117. W. C. Hueper. Experimental studies in metal carcinogenesis: IX. Pulmonary lesions in guinea pigs and rats exposed to prolonged inhalation of powdered metallic nickel. Arch. Pathol. *65*, 600-607 (1958).
118. F. W. Sunderman, Jr. The current status of nickel carcinogenesis. Ann. Clin. Lab. Sci. *3*, 156-180 (1973).
119. T. J. Lau, R. L. Hackett, and F. W. Sunderman, Jr. The carcinogenicity of intravenous nickel carbonyl in rats. Cancer Res. *32*, 2253-2258 (1972).

2

Alkylating Agents

ALEXEJ B. BORKOVEC and CHARLES W. WOODS Agricultural Research Center, U.S. Department of Agriculture, Beltsville, Maryland

I. CLASSIFICATION

The definition of an alkylating agent as an organic compound capable of introducing an alkyl group R into another molecule (HY) implies the existence of a structural entity R–X, in which the two moieties are linked with a labile bond. Following this definition, any alkyl-containing compound that reacts according to the general equation is an alkylating agent. With a few added restrictions concerning the

$$R{-}X + HY \rightleftharpoons R{-}Y + HX \quad (1)$$

reaction conditions, this simple classification would be useful for designating a large, but clearly defined group of organic reagents. Unfortunately, the present meaning of the term *alkylating agent* has become much broader and no general consensus exists as to its scope and limitations. The primary reason for this change was the realization that numerous toxicologically important compounds react by mechanisms similar to those encountered with alkylating agents. Because alkylation identified not only a certain structural feature of one of the reagents but also the process itself, the initially unambiguous meaning of the term *alkyl* (i.e., C_nH_{2n+1}) was gradually extended to a bewildering variety of organic moieties.

The first conference on Comparative Clinical and Biological Effects of Alkylating Agents [1], convened in 1957, had perhaps the greatest influence on the extended and simultaneously much loosened meaning and usage of the classification term. Subsequently, the distinction between alkylating and biological alkylating agents was sometimes made [2,3] to distinguish relatively simple reagents used in organic synthesis from more complex and pharmacologically interesting compounds, but such distinctions constitute a cure worse than the disease and do not restore the original clarity of the classification.

As will be seen in Section II, the mechanistic implications of the term alkylating agent also suffer from the same ambiguities discussed earlier. As a consequence, whether a given group of compounds is included among alkylating agents depends to some extent on the intentions and bias of the classifier. Because the present volume concerns primarily compounds with potential health hazards, our selection was guided by their toxicological characteristics and by the probability of their occurrence as environmental contaminants. The following categories and structurally defined groups were considered suitable for inclusion:

- Classical alkylating agents
  - Alkyl halides
  - Alkyl sulfates
  - Alkyl phosphates and thiophosphates
- Biological alkylating agents
  - Aziridines
  - Epoxides
  - Lactones
- Other alkylating agents
  - Diazoalkanes
  - Haloethers
  - Acrylates

The reasons for this classification and the overlap among the categories are discussed in some detail in the following sections on reaction mechanisms, practical application and potential hazards, and toxicological and physiological effects of these and related materials.

II. REACTION MECHANISMS

Because the way in which alkylating agents react is the most important guide in their classification and the basis for their existence as a special category of chemical compounds, a brief survey of the various mechanisms by which they are believed to alkylate other molecules will be given.

The generally accepted concept of alkylation is a special case of nucleophilic substitution reaction: the alkylating agent is the attacking species and the receptor is a moiety containing a nucleophilic center. Two fundamental mechanisms for the transfer of an electrophilic alkyl moiety to a nucleophilic receptor were formalized by Ingold [4]. The main difference between these mechanisms is the electronic and steric structure of the alkyl as it is transferred from the parent alkylating agent to the receptor. If the alkyl is first separated as a positively charged ion, a carbonium ion, which subsequently attaches itself to the receptor, the mechanism is unimolecular and the rate-determining reaction (2) is an ionization of the alkylating agent. Tho alkyl ion then reacts rapidly with any available nucle-

$$R{-}Y \;=\; R^{+} + X^{-} \tag{2}$$

$$R^{+} + H{-}Y \;=\; R{-}Y + H^{+} \tag{3}$$

ophile. If, on the other hand, the transfer of R proceeds gradually through an intermediate complex or transition state (4), the mechanism is bimolecular, and the alkylation tends to be more selective.

$$R{-}X + H{-}Y = [X{-}R{:}Y{-}H] = R{-}Y + H{-}X \tag{4}$$

Strictly speaking, RX refers to a monosubstituted alkane, and all the classical alkylating agents mentioned in Section I belong to this category. However, the mechanisms described in equations (2) to (4) are equally applicable to compounds more complex than the classical alkylating agents. Substitution of one or more hydrogen atoms of the alkyl moiety with other organic radicals or with atoms other than carbon leads to a great variety of structural types, which, as long as they follow the nucleophilic substitution mechanism in their reactions, can all be referred to as alkylating agents. Unfortunately, not even the reaction-mechanism criterion applies without exceptions. Diazoalkanes and related compounds are believed to alkylate via the corresponding carbene intermediates (5), and olefins, vinyl halides, and

$$RCH{=}N_2 \rightarrow R\bar{C}H + N_2 \tag{5}$$

acrylates frequently react by forming free radicals (6) rather than ionic intermediates. In view of these and the preceding considera-

$$RCH{=}CH_2 + Z\cdot \rightarrow R\dot{C}HCH_2Z \tag{6}$$

tions it is not surprising that the designation of a compound as an alkylating agent is ambivalent and frequently arbitrary. Nevertheless, its use is widespread and, as will be discussed later, probably more meaningful and justified on the basis of toxicology than on mechanistic and structural considerations. It is important, however, to realize that in a group as large and diverse as the alkylating agents, generalizations of any kind can be drawn, if at all, only after careful delimitation of the structural categories under discussion.

III. PRACTICAL APPLICATION AND POTENTIAL HAZARDS OF ALKYLATING AGENTS

Most categories of alkylating agents include industrial intermediates with yearly production volumes reaching millions of tons, whose economic importance is very high. However, the frequently high chemical reactivity which makes alkylating agents indispensable in industry or chemical laboratories precludes their direct use by the consumer; in fact, their appearance in consumer products or their presence in the human or animal environment invariably constitutes a problem with potentially serious consequences. This dominant characteristic of alkylating agents governs all their large-scale applications and confines their use to controlled operations in closed systems that can be monitored and appropriately regulated. In distinction to certain other hazardous or toxic industrial materials (e.g., fuels or pesticides), any introduction of an alkylating agent into the environment tends to be involuntary or accidental; if it does occur, the resulting contamination may present immediate problems or hazards, but in most instances the long-range problems of accumulation and persistence will be minimal. Therefore, the principal hazards associated with the industrial or laboratory use of alkylating agents is their presence, usually in very small quantities, in the immediate or close vicinity of the place of their production or utilization (i.e., in chemical production plants or in chemical laboratories). There are, however, exceptions to this generalization.

The extension of the concept of alkylating agents to compounds containing substituted alkyl groups happened primarily because of the advances in the chemotherapy of cancer [1,3,5]. The first, and initially the most important structural category was the nitrogen mustards, or 2-aminoethyl chlorides, which in their reactions with nucleophiles (7) conformed to the general mechanism of nucleophilic

$$R_2NCH_2CH_2-Cl + HY \rightarrow R_2NCH_2CH_2-Y + HCl \qquad (7)$$

substitution. By analogy, other aminoalkyl halides, aziridines, epoxides, episulfides, and alkanesulfonates were included in this extended class of cancer chemotherapeutic agents. Surveys of the constantly growing number of these materials and of their toxicological and pharmacological properties are conducted periodically by the U.S. Cancer Chemotherapy National Service Center* [6-8]. In another area of scientific research, the extended concept of alkylating agents is in frequent use. The induction of genetic mutations in living cells was discovered during World War II, when the effects of nitrogen and

---

*Present designation: Division of Cancer Treatment, National Cancer Institute, U.S. Department of Health and Human Services.

sulfur mustards, the infamous lethal gases used in World War I, were investigated [9]. Extensive experimental work with plants, insects, and other organisms followed and is still continuing. In plants, the purpose for inducing mutations has been the possibility of creating new mutant strains with improved agricultural or horticultural characteristics [10]. In insects, mutations were induced in the reproductive organs or gametes of adults to ensure their sterility or inability to reproduce [11-13]. The potential practical application or mutations induced by alkylating agents does not call for using large quantities of these materials or for introducing them freely into the environment, and similarly to chemotherapeutic agents, scientifically used mutagens do not constitute predictable hazards. Accidental small-scale exposures or local contamination are of course always possible, but such situations would require specific remedies that are beyond the scope and interest of this book.

It should be noted, however, that some of the categories of alkylating agents prominent in cancer therapy, plant mutagenesis, or insect chemosterilization have other, economically more important uses, and that such compounds are being produced and utilized in very large quantities. Perhaps the most important category is the epoxides, particularly ethylene and propylene oxide, which are used extensively as industrial intermediates. Less prominent are the lactones and aziridines, but because of the large production volumes of these and related volatile substances, their presence in and near the production facility becomes probable and may constitute hazards requiring precise determinations of their concentration and quantities.

In this chapter, the selection of compounds and classes of alkylating agents with specific analytical procedures was governed primarily by our estimate of the probability that a given compound or class may become hazardous to a large group of people or to the environment. Therefore, certain large and scientifically important classes (e.g., nitrogen mustards and alkanesulfonates) were omitted; on the other hand, certain classes were extended to include related compounds that may be hazardous in production and use. Among the latter, toxic fumigants widely used for disinfection and disinsection deserve special mention. The volatile epoxides, lactones, and various alkyl halides, particularly bromides, belong in this category. The intended function of these sterilizing agents is to kill all living organisms present on or within a given object without significantly changing the object's properties. Since their activity is best exerted in a gaseous state, ensuring optimal penetration and mobility, fumigation sterilization of nonporous and largely inorganic materials (e.g., surgical instruments, certain soils, and ceramic tiles or similar objects) raises only questions of the presence and persistence of the compound in the atmosphere close to the object. However, more complex and difficult questions arise when some of the fumigant becomes entrapped and is subsequently released over extended periods, or when it reacts with the treated object or its constituents. Among alkylating agents, the fumigation sterilants are exceptional in that they are used directly in the human environment without first being converted to other compounds. Consequently, their health hazards may be more frequently encountered than those of usually more toxic nitrogen mustards and other highly physiologically active research substances.

IV. TOXICOLOGY AND PHYSIOLOGICAL EFFECTS OF ALKYLATING AGENTS

The chemical reactivity of alkylating agents, which forms a basis for their classification, may be examined from a biochemical standpoint regarding their potential interaction with cellular constituents. The broad concept of a reaction mechanism in which compounds with electrophilic centers attack nucleophilic centers in substrate molecules includes biochemical alkylations of physiologically important compounds [3]. If these processes were sufficiently specific (i.e., if there were only a few nucleophilic cellular substrates receptive to alkylation), the physiological effects of alkylating agents could be defined and correlated with reactivity or some other measurable physicochemical characteristics of the agent. To a limited extent, such definitions and correlations are indeed possible, but the question of what constitutes a cellular substrate receptive to alkylation has no unique answer. Almost any cellular constituent containing nitrogen, oxygen, or sulfur can be alkylated, and the ubiquity of these nucleophilic centers in molecules composing living tissues makes indiscriminate and multiple alkylation a probable cause of acute toxicity of alkylating agents. Their lethal or near-lethal doses cause a variety of syndromes that are not sufficiently specific or indicative of specific biochemical reaction [14]. However, at much lower doses, the same materials exhibit a substantial selectivity, particularly in dividing cells, which may be expressed physiologically as mutagenicity, carcinogenicity, teratogenicity, or more broadly as cytostatic effects. It is this low level of exposure, frequently free of any observable pathological symptoms, that constitutes the main hazard of alkylating agents as environmental contaminants. On the other hand, the apparent specificity of certain alkylating compounds as cytostatic agents gave rise to a new category of drugs, the biological alkylating agents, applicable to the chemotherapy of cancer. Despite the immense research on the mechanism of biological effects induced by alkylating agents, no consensus exists with regard to the nature of the critical physiological substrate that is alkylated in vivo. Nevertheless, even without knowing the exact nature of the substrate, many investigators have successfully correlated the relationship between alkylating activity and specific physiological effects of antitumor agents [14], chemosterilants of insects

Table 1 Toxicity and Air Pollution Data of Frequently Used Alkylating Agents[a]

Compound	LD_{50} (mg/kg)	TLV (mg/m^3)	TOC (mg/m^3)
Acrylonitrile	82	45	3.7-51
Benzyl chloride	1,231	5	0.25
Diazomethane	301[b]	0.4	
sym-Dichloroethyl ether	75	90	>88
sym-Dichloromethyl ether	210	0.5[c]	
Dimethyl sulfate	440	5	
Epichlorohydrin	90	19	37.8
Ethylene dibromide	117-148	145	>200
Ethylene dichloride	680	200	23.2-450
Ethylene oxide	330	90	1,283
Ethylenimine	15	1	3.5
Glycidol	850	150	
Metepa	136-213		
Methyl iodide	0.15-0.22	29	
β-Propiolactone	50-100		
Propylene oxide	930	240	83
Propylenimine	19	5	
Styrene oxide	4,290		2
Tributyl phosphate	3,000		
Triethylenephosphoramide	37		
Triethylenethiophosphoramide	15[d]		
Trimethyl phosphate	840		
Vinyl chloride	650[e]	3	65,000
Vinylidene chloride	5,750[f]	50[c]	2,000

[a]LD_{50}, acute oral dose lethal to 50% of test rats; TLV, threshold limit value for employees' exposure (U.S.); TOC, threshold odor concentration.
[b]10 min inhalation lethal to rat.
[c]USSR norm.
[d]Intravenous administration.
[e]Inhalation, lowest reported lethal concentration (LCLo, mg/m^3).
[f]LDLo, dog.
Source: Data from Refs. 17 and 18.

and other organisms [11], and certain mutagens and carcinogens [15, 16]. To what extent these correlations apply to humans is one of the thorniest questions of present toxicology and one that will never be solved in the absence of reliable quantitation of each specific compound.

For a group as large and structurally heterogeneous as are the alkylating agents, toxicological generalizations are vague and of limited usefulness. Table 1 shows selected toxicological, regulatory, and human detection data on most alkylating agents described specifically in the following section. Even a cursory examination of the doses and concentrations of individual compounds producing comparable biological effects indicates immense differences defying a unified treatment. Some are severely acute poisons, others appear to be only mildly toxic or innocuous (the acute oral LD_{50} of ethyl alcohol in rats is 10,800 mg/kg). However, with the rapidly increasing number of alkylating agents showing mutagenic properties, the effects of chronic exposures to low concentrations of these materials deserve special attention. Mutagenicity itself is an extremely variable manifestation of interactions that are in turn limited and regulated by the concentration of the agent, conditions of its application, and the organism in which it is elicited. Although the qualitative aspects of mutagenesis, particularly those concerning species susceptibility, are very important for assessing human hazards, quantitative aspects of mutagenesis are perhaps of even greater significance and should never be disregarded.

V. ANALYTICAL PROCEDURES

Each category of alkylating agents listed in Section I contains a large number of compounds described in the chemical literature, but only a few of them are produced in commercially important quantities or are used with sufficient frequency to constitute a potential public hazard. In all instances where exposure of employees or the general public is suspected, the first and more pressing need is the quantitative determination of the pollutant. Although the most frequently encountered pollution problem is that of the concentration of vapors of the substance in the atmosphere, innumerable other problems may arise. Consequently, the analytical procedures mentioned in this section may not be universally applicable, and unless the references cited provide a specific answer, new procedures have to be developed. Since the most variable problem is the collection, isolation, and purification of the sample, several examples of different sampling techniques for a particular compound will be mentioned. Nevertheless, in many instances the specific problem of a user of this book will not exactly coincide with any of the methods described, and modifications will have to be introduced. It is hoped, however, that the variety of procedures described and the use of appropriate references will provide an adequate guide for developing procedures satisfactory for solving the specialized problem.

In recent years, the National Institute of Occupational Safety and Health (NIOSH) of the U.S. Department of Health and Human Services embarked on a long-range project of assembling and annually updating a Registry of Toxic Effects of Chemical Substances. This activity, mandated by the 1970 Occupational Safety and Health Act and the subsequently formed Occupational Safety and Health Administration (OSHA), U.S. Department of Labor, was accompanied by a compilation of sampling and analytical methods, some of which are now used in monitoring programs. Whenever applicable, the NIOSH analytical methods are mentioned and if possible supplemented by other procedures described in the chemical literature.

Because the chemical nomenclature and proper usage of chemical names is a frequent source of confusion, we selected a single system used for indexing by *Merck Index* [19], where synonyms, trade names, and other designations for each compound are cross-referenced. The metric system is used throughout the experimental section and all temperature data are in degrees Celsius.

A. Alkyl Halides

Methodology

In the classical concept of alkylating agents, alkyl halides conform to the general formula $C_nH_{2n+1}X$, where X is a halogen. However, the extended concept discussed earlier includes polyhalogenalkanes as well as compounds containing carbon-carbon double bonds and aromatic and aliphatic ring systems. Although a clear demarcation between alkylating and nonalkylating organic halogen compound is difficult to establish, aromatic compounds with a halogen directly attached to the aromatic ring are usually not included among alkylating agents.

NIOSH-recommended methods have been developed for 31 common alkyl halides. These methods depend on the concentration of the organic halide and are based on passing a stream of contaminated air through a small glass tube containing either activated charcoal or silica gel. The materials absorbed are eluted with an appropriate solvent, and the solution is analyzed by gas chromatography, usually with a flame ionization detector. Various sorbent tubes and portable pumps are available commercially from several suppliers. Some pumps are light in weight, battery operated, and can be suspended from the belt. The sorbent tube is connected to the pump by means of a flexible tube and is usually placed close to where breathing of the contaminated air occurs. The amount of organic vapor collected is a measure of personal exposure during the sampling period. The tubes need not be analyzed immediately but may be transported to another laboratory. Tables 2 and 3 list the solvents, columns, and temperatures used for analysis. A flame ionization detector is used for all these materials and charcoal sorbent tubes are commonly employed, except for sym-tetrabromoethane, which requires a silica gel tube [20].

Table 2 Conditions for Gas Chromatographic Analysis of Alkyl Halides

Name	NIOSH method	OSHA standard (ppm)	Sample volume (liter)	Sample rate (liter/min)	Eluent	GC column (Table 3)	Column temperature
Acetylene tetrabromide[a]	S117	1	100	1	Tetrahydrofuran	IX	105
Allyl chloride	S116	1	100	1	Benzene	V	160
Benzyl chloride	S115	1	10	0.2	Carbon disulfide	III	160
Bromoform	S114	0.5	10	0.2	Carbon disulfide	III	130
Carbon tetrachloride	S314	10	15	0.2	Carbon disulfide	I	60
Chlorobromomethane	S113	200	5	0.2	Carbon disulfide	III	80
Chloroform	S351	50 (ceiling)	15	1	Carbon disulfide	I	75
Chloroprene	S112	25 (skin)	3	0.01-0.05	Carbon disulfide	V	125
1,1-Dichloroethane	S123	100	10	0.2	Carbon disulfide	III	50
1,2-Dichloroethylene	S110	200	3	0.2	Carbon disulfide	III	60
Dichloromonofluoromethane	S109	100	3	0.01-0.05	Carbon disulfide	I	55
Dichlorotetrafluoroethane	S108	1000	3	0.01-0.05	Methylene chloride	VI	110
Difluorodibromomethane	S107	100	10	0.2	Isopropyl alcohol	III	60

Difluorodichloromethane	S111	1000	3	0.01-0.05	Methylene chloride	VI	110
Epichlorohydrin	S118	5	20	0.2	Carbon disulfide	IV	120
Ethyl bromide	S106	200	4	0.2	Isopropyl alcohol	III	60
Ethylene chlorohydrin	S103	5	20	0.2	5% isopropyl alcohol in carbon disulfide	III	130
Ethylene dibromide	S104	20	10	0.2	Carbon disulfide	III	130
Ethylene dichloride	S122	50	10	0.2	Carbon disulfide	X	70
Hexachloroethane	S101	1	10	0.2	Carbon disulfide	VIII	110
Methyl bromide	S372	20	11	0.75-1.0	Carbon disulfide	I	65
Methyl chloride	201	500	16	1	Methyl alcohol	VIII	170
Methyl chloroform	S328	350	6	0.2	Carbon disulfide	X	70
Methyl iodide	S98	5	50	1	Toluene	XI	190
Methylene chloride	S329	500	2.2	0.05	Carbon disulfide	I	60
Propylene dichloride	S95	75	10	0.2	Carbon disulfide	III	80
1,1,2-Trichloroethane	S134	10	10	0.2	Carbon disulfide	X	70
1,2,3-Trichloropropane	S126	50	10	0.2	Carbon disulfide	IV	160
Trichloroethylene	S336	100	10	0.2	Carbon disulfide	X	70
Trifluoromonobromoethane	S125	1000	1	0.05	Methylene chloride	V	160
Vinyl chloride	178	1	5	0.05	Carbon disulfide	II	60

[a] *Merck Index* name: sym-tetrabromoethane.

Source: Ref. 20, Vols. 1-3.

Table 3 Gas Chromatographic Columns Used in NIOSH Methods[a]

I	600 cm × 3.2 mm SS, 10% FFAP on Supelcoport (100-120 mesh)
II	600 cm × 3.2 mm SS, 10% SE-30 on Chromosorb W-AW DMCS (80-100 mesh)
III	300 cm × 3.2 mm SS, 10% FFAP on Chromosorb W-AW (80-100 mesh)
IV	300 cm × 32 mm SS, 10% FFAP on Chromosorb W-AW DMCS (80-100 mesh)
V	120 cm × 6.4 mm SS, Porapak Q (50-80 mesh)
VI	120 cm × 6.4 mm SS, Chromosorb 102 (80-100 mesh)
VII	90 cm × 3.2 mm SS, Porapak Q, N, or T (50-80 mesh)
VIII	300 cm × 3.2 mm glass, 3% OV-17 on Gas Chrom Q (100-120 mesh)
IX	90 cm × 6.4 mm glass, 5% SE-30 on Gas Chrom W (80-100 mesh)
X	300 cm × 3.2 mm SS, 10% OV-101 on Supelcoport (100-120 mesh)
XI	300 cm × 3.2 mm SS, Chromosorb 101

[a]SS, stainless steel.
Source: Ref. 20, Vols. 1-3.

Although this general technique is officially sanctioned and widely used, it suffers from a number of problems. The absorbent quality of coconut charcoal varies from lot to lot, and the desorption efficiency must be determined so that the analytical result may be corrected. Charcoal is also sensitive to high humidity, which decreases its absorptive capacity. High concentrations of other vapors may cause partial elution of the material of interest or cause interference with the gas chromatographic analysis. This can often be avoided by selecting a more suitable column. Very volatile halides may partially escape during elution, but desorption at dry ice temperature is reported to give higher recovery rates [21]. The capacity of the absorption tubes is limited and unless the sampling time is adjusted accordingly, breakthrough of the vapor may occur. The standard sorbent tube contains two sections of 100 mg and 50 mg of charcoal, which are desorbed and analyzed separately. If the smaller section, which is placed closest to the pump during sampling, contains more than 25% of that trapped by the larger section, it is probable that some sample was lost by breakthrough. Substitution of a more active charcoal with a higher capacity has been recommended for vinyl chloride, vinylidene chloride, and methyl chloride. Sorbent tubes containing 600 mg of charcoal are available commercially and can be used when higher than normal concentrations of vapor are expected.

Thermal desorption of the sorbent either directly onto the gas chromatographic column or into a plastic gas bag can be used to avoid problems with solvent desorption such as solvent impurities, high background or peak merging caused by large injection, and slow elution of solvent from the column. Vinyl chloride may be thermally desorbed by transferring the charcoal from the sorbent tube to a glass injection port liner and placing it in the 260 to 300° injection block. The volatile material is carried by the gas flow to the chromatographic column, which is maintained at 25° until desorption is completed. This concentrates the vinyl chloride into a narrow band. The oven temperature is then rapidly raised to 70° to elute the vinyl chloride [21]. More elaborate outboard tube ovens with valves arranged to switch the elution chamber in or out of the gas stream are available [22]. Sensitivity as low as 1 ppb may be obtained by this method since all of the material collected is available for analysis. This may also cause problems because repeat analysis of the same sample is not possible. Thermal desorption into a Saran gas bag has also been suggested to avoid problems with solvent desorption. Unfortunately, recoveries are inversely proportional to the quantity of material present in the charcoal [23]. Air samples have also been collected by the use of vacuum bottles or gas bags and analyzed by direct injection into a gas chromatograph. This eliminates the need for an expensive calibrated air pump, since the vapor concentration in the sample is independent of the sampling rate. Sensitivity is 30 to 50 ppb with 2 to 5 ml injections on Chromosorb 102 or Durapak (Carbowax 400 on Poracil) columns [21,24].

The detection of organic halides in water, particularly drinking water, is of utmost importance to public health. These materials may enter the water from waste discharge or landfill, chlorination of water, and leaching from plastic pipe. A variety of techniques have been developed to permit concentrating the pollutant from large quantities of water, separation from other collected materials, and quantification followed by identification. By means of a gas chromatograph equipped with a mass spectrometer for detection, pollutants may be identified and quantitatively determined to sub-ppb levels [25].

Alkyl halides have been isolated and identified by a general technique developed for volatile organics in water. A sample ranging from 5 to 500 ml is placed in a device similar to a gas washing bottle and purified helium or nitrogen is passed through the water to strip the volatile material. The exit gas is passed through an absorbent tube containing a porous polymer, usually Tenax GC, which traps the organic material. Fractionation can be achieved by conducting the gas purge first at 6°, then briefly at 95°, and for a longer period at 95°. The absorbed material is transferred by thermal desorption to a cold gas chromatographic column. Small quantities of absorbent can also be desorbed by means of the injection block. Chromosorb 101 and Tenax GC are usually satisfactory as gas chromatography column packings. A mass spectrometer is almost essential for peak detection because it provides identification as well as high sensitivity. Quantitative values are somewhat difficult to obtain by this method because of the uncertainty of complete extraction from the water and problems with desorption. Alkyl halides have been determined to 0.1 ppb [26-28].

Vinyl chloride has been determined without concentration in water to 0.1 ppb by gas chromatograph-mass spectrometry with a 1 ml injection. A dual column consisting of a 40 cm × 6 mm i.d. metal precolumn packed with 10% diglycerol on Chromsorb G NAW (60-80 mesh) followed by a 600 cm × 2 mm i.d. metal column packed with 5% SE-30 on Chromosorb W AW DCMS (60-80 mesh) was used [25].

Polyvinyl chloride and vinyl chloride-vinylidene chloride copolymer (Saran) have long been used for food packaging, plastic pipe, and molded parts. The monomers were originally believed not to migrate to food or liquid in contact with the polymer, but in 1973, liquor packaged in polyvinyl chloride bottles was found to contain the monomer. Sensitive analytical methods have since been developed to determine these and other alkyl halides in a wide variety of solids and liquids. Probably the most commonly used methods are gas chromatographic analyses of the sample neat, dissolved in a solvent, or of the head space gas above the sample. Alkyl halides are ideally suited for head space analysis because of their relatively high vapor pressures and only slight solubility in many of the liquids or solids in which they are determined. This technique depends on the analysis of the gas above a liquid or solid at equilibrium, and by comparison with similar standards, the quantity of analyte may be calculated. Greater sensitivity is achieved than with direct injection of a liquid or solid sample because 1000-fold greater quantities may be injected without causing interference from solvent impurities or background. Also, depending on the partition coefficient and the relative gas-liquid volumes, the analyte may be considerably concentrated in the gaseous phase. The system is often heated to accelerate the establishment of equilibrium and to increase the halide concentration in the gas. The injection of a gas also eliminates the need for disposable injection port liners, precolumns, and to a certain extent backflushing or temperature programming to purge the column of slowly eluting materials [21].

Vinyl chloride remaining unpolymerized in polyvinyl chloride has been determined by head space analysis of a 10% solution of the polymer in dimethyl acetamide. A Perkin-Elmer Multifract F-40 Automated Head-Space Analyzer equipped with a 180 cm × 3.2 mm stainless steel column packed with 0.4% Carbowax 1500 on Carbopak and a flame ionization detector was used. The polymer was placed in a septum-sealed vial with the solvent, and was dissolved by heating. The sample vials were placed on the instrument sample tray and equilibrated for at least 30 min at 90° before analysis. Peak heights obtained were compared with those obtained from similar samples made from monomer-free polymer and a known quantity of vinyl chloride to calculate the vinyl chloride concentration. The limit of detection was 50 ppb when the head space technique was used, or 1 to 2 ppm when a direct injection of the 10% polymer solution was employed [29]. Other gas chromatographic columns that have been used to determine residual vinyl chloride by direct injection of a tetrahydrofuran or dimethyl acetamide solution of the polymer are 300 cm × 3.2 mm stainless steel packed with Chromosorb 104 (60-80 mesh) at 100°, and 180 cm × 3.2 mm stainless steel packed with Porapak S (60-80 mesh) at 130°. A short precolumn was used with the latter packing and it was backflushed after each analysis to remove the solvent. A flame ionization detector was used with both columns. Vinyl chloride could be detected at 1 ppm but solvent impurities, particularly from tetrahydrofuran, were troublesome [30].

Head space analysis was used to determine vinyl chloride migration from the polymer into corn oil, 50% ethanol, 3% acetic acid, or heptane to 1 ppb or less. A 20 ml sample was placed in a nitrogen-flushed 35 ml bottle sealed with a Teflon-lined septum. After equilibration at 90° for 30 min, a 3 ml gas sample was removed with a hot gas syringe and the sample was analyzed on a 150 cm × 2 mm i.d. stainless steel column packed with Chromosorb 104 (60-80 mesh) at 95° with a 50 ml/min helium flow. Peak heights from a ionization detector were compared to those obtained from standards to quantify the results [31]. Vinylidene chloride migration from Saran film into food-simulating solvents was determined by a similar method. Samples of the film were sealed with the appropriate solvent in tin cans and held at 49°. Solvent samples were removed from the cooled can by means of a can-piercing device and placed in a septum-sealed vial. After equilibration at 90° for 30 min, a 1 to 2 ml gas sample was removed and analyzed on a 300 cm × 2 mm glass column packed with Chromosorb 104 (80-100 mesh) at 175° with 16 ml/min 5% argon in methane carrier gas. When an electron capture detector was used, the vinylidene chloride could be detected to 5 to 10 ppb [32].

Methylene chloride, ethylene dichloride, and trichloroethylene present in spice extracts have been isolated by a closed-system vacuum distillation techniques using toluene as a carrier. The distillate was analyzed by gas chromatography with electron capture detector on a 180 cm × 2 mm i.d. glass column packed with Porapak Q (80-100 mesh) or Porasil (100-150 mesh). Trans-1,2-dichloroethylene was used as an internal standard and trichloroethylene was detected to 30 ppb [33].

Analytical methods

Vinyl Chloride in Air. This method has been recommended by NIOSH for measuring vinyl chloride concentrations in workplace air for compliance with OSHA standards [34]. The method depends on trapping the vinyl chloride on activated charcoal, desorption of the captured material into carbon disulfide, and analysis of this solution by gas chromatography. The absorbent tubes, portable pump, and chromatography columns are commercially available (Supelco, Inc.; SKC, Inc.).

The sorbent tubes are 7 cm × 6 mm glass tubes, packed with 100 mg and 50 mg sections of 20-40 mesh activated charcoal that are flame sealed. The 50 mg charcoal section is used to determine whether breakthrough has occurred in the 100 mg section. Vinyl chloride, however, will migrate rapidly between these sections unless the exposed tube is stored at -20°. This problem may be avoided by using two tubes in series and combining both sections in each tube for analysis. The tubes are prepared for use by breaking the end seals so that an opening of not less than 2 mm is produced. Two tubes are linked together by means of short plastic tubing and connected to a calibrated pump. The air sample is drawn through the tubes at a flow rate of 50 ml/min for 100 min or less, depending on the expected concentration of vinyl chloride. A tube should be opened at the same time but without passing air for use as a blank. The tubes are capped with the plastic caps supplied and are transported to the laboratory. The tube may be shipped at ambient temperature but should be stored in the laboratory at -20°. Both charcoal sections of a tube are removed and placed in a 2 ml vial containing 1 ml of carbon disulfide. The charcoal must be added to the solvent to prevent local heating and loss of vinyl chloride. The vial is capped with a septum and held for 30 min with occasional agitation. The sample should be analyzed within 60 min after desorption. The desorbed vinyl chloride is analyzed by gas chromatography with a 600 cm × 3.2 mm stainless steel column packed with 10% SE-30 on Chromsorb W AWS (80-100 mesh) with 40 ml/min helium carrier. A flame ionization detector is used. A 5 μl sample is injected by means of the solvent flush technique. Standards are prepared by bubbling vinyl chloride through 5 ml of toluene in a weighed 10 ml flask. After 3 min about 100 to 300 mg should have been collected as determined by weighing the flask, and the solution is diluted to 10 ml with carbon disulfide. Dilutions are made so that standards containing between 0.2 and 1.5 μg/5 μl are obtained. Standards are stable for 3 days if stored at -20°. These standards are analyzed in the same manner as the samples and a plot of μg/ml versus peak area for a 5 μl injection is constructed. This allows direct reading of the weight of the vinyl chloride trapped in the sorbent tube. The efficiency of the desorption of the vinyl chloride from the charcoal will vary from batch to batch of charcoal and should be determined. A known concentration of vinyl chloride in air is prepared by injecting a known volume of vinyl chloride into a Tedlar bag containing a known volume of air. The concentration may be determined by injection of a gas sample into the gas chromatograph with a gastight syringe. This air is drawn through a sorbent tube with a calibrated pump and the tubes are desorbed and analyzed. Desorption efficiency is calculated from formula (8).

$$\text{Desorption efficiency} = \frac{\text{amount of VC}}{(\text{conc. VC in bag}) \times (\text{vol. sample})} \quad (8)$$

The concentration of vinyl chloride in air is calculated as follows. The weight found in the sample tube is read as μg/ml from the standard curve. This weight is then corrected by subtracting the blank, and the total is divided by the desorption efficiency to correct for this loss (9). Standardized concentration values expressed in mg/m^3 (10) or in ppm (11) can be obtained by appropriate conversions.

$$\text{Corrected weight} = \frac{\text{wt. sample - wt. blank}}{\text{desorption efficiency}} \quad (9)$$

$$mg/m^3 = \frac{\text{corrected weight } (\mu g)}{\text{vol. air (liters)}} \quad (10)$$

$$ppm = mg/m^3 \times \frac{24.45}{62.5} \times \frac{760}{p} \times \frac{t + 273}{292} \quad (11)$$

where

24.45 = molar volume at 25° and 760 mmHg
62.5 = molecular weight of vinyl chloride
p = pressure (mmHg) of air sampled
t = temperature of air sampled

Determination of Vinylidene Chloride in Food-Stimulating Solvents. Residual vinylidene chloride from Saran film that has migrated to corn oil or n-heptane can be determined by gas chromatographic analysis of the head space gas. A 20 ml solvent sample that had been stored in a sealed, tinned can with Saran film is removed with the aid of a can-piercing device (Alltech Assoc.) and a 30 ml syringe. The sample is transferred to a 35 ml screw-capped bottle having a Teflon-faced septum that had been flushed with nitrogen. After the sample is injected through the septum, the cap is loosened to relieve the pressure. The bottle is held in a 90° oil bath to equilibrate for 30 min and without removing the bottle, a 1 to 2 ml gas sample is removed with a gastight syringe that had been heated to 90° in a vacuum oven. The plunger is pumped several times to wet the barrel with the vapors and is held 30 sec after gas withdrawal to equilibrate the pressure between the bottle and the syringe. The syringe valve is closed before withdrawing the needle and the gas sample is immediately injected into the gas chromatograph. The peak area obtained is compared with those from known standards to calculate vinylidene chloride concentration. A stock standard solution of vinylidene chloride in heptane is prepared by transferring 100 μl of pure vinylidene chloride with a microliter syringe to 200 ml of heptane. This solution contains 625 ppm of the standard and is stable when stored under refrigeration. When diluted 1:10, a working standard is obtained from which head space standards are made by injecting the necessary quantities into 20 ml samples of corn oil or heptane in 35 ml bottles. The standard concentrations should span the expected concentrations of unknowns. Peak areas are used to quantitate chromatographic results. The gas chromatographic column is 300 cm × 2 mm, glass, packed with Chromosorb 104 (80-100 mesh) and operated at 175° with 16 ml/min of 5% argon in methane as carrier. An electron capture detector is used. A 2 to 3 ng injection of vinylidene chloride gives one-half scale deflection with a retention time of 4 min, and concentrations as low as 5 ppb can be detected [32].

B. Alkyl Sulfates

Methodology

Dimethyl sulfate collected from workplace air by absorption on a porous polymer resin has been determined to ppb levels by gas chromatography with a mass spectrometer as the detector. Tenax GC (60-80 mesh), Porapak Q (50-80 mesh), and Chromosorb 101 (60-80 mesh) have been tested and found satisfactory absorbents. After purification by extraction with acetone, 250 mg of the dried absorbent is packed in 10 cm tubes and held in place by glass wool. All volatile material is removed by heating at 220 to 250° for 24 hr in a slow stream of helium or nitrogen. Dimethyl sulfate is collected by drawing up to 10 liters of air through the absorption tube. The tube is then attached to a gas chromatograph so that the carrier gas passes through the tube. Heating the tube desorbs the collected material, which is carried by the gas stream to a metal capillary trap cooled in liquid nitrogen. This trap is then heated rapidly to transfer the sample to the chromatograph column. Sharper peaks without tailing are obtained by this technique than by desorption directly onto the column. The gas chromatography column used for dimethyl sulfate was a 3 m × 2 mm i.d. glass column packed with 5% DESGSE on

Chromosorb W (80-100 mesh) operated at 125° with a 20 ml/min flow of a helium carrier. As they emerge, peaks are detected and identified by means of a quadrupole mass spectrometer, and at least four mass fragment peaks should be used to identify the eluted material positively. Higher sensitivity may be obtained by single ion detection, but confidence in the identification is reduced. Storage of the absorption tube after sample collection can result in loss of dimethyl sulfate by reaction with other absorbed material. Sample tubes can be held for several days at -20° after being washed with dry helium to remove moisture [35].

Diethyl sulfate has also been collected and determined by a similar procedure using 2.5 g of Tenax GC in a 10 cm × 1.5 cm glass cartridge. The chromatography column was 3.6 m × 2.5 mm glass, packed with 2% DEGS on Supelcoport (80-100 mesh), and a flame ionization detector was used [36].

A colorimetric procedure sensitive to 0.15 μg/liter of dimethyl sulfate in air has been described. The 10 to 20 liter air sample is passed at a rate of 0.5 liter/min through two air scrubbers each containing 3 ml of pyridine. The dimethyl sulfate alkylates the pyridine to form N-methylpyridinium sulfate. To a 1 ml aliquot from each scrubber are added 2 ml of pyridine and 0.5 ml of 0.2 N sodium hydroxide, and the mixture is heated at 100° for 15 min. This hydrolyzes the pyridinium salt to gluconaldehyde, which reacts readily to form a colored Schiff base after 0.1 ml of aniline and 1 ml of acetic acid have been added. The sample is held in the dark for 30 min and absorbance is read at 484 nm [37].

C. Alkyl Phosphates and Thiophosphates

Methodology

Trialkyl and triaryl phosphates are readily separated and determined by gas chromatography. The flame photometric detector is often used because it combines high sensitivity with excellent selectivity for either phosphorus or sulfur. This reduces the usual background problems with low-level samples and eliminates the need for extensive cleanup procedure. Gas chromatograph-mass spectrometer combinations are also used and provide a highly sensitive system. Sufficient information is often obtained to identify the eluting material positively. Various trialkyl phosphates and thiophosphates have been determined by these methods as parts of a scheme to detect the mono and dialkyl esters from the hydrolysis or metabolism of pesticides and other phosphorus esters. Following isolation by ether extraction or absorption onto a resin, the mono and diesters are methylated with diazomethane to give the trialkyl esters, which can be chromatographed without thermal decomposition. The dialkyl esters can be extracted into ethyl acetate or 1:1 acetonitrile ether from blood, urine, or water after acidification with hydrochloric acid and saturation with sodium chloride [38]. These materials may also be concentrated from large volumes of water by absorption onto a macroreticular resin (XAD-4, Rohm and Haas). The resins are purified before use by extended extraction first with acetone and then with methanol. After acidification to pH 1.25 with hydrochloric acid, the water sample is passed through 100 ml of resin at a rate of 1 liter/hr. The phosphates are eluted from the resin with acetone and this solution is concentrated to a few milliliters under vacuum. Alkyl phosphates esters are extracted into ethyl acetate and completely esterified by treatment with diazomethane or diazoethane [39] and this product is then analyzed by gas chromatography. Greater sensitivity is claimed by cleanup of the crude alkylated mixture before gas chromatographic analysis. Trialkyl thiophosphates are easily extracted from an aqueous solution with hexane, and the phosphates are extracted with benzene. Further purification is achieved with liquid-solid chromatography on silica gel [40].

Gas chromatographic columns used to separate these triesters are 360 cm × 6.35 mm i.d. aluminum, packed with 20% Versamid 900 on Gas Chrom Q (60-80 mesh) [38], 1.8 m × 2 mm i.d. glass, packed with equal parts of 15% DC-QF-1 and 10% DC-200 on Gas Chrom Q (80-100 mesh), and for gas chromatograph-mass spectrometer a glass column packed with 3% OV-1 on Chromosorb W [39]. The limit of detection for these materials is about 2 ppb [39]. Degradation products of tributyl phosphate used in nuclear fuel processing have been determined by gas chromatography following methylation with diazomethane. A 1.4 m × 2 mm i.d. glass column containing 20% E-301 on Chromosorb W was used [41]. Tributyl phosphate, together with 32 other organic compounds, has been identified in Philadelphia drinking water. The contaminants were collected on a 5 cm × 11 cm column of XAD-2 (50-150 mesh) macroreticular resin. The water sample, after acidification to pH 4 with phosphoric acid, was passed through the column at a rate of 15 liters/hr. The organic material was eluted with ether and this solution was dried and concentrated. The residue was analyzed by gas chromatography with a 180 cm × 2.16 mm i.d. stainless steel column packed with 20% SE-30 on Gas Chrom Q (80-100 mesh); temperature was programmed from 80 to 200°. Peaks were detected and identified by an interfaced mass spectrometer [42]. Tributyl phosphate and triethyl phosphate were detected in groundwater under a land fill at levels of 1.7 and 0.3 μg/liter, respectively. The material was isolated by passing about 750 liters of water directly from the well through a 45.7 × 7.6 cm column of Nuchar C-190 (30 mesh) activated charcoal at a rate of 100 ml/min. The charcoal was then dried and extracted with chloroform in a Soxhlet apparatus. After concentration to 3 ml the sample was subjected to preliminary separation by liquid-solid chromatography on Silicar CC-7 and the fractions were analyzed by gas

Table 4 Sampling and Chromatographic Conditions for Phosphate Esters

	Tributyl phosphate	Tri-o-cresyl phosphate	Triphenyl phosphate
NIOSH method number	S208	S209	S210
OSHA limit (mg/m3)	5	0.1	3
Method range (mg/m^3)	2.7-12.6	0.029-0.170	1.25-6.99
Air sample (liters)	100	100	100
Rate (liters/min)	1.5	1.5	1.5
Filter	Cellulose ester	Cellulose ester	Cellulose ester
Eluent	10 ml ether	10 ml ether	10 ml ether
Column	OV-101 3% on Supelcoport (100-120 mesh) 180 × 0.32 cm i.d.	OV-101 3% on Supelcoport (100-120 mesh) 180 × 0.23 cm i.d.	OV-101 5% on Supelcoport (100-120 mesh) 180 × 0.32 cm i.d.
Column temperature (°C)	150	220	220

Source: Ref. 20, Vol. 3.

chromatography with either a 3% OV-1 on Gas Chrom Q (100-120 mesh) or a 3% Carbowax 20M on Gas Chrom Q (80-100 mesh) column. The peaks were detected and identified by mass spectroscopy [43]. Tributyl phosphate, tri-o-cresyl phosphate, and triphenyl phosphate present in air as aerosols may be readily determined by NIOSH-recommended methods. The sample is collected by drawing workplace air through a mixed cellulose ester membrane filter contained in a small plastic holder. The phosphate ester is eluted from the membrane with ethyl ether and determined by gas chromatography with a flame photometric detector. The filter, holder, and pump are commercially available (Millipore Corp.). Additional information is given in Table 4 [44-46]. The formation of a 1:1 complex of tributyl phosphate with nitric acid has been used as the basis of a titrimetric method for tributyl phosphate in hydrocarbon solvent used in uranium extraction. A sample is shaken with 10% sodium carbonate to remove dissolved uranium and then shaken several times with 8 N nitric acid. An aliquot of the organic phase is mixed with water and titrated with standard sodium hydroxide [47].

Analytical methods

Tributyl Phosphate. This method is recommended by NIOSH for measuring the concentration of tributyl phosphate in workplace air for compliance with OSHA regulations [44]. Tributyl phosphate present as an aerosol is collected by passing a known quantity of air through a membrane filter. The phosphate is extracted from the filter into ether and an aliquot is analyzed by gas chromatography. The filter device is a polystyrene cassette which contains a mixed cellulose ester membrane filter, 37 mm in diameter, with pore size 0.8 μm. The filter is supported by a cellulose pad which also serves to trap tributyl phosphate vapor. When operating at temperatures higher than 23°, it is necessary to use two of these cassettes in series to ensure complete collection of both aerosol and vapor. The cassettes are commercially available (Millipore Corp.). Air is drawn through the filter with a calibrated air pump at a rate of 1.5 liters/min until 100 liters of air has passed. This procedure will be satisfactory for an air concentration of phosphate ranging from 0.5 to 15 mg/m^3, but the sample size may be adjusted for higher or lower concentrations. After sampling, the cassettes are sealed until analysis with the plugs provided. A cassette which is carried through in the same manner as the other units but without passage of air should also be provided for use as a blank. The cassette is carefully opened and the filter and backup pad transferred with tweezers to a 56 g ointment jar with an aluminum-lined screw cap. Into each jar is pipetted 10 ml of ether. The jars are sealed and held for 30 min with occasional agitation and the samples are analyzed by gas chromatography with a flame photometric detector and a phosphorus filter. The column is 180 cm × 3.2 mm i.d. stainless steel packed with 3% OV-101 on Supelcoport (100-120 mesh) operated at 150° with 50 ml/min nitrogen carrier. A 5 μl sample is injected with a 10 μl syringe by means of the flush injection technique. The syringe is wetted with clean ether and 3 μl of ether is withdrawn. Then 0.2 μl of air is drawn up, and finally 5 μl of the sample. The plunger is withdrawn until this 5 μl sample is visible within the barrel. The sample volume must be between 4.9 and 5.0 μl. The amount of tributyl phosphate in the sample is read from a standard curve of peak area versus μg/10 ml of tributyl phosphate. Peak area is obtained most conveniently by means of an electronic integrator. The standards are prepared by diluting pure tributyl phosphate with ether and varying its concentration over the expected range of the air sample. Sample recovery from the membrane filter must be determined to eliminate this possible error. A known sample of tributyl phosphate is placed on a filter, the filter is air dried, and the material is extracted and analyzed. A correction factor is necessary if recovery is less than 95%.

D. Aziridines

Methodology

Aziridines, together with nitrogen mustards, constitute the majority of the category of biological alkylating agents. Research in cancer chemotherapy provided the impetus for synthesis of thousands of new compounds, most of them laboratory curiosities of limited shelflife and scientific interest. Nitrogen mustards, the larger of the two groups, have never achieved industrial importance, but aziridines, particularly the volatile ethylenimine and propylenimine, represent potentially useful intermediates in industrial organic synthesis. Other, more complex aziridines have been intermittently used in larger quantities, and because of their broad range of biological activities as cancer chemotherapeutic, insect sterilizing, and mutagenic agents, their detection is of considerable interest.

Titration with a standard acid is the simplest analytical method for basic aziridines. Satisfactory results are obtained in the absence of interfering bases by titration with a nonnucleophilic acid such as sulfuric or perchloric acid. This prevents ring opening, which can occur with a nucleophilic anion, leading to unrealistically high results. On the other hand, acid-induced polymerization of the aziridine has no influence on the titration, since the product is another secondary amine [48,49]. Other titrimetric methods usually involve a ring-opening reaction. The reaction of thiosulfate with an aziridine to give a Bunte salt is commonly used, but other reagents, such as bromide, thiocyanate, or pyridine, have been employed. These reactions are often carried out in the presence of a large excess of the nucleophile; the uptake of acid is then determined. Alternatively, a buffered solution may be used and the unused nucleophile back-titrated. Basic aziridines must be rapidly and completely protonated to prevent ring opening by nucleophilic attack of another basic aziridine. This is less important with negatively substituted aziridines because they have much less tendency to act as nucleophiles. The rate of reaction is increased by protonation of the aziridine nitrogen and the reaction is normally carried out at pH 4. Solvolysis of the aziridine ring does not consume acid and will cause low results [50]. The thiosulfate titration of aziridines is normally carried out by reacting the sample with a large excess of sodium thiosulfate. The pH is maintained at 4 during the reaction by frequent additions of standard sulfuric acid. A lower pH causes rapid decomposition of the thiosulfate without appreciably increasing the ring-opening reaction. With most aziridines, the reaction is complete within 30 min and the excess acid is back-titrated with standard base. Methyl orange indicator can be used for the pH 4 end point and phenolphthalein or phenol red for the back-titration, but more accurate results are obtained with the aid of a pH meter [51].

A procedure based on the reaction of ethylenimine and hydrobromic acid to give 2-bromoethylamine has been recommended as the best titrimetric method for basic aziridines. A sample containing 40 mEq of aziridine is neutralized with hydrochloric acid and mixed with 20 ml of saturated sodium bromide and 50 ml of 1 N hydrochloric acid. The mixture is boiled for 15 min, cooled, and back-titrated with standard sodium hydroxide to pH 4.8. This method is not applicable to water-insoluble or negatively substituted aziridines [50,52]. A similar method utilizing the reaction of hydriodic acid with an aziridine in nonaqueous solvent is suitable for almost any aziridine. The sample dissolved in chloroform, benzene, or acetone is mixed with an excess of tetraethylammonium iodide and titrated with standard perchloric acid in glacial acetic acid to a sharp crystal violet end point. The reaction with unreactive aziridines may be accelerated by the use of an excess of perchloric acid and back-titration with standard sodium acetate in acetic acid [53].

The highly nucleophilic thiocyanate ion has been used in methanol for the determination of sterically hindered aziridines. The sample in methanol is mixed with an excess of potassium thiocyanate and standard p-toluene sulfonic acid. Unlike thiosulfate, high acidity does not destroy the thiocyanate ion. The rate of ring opening is also faster, and the reaction mixture is back-titrated immediately with methanolic potassium hydroxide. Results obtained from the analysis of metepa were only slightly lower than those obtained in a thiosulfate titration, but analyses of other hindered aziridines were considerably lower than theoretical [54]. A novel method for water-insoluble aziridines is based on the reaction of pyridine with the aziridine ring in the presence of an excess of acid. An aziridine sample is dissolved in a 2.5-fold excess of 0.2 N pyridine hydrochloride in pyridine and held at room temperature for 30 min. After addition of water equal to twice the volume of pyridine, the excess acid is titrated with standard sodium hydroxide to a pH 10.5 end point [52].

Gas chromatography provides a rapid and sensitive analytical method for many volatile aziridines. Ethylenimine can be determined in air or water at levels as low as 2 to 5 ppm with a flame ionization detector or at higher levels with a thermal conductivity detector. Some column packings suitable for ethylenimine are 30% Dow Polyglycol E6000 on Celite (30-70 mesh), 30% Oronite Dispersant NI-W on Chromosorb W (80-100 mesh), 30% Triton X-100 on Gas Chrom P (100-200 mesh), and 15% Tergitol 35 on Chromosorb W (60-80 mesh) treated with potassium hydroxide. Peak tailing, which is also a problem with other amines, may be minimized by use of silanized support material and by treatment of the support with potassium hydroxide. Gas chromatography is also used to determine impurities in ethylenimine [50,52].

Nanogram quantities of phosphorus-substituted aziridines may be determined in air, water, and biological tissues by use of the flame photometric detector. Since this detector is sensitive only to phosphorus-containing substances when operated with a 526 nm filter, the need for cleanup of biological extracts is virtually eliminated [55]. Direct injection of these solutions greatly reduces the loss of sensitive materials because of isolation procedures. However, retention times may be temporarily changed by large, oily samples. Short, lighly loaded columns are often recommended to avoid decomposition of heat-sensitive aziridines. Bowman [56] has determined relative retention times for 19 phosphorus aziridines on 50 cm glass columns (4 mm i.d.) packed with Gas Chrom Q (80-100 mesh) with 5% liquid phase, such as Dexsil 300, OV-101, OV-17, OV-210, OV-225, and OV-25. Phosphorus aziridines containing thiophosphoryl groups (PS) chromatographed satisfactorily on all columns, but aziridines with phosphoryl groups (PO) tailed on all but those containing OV-225. Conditioning of the column can be achieved with 250 ng injections of the compound to be determined, until a 5 ng injection gives a constant response. This procedure is usually necessary for analysis of trace levels of phosphorus aziridines, particularly when phosphoryl groups are present. The OV-225-loaded column, which is the most polar among those mentioned earlier, does not tail with phosphoryl compounds, requires a minimum of conditioning, and is remarkably insensitive to contamination from crude biological materials. As an analytical procedure, gas chromatography is particularly useful because a qualitative as well as quantitative identification may be obtained simultaneously. Further confirmation at trace levels may be obtained by determining the p values for the material. These p values are defined as the fraction of material partitioning into the nonpolar phase of an equivolume immiscible binary solvent system. Values were determined for 19 aziridines in 11 solvent systems [55]. Gas chromatographic methods have been used for the determination of triethylenethiophosphoramide in boll weevils [57]; triethylenephosphoramide in fall army worm moths [55]; triethylenethiophosphoramide, bisazir, and P,P-bis(1-aziridinyl)-N-ethylphosphinothioic amide in mosquitoes [58,59]; and triethylenethiophosphoramide in spotted bollworms [60].

The most widely used colorimetric procedure for aziridines involves the reaction with 4-(4-nitrobenzyl)pyridine (NBP) to give a blue dye [61]. The reaction is not specific for aziridines and almost any alkylating agent will give the color. It has been used to detect nitrogen and sulfur mustards, alkyl halides, diethyl sulfate, alkanesulfonate esters, and various phosphorus, nitrogen, and silicon halides. One modification has been suggested as a general method to determine the presence of alkylating agents in air [62]. The reaction involved in the production of the blue dye is usually represented as an alkylation (12)

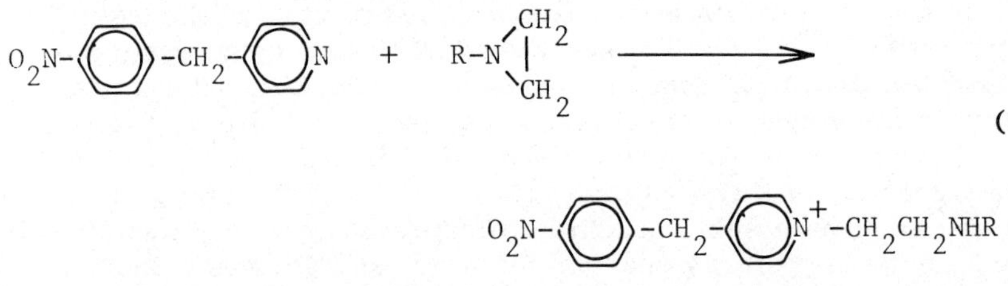

(12)

in which the nucleophilic NBP reacts at the carbon atom of the protonated aziridine. In the presence of base, the resulting intermediate yields a blue dye [50,63]. The reaction with aziridines is normally carried out at pH 4, usually in potassium hydrogen phthalate buffer. Water is often used as the reaction solvent, and acetone, methyl ethyl ketone, or ethanol serves as solvent for the NBP reagent. The mixture is heated on a steam or water bath for about 20 min, but it may be necessary to determine an optimum reaction period for a particular aziridine. After chilling in an ice bath, the color is produced by making the mixture alkaline and adding acetone or ethanol [61]. Various inorganic bases, such as potassium carbonate, sodium hydroxide, potassium hydroxide, or organic amines, may also be used, and increased color stability is claimed for some of these modifications. The dye has also been extracted into amyl acetate to avoid problems encountered with determinations of alkylating agents in biological fluids [64]. Since color stability may be a problem, the absorbance should be determined as rapidly as possible after development of the color. The absorption maximum usually occurs at 600 nm, but since this maximum may vary with different aziridines, it is worthwhile to determine the optimum wavelength for each specific compound. Interference can occur if competing nucleophiles, such as chloride or phosphate ion, are present. These react readily with the protonated aziridine and will cause low results. If the concentration of interfering ion is known, it may be possible to set up standards having equal concentrations and compensate for the interference [64]. Plasma proteins can also compete, and precipitation of these materials with trichloracetic acid and acetate buffer at pH 4 may be necessary [65]. This method will detect aziridines in concentrations as low as 1 μg/ml, and although it is less sensitive than gas chromatographic methods, it is easily carried out with most aziridines and with readily available or inexpensive equipment.

The quantitative reaction of ethylenimine in dilute aqueous solution with Folin's reagent (sodium 1,2-naphthoquinone-4-sulfonate with alkaline buffer) provides a sensitive method for the determination of aziridines unsubstituted on nitrogen [66]. The reaction goes to completion within a few minutes and the reaction product, 4-(1-aziridinyl)-1,2-naphthoquinone, is easily extracted into a small quantity of chloroform. This procedure eliminates interference from the product of ethanolamine and the reagent since all are insoluble in chloroform; however, it does not eliminate the interference of other primary and secondary amines. The absorbance may be measured at 420 nm or with increased sensitivity at 254 nm. Plant and laboratory air has been conveniently monitored for ethylenimine by passing the air through wash bottles containing buffered Folin's reagent followed by extraction with chloroform. Quantities as low as 0.2 ppm may be detected [67]. Interference from other amines may be eliminated by utilizing high-pressure liquid chromatography to separate the various 1,2-naphthoquinone derivatives. A 10 μm silica gel analytical column readily separates these products and the use of an ultraviolet (UV) detector at 254 nm allows detection of 5 ng/ml of ethylenimine [68].

Trace amounts of triethylenethiophosphoramide and triethylenephosphoramide in urine or serum have been determined by reaction with 2-naphthol and measurement of the product by fluorimetry. Triethylenethiophosphoramide and its metabolite triethylenephosphoramide may both be extracted from an aqueous sample into 10% methanol in chloroform, or alternatively, triethylenethiophosphoramide may be selectively removed by benzene. The reaction is carried out by heating the dry mixture of aziridine and 2-naphthol to 125 to 130° for 20 min. The product is hydrolyzed with hydrochloric acid to give 2-(2-naphthoxy)ethylamine, which is separated from the reagent by partition between ethylene dichloride and aqueous alkali. The fluorescent product is extracted into 1 N hydrochloric acid, and the fluorescence is measured at 355 nm with activation at 290 nm. Recovery from a spiked sample is greater than 90% at 50 ng/ml [69].

Analytical methods

Thiosulfate Titration of Propylenimine. An accurately-weighed sample of propylenimine containing approximately 2 mEq in 50 ml of water is titrated with 0.1 N sulfuric acid to pH 4.9. This volume of acid is not used in the calculation. To this solution is added 50 ml of 20% sodium thiosulfate solution and the mixture is warmed to 50°. The solution is titrated with 0.1 N sulfuric acid to pH 4 and kept between pH 4 and 5 by additions of the acid. After 30 min, the excess acid is titrated to pH 5.7 with a 0.1 N sodium hydroxide solution. A blank with 50 ml of the sodium thiosulfate solution is treated in the same manner. Propylenimine is equivalent to the acid titration less the base back-titration and the blank [70].

Thiosulfate Titration of Triethylenephosphoramide [52]. To an accurately weighed sample containing 1 mmol of triethylenephosphoramide is added 50 ml of a 20% sodium thiosulfate solution. This is titrated to pH 4 with 0.1 N sulfuric acid and kept at this pH for 30 min by adding additional acid solution as required. The solution is then back-titrated with 0.1 N sodium hydroxide solution to the break at about pH 8. The titration may also be carried out with methyl orange (pH 4) and phenol red (pH 8) indicators instead of a pH meter. A blank is run in the same manner with 50 ml of thiosulfate solution. The triethylenephosphoramide content of the sample is calculated usually as a weight percentage (13).

$$\text{Weight \%} = \frac{(ae - bf - ce - df) \times 173.1 \times 100}{\text{wt of sample (g)} \times 1000} \tag{13}$$

where

a = ml of sulfuric acid used for sample
b = ml of sodium hydroxide used for sample
c = ml of sulfuric acid used for blank
d = ml of sodium hydroxide used for blank
e = normality of sulfuric acid
g = normality of sodium hydroxide

Determination of Triethylenethiophosphoramide by Gas Chromatography. Boll weevils treated with tritheylenethiophosphoramide are homogenized in a glass tissue grinder with three successive portions (2 to 10 ml) of acetone and the supernatant liquid is filtered through a medium-porosity glass filter. The combined fractions are reduced in volume on a rotary evaporator (30°), and the final volume is adjusted with acetone to 1 ml for a single insect or 5 to 10 ml for 25 weevils. The acetone stops the metabolism of triethylenethiophosphoramide and the whole weevil in acetone, or the extract may be held at 0° for several weeks before analysis without appreciable loss. The extracts are analyzed for triethylenethiophosphoramide by gas chromatography with a flame photometric detector operated in the phosphorus mode. A 36 cm glass column (4 mm i.d.) containing 5% OV-225 on Gas Chrom Q (80-100 mesh) is used at 165°. Flow rates are as follows on a Hewlett-Packard 5710 instrument: nitrogen (carrier), 100 ml/min; hydrogen, 200; air, 50; and oxygen, 20. Results are recorded and calculated with a Hewlett-Packard Reporting Integrator, which automatically measures the area under the curve and compares this with a standard. As little as 2 ng of triethylenethiophosphoramide may be detected by this method [57].

Determination of Bisazir (P,P-bis(1-Aziridinyl)-N-Methylphosphinothioic Amide) in Air. Glass absorption tubes (15 mm o.d. × 15 mm long with 10 mm o.d. ends) are filled with 3 ml of Chromosorb 102 held in place with glass wool. The tubes are purged with a slow flow of helium at 200° overnight, washed with hexane, and dried with a stream of nitrogen. The air to be analyzed is drawn through the tube at a rate of 1 liter/min for 4 hr, or longer if the bisazir concentration is below 2 μg/m^3. The tube is capped on both ends with vinyl caps and stored under refrigeration until extraction. The absorbed bisazir is removed from the packing by percolating 50 ml portions of hexane through the tube three times. The combined fractions are concentrated on a rotary evaporator and the volume is adjusted to 1 ml with hexane. The bisazir in 10 μl aliquots is determined by gas chromatography with a 1 m × 2 mm i.d. glass column packed with 3% Dexil 410 on Gas Chrom Q (100-120 mesh). A flame photometric detector operated in the phosphorus mode is used. Oven temperature is 140°, and helium flow through the column in 20 ml/min. Results are corrected for the following losses: extraction, 5%; collection, 0.016% per liter of air passed; storage, 25% per week; concentration of extract, 11% [71].

Triethylenephosphoramide in Mexican Fruit Flies. Several hundred Mexican fruit flies that had been treated with triethylenephosphoramide at the pupal stage are killed by freezing and placed in chloroform (1 ml per 10 flies). The mixture is thoroughly shaken, filtered, and the residue is washed with chloroform. The combined filtrates are evaporated on a rotary evaporator to near dryness and the volume is adjusted with chloroform to equal 1 ml per 100 flies. A 1 ml aliquot is taken, evaporated to dryness, and dissolved in 1.5 ml of water. Duplicate aliquots of this solution estimated to contain 10 μg of triethylenephosphoramide are placed in 20 ml test tubes with water to a total volume of 3 ml. To each tube is added 1 ml of 5% 4-(4-nitrobenzyl)pyridine in acetone and 1 ml of 0.05 M potassium hydrogen phthalate. Duplicate tubes are also prepared containing 0, 5, 10, and 15 μg of triethylenephosphoramide in 3 ml of water and 1 ml each of the two reagents. A small boiling chip is placed in each tube and the tubes are heated together for 20 min in a boiling water bath. Then the tubes are held in an ice bath until color development. They are individually treated with 1 ml of 1 M potassium carbonate, 4 ml of acetone, and sufficient water to bring the volume to 10 ml. The blue solution is mixed gently and the absorbance relative to pure water is determined immediately at 600 nm. If the solutions are turbid because of insect material, they may be cleared by adding a small quantity of Hyflo Super-Cel and filtering. The absorbance from the blank is subtracted from the sample values. Plotting the net absorbance from the standard samples against concentration gives a straight line from which the unknown is read [72].

Ethylenimine in Air. A 250 ml gas bubbler equipped with an inlet tube having a No. 2 porosity sintered glass disk on its lower end is filled with 90 ml of water, 20 ml of Folin's reagent (0.138 g of potassium 1,2-naphthoquinone-4-sulfonate in 100 ml of water), and sufficient phosphate buffer solution (1.79 g of $Na_2HPO_4 \cdot 12H_2O$ in 50 ml of 0.1 N sodium hydroxide) to produce a pH of 10.2. Since the

Folin's reagent is sensitive to light, it should be freshly prepared and the bubbler bottle should be painted black or otherwise protected from light. Air is pulled through the tube at a rate not exceeding 10 liters/hr. The amount of air passed depends on the ethylenimine concentration: for air containing 1 to 5 ppm of the compound, 15 liters should be used. The contents of the scrubber is transferred to a separatory funnel and extracted twice with 20 ml portions of chloroform, the extracts are combined, and the volume is adjusted to 50 ml. A blank is carried out in the same manner, omitting only the air-washing step. A curve of absorbance versus concentration is obtained by the use of a known ethylenimine solution. This is prepared from pure ethylenimine to contain 25 μg/ml in distilled water containing a drop or two of 0.1 N sodium hydroxide to prevent carbon dioxide-initiated polymerization. Samples of 1, 2, 3, 5, and 10 ml are diluted to 100 ml, 20 ml of Folin's reagent is added, and the pH is adjusted to 10.2. This mixture is extracted twice with 20 ml of chloroform and the volume of the combined extracts is adjusted to 50 ml. Absorbance, determined in the same manner as the air sample extracts, is plotted versus concentration. The ethylenimine concentration of the air-washed sample may be read from this chart [67].

Colorimetric Determination of Ethylenimine. This procedure was developed to determine ethylenimine in the presence of other volatile primary and secondary amines in the pyrolyzate of polyethylenimine. The pyrolysis products are collected by passing the effluent airstream from the pyrolysis chamber through a loop of stainless steel tubing immersed in liquid nitrogen. The more volatile components of this condensate are then transferred to a gas-scrubbing bottle containing 50 ml of water, 10 ml of Folin's reagent, and 1 ml of buffer by means of an airstream while slowly heating the metal loop to 70°. The 1,2-naphthoquinone-amine derivatives are then removed from the solution by two extractions with 5 ml portions of chloroform. These are combined and analyzed by high-pressure liquid chromatography. The Folin's reagent is prepared daily by dissolving 0.1 g of sodium 1,2-naphthoquinone-4-sulfonate in 100 ml of water, and the buffer is 0.05 M trisodium phosphate (pH 11.7). Calibration standards are prepared by treating 50 ml samples containing 0.5 to 50 μg of ethylenimine with 10 ml of Folin's reagent and 1 ml of buffer. After holding for 3 min, the 4-(1-aziridinyl)-1,2-naphthoquinone is extracted with two 5 ml portions of chloroforms, which are subsequently combined. Standards may also be prepared by using appropriate quantities of pure 4-(1-aziridinyl)-1,2-naphthoquinone, which is readily synthesized [73]. The chloroform extracts are analyzed by high-pressure liquid chromatography on a 10 μm Micro Pak column (Varian, 50 cm × 2.2 mm i.d.), 1% isopropanol in methylene chloride at 80 ml/hr, and a UV detector at 254 nm. Sample sizes of 25 to 100 μl are used depending on the concentration, which is determined by comparing peak heights. The ethylenimine derivative is eluted in about 2.5 column volumes of solvent [68].

Colorimetric Determination of Triethylenethiophosphoramide and Triethylenephosphoramide. In a 25 ml centrifuge tube are placed 5 ml of urine, 0.25 ml of 0.5 M phosphate buffer (pH 7.4), and 15 ml of thiophene-free benzene, and the mixture is shaken for 40 min. Alternatively, 3 ml of plasma is treated with 0.5 ml of 15% tetrasodium edathamil before extraction. The tube is centrifuged, 10 ml of the benzene layer is removed and mixed with 2 ml of a 0.125% 2-naphthol solution in benzene, and the mixture is evaporated to dryness in a boiling water bath. The tube is then heated in an oil or wax bath at 125 to 130° for 20 min. After adding 4 ml of 2 N hydrochloric acid, the mixture is heated for 15 min in a boiling water bath. To the warm mixture is added 1 ml of 10 N sodium hydroxide solution and the tube is shaken. The mixture is extracted with 10 ml of ethylene chloride by shaking for 20 min, centrifuging, and by removing the aqueous layer. The organic phase is washed twice with 5 ml of 0.5 N sodium hydroxide. A 9 μl aliquot of the ethylene chloride layer is transferred to a clean tube and extracted with 2 ml of 1 N hydrochloric acid. The extract is washed with 15 ml of ethylene chloride, the aqueous layer transferred to a 1 cm square curvette, and the fluorescence is determined at 355 nm with activation at 290 nm. Known standards of triethylenethiophosphoramide in 0.9% saline are run at the same time as the unknown samples. Blanks with saline, urine, or plasma are also carried out and subtracted from the unknown and standard volumes. Unknown concentration of triethylenethiophosphoramide is calculated by direct proportionality.

Triethylenephosphoramide may be determined by the same procedure except that 10% methanol in chloroform is used for the initial extract instead of benzene. The methanol-chloroform extract will, however, extract triethylenethiophosphoramide, and if this is known to be present, a separate determination for this compound is carried out and subtracted from the result. The 2-naphthol may be purified by vacuum sublimation at 15 to 20 mmHg. Ethylene chloride is purified by passage through alumina and silica, followed by washing with 1 N sodium hydroxide and 1 N hydrochloric acid [69].

E. Epoxides

Methodology

Gas chromatographic methods are recommended by NIOSH and OSHA for monitoring levels of ethylene oxide, propylene oxide, glycidol, and epichlorohydrin in workplace air. These methods provide for collecting the epoxide by absorption onto activated charcoal contained in a glass sampling tube. The sample is later desorbed with a suitable

Table 5 Sampling and Chromatographic Conditions for Epoxides

	Ethylene oxide	Propylene oxide	Glycidol	Epichlorohydrin
NIOSH method number	S286	S75	S70	S118
OSHA limit (ppm)	50	100	50	5
Method range (mg/m^3)	20-270	25-720	15-450	2-60
Air sample (liters)	5	5	50	20
Rate (liters/min)	0.05	0.2	1	0.2
Absorbent	Charcoal	Charcoal	Charcoal	Charcoal
Eluent	CS_2	CS_2	THF	CS_2
Column (stainless steel)	Porapak QS 3 m × 3.2 mm	Porapak Q 120 cm × 6.4 mm	FFAP 10% 3 m × 3.2 mm	FFAP 10% 3 m × 3.2 mm
Column temperature (°C)	150	145	155	120

Source: Ref. 20, Vols. 2 and 3.

solvent and the epoxide concentration in the solution is determined by gas chromatography. The absorption tubes and calibrated air pumps are available commercially (Supelco, Inc.; SKC, Inc.). Additional information is given in Table 5 [74-77].

Tenax GC resin has been used to collect styrene oxide, propylene oxide, and glycidaldehyde from air. The absorbed epoxide is removed from the resin by a thermal desorption process in which the collecting tube is heated in a tube oven to 265°, and the epoxide is carried by a flow of helium to a nickel capillary tube trap cooled by liquid nitrogen. The trap is then connected to a gas chromatograph and heated rapidly to 175° to transfer the material to the column. The epoxide is analyzed on a 3.6 m × 2.5 mm i.d. silanized glass column packed with 2% DEGS on Supelcoport used with a flame ionization detector [36].

Direct injection of an air sample represents probably the simplest and most rapid gas chromatographic method for ethylene oxide in air.

For example, the concentration of ethylene oxide in fumigation chambers can be monitored by injecting a sample onto a 4 m × 6.3 mm column packed with 30% dioctylphthalate and operated at 50° with helium as carrier gas and a thermistor detector. The useful range of this method is 1 to 1000 mg/liter [78]. Ethylene oxide in sterilizing gas mixtures has also been determined by use of a 1.2 m × 6.4 mm glass column packed with Porapak R at 67° with a flame ionization detector [79]. Ethylene oxide is widely used as a means of sterilization for foods and materials that cannot tolerate high temperature and humidity. Since ethylene oxide and some of its degradation products are toxic, considerable effort has been given to residue analysis methods. Recent methods use either distillation or solvent extraction to remove the residue and gas chromatography of this solution or the head space gas. Ethylene oxide residues in a variety of plastics, rubber, and fabrics can be volatilized by heating to 100° in a closed vial. A sample of this head space air is analyzed by gas chromatography with 1.8 m × 3.2 mm stainless steel column packed with Porapak R (100-120 mesh) and operated at 150° with 25 ml/min helium gas carrier and a flame ionization detector. The limit of detection is 0.1 ppm when a 100 μl injection and a 100 mg sample are used. This method was compared to a dimethylformamide extraction technique. A polymer sample was extracted overnight and an aliquot of the extract analyzed by gas chromatography with a 1.8 m × 6.4 mm glass column packed with Porapak Q-S (100-120 mesh) and a flame ionization detector. Column temperature was held at 165° during elution of ethylene oxide and then raised to 215° to strip the column. Equivalent results are obtained with both methods; however, extraction of ethylene oxide from cotton was incomplete because this material does not swell in dimethylformamide. Acetone was reported to be a poor extracting solvent for ethylene oxide in polyester string, even after freeze grinding to increase the surface area. Results were only half of those obtained by head space analysis, even after 4 days of extraction [80].

Analysis of the ethylene oxide in air above an acetone extract has also been used to determine residues. A sample of powdered methyl methacrylate polymer is mixed with acetone in a septum-capped vial and after 10 min, a 1 ml sample of head space air is removed and analyzed by gas chromatography. Peak areas are compared to those obtained from standards with an equal amount of epoxide-free polymer and from acetone containing known quantities of ethylene oxide. The column used was 90 cm × 6.4 mm stainless steel packed with Chromosorb 101 (80-100 mesh) with a 30 ml/min helium flow at 120° with a flame ionization detector. A 1 ppm limit of detection is obtained with a 1 ml injection [81].

Numerous methods have been reported which involve the extraction of ethylene oxide from a solid with a solvent and analysis of this solution. Often few or no data are given on recovery or completeness of extraction because solid samples containing known quantities of ethylene oxide are difficult to prepare. If the solvent does not dissolve or at least swell the material, and if the material is not finely divided, complete extraction is difficult. Wheat flour that had been treated with ethylene oxide has been extracted with 5:1 acetone-water for 1 hr with a recovery of 92% and a limit of detection of 0.3 ppm. The extract was analyzed on a 2 m × 4.6 mm stainless steel column with 15% Ucon LB-550-X on Chromosorb W, helium carrier, and a flame ionization detector [82]. Ethylene oxide residues in dates were extracted with acetone and determined by gas chromatography on a 1.8 m × 3.2 mm glass column packed with Porapak R or 10% polyoxypropylene glycol on Chromosorb W. With a flame ionization detector, less than 1 ppm of ethylene oxide could be detected [83]. Grain sterilized with ethylene oxide was extracted with methanol for 24 hr and the extract was analyzed by gas chromatography. A 4 m × 4 mm glass column packed with 5% Carbowax 20M on Chromosorb T and equipped with a flame ionization detector was used. When temperature was programmed from 60 to 180°, the limit of detection was 1.7 ppm and the recovery at 25 ppm was 73% [84].

A rather lengthy procedure for the determination of ethylene oxide and ethylene chlorohydrin residues in rubber and plastics involves their extraction with a large volume of xylene. The chlorohydrin is removed by passage of the extract through a Florasil column and the ethylene oxide that passes through this column is converted to ethylene chlorohydrin on a Celite-hydrochloric acid packed column. This is collected from the eluate on another Florasil column and the absorbed chlorohydrin is eluted with ether; after concentration, it is determined by gas chromatography. A 1.8 m × 4 mm i.d. glass column with 20% Carbowax 20M on Gas Chrom Q (80-100 mesh) operated at 120° was used. With a flame ionization detector, the lower limit of detection is about 25 ng [85]. Trace quantities of ethylene oxide have been extracted from sterilized plastics and fabrics with acetone or tetrahydrofuran. The extract is analyzed by gas chromatography on a 1.8 m × 3.2 mm i.d. stainless steel column containing Chromsorb 102 (80-100 mesh). The column is operated at 100° for 9 min to elute ethylene oxide, then it is programmed to 200° to remove the acetone. The limit of detection is 0.7 ng with a 1 μl injection and a flame ionization detector [86].

A widely used colorimetric procedure for terminal oxiranes (epoxides) is based on hydrolyzing the epoxy ring to a corresponding glycol, oxidizing the glycol with periodic acid to formaldehyde, and treating the latter with chromotropic acid to form an intensely violet dye. Ethylene oxide has been determined by this method following distillation from nutmeg with water. The ethylene oxide was hydrolyzed with 0.25 N sulfuric acid at 98° for 1 hr. After neutralization with sodium hydroxide, an excess of sodium periodate was added and the solution was held 15 min at room temperature. Excess periodate was destroyed with sodium sulfite, and a 10 ml aliquot was treated with 40 ml of sulfuric acid and 50 mg of chromotropic acid. The absorbance temperature was measured at 570 nm and the color was stable for at least 48 hr [87]. Ethylene oxide and epichlorohydrin absorbed from an airstream into 40% sulfuric acid have been determined in this manner [88]. Ethylene oxide produced by hydrolysis of the pesticide aramite is determined by reaction with lepidine in diethylene glycol at 170°. The intense blue dye is measured at 610 nm. The reaction is sensitive to the presence of oxygen, water, and ethylenimine [89].

Glycidol used to sterilize milk of magnesia has been determined by esterification with 2,4-dinitrobenzenesulfonic acid and a reaction with piperazine to produce a dye that absorbs at 390 nm. The glycidol is isolated from the aqueous suspension by mixing with an equal amount of diatomaceous earth and by elution from a column with dichloroethane. Quantitative recoveries are obtained from 1 to 25 ppm in spiked samples [90]. Picric acid has been used as a reagent for propylene oxide, styrene oxide, and other oxiranes. A solution of the epoxide and picric acid in an ether-alcohol mixture is held at room temperature for 12 to 48 hr. After dilution with alkaline ethanol, the absorbance is measured at 490 nm [91].

Titrimetric methods for epoxides usually depend on a ring-opening reaction with a nucleophile. Hydrobromic acid, hydrochloric acid, mercaptans, thiosulfate, and sulfite have been used. Epoxides react rapidly with hydrobromic acid, particularly in glacial acetic acid, and direct titration is practical. Ethylene oxide and propylene oxide residues in rubber, tygon, and polyethylene have been titrated in this manner following isolation by distillation with chlorobenzene. Quantities between 1 and 70 mg were determined [92]. Free ethylene oxide in wheat and flour was removed by a stream of air and collected by passing the air through a bubbler containing 50% magnesium bromide in 0.1 N sulfuric acid. Excess acid was back-titrated with standard sodium hydroxide [82]. A somewhat more convenient method utilizes tetramethylammonium bromide in glacial acetic acid in place of the unpleasant and unstable hydrobromic acid. An excess of this reagent is used in acetone, benzene, chloroform, or chlorobenzene with the epoxide, and the mixture is titrated with standard perchloric acid to a crystal violet end point [53]. As little as 2 μEq of epichlorohydrin can be determined by this method [93].

The reaction of epoxides with an excess of dodecanethiol can be used as an analytical method when acid-base titrimetry is not possible. The reaction is complete at room temperature within 20 min in the presence of potassium hydroxide catalyst. Excess mercaptan is back-titrated with standard iodine solution [94]. Sodium thiosulfate will react with styrene oxide, glycidol, or other terminal epoxides at elevated temperature in aqueous solution. Either a small excess of standard thiosulfate is used and back-titrated with standard iodine solution, or a large excess may be employed and the amount of base liberated by the reaction titrated with standard acid [90,95]. Sodium sulfite has been used in the same manner to titrate ethylene oxide, propylene oxide, epichlorohydrin, glycidol, and styrene oxide [96].

Analytical methods

Ethylene Oxide Residue by Head Space Analysis. A 20 to 200 mg sample of plastic, rubber, or fabric is placed in a 8.8 ml screw-capped vial in which the original cap liner is replaced with a Teflon-faced septum, and the cap is drilled to allow access to the septum. The vial is heated in a 100° oven for 15 min and while still hot, a 100 μl sample of head space air is removed with a 100 μl gastight syringe. The air sample is immediately analyzed by gas chromatography. A duplicate sample is taken and analyzed. The cap on the vial is removed and the vial thoroughly flushed with nitrogen. The cap is replaced, and the vial is again heated and the head space gas analyzed as before. The sum of the average peak heights from the two heatings is used to determine ethylene oxide concentration. The septum of an 8.8 ml sample vial is pierced with two hypodermic needles, both attached to tygon tubing. One tube is connected to a tank containing ethylene oxide, and the other is placed under the surface of water. Ethylene oxide is passed at a rate of one bubble per minute for 15 min, and then both needles are removed from the septum. The concentration of ethylene oxide in this vial may be taken as 1.86 μg/μl. Samples are removed for dilution with a gastight 50 μl syringe. A small excess is drawn into the syringe, the needle is removed from the bottle, and while the needle is being held upward, the plunger is moved to the desired volume. A nitrogen-filled vial is pushed onto the needle and the ethylene oxide is injected. Dilutions are made to span the range of expected sample concentration. Samples are injected into the gas chromatograph in the same manner as the unknown samples. A plot of peak height versus micrograms of ethylene oxide per vial permits direct reading of total ethylene oxide in an unknown sample. The gas chromatograph is equipped with a flame ionization detector and a 1.8 m × 3.2 mm stainless steel column packed with Porapak R (100-120 mesh) and operated at 150° with 25 ml/min helium carrier [80].

Propylene Oxide in Air. This method has been recommended by NIOSH for measuring the concentration of propylene oxide in workplace air for compliance with OSHA standards [75]. Propylene oxide is trapped in activated charcoal contained in glass tubes, desorbed from the charcoal into carbon disulfide, and analyzed by gas chromatography. The sampling tubes and calibrated air pump are available commercially (Supelco, Inc.). The charcoal tubes are 7 cm long, 5 mm o.d., and 4 mm i.d. and contain two sections filled with 20-40 mesh activated coconut charcoal; the main section contains 100 mg and backup section contains 50 mg of the charcoal. A 2 mm urethane foam plug separates the two sections and a 3 mm foam plug is placed at the outlet end. The main charcoal section is held in place by a silylated glass wool plug at the front end. The purpose of the second section is to determine whether breakthrough has occurred on the main section. Appearance of more than 25% of the sample on this second section indicates that the sample may not have been completely collected, and a smaller volume of air should be sampled. The tubes are prepared for use by breaking the sealed ends so that an opening not less than 2 mm wide is obtained. The end containing the smaller charcoal section is attached to a tube leading to a pump and the tube is placed in an upright position to prevent channeling of the airstream. Air is drawn through the tube at a rate of 0.20 liter/min until 5 liters has been passed. The pump should be calibrated so that the flow rate is known within 5%. After 5 liters of air has passed, the tubes are capped with the supplied plastic caps. A blank should be provided by treating one tube in the same manner but without passage of air. The tubes are prepared for analysis by scoring and breaking the tube in front of the larger section. The glass wool is removed and the charcoal is placed in a 1 ml bottle furnished with a glass stopper or Teflon-lined cap. The foam plug is removed from the tube and the second charcoal section is placed in a second bottle. To each bottle is added 0.5 ml of carbon disulfide, the bottles are shaken occasionally over a 30 min period, and the samples are analyzed by gas chromatography with a flame ionization detector. The column used is 1.2 m × 6.4 mm stainless steel packed with Poropak Q (50-80 mesh) and operated at 145° with nitrogen carrier at 50 ml/min. A 5 μl sample is injected with a 10 μl syringe by means of the flush injection technique. The syringe is wetted with clean carbon disulfide and 3 μl of the solvent is withdrawn. Then 0.2 μl of air is drawn up, and finally 5 μl of the analytical sample. The plunger is withdrawn until this 5 μl sample is visible within the barrel. The volume of the sample should be between 4.9 and 5.0 μl. The amount of propylene oxide in the sample is calculated by comparing the area under the peak with that produced by a sample of known concentration. This is most conveniently obtained by the use of an electronic integrator and computer. Standards varying in concentration over the expected sample range should be prepared. It is most convenient to calculate concentrations as milligrams per 0.5 ml of carbon disulfide. Since equal volumes of unknown and standard are injected, results may be read directly as total material found. This result must be corrected for desorption efficiency, which is defined as the weight in milligrams recovered divided by the weight in milligrams absorbed, and should be determined at 0.5, 1, and 2 times the expected sample size. A 100 mg carbon section from an absorption tube is placed in a 5 cm × 4 mm i.d. glass tube that is flame sealed on one end, and the open end is capped with parafilm. The required quantity of propylene oxide contained in a 300 mg/ml hexane solution is applied to the charcoal with a microliter syringe inserted through the parafilm. The tube is capped with another layer of parafilm and let stand overnight to ensure complete absorption onto the charcoal. Duplicate tubes are prepared at all concentrations and a blank tube is treated in the same manner but without addition of sample. Standards are prepared concurrently by injecting identical amounts of propylene oxide into 0.5 ml of carbon disulfide. The tubes are desorbed with 0.5 ml of carbon disulfide and analyzed. The desorption efficiency at each concentration is calculated and plotted versus the amount of compound desorbed from the charcoal. The concentration of propylene oxide in air is calculated as follows. First the blank is subtracted from the volume found for each tube section; the larger section yields a larger blank. Then the two figures are added to give the total weight found and the sum is divided by the desorption efficiency to give the corrected weight per sample. This value, multiplied by 1000 and divided by the volume of the air sample, gives the result in mg/m^3.

F. Lactones

Methodology

The only lactone (i.e., the internal anhydride of a hydroxycarboxylic acid) that is of industrial significance and can be encountered as a contaminant or a pollutant is β-propiolactone.

Residues of β-propiolactone used to inactivate rabies virus or to sterilize delicate biological materials may be determined in either solid or liquid material. The β-propiolactone is extracted with chloroform which is partially removed in a Kuderna-Danish evaporator. After addition of butyric acid as an internal standard, the sample is analyzed by gas chromatography with Tenax GC or DEGS-phosphoric acid on Chromosorb W column. Some sample decomposition may occur on the DEGS-phosphoric acid column. Recovery rates for β-propiolactone added to aqueous protein solutions averaged 90% and 70% from solid protein. As little as 5 ppm may be detected in solid samples and 0.25 ppm in liquids [97,98].

β-Propiolactone in ambient air may be collected quantitatively by drawing the air through glass cartridges containing Tenax GC. The lactone and other absorbed materials are recovered from the Tenax by thermal desorption and determined by gas chromatography. The thermal desorption is accomplished by placing the cartridge in a heating block which is kept at 265° while nitrogen is passed through the Tenax to purge the absorbed material. The stream of nitrogen is then carried through a nickel capillary trap cooled with liquid nitrogen. By means of a valve system, this trap is placed in the carrier stream of a gas chromatograph, and the condensate is vaporized by rapidly heating the trap to 175°. The analytical column is 3.6 m × 2.5 mm i.d. silanized glass containing 2% DEGS on Supelcoport (80-100 mesh). Nitrogen is the carrier, a flame ionization detector is used, and the column temperature is programmed from 55 to 200° at 10°/min. The absorbent can be used repeatedly without losing its effectiveness, and absorbance is not affected by high humidity as often happens with activated charcoal. Losses during storage and transportation are less than 15% for β-propiolactone if the cartridges are contained in heavy-duty centrifuge tubes with Teflon-lined screw caps [36].

The purity of β-propiolactone, which often contains considerable acrylic acid or acetic anhydride, may be conveniently determined by thiosulfate titration. The reaction with an excess of standard thiosulfate is carried out in the presence of a limited amount of potassium phosphate (K_2HPO_4). After 10 to 20 min, excess thiosulfate is back-titrated with iodine solution to a starch end point. Results compared to those from cryoscopic analysis are lower by about 0.5% [99].

Analytical methods

Determination of β-Propiolactone. This method may be used to determine residues of β-propiolactone used to inactivate virus or sterilize biological materials [98]. A 20 ml sample of a protein solution is shaken with 10 ml of chloroform, and the resulting emulsion is separated by centrification for 30 min at 4000 rpm and 5°. The chloroform layer is removed and the extraction is repeated. The combined extracts are treated with 5 g of anhydrous sodium sulfate and filtered through a folded filter paper. A 10 ml aliquot is concentrated with a Kuderna-Danish apparatus to 2 ml. An internal standard of 100 μl of a 20 mg/ml solution of butyric acid in chloroform is added to the concentrated sample. The sample is analyzed by injection of 1 μl into a gas chromatograph equipped with a flame ionization detector and a 3 m × 3.2 mm stainless steel column packed with 15% DEGS and 3% phosphoric acid on Chromosorb W (100-120 mesh). The column is operated isothermally at 120° with 30 ml/min nitrogen carrier. Alternatively, a Tenax GC (60-80 mesh) column may be used at 130°. The weight of β-propiolactone (14) is calculated from the ratio of the areas under the sample and internal peaks, and from the detector response factor, which is 1.25.

$$\text{Weight (mg)} = \frac{1.25 \times \text{PL area} \times \text{BA (mg)}}{\text{BA area}} \tag{14}$$

where

PL area = area under β-propiolactone peak
BA area = area under butyric acid peak
BA (mg) = weight (mg) of butyric acid

G. Diazoalkanes

Methodology

Although several diazoalkanes are used in organic synthesis for alkylation reactions, only diazomethane has a wide industrial application as a methylating agent. All diazoalkanes are highly reactive and have to be generated from various precursors immediately before they are utilized.

Diazomethane may be determined in air in the range of 0.1 to 1.2 mg/m^3 by a NIOSH-recommended gas chromatographic procedure. The method depends upon the esterification of octanoic acid supported on XAD-2 resin by diazomethane to produce methyl octanoate. This ester is eluted with carbon disulfide and determined by gas chromatography. Recoveries of diazomethane are 90% at air concentrations of 0.2 ppm and 70% at 0.1 ppm [100]. Diazomethane in ether solution is widely used as a methylating agent for acids, alcohols, and other organic compounds. Concentration of these solutions may be easily determined by titrating an aliquot with 0.2 N benzoic acid in anhydrous ether until the solution is decolorized. A small excess of the acid is added, which is back-titrated with standard sodium hydroxide [101].

Analytical methods

Diazomethane in Air. Diazomethane is collected from a known volume of air by reaction with octanoic acid coated on XAD-2 resin. Before coating, the resin is washed in a column with 3 column volumes of methanol and 2 volumes of pentane and is dried at room temperature. The resin is coated with 1% octanoic acid by adding 0.1 g of the acid to a slurry of 10 g of the resin in 25 ml of acetone. The acetone is removed by evaporation under vacuum with a rotary evaporator. The absorption tubes are prepared by packing 100 mg and 50 mg portions of the coated resin which are separated and held in place with silylated glass wool in 7 cm × 4 mm i.d. glass tubes (SKC, Inc.). The ends of the tubing are flame sealed. A tube is prepared for air sampling by breaking the end seals to produce at least a 2 mm opening. The tube is attached to a calibrated air pump with a short length of tubing, with the 50 mg resin section closest to the pump. Nothing must be attached to the other end of the tube. The tube is held in an upright position to prevent channeling and 10 liters of air is passed at a rate of 0.2 liter/min. A tube to be used as a blank is opened at the same time and is treated in the same manner except that no air is passed. Both tubes are capped with plastic caps until analyzed. Each tube is scored with a file in front of the 100 mg section and the absorbent from each section is transferred to a separate 2 ml bottle. To each bottle is added 1 ml of carbon disulfide containing 5.6 μg/ml of tridecane used as an internal standard. The bottles are capped with Teflon-lined caps and held for 30 min with occasional agitation to desorb the methyl octanoate. The samples are then analyzed by gas chromatography. A series of standards are prepared with pure methyl octanoate in carbon disulfide varying in concentration over the expected range of the air samples. These standards are analyzed by gas chromatography in the same manner as the air samples. A curve is plotted of methyl octanoate (μg/ml) versus the peak area ratio of methyl octanoate to tridecane. Samples are analyzed on a gas chromatograph equipped with a flame ionization detector, a 15 cm × 3.2 mm stainless steel precolumn packed with 10% Carbowax 20M and 1.2% sodium hydroxide on Gas Chrom Q (80-100 mesh), and a 3 m × 3.2 mm stainless steel main column packed with 5% SP-1000 on Supelcoport (100-120 mesh). Column temperature is 95° and nitrogen is used as the carrier at 30 ml/min. Excess octanoic acid is collected in the precolumn, which should be replaced when background contamination or erratic operation is observed. All injections are 5 μl made with a 10 μl syringe operated by the solvent flush technique. The air concentration of diazomethane in mg/m^3 is calculated (15) from the total methyl octanoate found in the 100 mg and 50 mg sections less

$$mg/m^3 = \frac{\text{wt. methyl octanoate } (\mu g)}{\text{air volume} \times \text{recovery factor}} \times \frac{42.01}{158.2} \tag{15}$$

the blanks. Suggested recovery factors are 0.7 for 2 μg and 0.9 for 4 and 8 μg of diazomethane. The weight concentration can be converted to ppm (16) if desired.

$$\text{ppm} = \frac{mg}{m^3} \times \frac{24.45 \times 760 \times (t + 273)}{42.01 \times p \times 298} \tag{16}$$

where

p = air pressure (mmHg)
t = air temperature

H. Haloethers

Methodology

The development of methods for the identification and determination of sym-dichloromethyl ether (DCME) and chloromethyl methyl ether (CMME) to ppb levels was necessitated by the discovery that DCME is a potent human lung carcinogen. In practice, these volatile compounds present a hazard primarily as air contaminants. Although stable in humid air, they are rapidly destroyed in aqueous solution: the half life of DCME is less than 1 min in water but is greater than 20 hr in moist air [102].

Analysis at sub-ppb levels in air usually requires a concentration step, separation from other interfering material, and detection with a sensitive detector. A mass spectrometer is often used because it combines high sensitivity with sufficient information to identify the eluting material. Porous polymers such as Tenax GC, Chromosorb 101, and Porapak Q have been used to concentrate DCME and CMME from air. These absorbents are usually purified before initial use by extraction with methanol and acetone, and purged of all volatiles in a stream of nitrogen at an elevated temperature. The absorbents are packed in glass or metal tubes of a size determined by the desorption apparatus or sample volume. Following collection of the sample, the chloroethers are thermally desorbed onto a gas chromatography column. This has been accomplished by using heating tape [103], modified injection block [104], or an outboard tube oven [24]. The desorbed material is carried by the instrument carrier gas stream to the analytical column, which is kept at 25° until desorption is completed. This process concentrates the desorbed chloroether into a narrow band and gives a normal elution peak. Satisfactory chromatographic columns are 120 cm × 3.2 mm stainless steel packed with Chromosorb 101 at 130° [103], 360 cm × 2.5 mm i.d. glass packed with 2% DEGS on Supelcoport (80-100 mesh) [36], and 275 cm × 4 mm i.d. glass packed with 30% poly(ethyleneglycol)adipate on Celite AW (100-120 mesh) [104]. An automated procedure has been described for DCME that collects the sample on Tenax GC or Poropak Q, obtains a partial separation on a 10% DC-200 column, and obtains a final separation on a 7% OV-225 column. With a 7.5 liter air sample 0.1 ppb sensitivity is claimed when a flame ionization detector is used [105]. Derivatization of CMME and DCME may be used to improve the stability of the analyte and to increase detector sensitivity. The sodium salt of 2,4,6-trichlorophenol is used for this purpose in NIOSH method 220 [106] and in other recommended procedures because it is available in high purity and gives DCME and CMME derivatives that are readily analyzed by gas chromatography. The increase in chlorine content of the analyte produces a greatly enhanced response from the electron capture detector. Collection and derivatization is carried out simultaneously by passing the air containing CMME and DCME through a standard air impinger containing 10 ml of a solution of 2,4,6-trichlorophenol and sodium methoxide in methanol. After collection of the sample, the reagent is heated on a steam bath to complete the reaction; the cooled solution is diluted with water, and the derivatives are extracted into hexane [102]. DCME sensitivity may be increased by the use of equivalent quantities of reagents in the derivatizing solution, but then 2 N sodium hydroxide must be employed instead of water in the extraction step [107].

An on-column, gaseous derivatization is used in a rapid, automated method for CMME. A 2 to 5 ml air sample is injected by means of a loop onto a Chromosorb 101 precolumn. The CMME fraction is passed through a column containing the sodium salt of 2,4,6-trichlorophenol and OV-275 on glass beads where derivatization occurs. The derivative is immediately carried by the gas stream to a 150 cm × 3.2 mm stainless steel column packed with 0.1% OV-101 on GLC-100 textured glass beads. When the electron capture detector is used, a sensitivity of 1 ppm is obtained [108].

sym-Dichloroethyl ether and bis(2-chloroisopropyl)ether, unlike the 1-chloroethers, are not readily hydrolyzed in water. These compounds have been isolated and quantitatively determined in municipal drinking water by a solvent extraction-gas chromatographic method sensitive to 5 ng/liter. A 1-liter water sample is extracted three times with 60 ml portions of 15% ether in hexane and after drying, the extract is reduced in volume to 1 ml. A 50 μl aliquot is analyzed by gas chromatography with a chlorine-specific microcoulometric detector or with a Model 310 Hall detector. It is necessary to use two columns to eliminate interference from dichlorobenzene isomers. A 180 cm × 4 mm i.d. glass column packed with 4% SE-30 and 6% OV-210 on Gas Chrom Q (80-100 mesh) gives good separation of bis(2-chloroisopropyl) ether, and the same size column packed with 3% SP-1000 on Supelcoport (100-120 mesh) is suitable for bis(2-chloroethyl)ether [109].

Analytical methods

Chloromethyl Methyl Ether and sym-Dichloromethyl Ether in Air. This method is recommended by NIOSH for monitoring workplace air for compliance with OSHA standards [106]. The method involves the absorption and derivatization of the chloromethyl ethers and analysis of the derivatives by gas chromatography. The range of the method is 0.5 to 7.5 ppb. The derivatizing reagent is prepared by dissolving 25 g of sodium methoxide and 5 g of pure 2,4,6-trichlorophenol in 1 liter of distilled-in-glass methanol. The reagent is stable for 3 to 4 weeks if stored in a dark bottle. A 10 ml aliquot of the reagent is placed in each of two standard gas impingers having sintered glass inlet tubes. The two impingers are connected together and also to a rotometer with Teflon fittings and then to a calibrated vacuum pump. Air is drawn through the impingers at a rate of 0.5 liter/min for up to 2 hr, depending on the expected concentration of chloroethers. The reagent is transferred to screw-capped vials and heated on a steam bath (65 to 90°) for 5 min. To each cooled sample vial is then added a quantity of water equal to the reagent volume and 2 ml of hexane. The mixture is shaken for 5 min and allowed to separate. A 2 μl sample of the hexane layer is analyzed by gas chromatography. The gas chromatographic column used for both derivatives is a 1.83 m × 6.35 mm glass column packed with 0.1% OV-1 and 0.1% OV-17 on GLC-100 texture glass beads (100-120 mesh) at 140°. A ^{63}Ni electron capture detector is used. With nitrogen carrier gas flow set at 30 ml/min, the chloromethyl methyl ether derivative will elute after 5 min [107]. Standards of both chloromethyl methyl ether and sym-dichloromethyl ether are prepared by adding 2 μl of each to 50 ml of hexane. To 10 ml aliquotes of the derivatizing reagent in glass sample vials is added 10, 5, 2, 1, and 0 μl of the standard. This gives weights of 0.50, 0.25, 0.10, and 0.05 μg of dichloromethyl ether and 0.40, 0,20, 0.08, and 0.04 μg of chloromethyl methyl ether. The vials are heated on a steam bath for 5 min and are allowed to cool. Then to each vial is added 10 ml of water and 2 ml of hexane and the mixture is shaken for 5 min. A 2 μl aliquot of each hexane layer is analyzed. A standard curve for each chloromethyl ether is constructed by plotting peak height versus concentration in nanograms. The weight of each component may either be taken from the curve or calculated (17), and if necessary converted to concentration in ppb (18).

$$\text{Weight (ng)} = \frac{a \times b}{c} \qquad (17)$$

where

a = response for CMME or DCME in the sample
b = weight (ng) of CMME or DCME in the standard
c = response for CMME or DCME in the standard

$$\text{ppb (v/v)} = \frac{d \times 24.45}{v \times mw} \qquad (18)$$

where

d = weight (ng) of CMME or DCME
v = volume (liters) of air sampled
mw = molecular weight of CMME (80.5) or DCME (115)

sym-Dichloroethyl Ether in Air. This method has been recommended by NIOSH for monitoring the concentration of dichloroethyl ether in workplace air for compliance with OSHA standards [110]. Dichloroethyl ether is concentrated by absorption from an airstream on activated charcoal, desorbed with carbon disulfide, and this solution is analyzed by gas chromatography with a flame ionization detector. The useful range of the method is 10 to 270 mg/m^3. The sorbent tubes and calibrated air pump are commercially available (Supelco, Inc.; SKC, Inc.). The tubes are 7 cm × 6 mm, glass, and contain two sections of 20-40 mesh activated coconut charcoal in a 100 mg main section and a 50 mg backup section. The charcoal sections are held in place by silylated glass wool and are separated by a urethane foam plug. The purpose of the backup section is to detect breakthrough of the analyte from the main section. The tubes are prepared for use by breaking the end seals so that at least a 2 mm opening on both ends is produced. The sorbent tube is attached to a calibrated pump by a rubber tube with the 50 mg charcoal section closest to the pump, and the tube is held in an upright position during sampling to avoid channeling. Air is drawn through the tube at a rate of 1 liter/min for 15 min. The rate of flow may be checked with a rotometer or other airflow device, but this must be placed between the sorbent tube and the pump so that air can pass directly into the sorbent tube. After sampling, the tube is capped with the plastic caps provided and held until analysis. A tube to be used as a blank is treated in the same manner except that no air is passed. The tubes are prepared for analysis by scoring and breaking the tube in front of the larger section. The charcoal from each section is placed in separate 2 ml sample vials having Teflon-lined screw caps. To each vial is pipetted 1 ml of carbon disulfide and the samples are held for 30 min with occasional agitation. The solutions are then analyzed by gas chromatography with a 300 cm × 3.2 mm stainless steel column packed with 10% FFAP on Chromosorb W AW DMCS at 135° with a 50 ml/min stream of nitrogen carrier gas. A 5 μl injection is used with the solvent flush technique. Results are quantitized by comparing peak areas with those from standard samples. It is most convenient to express results as mg/ml because this gives the weight collected directly. No volume corrections are necessary if all injections are 5 μl. A standard curve is constructed by plotting area response versus mg/ml. The results taken from this curve must be corrected for desorption efficiency, which is defined as the weight recovered divided by the weight absorbed. A 100 mg charcoal section from the same lot of tubes used in the sampling is placed in a 64 mm × 4 mm i.d. glass tube sealed on one end and the other end capped with parafilm. The required quantity of dichloroethyl ether that is contained in a 0.337 g/ml hexane solution is applied to the charcoal with a microliter syringe. The needle is inserted through the parafilm cap and the tube is again capped with parafilm and held for 24 hr. Duplicate tubes are prepared at all concentrations and a blank tube is handled in the same manner. Standards are concurrently prepared by injecting the same volumes into 1.0 ml of carbon disulfide. The charcoal sections are desorbed with 1.0 ml of carbon disulfide and the solutions are analyzed. The desorption efficiency is calculated at each concentration and plotted versus the amount of analyte found at each concentration. The concentration of dichloroethyl ether in air is calculated in mg/m3 (19) or in ppm (20)

$$\mathrm{mg/m3} = \frac{\text{total wt. (mg)} \times 1000}{\text{de} \times \text{air volume (liters)}} \qquad (19)$$

where

de = desorption efficiency

$$\mathrm{ppm} = \frac{\mathrm{mg}}{\mathrm{m}^3} \times \frac{24.45 \times 760 \times (t + 273)}{\text{mol. wt.} \times p \times 298} \qquad (20)$$

where

p = air pressure (mmHg)
t = air temperature

Total weight represents the sum of contents of both absorbent sections less any value obtained in the blank. As mentioned earlier, this weight has to be corrected for desorption efficiency.

I. Acrylates

Methodology

The inclusion of acrylates among the alkylating agents is based primarily on the ubiquity of acrylonitrile, an industrial intermediate produced yearly in billion-pound quantities. In analogy to its structural analog vinyl chloride, acrylonitrile polymerizes easily, but its alkylating properties are expressed in cyanoethylating reactions, which are important in industrial and laboratory organic syntheses. Because of its wide utilization and high volatility (b.p. 77.3°), its vapors are potential air contaminants and pollutants.

NIOSH-recommended methods for acrylonitrile in air provide for the collection of the compound in a known volume of air by absorption onto activated coconut charcoal or Carbosieve B (pyrolized Saran) contained in a small glass tube. The absorbed material is removed from the absorbent by desorption with methanol, and this solution is analyzed by gas chromatography. The limit of detection is about 100 μg or 2 ppm in air if a 20 liter air sample is passed through the absorption tube. Columns used for the analysis are 1.8 m × 3.2 mm stainless steel packed with Porapak N (50-80 mesh) at 170° and 1.2 m × 6.4 mm stainless steel with Porapak Q (50-80 mesh) at 155° [111, 112].

A much more sensitive method involves passing a 1 liter sample through a 10 cm × 6.4 mm stainless steel column packed with Porapak N which quantitatively absorbs acrylonitrile as well as many other organic compounds. This tube is attached to the injection port of a gas chromatograph with the carrier gas flow through the tube. Heating to 200° for 5 min causes the acrylonitrile to be carried to the front part of the chromatographic column. The acrylonitrile and other pollutants are eluted by temperature programming at 15°/min to 200°. The column is 1.2 m × 3.2 mm stainless steel packed with Porapak N (80-100 mesh) and the detector is flame ionization. A sensitivity of 1 ppb with a 1 liter air sample is claimed [113].

Residual acrylonitrile remaining in polymeric material has been determined chromatographically by direct injection of a solution of the polymer with toluene as an internal standard. Both unknown and standard solutions are prepared by dissolving 0.5 g of the polymer in 5 ml of redistilled dimethylformamide and 1 ml of 0.5% toluene in dimethylformamide. Known amounts of acrylonitrile are added to the standard samples and 5 μl of the solutions is analyzed with a gas chromatograph equipped with a flame ionization detector. Two columns are used in series: a 90 cm × 3.2 mm 20% Tween 81 and a 3 m × 3.2 mm 10% Resoflex 446, both on Chromosorb W (30-60 mesh) at 120° with nitrogen carrier at 30 ml/min. Acrylonitrile, styrene, and butadiene may be determined to 10 ppm [114].

Acrylonitrile residues in polymer have been determined to 0.5 ppm levels by a head space analysis. This procedure involves analysis of the vapor above a solution of the polymer, and by means of standards, the calculation of the residue originally included in the polymer. The method allows injecting large samples without solvent interference and avoids the problem of column contamination with nonvolatile materials. The method is carried out by dissolving 0.5 g of the polymer in 5 ml of o-dichlorobenzene in a septum-sealed 24 ml bottle heated to 90°. After equilibrating at 90° for 30 min, the head space gas is analyzed with an automatic analyzer (Perkin-Elmer Multifract F-40). This gas chromatograph is equipped with a flame ionization detector and a 1.8 m × 3.2 mm stainless steel column packed with 0.4% Carbowax 1500 on Carbopack A (or 0.2% Carbowax 1500 on Carbopak C) operated at 100° with 30 ml/min helium carrier. Standards are prepared by dissolving monomer-free polymer in o-dichlorobenzene and adding known amounts of acrylonitrile by injection through the septum [29].

A method has recently been described for the colorimetric determination of acrylonitrile in water with a sensitivity to 5 ppm. The method depends on the formation of a yellow-colored complex produced by a reaction of pyridine in an alkaline hypochlorite solution with acrylonitrile. The color is stable for at least 20 min and is measured at 411 nm. Optimum color formation is obtained by selecting a final concentration of 75% pyridine, 25% water, 0.75% sodium hypochlorite, and 0.005 N lithium hydroxide. The color is developed by heating the reaction mixture at 60 to 65° for 20 min [115].

Various additions of certain reagents to the active double bond in acrylonitrile form the basis for several titrimetric methods. Sodium sulfite titration has been used to measure the amount of acrylonitrile monomer remaining in copolymer lattices. An excess of the reagent is employed, and the base liberated in the addition is titrated with standard acid. Acrylonitrile concentrations between 0.05 and 15% are determined directly [116]. The reaction of acrylonitrile with excess dodecanethiol has also been used. Excess thiol is back-titrated with standard iodine solution or titrated amperimeterically with silver nitrate [117].

Analytical methods

Acrylonitrile in Air. The acrylonitrile in a known volume of air is collected by passing an air sample through a small tube containing activated charcoal. The absorbed acrylonitrile is removed by extraction with methanol and then determined by gas chromatography. This method is described in NIOSH Method S156 [111]. The charcoal absorption tube is 7 cm × 6 mm and contains two sections of 20-40 mesh activated coconut charcoal. The tube contains a glass wool plug, 100 mg of charcoal, a urethane foam plug, 50 mg of charcoal, and a foam plug (in that order) and is flame sealed on both ends. The tubes and calibrated pump are commercially available (Supelco, Inc.). The tube is opened by breaking off enough of the seal at both ends to produce at least 2 mm openings. It is attached to a calibrated pump with a short length of tubing so that the smaller charcoal section is nearest the pump. During sampling, the tube is held upright to keep the charcoal evenly packed and to prevent channeling. Air is drawn through the tube at 0.20 liter/min until not more than 20 liters has passed. The size of the air sample must be adjusted to the concentration of acrylonitrile expected. The 100 mg section of charcoal will absorb at least 4 mg without appreciable leakage into the 50 mg section. The tube is capped with plastic caps until desorption and analysis. The tube is scored with a file in front of the 100 mg section and broken open. The charcoal from each section is transferred to separate 2 ml bottles and 1 ml of methanol is added to each sample. The bottles are capped with Teflon-lined caps and agitated periodically over a 30-min period. The solution is then analyzed by injecting a 5 μl aliquot into a gas chromatograph equipped with a flame ionization detector. The column used is 1.2 m × 6.4 mm stainless steel packed with Porapak Q (50-80 mesh) operated at 155° with nitrogen carrier at 50 ml/min. Duplicate analyses are made on all samples. The injection should be made with a 10 μl syringe by means of the solvent flush technique. First, 3 μl of clean methanol is drawn up, then 0.2 μl of air, and then 5 μl of sample. The plunger is drawn back until the complete sample is visible in the syringe barrel. The volume should be between 4.9 and 5.0 μl. Known standards covering the expected range are prepared by dilution of pure acrylonitrile with methanol. Standards are injected during the same time period as unknown samples. Acrylonitrile concentration is calculated by comparison of peak areas obtained from an electronic integrator. It may be necessary to include in the calculation a desorption efficiency factor because all the acrylonitrile may not desorb. This factor is determined by injecting into the charcoal, from a 100 mg section held in a small test tube, an amount of 0.239 g/ml acrylonitrile in hexane containing the same quantity of acrylonitrile that is expected to be captured from the air sampling. Also, tubes containing half and twice this amount and a blank are set up. The injection is made with a 10 μl syringe through a parafilm cap and the tube is sealed after the injection with more parafilm. All concentration levels are run in duplicate. After standing overnight, the charcoal is desorbed and analyzed in the same manner as the air samples. The desorption efficiency is calculated by dividing the average weight recovered by the weight added. A curve is plotted of desorption efficiency versus sample weight. The concentration of acrylonitrile in air is calculated as follows. The total acrylonitrile found is the sum of the 100 mg and 50 mg section results less the blank values. This total weight is divided by the desorption efficiency to give the corrected weight. Concentration in air is then calculated in mg/m^3 (21) or converted into ppm (22).

$$mg/m^3 - \frac{\text{corrected weight (mg)} \times 1000}{\text{air volume (liters)}} \tag{21}$$

$$ppm = mg/m^3 \times \frac{24.55}{mw} \times \frac{760}{p} \times \frac{t + 273}{298}$$

where

p = air pressure (mmHg)
t = air temperature
mw = molecular weight of acrylonitrile

REFERENCES

1. D. v. St. Whitelock (Ed.). Comparative clinical and biological effects of alkylating agents. Ann. N.Y. Acad. Sci. *68*(Art. 3), 657-1266 (1958).
2. L. A. Elson. *Radiation and Radiomimetic Chemicals*. Butterworth, London, 1963.
3. W. C. J. Ross. *Biological Alkylating Agents*. Butterworth, London, 1962.
4. C. K. Ingold. *Structure and Mechanism in Organic Chemistry*. Cornell University Press, Ithaca, N.Y., 1953.
5. B. L. Van Duren (Ed.). Biological effects of alkylating agents. Ann. N.Y. Acad. Sci. *163*(Art. 2), 589-1029 (1969).
6. Anonymous. A survey of alkylating agents. Cancer Chemother. Rep. *26*, 1-510 (1963).
7. L. H. Schmidt, R. Fradkin, R. Sullivan, and A. Flowers. Comparative pharmacology of alkylating agents. Cancer Chemother. Rep., Suppl. 2, Parts I-III, 1-1528 (1965).
8. J. S. Sandberg, H. B. Wood, Jr., R. R. Engle, J. M. Vendiffi, and A. Goldin. Methanesulfonates: the relationship of structure to antitumor activity. Cancer Chemother. Rep., Part 2, *3*, 137-229 (1972).
9. C. Auerbach. In *Chemical Mutagens* (A. Hollaender, Ed.), Vol. 3. Plenum Press, New York, 1973, pp. 1-19.
10. Anonymous. *Induced Mutations in Cross-Breeding*. Panel proceedings series, STI/PUB/447. International Atomic Energy Agency, Vienna, 1976.
11. A. B. Borkovec. *Insect Chemosterilants*. Interscience, New York, 1966.

12. A. B. Borkovec. Alkylating agents as insect chemosterilants. Ann. N.Y. Acad. Sci. *163*, 860-868 (1969).
13. A. B. Borkovec. Mechanism of action of alkylating and non-alkylating insect chemosterilants. ACS Symp. Ser. *2*, 130-135 (1974).
14. S. S. Sternberg, F. S. Philips, and J. Scholler. Pharmacological and pathological effects of alkylating agents. Ann. N.Y. Acad. Sci. *68*(Art. 3), 811-825 (1968).
15. L. Fishbein, W. G. Flamm, and H. L. Falk. *Chemical Mutagens*, Academic Press, New York, 1970.
16. A. Hollaender (Ed.). *Chemical Mutagens*, Plenum Press, New York, Vols. 1 and 2 (1971); Vol. 3 (1973).
17. H. E. Christensen (Ed.). *NIOSH Registry of Toxic Effects of Chemical Substances*. U.S. Government Printing Office, Washington, D.C., 1976.
18. K. Verschueren. *Handbook of Environmental Data on Organic Chemicals*. Van Nostrand Reinhold, New York, 1977.
19. M. Windholz (Ed.). *The Merck Index*, 9th ed. Merck & Co., Rahway, N.J., 1976.
20. *NIOSH Manual of Analytical Methods*, 3 vols. (D. G. Taylor, Coord.). DHEW (NIOSH) Pub. No. 77-157-A, B, C, 1977.
21. J. E. Purcell. Gas chromatographic analysis of vinyl chloride. Am. Lab. *7*, 99-109 (1975).
22. D. G. Parks, C. R. Ganz, A. Polinsky, and J. Schulze. A simple gas chromatographic method for the analysis of trace organics in ambient air. J. Am. Ind. Hyg. Assoc. *37*, 165-173 (1976).
23. W. L. Severs and L. K. Skory. Monitoring personal exposure to vinyl chloride, vinylidene chloride, and methyl chloride in an industrial work environment. J. Am. Ind. Hyg. Assoc. *36*, 669-676 (1975).
24. S. P. Levine, K. G. Hebel, J. Bolton, Jr., and R. E. Kugel. Industrial analytical chemists and OSHA regulations for vinyl chloride. Anal. Chem. *47*, 1075A-1080A (1975).
25. T. Fujii. Trace determination of vinyl chloride in water by direct aqueous injection gas chromatography-mass spectrometry. Anal. Chem. *49*, 1985-1987 (1977).
26. B. J. Dowty, D. R. Carlisle, and J. Laseter. New Orleans drinking water sources tested by gas chromatography-mass spectrometry. Environ. Sci. Technol. *9*, 762-765 (1975).
27. F. C. Kopfler, R. G. Melton, R. D. Lingg, and W. E. Coleman. GC/MS determination of volatiles for the National Organic Reconnaissance Survey (NORS) of drinking water. In *Identification and Analysis of Organic Pollutants in Water* (L. H. Keith, Ed.). Ann Arbor Science Publishers, Ann Arbor, Mich., 1977, pp. 87-104.

28. W. E. Coleman, R. D. Lingg, R. C. Melton, and F. C. Kopfler. The occurrence of volatile organics in five drinking water supplies using gas chromatography/mass spectrometry. In *Identification and Analysis of Organic Pollutants in Water* (I. H. Keith, Ed.). Ann Arbor Science Publishers, Ann Arbor, Mich., 1977, pp. 305-328.
29. R. J. Steichen. Modified solution approach for the gas chromatographic determination of residual monomers by head-space analysis. Anal. Chem. *48*, 1398-1402 (1976).
30. C. V. Breder, J. L. Dennison, and M. E. Brown. Gas-liquid chromatographic determinations of vinyl chloride in vinyl chloride polymers, food-simulating solvents and other samples. J. Assoc. Off. Anal. Chem. *58*, 1214-1220 (1975).
31. G. W. Diachenko, C. V. Breder, M. E. Brown, and J. L. Dennison. Gas-liquid chromatographic headspace technique for determination of vinyl chloride in corn oil and three food-simulating solvents. J. Assoc. Off. Anal. Chem. *60*, 570-575 (1977).
32. H.C. Hollifield and T. McNeal. Gas-solid chromatographic determination of vinylidene chloride in Saran film and three food-simulating solvents. J. Assoc. Off. Anal. Chem. *61*, 537-544 (1978).
33. B. D. Page and B. P. C. Kennedy. Determination of methylene chloride, ethylene dichloride, and trichloroethylene as solvent residues in spice oleoresins, using vacuum distillation and electron capture gas chromatography. J. Assoc. Off. Anal. Chem. *58*, 1062-1068 (1975).
34. *NIOSH Manual of Analytical Methods*, Vol. 1 (D. G. Taylor, Coord.). DHEW (NIOSH) Publ. No. 77-157-A, 1977, Method 178.
35. D. Ellgehausen. Determination of volatile toxic substances in the air by means of a coupled gas chromatograph-mass spectrometer system. Anal. Lett. *8*, 11-23 (1975).
36. E. D. Pellizzari, J. E. Bunch, R. E. Berkley, and J. McRae. Collection and analysis of trace organic vapor pollutants in ambient atmospheres. The performance of a Tenax GC cartridge sampler for hazardous vapors. Anal. Lett. *9*, 45-63 (1976).
37. D. Tomczyk and J. Bajerska. Spectrophotometric determination of small amounts of dimethyl sulfate in air. Chem. Anal. (Warsaw) *18*, 543-549 (1973).
38. M. T. Shafik and H. F. Enos. Determination of metabolic and hydrolytic products of organophosphorus pesticide chemicals in human blood and urine. J. Agric. Food Chem. *17*, 1186-1189 (1969).
39. C. G. Daughton, D. G. Crosby, R. L. Garnas, and D. P. H. Hsieh. Analysis of phosphorus-containing hydrolytic products of organophosphorus insecticides in water. J. Agric. Food Chem. *24*, 236-241 (1976).

40. M. T. Shafik, D. Bradway, and H. F. Enos. A cleanup procedure for the determination of low levels of alkyl phosphates, thiophosphates, and dithiophosphates in rat and human urine. J. Agric. Food Chem. *19*, 885-889 (1971).
41. A. Brignocchi and G. M. Gasparini. The gas chromatographic determination of the decomposition products of tributyl phosphate. Anal. Lett. *6*, 523-530 (1973).
42. I. H. Suffet, L. Brenner, and J. V. Radziul. GC/MS identification of trace organic compounds in Philadelphia drinking water. In *Identification and Analysis of Organic Pollutants in Water* (L. H. Keith, Ed.). Ann Arbor Science Publishers, Ann Arbor, Mich., 1977, pp. 375-397.
43. W. J. Dunlap, D. C. Shew, M. R. Scalf, R. L. Cosby, and J. M. Robertson. Isolation and identification of organic contaminants in ground water. In *Identification and Analysis of Organic Pollutants in Water* (L. H. Keith, Ed.). Ann Arbor Science Publishers, Ann Arbor, Mich., 1977, pp. 453-477.
44. *NIOSH Manual of Analytical Methods*. Vol. 3 (D. G. Taylor, Coord.). DHEW (NIOSH) Publ. No. 77-157-C, 1977, Method No. S 208.
45. *NIOSH Manual of Analytical Methods*. Vol. 3 (D. G. Taylor, Coord.). DHEW (NIOSH) Publ. No. 77-157-C, 1977, Method No. S 209.
46. *NIOSH Manual of Analytical Methods*. Vol. 3 (D. G. Taylor, Coord.). DHEW (NIOSH) Publ. No. 77-157-C, 1977, Method No. S 210.
47. R. J. Allen and M. A. DeSesa. New and improved analysis for tri-N-butyl phosphate. Nucleonics *15*(10), 88-98 (1957).
48. C. E. O'Rourke, L. B. Clapp, and J. O. Edwards. Reactions of ethylenimine: VIII. Dissociation constants. J. Am. Chem. Soc. *78*, 2159-2160 (1956).
49. D. H. Powers, Jr., V. B. Schatz, and L. B. Clapp. Reactions of ethylenimine: VII. Hammett ρ constants for ring opening with benzoic acids. J. Am. Chem. Soc. *78*, 907-911 (1956).
50. O. C. Dermer and G. E. Ham. *Ethylenimine and Other Aziridines*. Academic Press, New York, 1969.
51. E. Allen and W. Seaman. Method of assay for ethylenimine derivatives. Anal. Chem. *27*, 540-544 (1955).
52. Dow Chemical Co. Ethylenimine (brochure). Midland, Mich., 1965.
53. R. R. Jay. Direct titration of epoxy compounds and aziridines. Anal. Chem. *36*, 667-668 (1964).
54. R. C. Schlitt. Assay of aziridinyl compounds. Anal. Chem. *35*, 1063-1064 (1963).
55. M. C. Bowman and M. Beroza. Gas chromatographic determination of trace amounts of the insect chemosterilants tepa, metepa, methiotepa, hempa, and apholate and the analysis of tepa in insect tissue. J. Assoc. Off. Anal. Chem. *49*, 1046-1052 (1966).

56. M. C. Bowman. Analysis of insect chemosterilants. J. Chromatogr. Sci. *13*, 307-313 (1975).
57. P. H. Terry, D. G. McHaffey, and A. B. Borkovec. Uptake and residues of chemosterilants in boll weevils treated by fumigation or dipping. J. Econ. Entomol. *70*, 427-430 (1977).
58. J. A. Seawright, M. C. Bowman, and R. S. Patterson. Tepa and thiotepa: uptake, persistence, and sterility induced in pupae and adults of *Culex pipiens quinquofasciatus*. J. Econ. Entomol. *64*, 452-455 (1971).
59. J. A. Seawright, M. C. Bowman, and C. S. Lofgren. Thioaziridine chemosterilants: uptake, persistence, and sterility in pupae and adults of *Anopheles albimanus*. J. Econ. Entomol. *66*, 305-308 (1973).
60. D. Singh, M. K. K. Pillai, A. B. Borkovec, and P. H. Terry. Chemosterilization of *Earias fabia*. J. Econ. Entomol. *71*, 9-12 (1978).
61. J. Epstein, R. W. Rosenthal, and R. Ess. Use of γ-(4-nitrobenzyl)pyridine as analytical reagent for ethylenimines and alkylating agents. Anal. Chem. *27*, 1435-1439 (1955).
62. E. Sawicki, D. F. Bender, T. R. Hauser, R. M. Wilson, Jr., and J. E. Meeker. Five new methods for the spectrophotometric determination of alkylating agents including some extremely sensitive autocatalytic methods. Anal. Chem. *35*, 1479-1486 (1963).
63. T. J. Bardos, N. Datta-Gupta, P. Hebborn, and D. J. Triggle. A study of comparative chemical and biological activities of alkylating agents. J. Med. Chem. *8*, 167-174 (1965).
64. G. C. Butler, D. S. Kaushik, J. Maxwell, and J. G. P. Stell. The colorimetric estimation of thiotepa. J. Mond. Pharm. *10*, 359-364 (1967).
65. V. S. Mosienko, V. F. Novikova, and N. D. Dumbadze. Quantitative determination of chloroethylamines and ethylenimines in water and plasma with γ-(4-nitrobenzyl)pyridine. Lab. Delo, 430-431 (1976).
66. D. H. Rosenblatt, P. Hlinka, and J. Epstein. Use of 1,2-naphthoquinone-4-sulfonate for the estimation of ethylenimine and primary amines. Anal. Chem. *27*, 1290-1293 (1955).
67. T. R. Compton. Determination of traces of ethylenimine monomer in samples of air. Analyst *90*, 107-111 (1965).
68. D. E. Evans, R. J. Mayfield, and I. M. Russell. Rapid estimation of trace amounts of ethylenimine by high-pressure liquid chromatography. J. Chromatogr. *115*, 391-395 (1975).
69. L. B. Mellett and L. A. Woods. The comparative physiological disposition of thiotepa and tepa in the dog. Cancer Res. *20*, 524-532 (1960).
70. Interchemical Corporation. Propylene imine, (brochure). New York, 1966.

71. D. A. Carlson and K. D. Konyha. Chemosterilant co-distillation from water solution. Personal communication.
72. S. C. Chang and A. B. Borkovec. Determination of tepa residues on chemosterilized Mexican fruit flies. J. Econ. Entomol. *59*, 102-104 (1966).
73. W. Gauss and S. Petersen. Additional studies on ethylenimino quinones and related compounds. Angew. Chem. *69*, 252-257 (1957).
74. *NIOSH Manual of Analytical Methods*, Vol. 3. DHEW (NIOSH) Publ. No. 77-157-C, 1977, Method No. S 286.
75. *NIOSH Manual of Analytical Methods*, Vol. 2. DHEW (NIOSH) Publ. No. 77-157-B, 1977, Method No. S 75.
76. *NIOSH Manual of Analytical Methods*, Vol. 2. DHEW (NIOSH) Publ. No. 77-157-B, 1977, Method No. S 70.
77. *NIOSH Manual of Analytical Methods*. DHEW (NIOSH) Publ. No. 77-157-B, 1977, Method No. S 118.
78. T. Dumas. Determination of ethylene oxide in air by gas chromatography. J. Chromatogr. *121*, 147-149 (1976).
79. P. V. Allen and A. J. Vanderwielen. Determination of ethylene oxide in gas sterilants by Fourier transform infrared spectrometry. Anal. Chem. *49*, 1602-1606 (1977).
80. S. J. Romano, J. A. Renner, and P. M. Leitner. Gas chromatographic determination of residual ethylene oxide by head space analysis. Anal. Chem. *45*, 2327-2330 (1973).
81. L. A. Zagar. Determination of residual ethylene oxide in methyl methacrylate polymer powders by GLC. J. Pharm. Sci. *61*, 1801-1802 (1972).
82. S. C. Heuser and K. A. Scudamore. Fumigant residues in wheat and flour: solvent extraction and gas-chromatographic determination of free methyl bromide and ethylene oxide. Analyst *93*, 252-258 (1968).
83. S. Ben-Yehoshua and P. Krinsky. Gas chromatography of ethylene oxide and its toxic residues. J. Gas Chromatogr. *6*, 350-351 (1968).
84. K. Pfeilsticker, G. Fabricius, and G. Timme. Simultaneous gas-chromatographic determination of epoxyethane, ethylene chlorohydrin and ethanediol in grain. Z. Lebensm. Unters. Forsch. *158*, 21-25 (1975).
85. D. J. Brown. Determination of ethylene oxide and ethylene chlorohydrin in plastic and rubber surgical equipment sterilized with ethylene oxide. J. Assoc. Off. Anal. Chem. *53*, 263-267 (1970).
86. H. D. Spitz and J. Weinberger. Determination of ethylene oxide, ethylene chlorohydrin and ethylene glycol by gas chromatography. J. Pharm. Sci. *60*, 271-274 (1971).

87. R. E. Critchfield and J. B. Johnson. Colorimetric determination of ethylene oxide by conversion to formaldehyde. Anal. Chem. *29*, 797-800, (1957).
88. E. Sh. Gronsberg. Determination of ethylene oxide, epichlorohydrin, and ethylene glycol in the analysis of air. Khim. Prom., 508-509 (1961).
89. F. A. Gunther, R. C. Blinn, M. J. Kolbezen, and J. H. Barkley. Microestimation of 2 (p tert-butylphenoxy)isopropyl-2-chloroethyl sulfite residues. Anal. Chem. *23*, 1835-1842 (1951).
90. E. Ivashkiv and J. M. Dunham. Determination of trace amounts of glycidol in milk of magnesia. J. Pharm. Sci. *62*, 285-287 (1973).
91. J. A. Fioriti, A. P. Bentz, and R. J. Sims. The reaction of picric acid with epoxides: I. A colorimetric method. J. Am. Oil Chem. Soc. *43*, 37-41 (1966).
92. D. A. Gunther. Determination of absorbed ethylene and propylene oxides by distillation and titration. Anal. Chem. *37*, 1172-1773 (1965).
93. M. M. Chakrabarty, D. Bhattacharyya, and M. K. Kundu. A micro-titrimetric method for the determination of the oxirane functional group. Analyst *95*, 85-87 (1970).
94. B. J. Gudzinowicz. Quantitative determination of ethylene epoxide, and higher molecular weight epoxides using dodecanethiol. Anal. Chem. *32*, 1520-1522 (1960).
95. B. D. Sully. Determination of terminal epoxides, particularly styrene oxide. Analyst *85*, 895-897 (1960).
96. J. D. Swan. Determination of epoxides with sodium sulfite. Anal. Chem. *26*, 878-880 (1954).
97. M. O. Schmitz-Mosse. Analysis of β-propiolactone by gas-liquid chromatography. J. Chromatogr. *70*, 128-134 (1972).
98. D. Purggmayer and W. Stephan. Gas chromatographic trace analysis of β-propiolactone in sterilized serum proteins. Vox Sang. *31*, 191-198 (1976).
99. W. P. Tyler and D. W. Beesing. Chemical and cryoscopic analysis of β-propiolactone. Anal. Chem. *24*, 1511-1513 (1952).
100. *NIOSH Manual of Analytical Methods*, Vol. 3. DHEW (NIOSH) Publ. No. 77-157-C, 1977, Method No. S 137.
101. L. F. Fieser and M. Fieser. *Reagents for Organic Synthesis*, Vol. 1. Wiley, New York, 1968, p. 191.
102. J. C. Tou and G. J. Kallos. Possible formation of bis(chloromethyl)ether from the reactions of formaldehyde and chloride ion. Anal. Chem. *48*, 958-963 (1976).
103. *NIOSH Manual of Analytical Methods*, Vol. 1 (D. G. Taylor, Coord.). DHEW (NIOSH) Publ. No. 77-157-A, 1977, Method 213.
104. K. E. Evans, A. Mathias, N. Mellor, R. Silvester, and A. E. Williams. Detection and estimation of bis(chloromethyl)ether in

air by gas chromatography-high resolution mass-spectrometry. Anal. Chem. *47*, 821-824 (1975).

105. C. S. Frankel and R. F. Black. Automatic gas chromatographic monitor for the determination of parts-per-billion levels of bis(chloromethyl)ether. Anal. Chem. *48*, 732-737 (1976).
106. *NIOSH Manual of Analytical Methods*, Vol. 1 (D. G. Taylor, Coord.). DHEW (NIOSH) Publ. No. 77-157-A, 1977, Method 220.
107. R. A. Solomon and G. J. Kallos. Determination of chloromethyl methyl ether and bischloromethyl ether in air at the part per billion level by gas-liquid chromatography. Anal. Chem. *47*, 955-957 (1975).
108. G. J. Kallos, W. R. Albe, and R. A. Solomon. On-column reaction gas chromatography for determination of chloromethyl methyl ether at one part-per-billion level in ambient air. Anal. Chem. *49*, 1817-1820 (1977).
109. R. C. Dressmon, J. Fair, and E. F. McFarren. Determinative method for analysis of aqueous sample extracts for bis(2-chloro) ethers and dichlorobenzenes. Environ. Sci. Technol. *11*, 719-721 (1977).
110. *NIOSH Manual of Analytical Methods*, Vol. 3 (D. G. Taylor, Coord.). DHEW (NIOSH) Publ. No. 77-157-C, 1977, Method No. S 357.
111. *NIOSH Manual of Analytical Methods*, Vol. 3. DHEW (NIOSH) Publ. No. 77-157-C, 1977, Method No. S 156.
112. *NIOSH Manual of Analytical Methods*, Vol. 1. DHEW (NIOSH) Publ. No. 77-157-A, 1977, Method P & CAM No. 202.
113. J. W. Russell. Analysis of air pollutants using sampling tubes and gas chromatography. Environ. Sci. Technol. *9*, 1175-1178 (1975).
114. P. Shapras and G. C. Claver. Determination of residual monomers and other volatile components in styrene based polymers by gas chromatography. Anal. Chem. *36*, 2282-2283 (1964).
115. M. E. Hall and J. W. Stevens. Spectrophotometric determination of acrylonitrile. Anal. Chem. *49*, 2277-2280 (1977).
116. R. P. Taubinger. Direct determination of free acrylonitrile in aqueous copolymer latexes. Analyst *94*, 628-633 (1969).
117. D. W. Beesing, W. P. Tyler, D. M. Kurtz, and S. A. Harrison. Determination of acrylonitrile and α, β-unsaturated carbonyl compounds with dodecanethiol. Anal. Chem. *21*, 1073-1076 (1949).

3

Aromatic Amines and Azo Compounds

CHARLES R. NONY National Center for Toxicological Research,
U.S. Food and Drug Administration, Jefferson, Arkansas

I. INTRODUCTION

The majority of the analytical methods described in this chapter were developed for use in the aromatic amine program of the National Center for Toxicological Research (NCTR) during the past 8 years. Because of the stringent requirements placed on investigators engaged in small animal testing of hazardous substances, adequate chemical methods must be available for providing assurance of the identity, purity, and stability of the substance; its homogeneity, stability, and proper concentration in the dosage form; safe usage in the workplace; and safe disposal. Undoubtedly, the most important requirement in toxicological research is the evaluation of the various chemical aspects of an experiment *prior* to the initiation of animal tests, if such tests are to be valid.

In toxicological experiments, the test substance is usually administered to an animal by gavage, injection, inhalation (as particles, aerosols, or vapors), application to the skin, or orally as a solid or liquid. Oral administration of the substance via the diet or drinking water is most convenient for long-term experiments with large numbers of animals receiving multiple doses. Although oral doses may be given in the form of a liquid, pellet, granule, emulsion, agar block, and so on, thus far only granular laboratory chow and drinking water have been used as vehicles for dosing animals in large-scale tests at the NCTR. Therefore, most of the methods that follow feature these two substrates when determining the concentration of the test substance, usually at residue levels. Other substrates amenable to these methods are blood and urine from mice and rats and various microbiological media used in experiments to study biodegradation of test substances.

Because of the potential hazard of occupational exposure to carcinogenic test compounds, especially by workers who prepare dosed animal diets, the NCTR has established an ongoing surveillance program for monitoring human urine samples using the methods discussed to signal any exposure that may occur. So that the environment outside the NCTR would be protected from any hazardous substances, a system for the removal of carcinogens from wastewater was developed, fabricated, and installed, and is monitored by employing the methods described.

This chapter is directed toward the analytical methodology of selected aromatic amines that are known to cause, or are suspected of causing, cancer in humans. In etiological studies of workers in the chemical industry, the three aromatic amines 2-naphthylamine, benzidine, and 4-aminobiphenyl, have been established as human bladder carcinogens as a result of prolonged occupational exposure. Although there are many other causes of bladder cancer, the aromatic amines have dominated this field. In an excellent review of bladder cancer by J. M. Price [1] it was stated that bladder cancer is unique among the many forms of cancer that afflict humans in being the only form of human cancer in which one may name with confidence a specific chemical as the causal agent. The reason for this is the relatively pure form in which the chemicals appear in the environment. Most other recognized human carcinogens occur in mixtures such as oils, tars, soot, or smoke. If estimates are correct that 60% or more of all human cancers are due to environmental agents, about 500,000 cases per year may be involved [2]. This would include the relatively small number of industrial workers who may be occupationally exposed to high levels of concentrated chemicals and products ranging upward to the relatively large number of consumers who may be exposed to diluted forms of hazardous chemicals and products.

In contrast to pure forms and mixtures, chemical carcinogens and/or suspect chemicals are present in chemically combined forms, for example, benzidine or 3,3'-dichlorobenzidine, present in a large number of commercial azo dyes and pigments. Presumably, there would be no problem if the dye or pigment were pure and remained intact; however, studies with rhesus monkeys [3] that were fed four benzidine dyes indicated that the benzidine moiety was released in each case through metabolic reduction, as evidenced by chemical analysis of the urine. Not only was the free amine found, but also a metabolite of benzidine, monoacetylbenzidine. This naturally leads one to speculate about what might occur if a worker in the dye industry were to accidentally ingest or inhale some quantity of a benzidine dye. Since the aromatic amine moieties seem to play a most important role when assessing the extent or effects of a suspected exposure, the methods described in this chapter for dyes emphasize the impurities and/or the breakdown products rather than the dye molecule per se. A number of conventional methods for the analysis and identification of a given synthetic dye are presented in an excellent book edited by Venkataraman [4].

It is hoped that the reader will find that the compounds discussed in this chapter are fairly typical of chemicals used as model carcinogens in cancer research; intermediates in the dye and pigment industries; finished dyes and pigments used in the paper, textile, leather, plastics, and paint industries; and one naturally occurring compound, cycasin, that is a toxic constituent of cycad seeds used as a source of food and medicines in many parts of the world [5].

II. AROMATIC AMINES

A. 2-Acetylaminofluorene (2-AAF) and 2-Aminofluorene (2-AF) [6]

General description of method

Procedures are described for determining residues of 2-AAF in laboratory chow and six different microbiological media by spectrophotofluorescence (SPF) and gas chromatography (GC). The salient elements of the SPF method are: extraction, a rapid cleanup on alumina, acid hydrolysis of 2-AAF to 2-AF, further cleanup by organic solvent extraction of interferences from the aqueous amine hydrochloride, conversion of the hydrochloride to the free base (2-AF) and its extraction, and finally quantification of 2-AAF as 2-AF by SPF. In the GC method, the extract is cleaned up by solvent partitioning followed by silica gel chromatography with residues being determined directly as 2-AAF. Additional data are presented concerning partition values (p values); GC and SPF characteristics; adsorption liquid chromatographic properties of 2-AAF, 2-AF, and fluorene; and solubility values for 2-AAF in various solvents.

Introduction

2-Acetylaminofluorene (2-AAF; N-2-fluorenylacetamide) is a carcinogen that has been widely studied and is known to produce tumors in specific organs [7,8]. As part of a long-term, low dose study of 2-AAF in mice, an analytical method was required for monitoring residues of the compound added to the animal's diet to ensure the requisite dosage as well as the homogeneity and stability of 2-AAF in the diet. In addition, microbiological systems that will degrade 2-AAF and thus destroy its carcinogenic activity were being sought, and a method for analyzing traces of the compound in the growth media was required. Formulas of 2-AAF and two of its degradation products, 2-aminofluorene (2-AF) and fluorene, are shown in Figure 1.

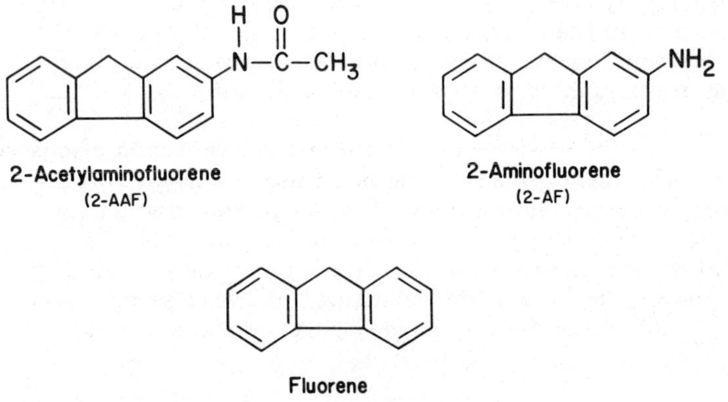

Figure 1 Formulas of 2-AAF, 2-AF, and fluorene. (From Ref. 6.)

Several methods for determining residues of 2-AAF have been reported. Westfall [9] devised a colorimetric method for estimating 2-AF in biological material by diazotizing the amino group and coupling with sodium 2-naphthol-3,6-disulfonate. Later, Westfall and Morris [10] used the method to analyze for 2-AAF after hydrolyzing it to 2-AF; their reagent blanks for tissue extracts were equivalent to 1 to 5 μg of 2-AF. Sandin et al. [11] determined the molar extinction coefficient and absorption maximum of 2-AAF to be 4.46 at 288 nm, respectively. Irving [12] determined 2-AAF and 2-AF in urine extracts by ultraviolet (UV) absorption after separating them by solvent partitioning. The analysis of 2-AAF and its degradation products (particularly the hydroxylated metabolites) has depended mostly on the use of ^{14}C-labeled material [13,14]. None of these procedures, however, were sufficiently specific and sensitive for the substrates of interest; therefore, the following procedures were developed. All temperature data are in degrees Celsius.

Experimental

Materials. Fluorene (m.p. 114 to 115°) and 2-AF (m.p. 126 to 127°) were purchased from Eastman Organic Chemicals, Rochester, New York. The 2-AAF (m.p. 193 to 195°) was purchased from Aldrich Chemical Co., Milwaukee, Wisconsin. The fluorene and 2-AAF were used as received since they contained no extraneous GC peaks and recrystallization failed to change their GC or SPF response. The 2-AF (light brown) was recrystallized from methanol-water prior to use; although a white crystalline product was obtained, the melting point remained essentially unchanged. Purification of the 2-AF removed extraneous GC peaks and enhanced the GC and SPF responses by about 5%.

Adsorbents were silica gel (No. 3405) from J. T. Baker Chemical Co.; basic alumina, Brockman activity I (No. A-941), and Hyflo Super-Cel (No. H-333) from Fisher Scientific Co.; charcoal (Darco KB) from Atlas Chemical Industries, Wilmington, Delaware. The silica gel was dried overnight at 130°, adjusted to 7% moisture with buffer pH 7 (Fisher Scientific Co., No. SO-B-108), mixed well, and allowed to stand overnight prior to use. The other adsorbents were used as received. The sodium sulfate was anhydrous. All reagents were CP grade and solvents were pesticide grade. The laboratory chow (Type 5010-C, Ralston Purina Co., St. Louis, Missouri) contained about 6% fat and had a pH of 5.5; 93.3% was not volatile at 110° overnight. All ingredients for the microbiological culture media were purchased from Difco Laboratories, Detroit, Michigan. The media were prepared in accordance with the directions supplied by the manufacturer except that the proteose peptone was a 2% aqueous solution of Bacto-Proteose Peptone No. 3.

Preparation of Samples for Analysis by Gas Chromatography

Laboratory chow. A 20 g portion of the sample was deactivated by the addition of 20 ml of distilled water, then extracted with 100 ml of chloroform-methanol (9:1, v/v) in a 150 ml bottle sealed with a Teflon-lined cap by using an Eberbach shaker (Curtin Scientific Co., No. 205-575) operated for 2 hr at 200 excursions/min. The supernatant was then percolated through a plug of anhydrous sodium sulfate (25 mm diam × 30 mm thick), and 50 ml of the extract (equivalent to 10 g of sample) was evaporated to dryness on a 60° water bath under water pump vacuum. The residue was dissolved in 10 ml of acetonitrile and extracted twice with 20 ml portions of hexane, then the acetonitrile phase was evaporated to dryness as described. The residue was dissolved in 20 ml of benzene by using the 60° water bath and a Teflon policeman, and the solution was reserved for subsequent silica gel cleanup.

A silica gel column was prepared by adding successively to a 12 mm i.d. glass tube (Kontes No. 420,000) a plug of glass wool, 5 g of sodium sulfate, 5 g of silica gel (7% buffer, pH 7), and 5 g of sodium sulfate. The column was washed with 20 ml of benzene and the eluate discarded. The benzene solution of the chow extract was added to the column and after it had percolated into the adsorbent, the container and the column were washed with five 10 ml rinses of 2% acetone in benzene (the combined eluates contain residues of fluorene and 2-AF if any were present in the extractive). Finally, the column was eluted with 60 ml of 5% acetone in benzene (this eluate contains 2-AAF). The fractions were then evaporated to dryness as described and the residues dissolved in an appropriate volume of chloroform (e.g., 2 to 5 ml) for injection into the GC.

Microbiological media. Twenty milliliters of the medium was mixed with 1 g of sodium chloride in a 125 ml separatory funnel, extracted three times with 10 ml portions of chloroform, and each portion successively percolated through a plug of sodium sulfate (25 mm diam. × 10 mm thick). The combined extracts were evaporated to dryness as described; the residue was dissolved in 20 ml of benzene and reserved for silica gel cleanup.

A silica gel column was prepared as described for analysis of the laboratory chow except that 2 g of silica gel was used and the column was washed with 10 ml of benzene prior to use. The benzene solution of the extract was added to the column, allowed to percolate into the adsorbent, then the container and the column were washed twice with 10 ml portions of 2% acetone in benzene (the combined eluates contain fluorene and 2-AF). The column was then eluted with 20 ml of 8% acetone in benzene (contains residues of 2-AAF). The fractions were evaporated to dryness as described and the residue dissolved in chloroform (about 1 to 2 ml) for injection into the GC.

Preparation of Samples for Analysis by Spectrophotofluorescence

Laboratory chow. A 3 g portion of the sample was deactivated by the addition of 3 ml of distilled water, then extracted on the shaker as previously described except with 15 ml of chloroform-methanol (9:1, v/v) in a culture tube (20 × 150 mm) sealed with a Teflon-lined cap. The supernatant was decanted through a plug of sodium sulfate (15 mm diam × 10 mm thick) and the percolate centrifuged at 1000 rpm for 10 min. Five milliliters of the extract (1 g equivalent of chow) was then added to a column (Kontes No. 420,000) consisting of 2 g of basic alumina supported by a plug of glass wool. The column was washed twice with 2 ml portions of chloroform and the total effluent collected in a culture tube, then evaporated to near dryness with a jet of dry air and finally to dryness with water pump vacuum and a 60° water bath. Hydrolysis of 2-AAF to 2-AF was then accomplished by adding 4 ml of methanol and 2 ml of concentrated HCl to the dry residue and heating it in the sealed tube at 85° for 2 hr by using a tube heater (Kontes No. 720,000). After the tube had cooled, 3 ml of distilled water was added and the contents extracted three times with 7 ml portions of benzene; each portion of benzene was carefully withdrawn and discarded by using a 10 ml syringe and cannula. Next, 4 ml of 10 N sodium hydroxide was added and the contents extracted three times with 7 ml portions of benzene. Each portion was successively percolated through a plug of sodium sulfate (15 mm diam × 10 mm thick) and collected in a 50 ml glass-stoppered flask containing a boiling bead and 1 drop of diethylene glycol to serve as a "keeper." The contents were evaporated just to dryness under water pump vacuum at 60° and the residue dissolved in an appropriate volume of methanol (5 ml or more) for SPF analysis.

Microbiological media. Ten milliliters of the medium in a culture tube containing 1 g of sodium chloride was extracted with two 10 ml portions of benzene, which were successively percolated through a plug of sodium sulfate (15 mm diam × 10 mm thick). The total extractive was then percolated through a 2 g alumina column and the benzene effluent discarded. The column was then washed with 5 ml of chloroform-methanol (9:1, v/v) and two 2 ml portions of chloroform; the combined washings were evaporated, hydrolyzed, extracted, and prepared for SPF analysis as described for laboratory chow except that only two extractions of the acid phase were required.

Solubility and p-Value Determinations. The solubility of 2-AAF in several solvents was determined by preparing supersaturated solutions (5 ml) in 10 ml flasks by alternately heating them in a water bath at 50° and shaking them with a vortex mixer during a period of 4 hr. The solutions were then mechanically shaken at ambient temperature (25 ± 2°) for 6 days. The supernatant was decanted into glass-stoppered tubes and centrifuged at 2000 rpm for about 4 hr. Portions of the supernatant were appropriately diluted and analyzed by GC.

Extraction p values for the three compounds in several immiscible binary solvent systems were determined by GC as described by Bowman and Beroza [15,16].

Gas Chromatographic Analysis. A Hewlett-Packard Model 5750 gas chromatograph with a flame ionization detector (FID) was fitted with a 100 cm glass column (4 mm i.d., 6 mm o.d.) containing 10% OV-101 (w/w) on 80-100 mesh Gas Chrom Q (Applied Science Lab, State College, Pennsylvania) and operated under the following conditions after preconditioning the column overnight at 275°: helium carrier gas, 75 ml/min; column, 250°; injection port, 275°; detector, 290°. Under these conditions, retention times (t_R) for fluorene, 2-AF, and 2-AAF were 0.55, 1.45, and 3.60 min, respectively.

Five milliliters of the cleaned-up extract dissolved in chloroform was injected for analysis. Quantification of the unknown was based on the peak height of known amounts of standard; peak height to about 1×10^{-8} AFS was proportional to concentration of sample. Initial conditioning of the GC column by repeatedly injecting 2-AAF and extracts was required for reproducible, linear, and sensitive responses.

Spectrophotofluorometric Analysis. An Aminco-Bowman instrument (American Instrument Co., Silver Spring, Maryland) equipped with a xenon lamp and a 1P28 detector was used with 1 cm cells and a 2-2-2 mm slit program to measure fluorescence. Excitation and emission maxima for the three compunds were: 2-AAF; λ_{Ex} = 296 nm, λ_{Em} = 328 nm; 2-AF: λ_{Ex} = 297 nm, λ_{Em} = 366 nm; fluorene: λ_{Ex} = 266 nm, λ_{Em} = 307 nm. All dilutions were made with methanol. During operation, the instrument was calibrated frequently to produce a relative intensity (RI) of 5.0 with a solution of 0.3 μg of quinine sulfate/ml of 0.1 N sulfuric acid (λ_{Ex} = 350, λ_{Em} = 450). Readings were corrected for the solvent blank and RI was plotted versus concentration of the three compounds on log-log paper to produce standard curves.

All samples were diluted to contain extract equivalent to 0.2 g of chow/ml or to 2 g of medium/ml or diluted further as required. To make certain that the RI is within the linear range of the standard curve and thus unaffected by concentration quenching, samples were diluted with an equal volume of solvent; the RI of the diluted samples should be about half that of the undiluted solution. If it was not, dilution was continued until RI was halved by dilution. After the untreated control sample (diluted in the same manner as the unknown) was subtracted, concentration in μg/ml was determined from the standard curve. Since residues of 2-AAF are analyzed as 2-AF, the analytical results are multiplied by a factor 1.23 to express them as 2-AAF.

Results and discussion

In studies concerning the efficiency of extracting residues of 2-AAF from aged samples of spiked chow, higher recoveries were obtained from portions shaken at room temperature than from those extracted in a Soxhlet apparatus. The addition of water to deactivate the sample greatly enhanced recovery (up to 30% enhancement), particularly from autoclaved samples. The reason for lower recoveries from the Soxhlet extractions is not known; however, the prolonged exposure of the sample at the reflux temperature of the solvent may have caused partial degradation and/or conjugation of the residue.

Recoveries from chow spiked with 5, 50, and 250 ppm of 2-AAF and analyzed by the GC procedure (partitioning and silica gel cleanup) averaged 63, 87, and 97%, respectively. Samples from the GC analysis were not sufficiently clean for SPF. However, a satisfactory additional cleanup was achieved by adding a benzene solution (5 ml) of the GC sample to a column (12 mm i.d.) containing 1.25 g of Darco KB-Hyflo Super-Cel (1:4, w/w) and eluting the 2-AAF with 25 ml of benzene-acetone (1:1, v/v); the eluate was evaporated to dryness and analyzed by SPF as 2-AAF per se as described. This cleanup further reduced recoveries to about 52, 67, and 69% for the 5, 50, and 250 ppm samples, respectively. Sensitivities (based on twice the interference from untreated samples) of both the GC and SPF procedures for chow and the GC procedure for biological media were about 1 and 0.1 ppm, respectively. Figure 2 shows typical gas chromatograms of the analytical standards and extracts of chow and a biological growth medium (Rogosa). A comparison of Figure 2B (solvent partitioning only) and 2C illustrates the reduction in interference accomplished by the silica gel chromatography; the 2-AAF residues in chow (Fig. 2D) could not be analyzed without the silica gel cleanup.

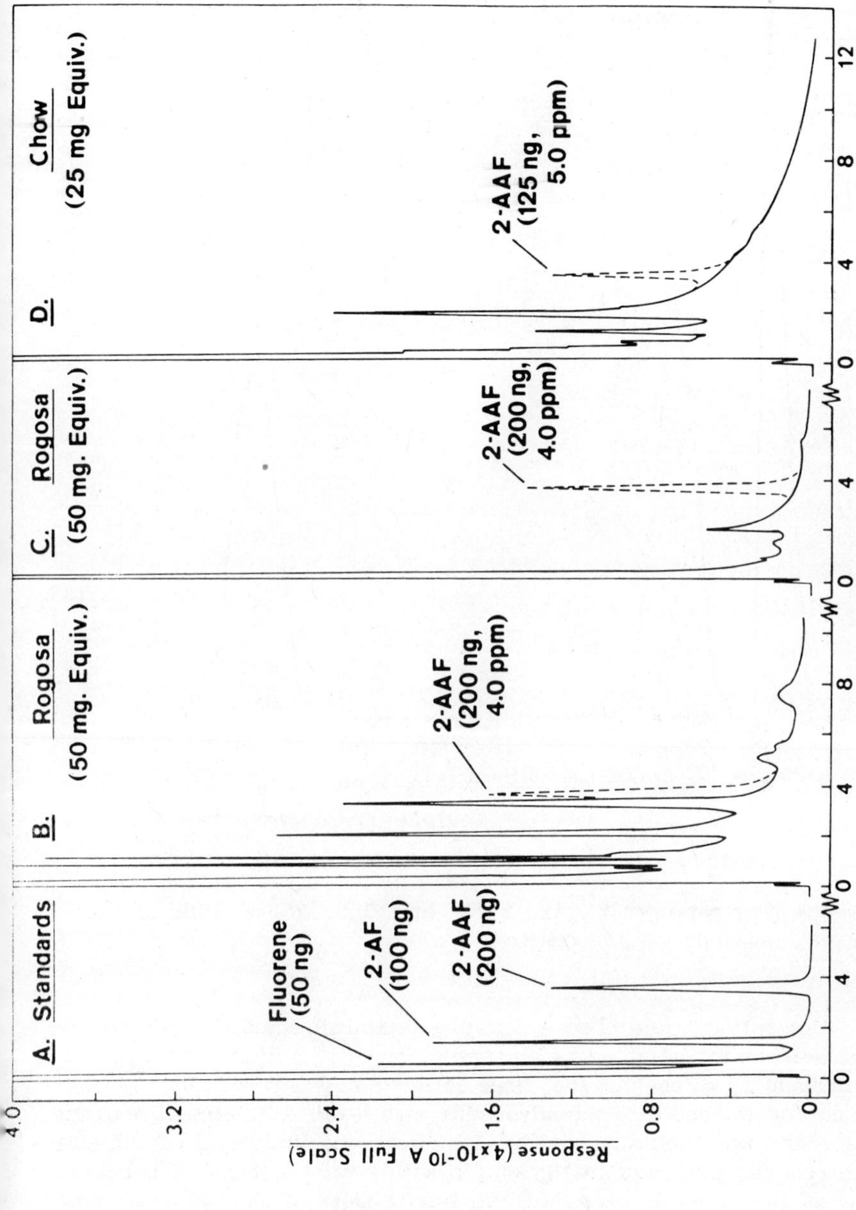

Figure 2 Gas chromatograms of 2-AAF and two of its analogs. Solid lines in chromatograms (B), (C), and (D) are unspiked extracts carried through the method [exception: (B) was not cleaned up with silica gel]; dashed lines are the same solutions spiked with 2-AAF. (From Ref. 6.)

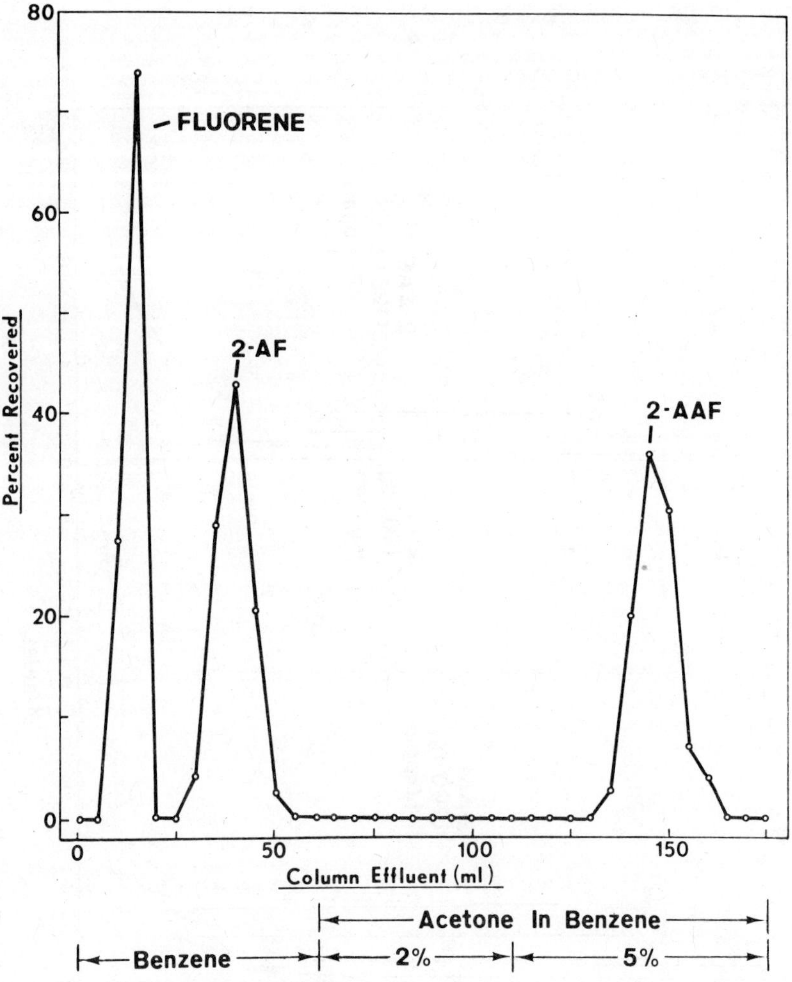

Figure 3 Separation of 2-AAF, 2-AF, and fluorene by liquid chromatography on silica gel. (From Ref. 6.)

Adsorption liquid chromatography of the three compounds on silica gel was investigated as a cleanup for GC. A 1 ml solution containing 500 μg of each of the three compounds was placed on the column and washed into the adsorbent with a few milliliters of benzene. This eluate was then analyzed by gas chromatography of 5 ml aliquots as the column was sequentially eluted with a total of 60 ml of benzene, 50 ml of 2% acetone in benzene, and finally 65 ml of 5% acetone in benzene. As shown in Figure 3, fluorene and 2-AF were completely

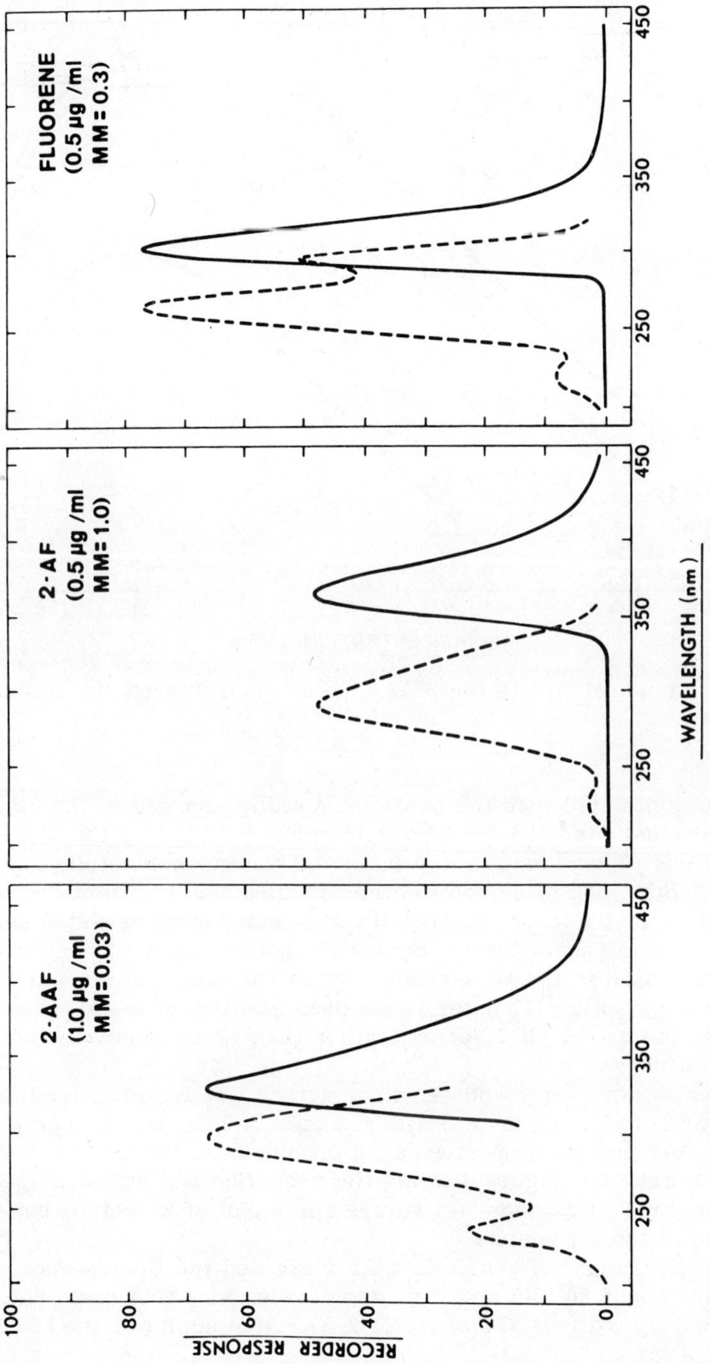

Figure 4 Excitation (dashed line) and emission (solid line) spectra of 2-AAF, 2-AF, and fluorene in methanol. (From Ref. 6.)

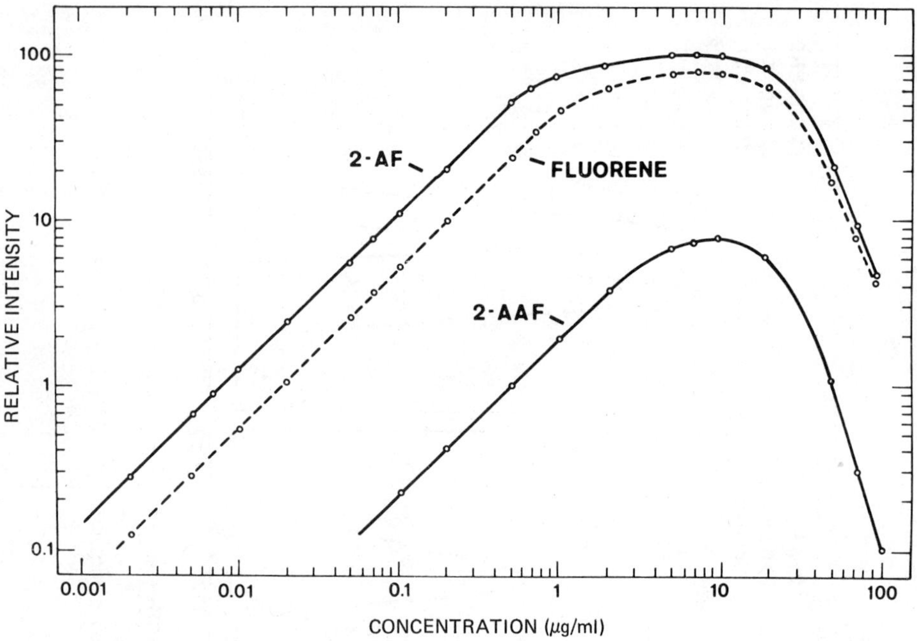

Figure 5 Standard curves for 2-AAF, 2-AF, and fluorene in methanol. (From Ref. 6.)

separated and eluted with the benzene, nothing emerged in the 2% acetone effluent, and the 2-AAF was completely eluted by the 5% acetone mixture. These results may be useful for metabolic studies or for the adaption of the method to other substrates. In studies with spiked extracts, it was found that the 2% acetone mixture eluted much of the interfering materials but no 2-AAF; accordingly, this solvent mixture was used in the GC cleanup. When the silica gel was partially deactivated by adding 7% water, some decomposition of 2-AAF was observed; the use of pH 7 buffer, rather than water alone, corrected the difficulty.

Later, a more rapid and sensitive method was required for the analysis of 2-AAF residues in smaller samples. The strong fluorescence of 2-AF and its properties as an organic base formed the basis of the SPF method. Figure 4 shows the excitation and emission spectra of the three compounds and Figure 5 is a plot of RI versus concentration of the compounds.

Acid hydrolysis of 2-AAF to 2-AF increased the fluorescence of the residue about 50-fold and provided a sensitivity that could not be obtained by a direct SPF assay of 2-AAF. In addition, the acid

Table 1 SPF and GC Analysis of Extracts of Laboratory Chow Spiked with 2-AAF

Added		Recovered($\bar{x}$ ± SE)[a]	
ppm	μg[b]	μg[b]	%
		SPF Analysis	
0	0	0.243 ± 0.022	-
2.0	2.0	1.53 ± 0.03	76.5 ± 1.5
20	20	17.3 ± 0.1	86.5 ± 0.5
200	200	170 ± 1.3	85.0 ± 0.7
		GC Analysis[c]	
20	20	16.8 ± 0.3	84.2 ± 1.5
200	200	165 ± 2.6	82.3 ± 1.3

[a]Mean of four samples.
[b]Per gram of sample.
[c]Methanol solutions from the SPF analysis were evaporated to dryness, dissolved in chloroform, and the 2-AF analyzed by GC.
Source: Ref. 6.

hydrolysis of the acetyl group followed by the organic solvent extraction of the aqueous phase containing 2-AF as the amine hydrochloride provided a cleanup far superior to that obtained in the GC method. Therefore, the SPF procedure is preferred to GC for analyzing low levels of residues.

Quadruplicate samples of lab chow untreated and spiked with 2-AAF at 2, 20, and 200 ppm were analyzed by the SPF procedure; the results are presented in Table 1. Based on twice the SPF reading obtained from the untreated chow, the limit of sensitivity would be set at about 0.5 ppm, but because its fluorescence was highly reproducible and the excitation and emission maxima from the chow did not correspond to those of 2-AF, identification and estimation of residues as low as the 0.1 ppm level may be possible.

Four replicates of the six microbiological media untreated and spiked with 2-AAF at 0.10 and 1.0 ppm were also analyzed by the SPF method and the results are presented in Table 2. Limits of sensitivity (based on twice the SPF reading of the untreated medium) varied from about 14 ppm from Rogosa to 52 ppb for the thioglycolate medium. Again, the fluorescence of the untreated samples was highly reproducible and did not correspond to that of 2-AF.

The SPF procedure for both chow and media detects residues of 2-AAF and 2-AF. Recoveries of 2-AF are generally about 10% lower

Table 2 SPF Analysis of Six Different Biological Growth Media Spiked with 2-AAF at 0.0, 0.1, and 1.0 ppm

	Added		Recovered ($\bar{x}$ ± SE)[a]	
Biological medium	ppm	μg[b]	μg[b]	%
Rogosa	0	0	0.057 ± 0.003	-
	0.10	1.00	0.805 ± 0.024	80.5 ± 2.4
	1.00	10.0	8.76 ± 0.155	87.6 ± 1.6
Lactobacillus MRS	0	0	0.067 ± 0.005	-
	0.10	1.00	0.846 ± 0.012	84.6 ± 1.2
	1.00	10.0	8.79 ± 0.113	87.9 ± 1.1
Brain heart infusion	0	0	0.200 ± 0.005	-
	0.10	1.00	0.901 ± 0.013	90.1 ± 1.3
	1.00	10.0	9.07 ± 0.229	90.7 ± 2.3
Proteose peptone	0	0	0.114 ± 0.008	-
	0.10	1.00	0.702 ± 0.020	70.2 ± 2.0
	1.00	10.0	8.25 ± 0.286	82.5 ± 3.9
Trypticase soy dextrose	0	0	0.127 ± 0.003	-
	0.10	1.00	0.864 ± 0.153	86.4 ± 1.5
	1.00	10.0	8.73 ± 0.090	87.3 ± 0.9
Thioglycolate	0	0	0.234 ± 0.012	-
	0.10	1.00	0.897 ± 0.031	89.7 ± 3.2
	1.00	10.00	8.89 ± 0.106	88.9 ± 1.1

[a]Mean of four samples.
[b]Per 10 ml of medium.
Source: Ref. 6.

than 2-AAF, probably because of its greater volatility. Studies with chow and media spiked with 2-AAF and autoclaved have indicated that the compound is stable; however, if residues of 2-AF are sought, the analysis may be performed by omitting the 2-hr hydrolysis at 85° and immediately extracting the acidified extract at ambient temperature to remove any residues of 2-AAF before hydrolysis occurs. The behavior of the hydroxylated metabolites of 2-AAF in the analytical procedure is not known since analytical standards are not available. However, any residues of these compounds extracted by the procedure might be lost during the adsorption column cleanup. For example, N-OH-2-AAF is apparently irreversibly sorbed by alumina and silica gel on thin layer plates [17].

The SPF method for media, with minor modifications, has been applied to the analysis of 2-AF and 2-AAF at the low-ppb level in wastewater, human urine, fixatives, and other aqueous substrates.

The possibility of analyzing for traces of the compounds by preparing electron-capturing derivatives was investigated. When the three compounds were dissolved in 1 ml of chloroform and reacted with 50 μl of liquid bromine for 5 min at ambient temperature, derivatives with high electron-capturing properties were obtained. Presumably, two bromine atoms were added to the fluorene ring of each compound. Unfortunately, this technique had to be rejected because cleaned-up extracts of the brominated samples contained electron-capturing interferences.

Solubility data for 2-AAF in the common organic solvents and in vegetable oils were required before analytical method development and the formulation of animal diets could be undertaken; such values could not be found in the literature. The results of our determinations were as follows:

Solvent	Solubility of 2-AAF (mg/ml) at 25 ± 2°C
Acetone	42.0
Acetonitrile	16.3
Benzene	27.4
Chloroform	36.0
Corn oil	2.26
Dimethyl sulfoxide	>200
Ethyl acetate	56.6
Ethyl alcohol (95%)	22.2
Hexane	0.02
Methyl alcohol	24.2
Peanut oil	2.46
Propylene glycol	11.1
Soybean oil	2.00
Water	0.007

Partition values (the fraction of solute partitioning into the nonpolar phase of an equivolume immiscible binary solvent system) are useful in developing extraction and cleanup procedures and in confirming the identities of GC peaks [15,16,18,19]. The following values were obtained for the compounds: (1) in chloroform-aqueous NaOH, HCl, or H_2SO_4 (0.001, 0.1, or 10 N), fluorene and 2-AAF are 1.0; (2) in chloroform-aqueous NaOH (0.001, 0.1, or 10 N), aqueous HCl, or H_2SO_4 (0.001 N), 2-AF is 1.0; (3) in chloroform-aqueous HCl or H_2SO_4 (10 N), 2-AF is 0.01 or less; and (4) in chloroform-aqueous HCl or H_2SO_4 (0.1 N), 2-AF was about 0.17. Values for 2-AAF were determined in several other solvent systems as follows: hexane-acetonitrile, 0.008; chloroform-water, 1.0; chloroform-60% methanol (40% water), 0.94; hexane-dimethylformamide, 0.004; benzene-water, 1.0; and hexane-80% acetone (20% water), 0.24.

The analysis of 2-AAF in wastewater via SPF is discussed in Section II.G. A procedure for determining 2-AF and 2-AAF in human urine and wastewater via EC-GC of pentafluoropropionyl derivatives is presented in Section II.H.

B. 4-Ethylsulfonylnaphthalene-1-Sulfonamide (ENS) [20]

General description of method

Procedures are described for the analysis of ENS residues in laboratory chow, blood, human urine, wastewater, and microbiological media employing spectrophotofluorescence (SPF) and/or gas chromatography (GC). Extensive cleanup is required for the SPF procedures, resulting in adequate sensitivity and specificity. The acidic property of ENS formed the basis of the cleanup and derivatization procedures. The GC methods require only an extraction cleanup followed by methylation of the ENS with diazomethane and subsequent analysis by using a flame photometric detector operated in the sulfur mode. Additional information is presented concerning the relative efficiencies of several solvent extraction systems, solubility values for ENS in water and hexane, partition values (p values) for ENS in several solvent systems, optimization of the methylation reaction of ENS with diazomethane, and the efficacy of the SPF method by analysis of urine from a dog dosed with [^{14}C]ENS.

Introduction

4-Ethylsulfonylnaphthalene-1-sulfonamide (ENS or 4-ENS), a known carcinogen administered as a single dose, induced epithelial hyperplasia of the bladder in mice [21]; prolonged dietary dosing with ENS produced a greater degree of epithelial hyperplasia and frequently, bladder tumors [22,23]. More recent investigations [24,25] indicated that most of these effects resulted from an alteration of urinary pH and irritation from calculi induced by ENS rather than from direct action of the chemical on the bladder epithelium. Since toxicological tests with ENS were planned at our laboratory and no suitable procedure could be found in the literature, the following procedures were developed to satisfy our requirements. The formula of ENS is shown in Figure 6.

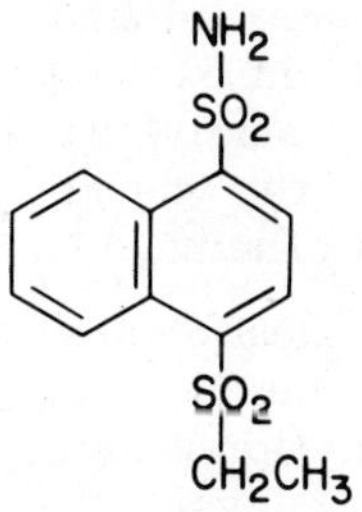

Figure 6 Formula of ENS. (From Ref. 20.)

Experimental

Materials. The 4-ENS (m.p. 199 to 200°), purchased from Pfaltz and Bauer, Inc., Flushing, New York, was used as received since it contained no extraneous GC peaks and recrystallization failed to change its GC or SPF response.

Adsorbents were silica gel (No. 3405) from J. T. Baker Chemical Co., and acid alumina, Brockman Activity I (No. A-948) from Fisher Scientific Co. The silica gel, used as received, contained 3.7% moisture. The sodium sulfate was anhydrous. All reagents were CP grade and solvents were pesticide grade. The laboratory chow (Type 5010-C, Ralston Purina Co., St. Louis, Missouri) contained 6% fat, had a pH of 5.5, and 6.7% was volatile at 110° overnight. Ingredients for the microbiological culture media were purchased from Difco Laboratories, Detroit, Michigan, and prepared in accordance with the directions supplied by the manufacturer. The ethereal diazomethane reagent was prepared from Diazald by using the reagent, kit, and instructions supplied by the manufacturer (Aldrich Chemical Co., Milwaukee, Wisconsin), then stored at -10° until used.

Preparation of Samples for Analysis by Spectrophotofluorescence

Laboratory chow. Two extraction methods were employed to determine the relative efficiencies of recovering residues of ENS.

1. A portion of the sample was deactivated by the addition of 20 ml of distilled water, then extracted with 100 ml of chloroform-methanol (9:1, v/v) in a 250 ml glass-stoppered bottle by shaking for 2 hr at 200 excursions/min on an Eberbach shaker (Curtin Scientific Co., No. 205-575). The supernatant was then percolated through a plug of anhydrous sodium sulfate (25 mm diam × 30 mm thick), centrifuged at 2000 rpm for 10 min, carefully decanted through a plug of glass wool, and stored in a tightly sealed container for subsequent cleanup.
2. A 20-g sample was tightly wrapped in Whatman No. 1 filter paper, placed in a Soxhlet apparatus (W. H. Curtin Co. No.

087.486), and extracted with 100 ml of chloroform-methanol (9:1, v/v) for 2 hr at the rate of about 30 solvent exchanges per hour. The extract was then quantitatively percolated through a plug of sodium sulfate as described, the volume adjusted to 100 ml, and stored for subsequent cleanup.

A 10 ml aliquot of the chow extract from the mechanical or Soxhlet procedure was pipetted into a 30 ml culture tube containing 10 ml of 1 N NaOH, sealed with a Teflon-lined cap, shaken vigorously for 2 min, then centrifuged at 1500 rpm for 10 min. The chloroform layer (bottom) was withdrawn and discarded by using a 10 ml syringe and cannula. The aqueous layer was extracted twice more with 10 ml portions of chloroform, which were also discarded. The aqueous phase was then made strongly acid by the addition of 2 ml of concentrated HCl and extracted three times with 10 ml portions of chloroform, successively percolating them through a plug of anhydrous sodium sulfate. The combined extracts were evaporated to dryness on a 60° water bath under water pump vacuum and reserved for subsequent column cleanup.

Two glass columns (12 mm i.d., Kontes No. 420,000) were prepared by adding successively a plug of glass wool, 5 g of sodium sulfate, the adsorbent, and 5 g of sodium sulfate. In one column, the adsorbent was 2 g of silica gel (as received) and in the other 1 g of acid alumina (Brockman activity I). The columns were arranged in tandem and prewashed by adding 10 ml of benzene-5% acetone to the one on top, which contained the silica gel; the lower column (alumina) was then removed. The dry extract from the solvent partitioning step was then dissolved in 5 ml of benzene-5% acetone and added to the silica gel column. The container and column were washed with three additional 5 ml portions of the same solvent and the eluant discarded. The columns were again placed in tandem and 20 ml of benzene-10% acetone was added to elute the ENS from the silica gel column onto the alumina. The silica gel column and the effluent from the alumina column were discarded. Finally, the alumina column was eluted with 25 ml of chloroform-methanol (9:1, v/v). The effluent was collected, evaporated to dryness as described, and the residue dissolved in an appropriate volume of acetonitrile for SPF analysis.

Microbiological media. Ten milliliters of the medium was added to a 30 ml culture tube containing 1 g of NaCl; 0.2 ml of concentrated HCl and 10 ml of benzene were added, then the tube was sealed, shaken, and centrifuged. The benzene layer was carefully withdrawn by using a syringe and cannula and added to a dry acid alumina column prepared as described for chow. The extraction was repeated with two additional 10-ml portions of benzene and the eluate from the column was discarded. The residue of ENS was eluted from the alumina column by using 20 ml of chloroform-methanol (9:1, v/v). The column effluent was evaporated to dryness and the residue dissolved in acetonitrile for SPF analysis.

Wastewater. Fifty milliliters of the sample was added to a 70 ml culture tube containing 2 g of NaCl; 0.5 ml of concentrated HCl and 15 ml of benzene were then added and the tube was sealed, shaken, and centrifuged. The benzene layer was removed, added to an alumina column, and the extraction was repeated with two additional 15 ml portions of benzene. The ENS on the alumina was then eluted, evaporated, and prepared for SPF analysis as described for media.

Blood. Procedures employing no hydrolysis of the substrate prior to the extraction of ENS residues as well as acid or alkaline hydrolysis were used.

1. *No hydrolysis.* Six milliliters of distilled water, 1 ml of concentrated HCl, and 1 g of NaCl were added to a 20 ml culture tube containing 1 ml of whole blood. The contents were mixed and extracted twice with 10 ml portions of benzene, cleaned up on an alumina column, and prepared for SPF analysis as described for media.
2. *Acid hydrolysis.* Samples were analyzed as for no hydrolysis except that the mixture in the sealed tube was held in a 80° heating block for 2 hr with frequent shaking, then cooled prior to the extraction with benzene.
3. *Alkaline hydrolysis.* Samples were analyzed as for no hydrolysis except that 1 ml of 10 N NaOH was substituted for the HCl. The mixture was then held at 80° for 2 hr, cooled, and acidified with 2 ml of concentrated HCl. The mixture was then extracted, cleaned up, and prepared for SPF analysis as described.

Urine. Procedures utilizing acid or alkaline hydrolysis prior to extraction as well as no hydrolysis were tested.

1. *No hydrolysis.* Analyses were performed exactly as described for wastewater.
2. *Acid hydrolysis.* Analyses were performed as described for wastewater except that the acidified mixture was heated at 80° for 2 hr in a water bath, then cooled prior to the extraction with benzene.
3. *Alkaline hydrolysis.* These analyses were also performed as described for wastewater except that 0.5 ml of 10 N NaOH was substituted for the HCl; the mixture was heated at 80° for 2 hr, cooled, and acidified with 1 ml of concentrated HCl prior to extraction with benzene.

Preparation of Samples for Analysis by Gas Chromatography. A 25 ml aliquot of the chow extract from the mechanical or Soxhlet procedure was pipetted into a 50 ml culture tube containing 10 ml of 1 N NaOH, tightly sealed with a Teflon-lined cap, vigorously shaken for 2 min, and centrifuged at 1500 rpm for 10 min. The chloroform layer was withdrawn and discarded and the aqueous layer extracted with two additional 10 ml portions of chloroform which were also discarded. The aqueous phase was acidified by adding 2 ml of concentrated HCl, then extracted with three 10 ml portions of chloroform, successively percolating them through a plug of sodium sulfate. The combined extracts were evaporated to dryness under water pump vacuum in a 60° water bath. The ENS was then methylated by adding 5 ml of ethereal diazomethane reagent to the dry residue and allowing the mixture to stand tightly sealed, overnight, in the dark at ambient temperature. The solvent was then evaporated under water pump vacuum in a 60° bath and the residue dissolved in an appropriate volume of chloroform for injection into the GC.

Spectrophotofluorometric Analysis. An Aminco-Bowman instrument (American Instrument Co., Silver Spring, Maryland) equipped with a xenon lamp and a 1P28 detector was used with 1 cm cells and a 2-2-2 mm slit program to measure fluorescence. Excitation and emission maxima for ENS were λ_{Ex} = 308 nm, λ_{Em} = 380 nm. All dilutions were made in acetonitrile. The instrument was frequently calibrated to produce a relative intensity (RI) of 5.0 with a solution of 0.3 μg of quinine sulfate/ml of 0.1 N sulfuric acid (λ_{Ex} = 350 nm, λ_{Ex} = 450 nm). Readings were corrected for the solvent blank and RI was plotted versus concentration of ENS on log-log paper to produce a standard curve.

To ensure that the RI was within the linear range (about 0.3 μg/ml or less) of the standard curve and thus unaffected by concentration quenching, samples were diluted with an equal volume of solvent to ascertain whether the RI was about half that of the undiluted solution. If it was not, dilution was continued until RI was halved by dilution. The RI of the untreated control sample was then subtracted from that of the unknown and concentration in μg/ml was determined from the standard curve.

Gas Chromatographic Analysis. A Hewlett-Packard Model 5750 gas chromatograph equipped with a flame photometric detector (Tracor Inc., Austin, Texas) fitted with a water-cooled adapter was operated in the sulfur mode (394 nm filter). The 100 cm glass column (4 mm i.d.) contained 5% Dexsil 300 GC (w/w) on Gas Chrom Q (80-100 mesh) and was operated isothermally at 280°; it was conditioned overnight at 350° prior to use. Flow rates of the gases in ml/min were: nitrogen (carrier) 160; hydrogen, 200; oxygen, 40. Temperatures of the injection port and the detector were 300 and 280°. Under the stated conditions, retention times (t_R) for ENS, its monomethyl, and its dimethyl derivatives were 2.25, 1.95, and 1.70 min, respectively. Two sulfur-containing pesticide reference compounds, coumaphos [0-(3-chloro-4-methyl-2-oxo-2H-1-benzopyran-7-yl)O,O-diethylphosphorothioate] and Dition [2-(2,4-dihydroxyphenyl)-1-cyclohexene-1-

carboxylic acid-δ-lactone o,o-diethylphosphorothioate] had t_R values of 1.40 and 2.55 min. All injections were made in 25 μl of chloroform.

Derivatization, p Values, and Solubility Determinations. Because of the unusually slow methylation reaction of ENS with ethereal diazomethane (about 12 mg of diazomethane/ml of reagent), rate studies at three temperatures were performed to optimize conditions of the reaction. Three flasks, each containing 120 μg of ENS and 30 ml of the diazomethane reagent were stored either in a freezer (-10°), refrigerator (5°), or in the dark at ambient temperature (25°). Samples (2 ml) were taken immediately and 0.25, 0.50, 0.75, 1, 2, 3, 4, 5, 6, 7, and 24 hr later at each temperature. The diazomethane reagent was immediately evaporated under water pump vacuum at ambient temperature to stop the reaction and the residue dissolved in 2 ml of chloroform for GC analysis. The percent of ENS derivatized (as the monomethyl, dimethyl, and total of both derivatives) was plotted versus reaction time.

The water solubility of ENS at 25 ± 2° was determined by SPF as described by Bowman and King [6].

Extraction p values for ENS were determined in several immiscible binary solvent systems by SPF in the manner described by Bowman and Beroza [18].

Recovery Experiments. Quadruplicate samples (20 g) of chow for the mechanical extraction procedure were separately spiked with 1 ml of chloroform containing the appropriate amount of ENS to yield residues of 0, 1, 5, 10, and 20 ppm. After the addition of 20 ml of water and 99 ml of chloroform-methanol (9:1, v/v), the samples were extracted and analyzed in the usual manner. It should be noted that some of the methanol from the mixed solvent remains in the water; therefore, each 5 ml aliquot of the extract is equivalent to 1.088 g of sample. This factor must be used in calculating the residue results. Additional samples of chow were spiked with 10 ppm of ENS and mechanically extracted with several other mixed solvent systems to check the efficiency of extraction. Quadruplicate samples for the Soxhlet extractions were also spiked as described for the mechanical procedure, except that the solvent containing the ENS was pipetted directly onto the chow on the filter paper; the sample was then wrapped, inserted into the apparatus, and extracted as described.

Quintuplicate samples of both biological media were separately spiked with 100 μl of methanol containing the appropriate amount of ENS to produce residues of 0, 0.1, and 1.0 ppm. The samples were allowed to stand in the refrigerator (5°) overnight prior to extraction. Samples (1 ml) of whole rat blood were spiked in the same manner at 0 and 10 ppm held at 5° overnight, and analyzed as described. Wastewater and urine samples (50 ml) were spiked at 0 and 20 ppb by adding 1 ml of methanol containing the appropriate amount of ENS, held at 5° overnight, and analyzed as described.

Assays of Urine from a Dog Dosed with [^{14}C]ENS. This experiment was performed to determine the efficacy of our SPF assay of urine from an animal dosed with ENS, since it is recognized that residues resulting from the metabolic process may behave differently from those spiked directly into the substrate.

The Division of Molecular Biology at NCTR was engaged in metabolic studies with an 11-month-old female beagle (10 kg), which was given a single oral dose of 41.3 mg of [^{14}C]ENS (18.2 μCi/mg) and the urine was subsequently collected at 24 hr intervals. Portions of these samples previously assayed radiometrically (total equivalents of ENS) were used to evaluate our procedure.

To determine free ENS by SPF, a 1 ml sample of urine, 9 ml of water, 0.5 g of NaCl, and 0.1 ml of concentrated HCl were mixed in a 20 ml culture tube and extracted with three 5 ml portions of benzene. The extraction and cleanup of free ENS and hydrolyzed conjugates were done as described for media. The aqueous phase was then subjected consecutively, first to alkaline and then to acid hydrolysis at 80° for 2 hr to evaluate the possibility of assaying conjugated ENS. Tests were also made to determine the effect of reversing the order of hydrolysis. The hydrolysis procedures were as follows:

1. Alkaline hydrolysis followed by acid hydrolysis; the aqueous phase was made alkaline by adding 0.2 ml of 10 N NaOH, heated, cooled, acidified with 0.2 ml of concentrated HCl, and extracted.
2. Acid hydrolysis followed by alkaline hydrolysis; the aqueous phase, already acid, was heated, cooled, and extracted. Then after the addition of 0.2 ml of 10 N NaOH, the sample was heated, cooled, acidified with 0.2 ml of concentrated HCl, and extracted.

Samples of water and untreated urine, unspiked and spiked with 10 ppm of ENS, were carried through the entire SPF procedure.

Results and discussion

In preliminary studies to select an efficient solvent system for mechanically extracting residues of ENS from chow, samples were spiked with 10 ppm and analyzed by GC. Samples of chow for the chloroform-methanol (9:1, v/v), benzene, and benzene-methanol (9:1, v/v) extractions were deactivated with an equal weight of water prior to extractions. Results of these tests were as follows:

Solvent (v/v)	ENS recovered (%)
Chloroform-methanol (9:1)	84.9
Benzene	52.9
Benzene-methanol (9:1)	58.2

Solvent (v/v)	ENS recovered (%)
Acetone-water (2:1)	86.4
Acetone-water (5:1)	67.3
Acetonitrile-water (2:1)	59.5
Acetonitrile-water (5:1)	52.5

The mechanical extraction with chloroform-methanol (9:1, v/v) was essentially as efficient as any solvent tested; therefore, it was adopted for use because the solvent was directly extractable with aqueous alkali for the initial cleanup step. A Soxhlet extraction of chow spiked with 10 ppm of ENS employing chloroform-methanol (9:1, v/v) yielded a recovery of 99.1%. Samples of chow were, therefore, spiked with ENS at several levels, extracted by using both methods, and assayed by SPF and GC to evaluate the analytical procedure.

The SPF procedure is highly sensitive and it is the method of choice, especially where ultralow residues of ENS are sought in the presence of low-level interferences. Nevertheless, some type of cleanup is usually necessary prior to SPF analysis of most substrates and in the case of chow (high-level interferences) the extensive multi-step procedure previously described was required. The excitation and

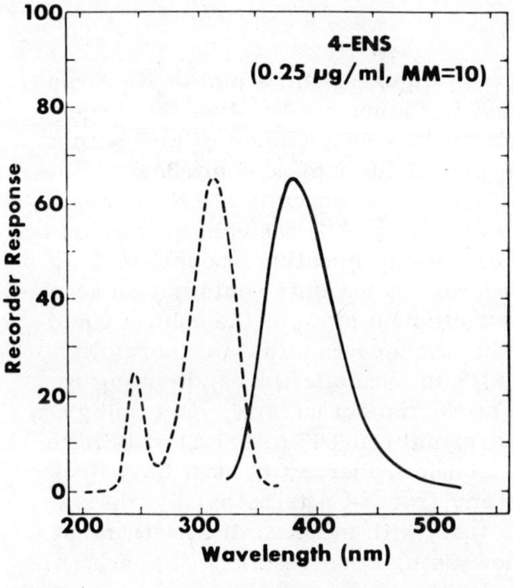

Figure 7 Excitation (dashed line) and emission (solid line) spectra of ENS in acetonitrile (MM denotes instrument meter multiplier setting). (From Ref. 20.)

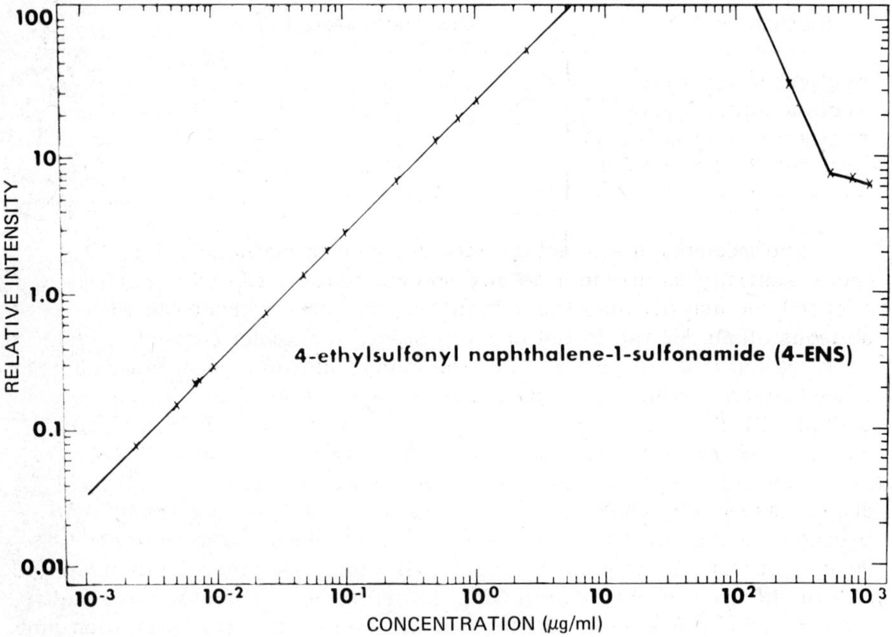

Figure 8 Standard curve for ENS in acetonitrile. (From Ref. 20.)

emission spectra of ENS is shown in Figure 7 and a plot of RI versus concentration of ENS is presented in Figure 8. Relative fluorescent intensity is directly proportional to the concentration of ENS within the range of about 2 ng to 3 μg per milliliter of acetonitrile.

The gas chromatography of microgram amounts of ENS per se was accomplished with difficulty and only after the column was conditioned with the compound by repeatedly injecting amounts of 5 μg or more. Reproducible GC of submicrogram amounts could not be accomplished, probably because the conditioned state of the column could not be maintained by injecting the smaller amounts. We therefore sought a means of derivatizing ENS to eliminate the conditioning requirements and permit analysis at the nanogram level. One milligram of ENS heated in a sealed tube overnight at 80° with 1 ml of BSA reagent [N,O-bis(trimethylsilyl)acetamide, Pierce Chemical Co., Rockford, Illinois] failed to produce any trace of a trimethylsilyl derivative of the compound; however, tests with ethereal diazomethane at room temperature indicated a slow methylation reaction. Experiments were therefore initiated to optimize the process for use in quantitative determinations of ENS. Results of the reaction rate studies with ENS and diazomethane at three temperatures are illustrated in Figure 9.

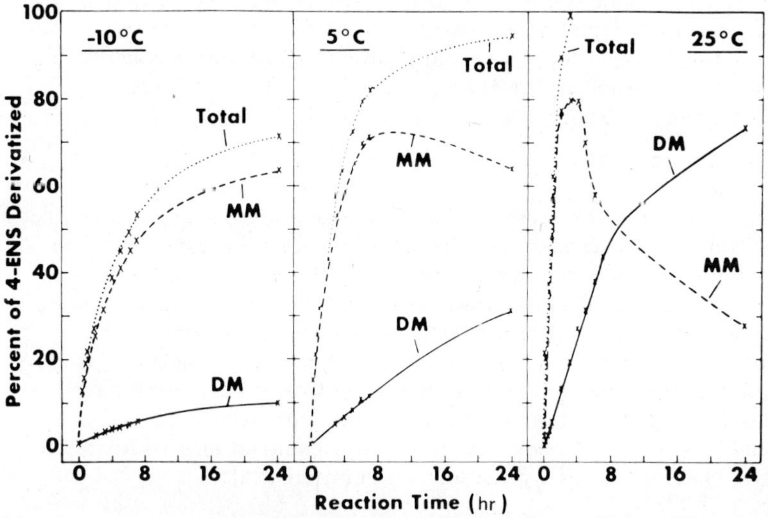

Figure 9 Rate of methylation of ENS with diazomethane at three temperatures (MM and DM denote monomethyl and dimethyl derivatives). (From Ref. 20.)

The reaction of ENS with diazomethane resulted in the formation of two compounds, presumed to be its monomethyl (MM) and dimethyl (DM) derivatives. This assumption is based on the GC retention times of the compounds and the rates of their formation. If two consecutive reactions occur to produce the dimethyl derivative via the monomethyl derivative, the overall reaction is of the form

$$A \xrightarrow{k_1} B \xrightarrow{k_2} C \tag{1}$$

where A is ENS and B and C are the monomethyl and dimethyl derivative of ENS, respectively. The applicable simultaneous differential rate equations are

$$\frac{-dx}{dt} = k_1 x \tag{2}$$

$$\frac{-dy}{dt} = -k_1 x + k_2 y \tag{3}$$

$$\frac{dz}{dt} = k_2 y \tag{4}$$

where x, y, and z are the respective concentrations of A, B, and C; t is the time; and k_1 and k_2 are the reaction rates of compounds A and

B, respectively. The solution of these equations, based on the assumption that only irreversible first-order steps are involved, is found in general textbooks [26]. The data indicate that this assumption is valid for this reaction under the specified conditions. Equation (2) can be integrated directly, giving

$$x = x_0 \exp(-k_1 t) \tag{5}$$

where x_0 is the initial concentration. Because of the large molar excess (21,400:1) of diazomethane to ENS used in this work, the concentration of ENS declined exponentially with time as occurs in any first-order reaction; that is, there was no apparent effect on rates due to the competition of ENS and monomethyl ENS for diazomethane.

Plots of log x versus time for the first hour of reaction, which exhibited excellent linearity at all three temperatures, were extrapolated and the time, τ, at which the ENS concentration had decreased to one-half the original concentration was measured and used to calculate the reaction rates by use of the relation [26]

$$k = \ln \frac{2}{\tau} \tag{6}$$

The reaction rates were found to be 0.17, 0.38, and 0.95 μg/ml per hour at -10, 5, and 25°, respectively. Another observation of the agreement between theory and these experimental data is that the plot of ln k versus the reciprocal of the absolute temperature gives a linear relationship as predicted by the Arrhenius equation [26]

$$k = A \exp\left(\frac{-E_a}{RT}\right) \tag{7}$$

where E_a is the activation energy, R is the gas constant, T is the absolute temperature, and A is a constant of integration.

At 25° the reaction of ENS is essentially complete (>98%) after 3 hr (Fig. 9). As the concentration of ENS asymptotically approaches zero, the formation of MM decreases and its conversion to DM continues causing its net concentration to decrease. At 5 and 25° the concentration of MM reached a maximum when its rate of formation equaled its rate of reaction. At -10° even after 24 hr, sufficient unreacted ENS remained so that no maximum for MM was observed.

These data indicate that 4 hr at 25° is adequate for essentially complete conversion of ENS to the monomethyl and dimethyl derivatives. Although at lower temperatures the diazomethane is more stable and available to react for a longer period of time, the decrease in reaction rate negates these advantages. We therefore adopted an overnight reaction (about 16 hr) at ambient temperature in order to produce a higher proportion of the dimethyl derivatives since its response (peak height) is 1.27 greater than the monomethyl derivative.

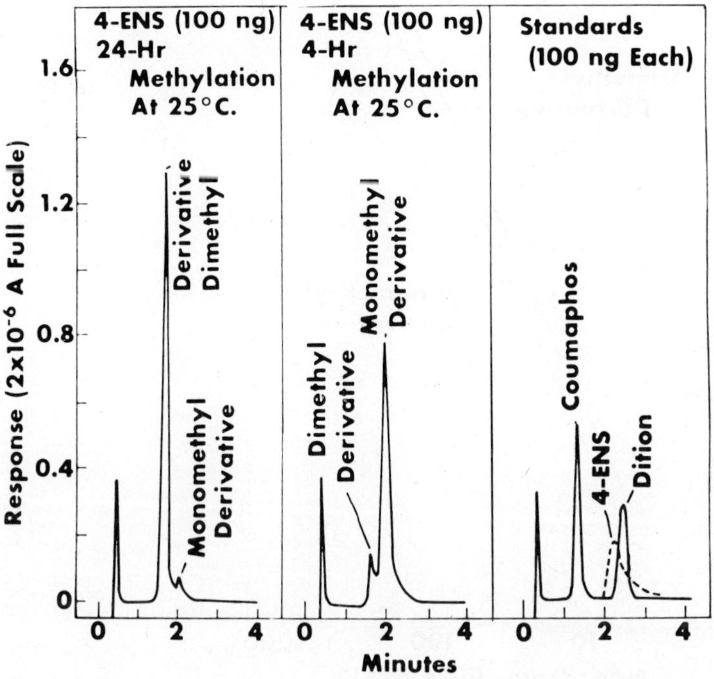

Figure 10 Typical gas chromatograms of methylated ENS, reference compounds, and ENS per se injected in 25 μl of chloroform. (From Ref. 20.)

Calculations of ENS residues via GC were accomplished in the following manner. A standard sample of ENS was reacted with diazomethane at ambient temperature for 24 hr as previously described and a series of dilutions was made to allow 25 μl injections containing 7.5 to 500 ng equivalents of ENS. The detector response of each peak (MM and DM derivatives) was plotted on log-log paper versus total nanogram equivalents of ENS, and in each case was found to be linear with identical slopes. The plots are represented by an equation of the form

$$\log n = m \log R + k \quad (8)$$

where n represents nanograms injected; R the detector response (amp); m the slope; and k the arbitrary constant.

The slope for both lines was determined to be 0.524 compared to 0.5, which would be expected from previous studies of the flame photometric detector operated in the S mode [27]; that is, the plot of amount injected versus the square root of the detector response would be linear.

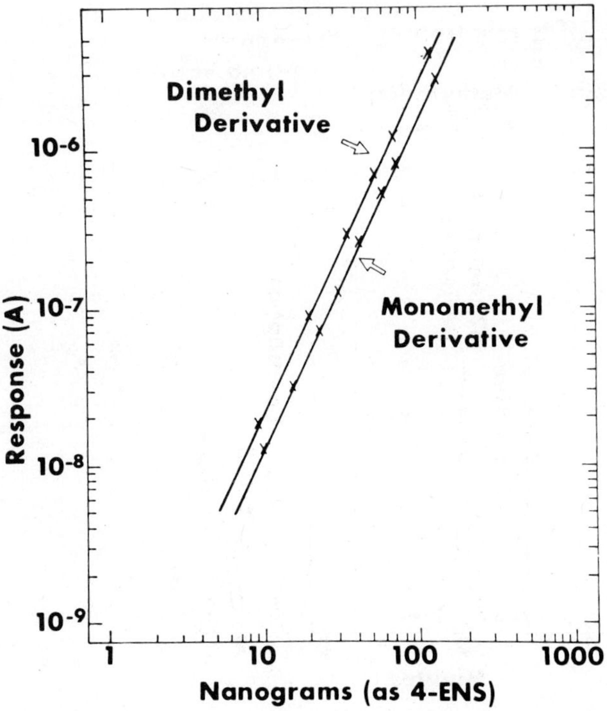

Figure 11 Standard curves for the monomethyl and dimethyl derivatives of ENS with the flame photometric detector (394 nm filter). (From Ref. 20.)

GC responses from samples, methylated at 25° for 4 hr (mostly MM) and 24 hr (mostly DM), as illustrated in Figure 10, were used to set up simultaneous equations to determine the relative response for each derivative of ENS. Each peak height was first converted to an arbitrary concentration, using values from the MM curve already described, in order to obtain values linearly related to concentration. These linear values, M and D, were then employed in the following equations:

$$aM_1 + bD_1 = 100 \text{ ng ENS} \quad (9)$$

$$aM_2 + bD_2 = 100 \text{ ng ENS} \quad (10)$$

where a and b are constants which are the detector response factors of the two derivatives. By equating the sum to 100 ng of ENS, actual concentrations in nanogram equivalents of ENS are calculated for each derivative. The ratio of the DM to MM response (b/a) was found to be 1.27. These results were then used to calculate actual response curves of the MM and DM derivatives (Fig. 11). Calculations performed on samples intermediate to those at 4 and 24 hr confirmed the validity of this method of calculation, since the sum of MM and DM remained constant. Total residues of ENS in all samples were obtained by summing the nanogram equivalents of the two derivatives.

Dition can be used as a stable reference standard for the detector response, but since the slope of its curve is 0.482, the same amount should always be injected.

Results from assays of chow spiked with ENS at various levels, extracted by two procedures and assayed by both SPF and GC, are presented in Table 3. Soxhlet extractions yielded higher recoveries of ENS residues in all instances; however, the SPF background of untreated control samples was also higher due to the more rigorous extraction. Recoveries from the GC method were also superior to those via SPF because of the minimal cleanup required for GC. Most of the losses of ENS in the SPF procedure occurred at the alumina adsorption step. Both methods are of about equal sensitivity and require about the same amount of time; however, less labor is required for the GC method. On the other hand, the GC procedure has the disadvantage of requiring regular preparation of diazomethane. Any combination of the two extraction and analytical procedures are considered acceptable for the analysis. In cases where maximum recovery, sensitivity, and specificity are required, the Soxhlet-GC procedure is recommended. It should also be noted that even after the rigorous cleanup for SPF analysis, some concentration quenching occurs in the untreated controls; therefore, for the purpose of correcting SPF readings, both the spiked and unspiked samples must be diluted identically.

Results from SPF assays of biological media are presented in Table 4. Limits of sensitivity (twice background) for the 10 ml samples were about 1 and 4 ppb for trypticase soy dextrose and brain heart infusion media. Recoveries at 0.10 and 1.0 ppm and precision were excellent.

Table 5 lists the results of SPF assays of urine, wastewater, and blood. Urine spiked with 20 ppb of ENS (no hydrolysis) yielded 98% recoveries and a control background of about 18 ppb; with alkaline hydrolysis the recovery dropped to 76% with a background of 38 ppb. Assays of urine after acid hydrolysis could not be accomplished because a purple-colored interference was produced by the reaction of the acid with the unspiked substrate. Wastewater spiked with 20 ppb of ENS gave recoveries of 80% while the control background was about 1 ppb. Sensitivity could easily be increased by extracting larger samples. Recoveries of ENS from blood spiked at 10 ppm were 31, 51, and 81% by procedures employing no hydrolysis, alkaline hydrolysis, and acid hydrolysis, respectively. The acid hydrolysis procedure with its control background of 38 ppb is therefore the preferred method.

Table 3 SPF and GC Analysis of Extracts of Laboratory Chow Spiked with ENS and Extracted by Two Procedures

Extraction procedure	Added ppm	Added μg[b]	Milligram equivalents of chow/analysis[c]	Recovered ($\bar{x}$ ± SE)[a] ppm	Recovered ($\bar{x}$ ± SE)[a] %
			SPF Analysis		
Mechanical	0	0	40	0.278 ± 0.005	-
			20	0.328 ± 0.026	-
			10	0.341 ± 0.010	-
			5	0.426 ± 0.015	-
	1.0	20	40	0.686 ± 0.026	68.6 ± 2.6
	5.0	100	20	3.91 ± 0.13	78.2 ± 2.6
	10.0	200	10	7.46 ± 0.07	74.6 ± 0.7
	20.0	400	5	15.7 ± 0.1	78.5 ± 0.5
Soxhlet	0	0	40	0.739 ± 0.041	-
			20	0.790 ± 0.026	-
			10	0.909 ± 0.043	-
			5	0.938 ± 0.044	-
	1.0	20	40	0.783 ± 0.004	78.3 ± 4.4
	5.0	100	20	4.22 ± 0.21	84.4 ± 4.2
	10.0	200	10	8.25 ± 0.66	82.5 ± 6.6
	20.0	400	5	16.9 ± 0.6	84.5 ± 3.3
			GC Analysis		
Mechanical	0	0	125	< 0.15	-
	1.0	20	125	0.864 ± 0.040	86.4 ± 4.0
	5.0	100	25	4.05 ± 0.19	81.0 ± 3.8
	10.0	200	12.5	8.70 ± 0.13	87.0 ± 1.3
	20.0	400	6.25	17.1 ± 0.3	85.5 ± 1.5
Soxhlet	0	0	125	< 0.15	-
	1.0	20	125	1.00 ± 0.023	100 ± 2.3
	5.0	100	25	4.48 ± 0.03	89.6 ± 0.6
	10.0	200	12.5	8.50 ± 0.33	85.0 ± 3.3
	20.0	400	6.25	17.7 ± 0.4	88.5 ± 2.0

[a]Mean of four samples.
[b]Per 20 g of chow.
[c]Per milliliter for SPF readings or per 25 μl injection for GC.
Source: Ref. 20.

Table 4 SPF Analysis of Extracts of Biological Media Spiked with ENS

Biological medium	Added ppm	Added μg[b]	Milligram equivalents of medium/ analysis[c]	(Recovered ($\bar{x}$ ± SE)[a] ppm	(Recovered ($\bar{x}$ ± SE)[a] %
Brain	0	0	1000	0.0380 ± 0.0018	-
heart	0.10	1.0	1000	0.0912 ± 0.0015	91.2 ± 1.5
infusion	1.00	10.0	200	0.908 ± 0.011	90.8 ± 1.1
Trypticase	0	0	1000	0.0138 ± 0.0004	-
soy	0.10	1.0	1000	0.0998 ± 0.0019	99.8 ± 1.9
dextrose	1.00	10.0	200	0.863 ± 0.027	86.3 ± 2.7

[a]Mean of five samples.
[b]Per 10 ml of medium.
[c]Per milliliter for SPF readings.
Source: Ref. 20.

The development of analytical methodology for metabolites of ENS was not undertaken because metabolism studies employing [^{14}C]ENS were incomplete and analytical standards were not available [28].

The results of SPF and radiometric assays of untreated urine and that from the dog dosed with [^{14}C]ENS are presented in Table 6. Recoveries via SPF of unlabeled ENS from water and untreated urine spiked with 10 ppm of ENS were 98.5 and 94.1%, respectively. Recovery of ENS, even from a sample of urine spiked directly with the compound and extracted within the hour, was enhanced by hydrolysis, which indicated that some conjugation had already occurred.

The total recovery of ENS (free + conjugated) from treated urine by the SPF method was 58.8 ± 1.2% of that indicated by radiometric assays at all sampling intervals. On the other hand, free ENS (no hydrolysis) varied from 37 to 52%, which indicated that hydrolysis is necessary for higher and more consistent results. Radiometric and SPF assays of the free and hydrolyzed fractions from the SPF procedure were essentially identical. About 41% of the radioactivity in the treated urine was not extractable as free ENS or after alkaline and acid hydrolysis under the rather mild conditions employed. Although the order in which the alkaline and acid hydrolysis were performed had little effect on the total hydrolyzable residues recovered, both types of hydrolyses were required for optimum recovery. The nature of the unextractable radioactive material, and whether a m

Table 5 SPF Analysis of Extracts of Urine, Wastewater, and Whole Rat Blood Spiked with ENS

Added		Type of	Milligram equivalents of substrate/	Recovered[a]	
ppm	μg[b]	hydrolysis	analysis[c]	ppm	%
			Urine		
0	0	None	5000	0.0184	-
0.020	1.0	None	5000	0.0196	98
0	0	Alkaline	5000	0.0380	-
0.020	1.0	Alkaline	5000	0.0152	76
0	0	Acid	5000	d	d
0.020	1.0	Acid	5000	d	d
0.200	10.0	Acid	5000	d	d
			Wastewater		
0	0	None	5000	0.0010	-
0.020	1.0	None	5000	0.0160	80
			Whole Rat Blood		
0	0	None	200	0.022	-
10.0	10.0	None	20	3.14	31
0	0	Alkaline	200	0.051	-
10.0	10.0	Alkaline	20	5.10	51
0	0	Acid	200	0.038 ± 0.0031	-
10.0	10.0	Acid	20	8.13 ± 0.17	81.3 ± 1.7

[a]Mean of duplicate samples except rat blood (acid hydrolysis) is mean of four samples.
[b]Per 50 ml of urine and wastewater; per milliliter of rat blood.
[c]Per milliliter for SPF reading.
[d]Development of purple-colored product upon acid hydrolysis of unspiked urine prevented the assay via SPF.
Source: Ref. 20.

rigorous hydrolysis will increase the recovery, are not known but are currently being investigated. Nevertheless, the results of this study demonstrate the usefulness of the SPF procedure for determining traces of unlabeled ENS in a biological substrate.

Table 6 SPF and Radiometric Analysis of Urine Taken at Various Intervals from a Dog Treated with [^{14}C]ENS

Sample	Total ENS equivalents (ppm) (radiometric assay)	ENS recovered (ppm), SPF assays			
		Free (no hydrolysis)	After hydrolysis[a] Alkaline	After hydrolysis[a] Acid	Total
Water[b] (control)	-	0.10	0.08 (0.06)	0.06 (0.13)	0.24
Water[c] (spiked at 10 ppm)	-	9.32	0.51 (0.01)	0.02 (0.44)	9.85
Urine[b] (control)	-	0.18	0.15 (0.12)	0.21 (0.36)	0.54
Urine[c] (spiked at 10 ppm)	-	8.62	0.67 (0.01)	0.12 (0.79)	9.41
Treated urine[c] (0-1 day)	41.57	15.5	8.23 (6.02)	1.08 (1.72)	24.8
Treated urine[c] (1-2 days)	30.25	11.5	5.73 (5.19)	0.60 (1.49)	17.8
Treated urine[c] (2-3 day)	5.19	2.70	0.29 (0.00)	0.00 (0.13)	2.99
Treated urine[c] (3-4 day)	10.15	4.97	0.87 (0.16)	0.16 (0.078)	6.00

[a]Alkaline hydrolysis performed prior to acid hydrolysis. Data for alkaline hydrolysis subsequent to acid hydrolysis are given in parentheses.
[b]Excitation and emission maxima did not correspond to those of ENS.
[c]Appropriate control has been subtracted for SPF data.
Source: Ref. 20.

Partition values for ENS were as follows:

Solvent system	p Value
Benzene-water	0.62
Chloroform-water	0.94
Chloroform-60% methanol (40% water)	0.80
Chloroform-aqueous Na_2CO_3 (saturated)	0.18
Chloroform-aqueous $NaHCO_3$ (saturated)	0.94
Chloroform-aqueous NaOH (1 or 4 N)	0.00

The following systems all gave p values of 0.00: hexane-water, -acetonitrile, or -80% acetone (20% water); isooctane-dimethyl sulfoxide (DMSO), -90% DMSO (10% water), -dimethylformamide (DMF), or 85% DMF (15% water); and heptane-90% ethanol (10% water). The solubilities of ENS at 25 ± 2° in water and hexane were found to be 113 and 0.031 ppm, respectively.

C. Benzidine, 3,3'-Dimethylbenzidine, and 3,3'-Dimethoxybenzidine [29]

General description of method

Spectrophotofluorometric (SPF) methods are described for the trace analysis of benzidine, 3,3'-dimethylbenzidine, 3,3'-dimethoxybenzidine, and their dihydrochloride salts in microbiological growth media, wastewater, potable water, human urine, and rat blood. The salient elements of the methods for these known or suspected carcinogens are: extraction of the residues as the free amine with benzene, rapid cleanup on an alumina column, and quantification of the free amine in methanol via SPF. Potable water solutions of the salts are diluted with buffer (pH 4) and quantified directly by SPF. Ancillary analytical information concerning the solubility and stability of these compounds, p values, gas chromatographic analysis of the free amines, and thin layer chromatographic data in 10 solvent systems are also presented.

Introduction

Urinary bladder tumors in human subjects exposed to chemicals utilized in the synthesis of dyes were first reported by Rehn [30] in 1895. Rehn called the lesions "aniline tumors"; however, subsequent research proved that aniline was not the causative agent, and other aromatic amines, such as benzidine and its congeners, were then indicated. The toxicological effects of compounds in the benzidine family have been widely studied for several years, and in 1974 the

U.S. Department of Labor called for the regulation of benzidine, 3,3'-dichlorobenzidine, and 4-aminobiphenyl by placing them on the list of chemical compounds known to cause, or suspected to cause human cancer from occupational exposure [31]. A comprehensive overview of the literature and problems associated with the use of benzidine and its congeners was reported by Haley [32].

Before proposed long-term feeding studies with benzidine, 3,3'-dimethylbenzidine (diorthotoluidine), and 3,3'-dimethoxybenzidine (dianisidine) could be initiated at the National Center for Toxicological Research (NCTR), analytical methods were sought to satisfy all the experimental requirements previously discussed (e.g., purity, dose level verification, urine monitoring, etc.). In addition, a procedure was also needed for evaluating the microbiological systems which were being tested in an attempt to discover a means of destroying the carcinogenic effects of the chemicals. The formulas of the three compounds and their abbreviations are shown in Figure 12. To improve their water solubility and chemical stability and reduce volatility, the chemicals are administered to the animals as aqueous solutions of dihydrochlorides; therefore, analytical methods for these salts were also required.

Several colorimetric methods for benzidine, based on diazotization and coupling reactions, have been reported [33-35]; also, Chloramine-T reagent was employed to determine benzidine and its congeners [36,37]. Clayson et al. [38] reported a qualitative method for benzidine and its metabolites based on reverse-phase paper chromatography. Rinde [39] used 2,4,6-trinitrobenzenesulfonic acid and fluorescamine to detect benzidine on thin layer chromatographic plates; spectrophotometric and fluorimetric methods employing these reagents were also used to quantitate benzidine excretion following feeding of benzidine dyes. None of these methods, however, provide the sensitivity, specificity, accuracy, and precision required for our use; therefore, the following procedures were developed.

Experimental

Materials. Benzidine (m.p. 127 to 129°) was purchased from Fisher Scientific Co., and the benzidine·2HCl was Matheson, Coleman, Bell chemical No. B-260. The 3,3'-dimethylbenzidine (m.p. 129 to 131°) and 3,3'-dimethoxybenzidine·2HCl were purchased from Pfaltz and Bauer Co., Flushing, New York. The 3,3'-dimethylbenzidine·2HCl was prepared from the corresponding amine (2 g in 50 ml of benzene) by bubbling an excess of anhydrous HCl through the solution to precipitate the salt; the 3,3'-dimethoxybenzidine (m.p. 137 to 139°) was prepared from an aqueous solution of the corresponding salt by making it strongly alkaline with NaOH and extracting the free amine with benzene. All six chemicals were vacuum dried overnight at 60° prior to use. The high purity of the amines was demonstrated by

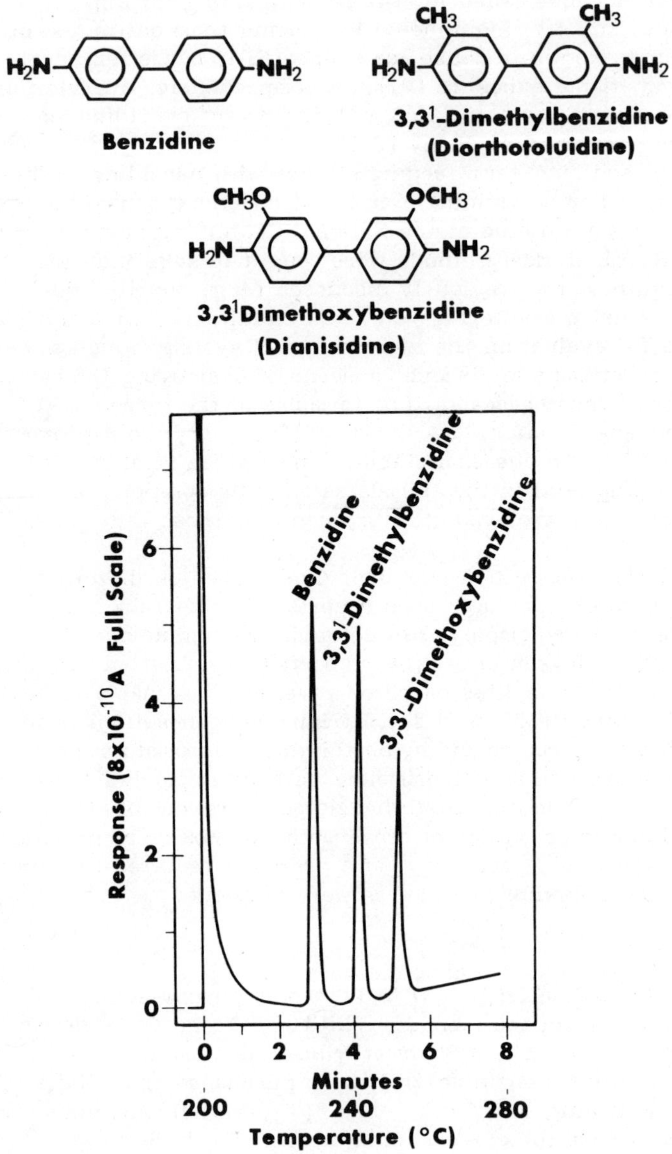

Figure 12 Top: Formulas of benzidine; 3,3'-dimethylbenzidine; and 3,3'-dimethoxybenzidine. Bottom: A typical temperature-programmed chromatogram of 500 ng amounts of the three compounds injected in 5 μl of chloroform. (From Ref. 29.)

the absence of extraneous GC peaks; the salts, after conversion to the free amines, were also free of extraneous GC peaks and yielded the correct amount of product.

The adsorbent (basic alumina, Brockman activity I) from Fisher Scientific Co. (No. A-941) was used as received. Sodium sulfate was anhydrous; all reagents were CP grade; and all solvents were pesticide grade. Ingredients for the microbiological culture media were purchased from Difco Laboratories, Detroit, Michigan, and the media were prepared in accordance with the instructions supplied by the manufacturer. The TLC plates (20 × 20 cm, Fisher No. 6-601A), precoated with Silica Gel GF (250 μm thick), were activated in an oven at 130° for 1 hr and allowed to cool in a desiccator prior to use. All culture tubes were of borosilicate glass and equipped with Teflon-lined screw caps. The buffer (pH 4, potassium biphthalate, 0.05 M) was Fisher Chemical No. SO-B-98.

Preparation of Samples for SPF Analysis

Microbiological growth media. Ten milliliters of the trypticase soy dextrose (TSD) or brain heart infusion (BHI) medium was added to a 30 ml culture tube and 1 g of NaCl, 0.2 ml of 10 N NaOH, and 10 ml of benzene were added. The tube was sealed, shaken vigorously for 2 min, and centrifuged for 10 min at 2000 rpm. The benzene layer was carefully withdrawn by using a syringe and cannula and percolated through a plug of sodium sulfate (25 mm diam × 10 mm thick) in tandem with a glass column (12 mm i.d., Kontes No. 420,000) prepared by adding successively a plug of glass wool, 5 g of sodium sulfate, 1 g of basic alumina, and 5 g of sodium sulfate. The medium was extracted with two additional 10 ml portions of benzene, which were successively percolated through the plug and column. Finally, the column was washed with 10 ml of dichloromethane-10% methanol to ensure complete elution of the free amine residue from the column. The combined eluates, after the addition of 1 drop of diethylene glycol to serve as a keeper, were evaporated just to dryness by using water pump vacuum and a 60° water bath. The dry residue was dissolved in an appropriate amount of methanol for SPF analysis as the free amine.

Wastewater. One hundred milliliters of the sample, 2 g of NaCl, and 0.5 ml of 10 N NaOH were added to a 160 ml culture tube. The sample was then shaken, centrifuged, cleaned up, and prepared for analysis as described for media. Exception: three 15 ml portions of benzene were used for the extraction.

Urine. Procedures utilizing alkaline hydrolysis or acid hydrolysis prior to extraction, as well as no hydrolysis, were tested:

1. *No hydrolysis.* Analyses were performed exactly as described for wastewater.

2. *Alkaline hydrolysis.* Analyses were performed exactly as described for wastewater except that the alkaline solution in the tube was sealed, heated in a water bath at 80° for 2 hr, then cooled prior to the extraction with benzene.
3. *Acid hydrolysis.* These analyses were also performed as described for wastewater, except that 0.5 ml of concentrated HCl was substituted for the 10 N NaOH; then the mixture was heated at 80° for 2 hr, cooled, and made alkaline with 1 ml of 10 N NaOH prior to extraction with benzene.

Blood. Procedures employing no hydrolysis of the sample prior to extraction, as well as alkaline or acid hydrolysis, were tested:

1. *No hydrolysis.* Six milliliters of distilled water, 1 ml of 10 N NaOH, and 1 g of NaCl were added to a 20 ml culture tube containing 1 ml of whole rat blood. The contents were mixed and then extracted with three 10 ml portions of benzene, cleaned up, and prepared for SPF analysis as described for media.
2. *Alkaline hydrolysis.* Samples were analyzed as for no hydrolysis except that the mixture in the sealed tube was held in an 80° heating block for 2 hr with frequent shaking, then cooled prior to extraction with benzene.
3. *Acid hydrolysis.* Analyses were performed as for no hydrolysis except that 1 ml of concentrated HCl was substituted for the NaOH and the sealed tube was then heated at 80° for 2 hr, cooled, and made alkaline by adding 2 ml of 10 N NaOH. The mixture was then extracted, cleaned up, and prepared for SPF analysis as described.

Potable water. Aqueous solutions of the dihydrochloride salts slated for use as the animals' drinking water to administer the proper dosage of test chemical are assayed for proper concentration after sequential dilutions with water containing 2% (v/v) of buffer (pH 4). The fluorescence of the diluted sample (e.g., 1 ppm) is compared directly with that of a standard solution prepared in the same manner.

Recovery experiments. Triplicate samples of both biological media were separately spiked with 100 μl of methanol (or water) containing the appropriate amount of the free amine (or its salt) to produce residues of 0, 0.1, and 1.0 ppm. The samples were allowed to stand in the refrigerator (5°) overnight prior to extractions. Samples (1 ml) of whole rat blood were spiked in the same manner at 0 and 10 ppm, held at 5° overnight, and analyzed as described. Wastewater and urine samples (100 ml) were spiked at 0 and 20 ppb by adding 1 ml of methanol (or water) containing the appropriate amount of the test compound, held at 5° overnight, and analyzed as described.

Stability of Aqueous Solutions of the Test Compounds. Aqueous solutions of the three amines (about 50 ppm) and of their dihydrochloride salts (about 50 and 500 ppm) were prepared for use in tests to determine the chemical stability of the test compounds under simulated animal test conditions. The animal drinking water dispenser for each cage (four mice per cage) consisted of a glass bottle (500 ml, 62 mm square × 180 mm high) fitted with a No. 8 rubber stopper and a stainless steel "sipper tube" (8 mm o.d. × 90 mm long) containing a steel ball to serve as a valve. Triplicate dispensers, each containing 375 ml of the various test solutions, were placed in cages and exposed to ambient conditions (25 ± 2° and continuous fluorescent lighting) in the animal room. Samples (10 ml) were taken from each dispenser immediately and 1, 2, 4, 8, and 16 days later. The pH of each sample was determined and solutions of the salts were diluted and analyzed as described for potable water. Solutions of the free amines were diluted with methanol to an appropriate concentration (e.g., 0.5 μg/ml) and the fluorescence related to standards of the free amines diluted in the same manner.

Gas Chromatographic Analysis. A Hewlett-Packard Model 5750 gas chromatograph equipped with a flame ionization detector (FID) was fitted with a 100 cm glass column (4 mm i.d., 6 mm o.d.) containing 10% OV-101 (w/w) on Gas Chrom Q (80-100 mesh) and operated with a helium carrier flow of 100 ml/min. The injection port and detector temperatures were 275 and 290°, respectively. The column oven was operated isothermally for the quantitative analysis of the individual free amines (e.g., p-value determinations) as follows: benzidine (215°); 3,3'-dimethylbenzidine (235°); and 3,3'-dimethoxybenzidine (240°); under these conditions, their retention times (t_R) were 2.35, 2.25, and 2.70 min, respectively. In assays concerning the GC purity of the free amines, the oven was temperature programmed from 200 to 280° at the rate of 10°/min. A typical temperature-programmed chromatogram of the three compounds is shown in Figure 12.

Spectrophotofluorescence Analysis. An Aminco-Bowman instrument (American Instrument Co., Silver Spring, Maryland), equipped with a xenon lamp and a 1P28 detector, was used with 1 cm^2 cells and a 2-2-2 mm slit program to measure fluorescence. All dilutions of the free amines were freshly prepared in methanol and those of the salts were in water-2% buffer (pH 4). Excitation (λ_{Ex}) and emission (λ_{Em}) wavelengths (nm) and relative intensities (RI) were:

Compound	λ_{Ex} (nm)	λ_{Em} (nm)	RI (μg/ml)
Benzidine	295	396	33.5
Benzidine·2HCl	302	410	7.45
3,3'-Dimethylbenzidine	300	384	51.8
3,3'-Dimethylbenzidine·2HCl	310	410	12.2

Compound	λ_{Ex} (nm)	λ_{Em} (nm)	RI (μg/ml)
3,3'-Dimethoxybenzidine	312	380	64.3
3,3'-Dimethoxybenzidine·2HCl	318	422	8.25

The instrument was frequently calibrated to produce a RI of 5.0 with a solution of 0.3 μg of quinine sulfate/ml of 0.1 N sulfuric acid (λ_{Ex} = 350, λ_{Em} = 450). Readings were corrected for solvent blanks and RI was plotted versus concentration of the six compounds on log-log paper to produce a standard curve.

To ensure that the RI was within the linear range of the standard curve and thus unaffected by concentration quenching, samples were diluted with an equal volume of solvent to ascertain whether the RI was about half of the undiluted solution. If it was not, dilution was continued until RI was halved by dilution. Extracts of wastewater and urine, medium, and blood for SPF analysis were first diluted to contain 10, 1, and 0.2 g equivalents of sample per milliliter, respectively; further dilutions were made as required to make certain that the RI was within the linear range of the standard curve. The RI of the untreated control samples was then subtracted from that of the unknown and concentration (μg/ml) was determined from the standard curve. In the instances where salts are assayed as the free amines, the analytical results for benzidine, 3,3'-dimethylbenzidine, and 3,3'-dimethoxybenzidine are multiplied by the factors 1.40, 1.34, and 1.30, respectively, to express them on the proper basis.

Solubility, p Value, and TLC Determinations. The solubilities of benzidine, 3,3'-dimethylbenzidine, 3,3'-dimethoxybenzidine, and their salts in water at 25 ± 2° were determined by SPF as described by Bowman and King [6].

Extraction p values for the three amines were determined in several solvent systems by GC in the manner described by Bowman and Beroza [18].

The TLC determinations were made by using a Gelman Model 51325-1 apparatus and activated glass plates precoated with silica gel GF. The plates were spotted with 5 μl (5 μg) of methanol solutions of the free amines or anthracene (reference compound). After the developing solvent had ascended 13 cm above the spotting line (about 25 min), the plates were removed and the solvent allowed to evaporate. The spots were made visible by viewing them under ultraviolet light (254 nm) and the R_f values calculated.

Results and discussion

In preliminary studies of the analytical chemical properties of these compounds, the free amines were found to gas-chromatograph well

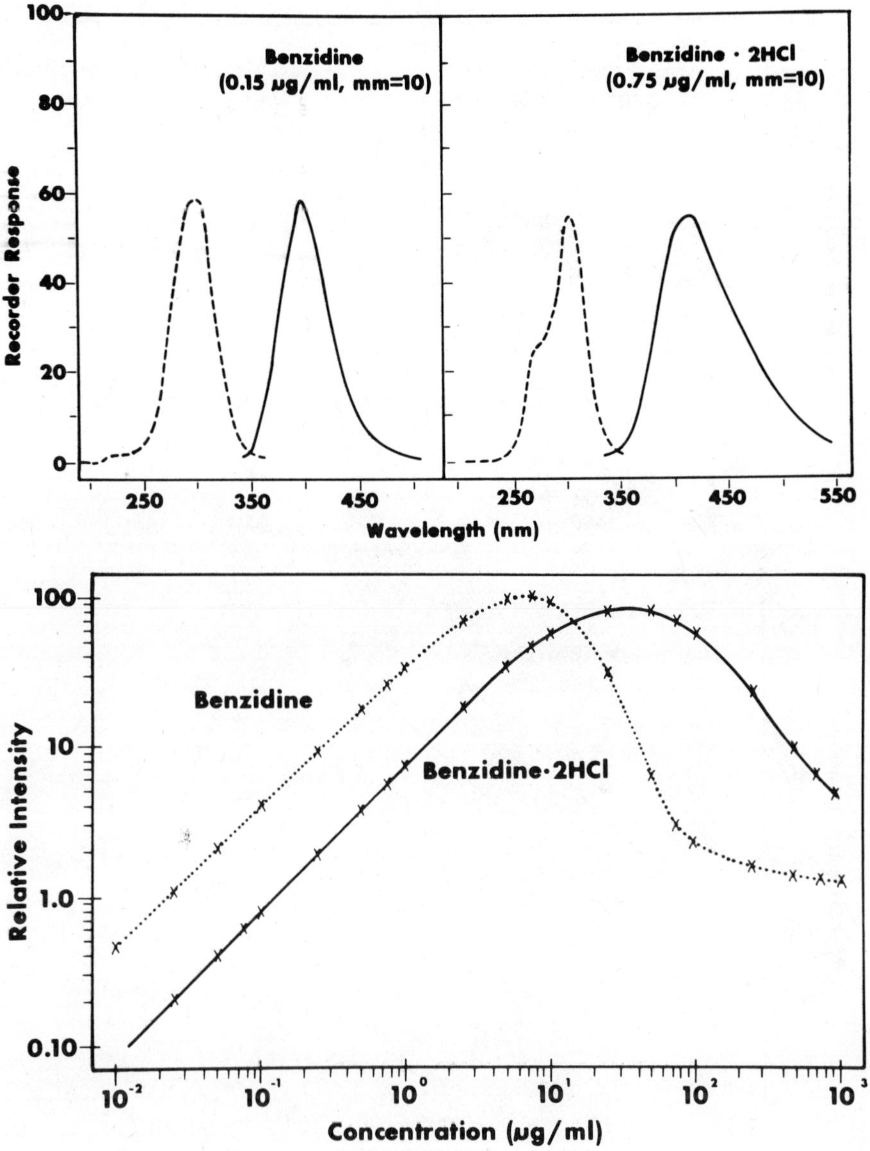

Figure 13 Top: Excitation (dashed line) and emission (solid line) spectra of benzidine and its dihydrochloride salt. Bottom: Standard curves for the two compounds. (From Ref. 29.)

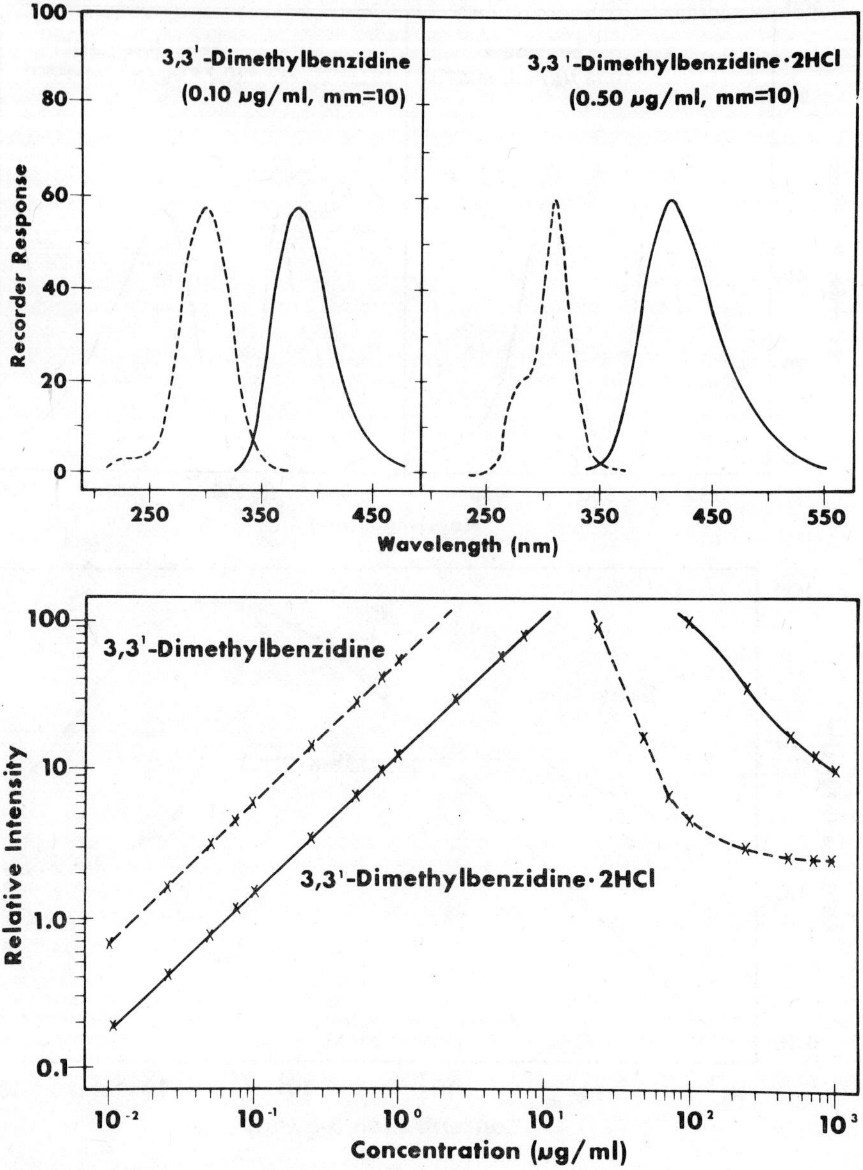

Figure 14 Top: Excitation (dashed line) and emission (solid line) spectra of 3,3'-dimethylbenzidine and its dihydrochloride salt. Bottom: Standard curves for the two compounds. (From Ref. 29.)

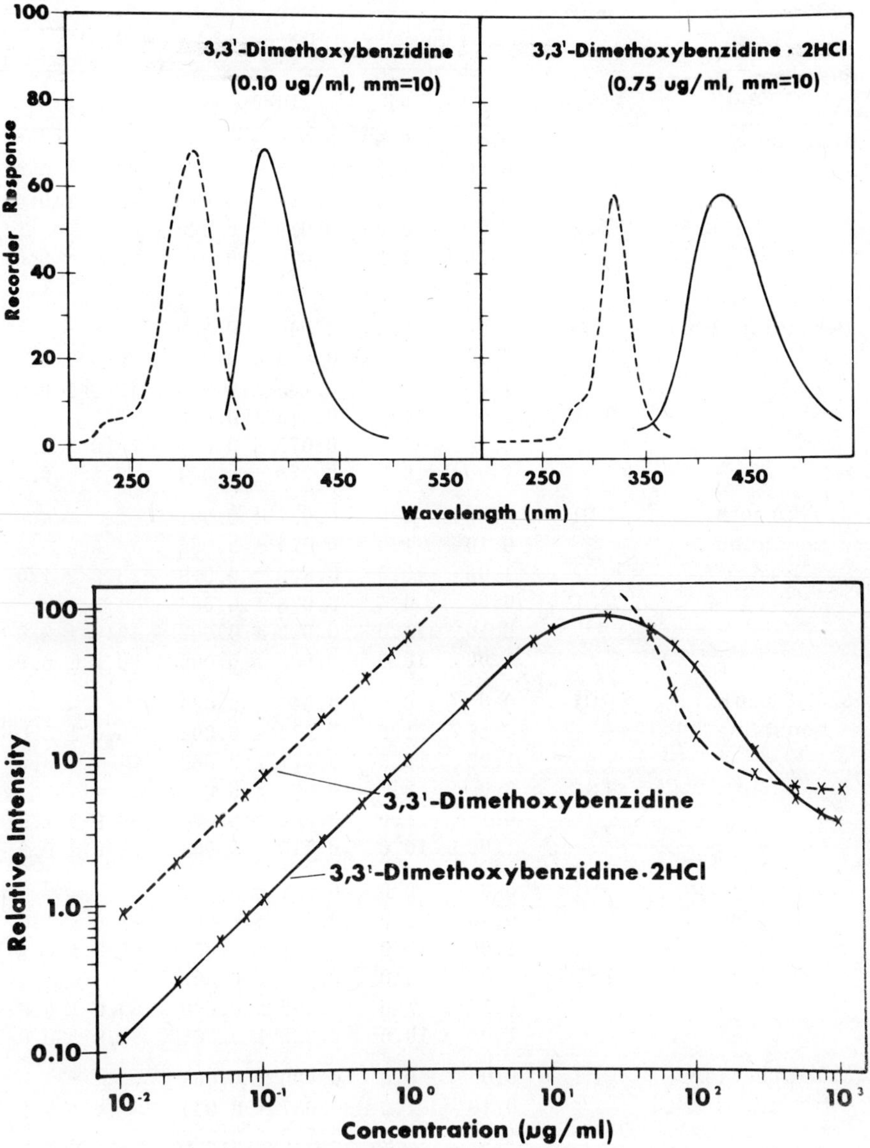

Figure 15 Top: Excitation (dashed line) and emission (solid line) spectra of 3,3'-dimethoxybenzidine and its dihydrochloride salt. Bottom: Standard curves for the two compounds. (From Ref. 29.)

Table 7 Analysis of Two Biological Growth Media Spiked with Benzidine, Two Congeners, and Their Salts at 0, 0.10, and 1.0 ppm

		Added[a]		Recovered ($\bar{x}$ ± SE)[b]	
Compound	Medium	ppm	μg	ppm	%
Benzidine	BHI	0.0	0.0	0.040 ± 0.000	
		0.10	1.0	0.070 ± 0.000	70.0 ± 0.0
		1.00	10.0	0.780 ± 0.004	78.0 ± 0.4
	TSD	0.0	0.0	0.019 ± 0.000	-
		0.10	1.0	0.075 ± 0.000	75.0 ± 0.0
		1.00	10.0	0.787 ± 0.012	78.7 ± 1.2
Benzidine·2HCl	BHI	0.0	0.0	0.040 ± 0.000	-
		0.10	1.0	0.073 ± 0.002	73.0 ± 2.0
		1.00	10.0	0.795 ± 0.000	79.5 ± 0.0
	TSD	0.0	0.0	0.019 ± 0.002	-
		0.10	1.0	0.073 ± 0.001	73.0 ± 1.0
		1.00	10.0	0.778 ± 0.004	77.8 ± 0.4
3,3'-Dimethyl-benzidine	BHI	0.0	0.0	0.037 ± 0.001	-
		0.10	1.0	0.074 ± 0.005	74.0 ± 5.0
		1.00	10.0	0.839 ± 0.010	83.9 ± 1.0
	TSD	0.0	0.0	0.029 ± 0.004	-
		0.10	1.0	0.073 ± 0.002	73.0 ± 2.0
		1.00	10.0	0.902 ± 0.009	90.2 ± 0.9
3,3'-Dimethyl-benzidine·2HCl	BHI	0.0	0.0	0.045 ± 0.004	-
		0.10	1.0	0.070 ± 0.002	70.0 ± 2.0
		1.00	10.0	0.777 ± 0.006	77.7 ± 0.6
	TSD	0.0	0.0	0.036 ± 0.003	-
		0.10	1.0	0.064 ± 0.001	64.0 ± 1.0
		1.00	10.0	0.710 ± 0.003	71.0 ± 0.3
3,3-Dimethoxy-benzidine	BHI	0.0	0.0	0.031 ± 0.003	-
		0.10	1.0	0.078 ± 0.001	78.0 ± 1.0
		1.00	10.0	0.923 ± 0.007	92.3 ± 0.7
	TSD	0.0	0.0	0.019 ± 0.001	-
		0.10	1.0	0.055 ± 0.000	55.0 ± 0.0
		1.0	10.0	0.829 ± 0.008	82.9 ± 0.8
3,3'-Dimethoxy-benzidine·2HCl	BHI	0.0	0.0	0.030 ± 0.003	-
		0.10	1.0	0.057 ± 0.005	57.0 ± 5.0
		1.00	10.0	0.715 ± 0.002	71.5 ± 0.2
	TSD	0.0	0.0	0.027 ± 0.003	-
		0.10	1.0	0.052 ± 0.001	52.0 ± 1.0
		1.00	10.0	0.770 ± 0.006	77.0 ± 0.6

[a] Per 10 ml of sample.
[b] Mean and standard error from triplicate assays; spiked samples are corrected for controls. Controls and 0.10 ppm samples contained 1 g equivalent of medium/ml for SPF reading; the 1.0 ppm samples contained 0.2 g equivalent/ml.
Source: Ref. 29.

with minimal column conditioning; the three compounds were also readily separated (Fig. 12) and quantified. GC analysis was therefore employed for p-value determinations and purity assays; however, the FID lacked the sensitivity and specificity required for trace analysis of residues in a variety of substrates. The possibility of oxidizing the free amines to their corresponding dinitro analogs was investigated, since these derivatives might then be assayed by electron capture GC with higher sensitivity and specificity. The use of m-chloroperbenzoic acid, hydrogen peroxide, and potassium permanganate under various reaction conditions, however, produced no more than a 20% yield of the derivative. The portion of the free amines not derivatized remained unchanged or was converted to products that did not emerge from the gas chromatograph, depending on the severity of the oxidation reaction.

Tests pertaining to the SPF properties of the compounds revealed that all six fluoresce strongly. The RI values of the free amines in methanol were about five times greater than those of the salts in aqueous buffer. Limits of detection and linearity of the amines and salts were about 2 and 10 ng/ml, respectively. As expected, the SPF response of aqueous solutions of the salts varied with pH, and assays of these compounds diluted with water alone were not reproducible. This problem was overcome by using an aqueous solution containing 2% buffer (v/v, pH 4) for dilutions and SPF measurements. Excitation and emission spectra and standard curves for the six compounds are presented in Figures 13 to 15. SPF was selected for subsequent assays because of its high sensitivity and the specificity afforded of the characteristic excitation and emission maxima of each compound. Determination of the three amines or the three salts in admixture was attempted by measuring RI at the excitation and emission maxima for each compound and calculating the amount of each constituent by using simultaneous equations. However, this was not successful because of the large differences in specific RI and extensive overlap of the spectra.

Results from the assays of microbiological growth media are presented in Table 7. Recoveries averaged 68 and 80% for samples spiked with 0.10 and 1.0 ppm, respectively. The SPF background for unspiked BHI and TSD media was about 0.04 and 0.02 ppm. Lowest recoveries were obtained with 3,3'-dimethoxybenzidine and its salt. Assays of samples of wastewater (collected from the decontamination of control animal cages) separately spiked with 20 ppb of each compound gave recoveries averaging 75% (Table 8). The precision was excellent and the control background was about 4 ppb.

Table 9 lists the results of SPF assays of whole rat blood spiked with 10 ppm of the six compounds. Recoveries without hydrolysis of the sample and after alkaline or acid hydrolysis averaged about 14, 19, and 63%, respectively. Acid hydrolysis is, therefore, required to re-

Table 8 Analysis of Wastewater Spiked with Benzidine, Two Congeners, and Their Salts at 0 and 20 ppb

	Added[a]		Recovered ($\bar{x}$ ± SE)[b]	
Compound	ppb	μg	ppb	%
Benzidine	0	0.0	4 ± 1	-
	20	2.0	17 ± 0	85
Benzidine·2HCl	0	0.0	4 ± 1	-
	20	2.0	15 ± 1	75
3,3'-Dimethylbenzidine	0	0.0	4 ± 1	-
	20	2.0	15 ± 0	75
3,3'-Dimethylbenzidine·2HCl	0	0.0	3 ± 1	-
	20	2.0	13 ± 1	65
3,3'-Dimethoxybenzidine	0	0.0	3 ± 0	-
	20	2.0	16 ± 0	80
3,3'-Dimethoxybenzidine·2HCl	0	0.0	3 ± 0	-
	20	2.0	14 ± 1	70

[a]Per 100 ml of sample.
[b]Mean and standard error from triplicate assays; spiked samples are corrected for controls. Samples contained 10 g equivalents of water/ml for SPF reading.
Source: Ref. 29.

cover a substantial portion of the residue; the control background was about 0.15 ppm. Recovery of the compounds from blood varied inversely with their polarity.

Data from human urine spiked with 20 ppb of the compounds are presented in Table 10. Recoveries of the free amines from urine without hydrolysis and after alkaline hydrolysis were 90 and 68%, respectively; those for the salts were 38 and 57%. It is apparent that the procedure employing no hydrolysis should be used when residues of the free amines are sought, since alkaline hydrolysis diminished the recovery by about 20%. On the other hand, alkaline hydrolysis enhanced the recovery of the salts by about 20%; the reason for this behavior is not fully understood. Acid hydrolyses of urine were also performed; however, formation of a purple-colored product in both control and spiked samples prevented the assay by SPF.

Table 9 Analysis of Whole Rat Blood Spiked with Benzidine, Two Congeners, and Their Salts at 0 and 10 ppm

Compound	Hydrolysis	Added[a] ppm	Added[a] μg	Recovered ($\bar{x}$ ± SE)[b] ppm	Recovered ($\bar{x}$ ± SE)[b] %
Benzidine	None	0.0	0.0	0.051 ± 0.013	-
		10.0	10.0	0.668 ± 0.216	6.7 ± 2.2
	Alkaline	0.0	0.0	0.063 ± 0.013	-
		10.0	10.0	2.52 ± 0.34	25.2 ± 3.4
	Acid	0.0	0.0	0.048 ± 0.005	-
		10.0	10.0	7.39 ± 0.09	73.9 ± 0.9
Benzidine·2HCl	None	0.0	0.0	0.045 ± 0.007	-
		10.0	10.0	0.563 ± 0.108	5.6 ± 1.1
	Alkaline	0.0	0.0	0.086 ± 0.028	-
		10.0	10.0	2.49 ± 0.31	24.9 ± 3.1
	Acid	0.0	0.0	0.052 ± 0.008	-
		10.0	10.0	7.57 ± 0.125	75.7 ± 1.2
3,3'-Dimethylbenzidine	None	0.0	0.0	0.152 ± 0.052	-
		10.0	10.0	1.58 ± 0.13	15.8 ± 1.3
	Alkaline	0.0	0.0	0.276 ± 0.044	-
		10.0	10.0	2.16 ± 0.10	21.6 ± 1.0
	Acid	0.0	0.0	0.223 ± 0.006	-
		10.0	10.0	6.55 ± 0.09	65.5 ± 0.9
3,3'-Dimethylbenzidine·2HCl	None	0.0	0.0	0.152 ± 0.052	-
		10.0	10.0	2.85 ± 0.19	28.5 ± 1.9
	Alkaline	0.0	0.0	0.276 ± 0.044	-
		10.0	10.0	2.11 ± 0.06	21.1 ± 0.6
	Acid	0.0	0.0	0.223 ± 0.006	-
		10.0	10.0	6.04 ± 0.37	60.4 ± 3.7
3,3-Dimethoxybenzidine	None	0.0	0.0	0.128 ± 0.049	-
		10.0	10.0	0.464 ± 0.098	4.6 ± 1.0
	Alkaline	0.0	0.0	0.236 ± 0.034	-
		10.0	10.0	1.19 ± 0.47	11.9 ± 4.7
	Acid	0.0	0.0	0.192 ± 0.006	-
		10.0	10.0	5.35 ± 0.06	53.5 ± 0.6
3,3'-Dimethoxybenzidine·2HCl	None	0.0	0.0	0.128 ± 0.049	-
		10.0	10.0	2.10 ± 0.20	21.0 ± 2.0
	Alkaline	0.0	0.0	0.236 ± 0.034	-
		10.0	10.0	1.01 ± 0.18	10.1 ± 1.8
	Acid	0.0	0.0	0.192 ± 0.006	-
		10.0	10.0	4.64 ± 0.14	46.4 ± 1.4

[a]Per milliliter of sample.
[b]Mean and standard error from triplicate assays; spiked samples are corrected for controls. Control and spiked samples contained 200 and 20 mg equivalents of blood/ml, respectively, for the SPF readings.
Source: Ref. 29.

Table 10 Analysis of Human Urine Spiked with Benzidine, Two Congeners, and Their Salts at 0 and 20 ppb

Compound	Hydrolysis[c]	Added[a]		Recovered ($\bar{x} \pm$ SE)[b]	
		ppb	μg	ppb	%
Benzidine	None	0	0.0	5 ± 0	-
		20	2.0	18 ± 1	90
	Alkaline	0	0.0	6 ± 1	-
		20	2.0	13 ± 1	65
Benzidine·2HCl	None	0	0.0	5 ± 0	-
		20	2.0	7 ± 1	35
	Alkaline	0	0.0	6 ± 1	-
		20	2.0	11 ± 1	55
3,3'-Dimethyl-benzidine	None	0	0.0	5 ± 0	-
		20	2.0	18 ± 1	90
	Alkaline	0	0.0	6 ± 1	-
		20	2.0	14 ± 1	70
3,3'-Dimethyl-benzidine·2HCl	None	0	0.0	5 ± 0	-
		20	2.0	8 ± 1	40
	Alkaline	0	0.0	6 ± 1	-
		20	2.0	11 ± 2	55
3,3'-Dimethoxy-benzidine	None	0	0.0	4 ± 1	-
		20	2.0	18 ± 2	90
	Alkaline	0	0.0	5 ± 1	-
		20	2.0	14 ± 1	70
3,3'-Dimethoxy-benzidine·2HCl	None	0	0.0	4 ± 0	-
		20	2.0	8 ± 1	40
	Alkaline	0	0.0	5 ± 1	-
		20	2.0	12 ± 1	60

[a]Per 100 ml of sample.
[b]Mean and standard error of triplicate assays; spiked samples are corrected for controls. Control and spiked samples contained 10 g equivalents of urine/ml for the SPF readings.
[c]Development of purple-colored product upon acid hydrolysis of unspiked urine prevented the assay via SPF.
Source: Ref. 29.

Table 11 Stability of Aqueous Solutions of Benzidine and Its Dihydrochloride After Exposure to Simulated Animal Test Conditions for 16 Days

Sampling interval (days)	Concentration and pH of solution indicated[a]					
	Benzidine		Benzidine·2HCl			
	50 ppm solution		50 ppm solution		500 ppm solution	
	ppm	pH	ppm	pH	ppm	pH
0	54.0 ± 0.0	6.70 ± 0.10	49.7 ± 0.2	3.95 ± 0.01	507 ± 3	3.30 ± 0.02
1	52.0 ± 0.2	6.35 ± 0.15	49.6 ± 0.2	3.95 ± 0.01	496 ± 2	3.26 ± 0.01
2	53.8 ± 2.9	6.65 ± 0.12	49.7 ± 0.3	4.00 ± 0.21	493 ± 3	3.25 ± 0.02
4	52.8 ± 0.5	6.45 ± 0.10	49.4 ± 0.5	4.07 ± 0.02	498 ± 4	3.34 ± 0.02
8	50.2 ± 0.7	6.35 ± 0.30	49.9 ± 0.1	4.10 ± 0.02	504 ± 4	3.35 ± 0.05
16	47.8 ± 0.7	6.25 ± 0.18	48.9 ± 0.2	3.98 ± 0.07	497 ± 4	3.35 ± 0.03

[a]Mean and standard error from triplicate assays.
Source: Ref. 29.

Results of 16-day stability studies with aqueous solutions of benzidine (50 ppm) and its salt (50 and 500 ppm) under simulated animal test conditions are presented in Table 11.

The solutions of the salt were essentially stable, with a decrease in concentration of less than 2% during the test period, whereas the free amine declined about 11%. In similar tests, 3,3'-dimethylbenzidine and its salt declined about 9%, and 3,3'-dimethoxybenzidine and its salt declined about 64 and 9%, respectively. The results in Table 11 illustrate the excellent precision of the SPF procedure for the analysis of these compounds in potable water.

Partition values (the fraction of solute partitioning into the non-polar phase of an equivolume immiscible binary solvent system) are useful in developing extraction and cleanup methods and for confirmatory tests.

The following values were obtained for the three free amines by using gas chromatography:

	p Value		
Solvent system	Benzidine	3,3'-Dimethyl-benzidine	3,3'-Dimethoxy-benzidine
Hexane-acetonitrile	0.02	0.01	0.03
Hexane-80% acetone (20% water)	0.08	0.16	0.15
Chloroform-water	1.0	1.0	1.0
Chloroform-60% methanol (40% water)	0.85	0.96	0.97
Chloroform-aqueous NaOH (5.0, 0.5, or 0.05 N)	1.0	1.0	1.0
Chloroform-aqueous HCl (5.0, 0.5, or 0.05 N)	0.00	0.00	0.00
Hexane-dimethylformamide	0.00	0.00	0.00

Solubility data for the three amines and their dihydrochloride salts were required before analytical method development or formulation of the spiked animal drinking water could be undertaken; precise values could not be found in the literature. Results of our determinations via SPF were as follows:

Compound	Solubility in water (mg/ml) at 25 ± 2°
Benzidine	0.52
Benzidine·2HCl	61.7
3,3'-Dimethylbenzidine	1.3
3,3'-Dimethylbenzidine·2HCl	76.7
3,3'-Dimethoxybenzidine	0.06
3,3'-Dimethoxybenzidine·2HCl	41.4

TLC R_f values for the three free amines and anthracene (included as a reference compound) in 10 solvent systems are reported in Table 12. These data are useful in the development of cleanup procedures and for the separation and identification of the compounds in admixture. The three compounds were separated by using 10% acetone or methanol in chloroform or benzene. Aqueous solutions of the salts spotted and developed as described gave R_f values identical to those of the free amines in all the solvent systems tested.

At the onset of animal tests with benzidine·2HCl-treated drinking water, routine monitoring of the air and work areas was also initiated to signal any accidental exposure of our personnel to traces of the compound. Air samples were collected by using a Model No. EMWL-2000H High Volume Air Sampler (General Metal Works, Inc., Cleves, Ohio) equipped with a No. 3000 (20 × 25 cm) fiberglass filter (retains 99.9% of particles larger than 0.3 μm in diameter) and operated continuously during the workday with an air flow of 1.42 m^3/min; the filter was removed weekly for chemical analysis and a new one was installed. For analysis, the filter was cut into small pieces, mechanically shaken with 250 ml of 0.1 N HCl for 1 hr, filtered, made alkaline with 5 ml of 10 N NaOH, and extracted three times with 25 ml portions of chloroform. The combined chloroform extracts successively percolated through a plug of sodium sulfate were evaporated to dryness in the presence of 1 drop of keeper; the dry residue was dissolved in benzene for cleanup and analysis as described for wastewater. The SPF background of a new filter is equivalent to about 0.4 μg of benzidine, whereas after a week in the sampling device, it averages about 10 μg. This background fluorescence has not exhibited the characteristic excitation and emission maxima of the compound sought and, thus far, all filters except those spiked in the laboratory have contained no detectable residues of the test chemical.

The monitoring of work areas (cages, floors, benches, apparatus, etc.) suspected of being contaminated with benzidine·2HCl (or benzidine) is accomplished by using kits consisting of a cotton applicator and a 5 ml culture tube containing exactly 2 ml of the aqueous buffer. The applicator is moistened with the aqueous buffer and used

Table 12 TLC R_f Values of Benzidine, 3,3'-Dimethylbenzidine, 3,3'-Dimethoxybenzidine, and Anthracene in 10 Solvent Systems

Solvent system (v/v)	R_f values (× 100) of compound indicated			
	Benzidine	3,3'-Dimethyl-benzidine	3,3'-Dimethoxy-benzidine	Anthracene
Chloroform	10	14	11	100
Chloroform-ethyl acetate (9:1)	20	29	29	92
Chloroform-diethyl ether (9:1)	21	32	32	100
Chloroform-acetone (9:1)	24	33	38	83
Chloroform-methanol (9:1)	70	80	85	97
Benzene	2	2	2	69
Benzene-ethyl acetate (9:1)	9	11	13	73
Benzene-diethyl ether (9:1)	6	10	11	75
Benzene-acetone (9:1)	16	21	26	76
Benzene-methanol (9:1)	33	45	50	81

Source: Ref. 29.

to swab a specific area, then the applicator is vigorously stirred in the buffer after each of several subsequent swabbings of the same area. The tube and contents are then centrifuged at 2000 rpm for 10 min to remove any suspended material. One milliliter of the supernatant is either analyzed directly or appropriately diluted as described for the analysis of potable water. Background fluorescence is generally equivalent to 0.10 μg of benzidine; areas contaminated with as little as 0.30 μg of the salt are readily detected and the identity of the chemical confirmed by its characteristic excitation and emission maxima.

D. 3,3'-Dichlorobenzidine [40]

General description of method

Gas chromatographic methods are described for the trace analysis of 3,3'-dichlorobenzidine and its dihydrochloride salt in animal chow, wastewater, and human urine. Salient elements of the method for these known carcinogens in chow are: extraction of the residues as the free amine and a cleanup via acid-base liquid-liquid partitioning with benzene followed by a silica gel column. With wastewater and human urine, residues are adsorbed by percolating the sample through a column of XAD-2, eluted with acetone, and cleaned up with acid-base partitioning and a silica gel column. Residues are assayed by gas chromatography (GC) either as the free amine or after conversion to the pentafluoropropionyl (PFP) derivative by using an electron capture (EC) or a rubidium-sensitized thermionic-type (N/P) detector. Minimum detectable residues in chow, wastewater, and human urine are about 3 ppb, 18 ppt, and 60 ppt, respectively, as determined by EC-GC of the PFP derivative.

Introduction

Benzidine and certain related 3,3'-disubstituted analogs such as 3,3'-dichlorobenzidine (3,3'-dichloro-4,4'-diaminobiphenyl), hereafter referred to as DiClBzd, have been used for more than 60 years as intermediates in the manufacture of organic pigments [36,37,41] and the toxicological effects of compounds in the benzidine family were widely studied for many years. In 1974 the U.S. Department of Labor called for the regulation of benzidine and DiClBzd by placing them on a list of 14 chemical compounds known to cause, or suspected of causing cancer from occupational exposure. An excellent review of the literature and problems associated with the use of benzidine and its congeners was reported by Haley [32].

Since toxicological tests with DiClBzd are proposed at our laboratory, analytical methodology is required. Colorimetric methods for benzidine and other aromatic amines based on diazotization and coupling reactions have been reported [34,35]; however, DiClBzd was not included. Other researchers [36,37] used Chloramine-T reagent to determine benzidine, DiClBzd, and congeners. Clayson et al. [38] quantitated benzidine and its metabolites via reverse-phase paper chromatography, but DiClBzd was not studied. Sawicki et al. [42] studied the fluorometric behavior of 45 polynuclear aromatic amines and heterocyclic imines; later, Bowman et al. [29] and Holder et al. [43] reported sensitive spectrophotofluorescent procedures for benzidine, its congeners, and other aromatic amines in a variety of substrates. DiClBzd was not included in any of these studies, probably because of its low fluorescence. Since no suitable method could be found in the literature, the following procedures were developed for the trace

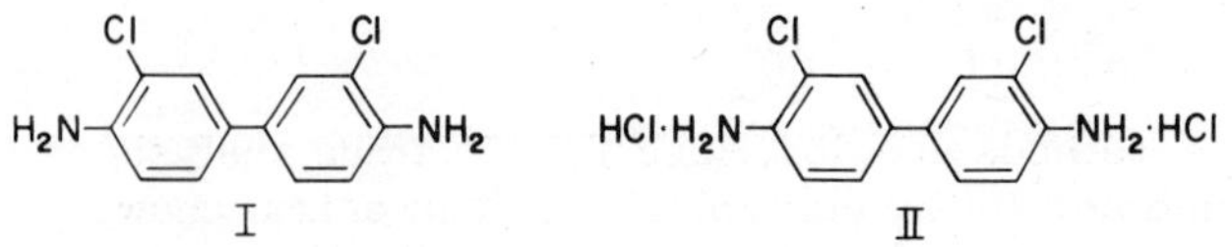

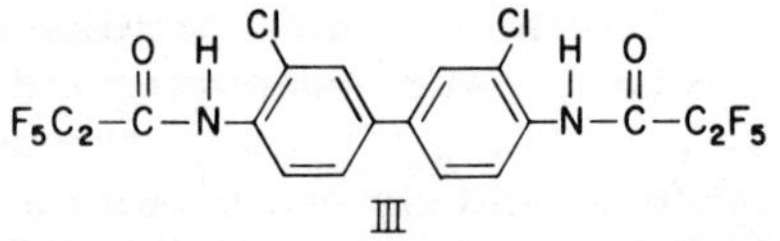

Figure 16 Formulas of 3,3'-dichlorobenzidine (I), its dihydrochloride salt (II), and its pentafluoropropionyl (PFP) derivative (III). (From Ref. 40.)

analysis of DiClBzd in our substrates. The formulas of DiClBzd (I), its dihydrochloride salt (II), and its pentafluoropropionyl (PFP) derivative (III) are presented in Figure 16.

Experimental

Materials. The DiClBzd·2HCl (Lot No. 12414, Pfaltz and Bauer Co., Flushing, New York) was washed several times with aqueous 1 N HCl, filtered, and dried in a vacuum oven at ambient temperature for 3 days. DiClBzd was prepared by dissolving DiClBzd·2HCl in aqueous 1 N NaOH and extracting the free amine with benzene; the solvent was then evaporated and the product dried overnight in a vacuum oven at 60°. The DiClBzd contained no extraneous GC peaks (via EC, N/P, and flame ionization detection). The DiClBzd·2HCl, after conversion to the free amine, was also free of extraneous GC peaks and yielded the correct amount of product.

Silica gel (No. 3405, J.T. Baker Chemical Co., Phillipsburg, New Jersey) was heated in an oven at 130° and stored in a desiccator prior to use. The silica gel was then partially deactivated with 4% water for use in the analytical procedure by adding 24 g of the dry material to a glass-stoppered bottle containing 1.0 ml of water dispersed on its inner surface; the contents were mixed well and allowed to stand for 24 hr with occasional shaking prior to use.

The XAD-2 resin, about 450 g (No. 3409, Mallinckrodt Chemical Co., St. Louis, Missouri), was transferred to a 2000-ml flask and washed by swirling it with 500 ml of distilled water for about 1 min; the supernatant was then decanted and discarded. The process was repeated by using three additional 500 ml portions of water followed by five 200 ml portions of acetone. The resin was transferred to a Büchner funnel to remove most of the acetone, then dried overnight in an oven at 70°.

Trifluoroacetic anhydride (TFA) (No. 67364) and pentafluoropropionic anhydride (PFP) (No. 65193) were obtained from Pierce Chemical Co., Rockford, Illinois; the heptafluorobutyric anhydride (HFB) (No. 270085) was obtained from Regis Chemical Co., Morton Grove, Illinois. The 1 g ampules were opened immediately prior to use and a 50 μl Hamilton syringe was used to withdraw the derivatizing agent from the vial and deliver it into the reaction vessel.

Trimethylamine (TMA) reagent was prepared by dissolving 2.0 g of the hydrochloride salt in 5 ml of 5 N NaOH and extracting the free amine with four 5 ml portions of benzene which were successively percolated through a plug of sodium sulfate (about 25 mm diam × 20 mm thick); the volume of the combined extracts was adjusted to 20 ml with benzene. This stock solution (about 1 M) was stored at 5°; portions were diluted 20-fold with benzene immediately prior to use.

The buffer solution (pH 6.0) was prepared by dissolving 136 g of KH_2PO_4 in 900 ml of distilled water and adjusting the pH to exactly 6.0 with 10 N NaOH. The volume was then adjusted to exactly 1 liter.

The keeper solution was paraffin oil (No. 01762, Applied Science Lab., State College, Pennsylvania), 20 mg/ml of benzene.

The animal chow (Laboratory Chow, Type 5010-C, Ralston Purina Co., St. Louis, Missouri) contained 6% fat, had a pH of 5.5, and 6.7% was volatile at 100° overnight.

All solvents were pesticide grade and all reagents were CP grade.

Preparation of Cleanup Columns

Silica gel. Columns (12 mm i.d., No. 420,000, Kontes Glass Co., Vineland, New Jersey) equipped with a 50 ml reservoir were prepared by successively adding a plug of glass wool, 2 g of Na_2SO_4, 2 g of silica gel (4% water), and 2 g of Na_2SO_4. A separate drying tube containing a plug of Na_2SO_4 (about 25 mm diam × 15 mm thick) was placed at the top of each column. The columns and drying tubes were prepared immediately prior to use and washed with five 5 ml portions of benzene which were discarded. (Note: The silica gel must be evaluated prior to use to provide assurance that DiClBzd elutes as indicated in the procedure. The container is kept tightly sealed to avoid changes in moisture content.)

XAD-2. Columns (12 mm i.d.), as previously described, were prepared by inserting a ball of glass wool (about 3 mm diam) into the stem to support the resin and to restrict the solvent flow; 2 g of the dry XAD-2 resin was then added to the column by using 5 ml of acetone. After a plug of glass wool was placed on top of the resin to hold it in place, the column was washed with five additional 5 ml portions of acetone followed by 5 ml portions of distilled water prior to use.

Preparation of Samples for Analysis

Animal chow. A 2 g portion of animal chow weighed into a 100 ml glass-stoppered flask was made alkaline by adding 5 ml of aqueous 0.2 N NaOH; 50 ml of benzene was added and the sample was mechanically extracted for 2 hr on a reciprocating shaker (No. 6000, Eberbach Corp., Ann Arbor, Michigan) at a rate of 200 excursions/min. The supernatant extract was decanted into a 50-ml culture tube and centrifuged at 1200 rpm for 15 min to remove any suspended particles of chow (Note: All culture tubes were borosilicate glass equipped with Teflon-lined screw caps.) A 25 ml portion of the extract (1 g equivalent of sample) was transferred to a 50 ml round-bottom flask and evaporated to dryness by using a 60° water bath and water pump vacuum. The residue was dissolved in 5 ml of benzene, transferred to an 18 ml culture tube containing 5 ml of 4 N HCl, vigorously shaken by hand for 5 min, and the benzene layer was discarded. Two additional 5 ml portions of benzene were used sequentially to wash the flask and to extract the acid phase in the tube; the benzene layers were discarded. (Note: At this point the sample may be stored in a refrigerator overnight.)

Eight milliliters of benzene and 3 ml of 10 N NaOH were then added to the tube; the contents were vigorously shaken by hand for 5 min and then centrifuged at 1000 rpm for 2 to 5 min to separate the layers. The benzene layer (contains DiClBzd) was withdrawn and transferred to a silica gel column and two additional extractions with 8 ml portions of benzene were performed in the same manner. Finally, the column was washed with three 5 ml portions of benzene. All effluent from the column except the first 5 ml was collected in a 50 ml round-bottom flask containing 0.5 ml of keeper solution, evaporated to dryness under water pump vacuum at 60° as described, and the residue was dissolved in an appropriate volume of benzene (e.g., 1 ml) for direct analysis via EC-GC or N/P-GC or for derivatization of PFP-DiClBzd prior to GC analysis.

Wastewater. The sample of wastewater (100 ml) was allowed to percolate through an XAD-2 column prepared as described and two 10 ml portions of distilled water were used successively to wash the sample container and the column; the column was then washed with an additional 80 ml of distilled water and a rubber bulb was used to force most of the water from the resin. The DiClBzd and/or DiClBzd·2HCl residues were eluted from the column by using four 4 ml portions of acetone and the effluent was collected in an 18 ml culture tube; a rubber bulb was used to force most of the acetone from the resin.

One milliliter of 12 N HCl was added and the tube was vigorously shaken by hand for 5 min. The contents of the tube were concentrated to about 4 ml using a tube heater (Kontes No. 720,000) set at 60° and a gentle stream of nitrogen. Benzene (4 ml) and 0.5 ml of

12 N HCl were added, the contents were shaken for 2 min, and the benzene layer was discarded. The extraction was repeated with two additional 4 ml portions of benzene, which were also discarded. Next, 2 ml of 10 N NaOH and 5 ml of benzene were added, the contents were shaken for 5 min, and the benzene layer was transferred to a silica gel column. The contents of the tube were extracted with two additional 5 ml portions of benzene, which were successively added to the column. The column was eluted with five additional 5 ml portions of benzene and all the effluent except the first 5 ml was collected in a 50 ml round-bottom flask containing keeper and evaporated to dryness as described for chow and the residue was dissolved in an appropriate volume of benzene (e.g., 2 ml) for direct analysis or for derivatization to PFP-DiClBzd prior to GC analysis.

Urine. A sample of 100 ml of human urine was percolated through XAD-2, the column was washed with water, the residues were eluted with acetone, and the acetone eluate was concentrated using a tube heater and a stream of nitrogen exactly as described for wastewater except that the volume of the acetone eluate was concentrated to about 2 ml. Benzene (2 ml) was added, the contents were shaken for 2 min, and the benzene layer was discarded; the extraction was repeated with two additional 2 ml portions of benzene, which were also discarded. Benzene (4 ml) and 1.5 ml of 10 N NaOH were added to the acid phase, the contents were shaken for 5 min and centrifuged to separate the layers, and the benzene layer was transferred to a silica gel column. The extraction was repeated twice with 3 ml portions of benzene, which were also added to the column. Finally, the column was eluted with five 6 ml portions of benzene and all of the effluent except the first 5 ml was collected, evaporated to dryness, and the residues were dissolved in benzene for analysis as described for wastewater.

Gas Chromatographic Analysis

EC detection. A Hewlett-Packard (Palo Alto, California) Model 5750B instrument equipped with a ^{63}Ni EC detector (Tracor Inc., Austin, Texas) and a 100 cm glass column (4 mm i.d.) containing 5% OV-101 on 80-100 mesh Gas Chrom Q, conditioned at 275° overnight prior to use, was operated at 215° in the dc mode with nitrogen carrier flow of 160 ml/min. The detector temperature was 270° and the injection port was 235°. Under these conditions, the retention time (t_R) of DiClBzd was 2.35 min and its TFA, PFP, and HFB-derivatives were 2.10, 2.00, and 2.45 min, respectively. The t_R of a reference standard of p,p'-DDT used to monitor the performance of the EC-GC system was 1.85 min.

N/P detection. A Perkin-Elmer (Norwalk, Connecticut) Model 3920B instrument equipped with a rubidium-sensitized N/P detector and a 90 cm glass column (2 mm i.d.) containing 5% OV-101 on 80-100 mesh Gas Chrom Q, conditioned at 275° overnight prior to use, was operated at 245° with a nitrogen carrier gas flow of 15 ml/min. The injection port and interface (transfer line and detector) temperatures were 250 and 260°, respectively. Gas flow for hydrogen and air were 1.1 and 64 ml/min, respectively. The temperature controller for the rubidium bead was set at 525. Under these conditions, the t_R values for DiClBzd, and its PFP derivative, and p,p'-DDT were 2.80, 2.30, and 2.20 min, respectively.

All injections were in 5 μl of benzene. Samples of unknown residue content were quantitated by relating peak heights to those of a known amount of the compound. DiClBzd or DiClBzd·2HCl were expressed in terms of the other by using the following factor: DiClBzd × 1.29 = DiClBzd·2HCl.

Derivatization of DiClBzd

Preparation of various derivatives for EC-GC evaluation. TFA, PFP, and HFB derivatives of DiClBzd were prepared by our modifications of the procedure described by Walle and Ehrsson [44] and Ehrsson et al. [45]. TMA solution (0.5 ml of 0.05 M) was added to an 8 ml culture tube containing the DiClBzd (1 μg or less) dissolved in exactly 1.5 ml of benzene (total benzene = 2.0 ml) and followed by 50 μl of the appropriate fluorinated anhydride reagent. The tube was sealed, shaken, heated in a 50° water bath for 15 min, cooled, and the reaction was terminated by the addition of 1 ml of phosphate buffer (pH 6.0). The tube was shaken for 1 min, centrifuged for 1 min at 1000 rpm, and the lower aqueous layer was discarded; the extraction was repeated with an additional 1 ml portion of buffer. The upper benzene layer was transferred to a dry 8 ml culture tube containing 0.5 g of Na_2SO_4, shaken, and either injected directly into the GC or after appropriate dilution with benzene.

Derivatization of cleaned-up extracts for analysis. Appropriate portions of the cleaned-up extracts of chow, wastewater, or human urine were adjusted to exactly 1.5 ml of benzene in an 8 ml culture tube and subjected to derivatization by using TMA solution and PFP reagent. For example, with extracts of wastewater or human urine, 50 g equivalents were derivatized and with chow containing 1 ppm of residue or less, a 0.5 g equivalent was used. Correspondingly smaller amounts of chow extract were derivatized for samples containing higher levels of DiClBzd or its salt; however, such samples may also be analyzed without being derivatized.

Recovery Experiments

Animal chow. Triplicate 2 g samples of chow were spiked with 0, 0.01, 0.10, 1.0, 10, 100, and 1000 ppm of DiClBzd·2HCl by adding an appropriate amount of the chemical in 1 ml of methanol. The solvent was then removed by using a 60° water bath and water pump vacuum to simulate the conditions under which bulk amounts of the diet will be prepared for use in animal tests. The samples were then allowed

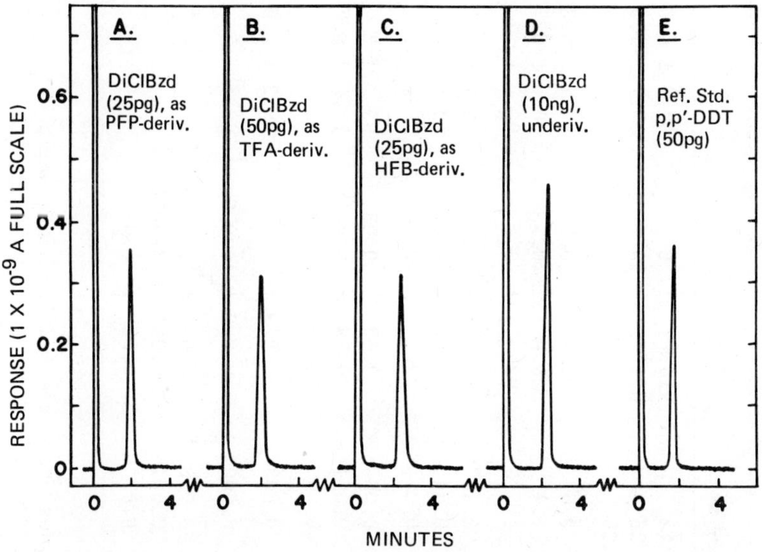

Figure 17 Electron capture gas chromatograms. (A), (B), and (C) are pentafluoropropionyl, trifluoroacetyl, and heptafluorobutyryl derivatives of DiClBzd; (D) is DiClBzd per se; and (E) is a p,p'-DDT reference standard. All injections are in 5 μl of benzene. (From Ref. 40.)

to cool, extracted, cleaned up, and assayed to determine the accuracy and precision of the procedure.

Wastewater and urine. Triplicate 100 ml samples of wastewater or human urine in 180 ml culture tubes were spiked with 0, 0.10, 1.0, 10, or 20 ppb of DiClBzd or DiClBzd·2HCl by adding an appropriate amount of the chemical in 0.5 ml of methanol. The tubes were sealed, mixed, and allowed to stand overnight at 5° prior to analysis.

Results and discussion

In feeding studies with carcinogens administered to large numbers of mice at our laboratory, animals are dosed either via their drinking water or their diet, and the use of drinking water is generally the method of choice if the chemical is sufficiently soluble and stable. Unfortunately, solubilities of DiClBzd and DiClBzd·2HCl in water at 25 ± 2° which were approximated at 3.0 and 30 ppm, respectively, precluded the use of this medium. However, the solubility of DiClBzd·2HCl (preferred to DiClBzd because of its lower volatility) in 95% ethanol at 25 ± 2°, which was approximated at 12.6 mg/ml, was sufficient to permit the use of the solvent in the preparation of dosed diet.

Table 13 Gas Chromatographic Analysis of 3,3'-Dichlorobenzidine Dihydrochloride in Animal Chow Spiked at Various Levels as Determined by Three Procedures

Added[a]			Equivalents of chow/	Recovered ($\bar{x}$ ± SE)[b]		
μg	ppm	Procedure	analysis	μg	ppm	%
2000	1000	EC-underiv.	10 μg	1830 ± 12	914 ± 6	91.4 ± 0.6
		EC-PFP-deriv.	33.3 ng	1780 ± 26	891 ± 13	89.1 ± 1.3
		N/P-underiv.	1.0 mg	1880 ± 20	940 ± 10	94 ± 1
200	100	EC-underiv.	100 μg	185 ± 0.6	92.7 ± 0.3	92.7 ± 0.3
		EC-PFP-deriv.	500 ng	181 ± 1.4	90.4 ± 0.7	90.4 ± 0.7
		N/P-underiv.	1.0 mg	184 ± 4	92 ± 2	92 ± 2
20.0	10.0	EC-underiv.	1.0 mg	18.1 ± 0.38	9.07 ± 0.19	90.7 ± 1.9
		EC-PFP-deriv.	5.0 μg	17.9 ± 0.34	8.95 ± 0.17	89.5 ± 1.7
		N/P-underiv.	1.0 mg	18.2 ± 0.2	9.1 ± 0.1	91 ± 1
2.0	1.00	EC-underiv.	5.0 mg	1.38 ± 0.06	0.69 ± 0.03	69 ± 3
		EC-PFP-deriv.	25.0 μg	1.57 ± 0.014	0.785 ± 0.007	78.5 ± 0.7
		N/P-underiv.	5.0 mg	1.56 ± 0.06	0.78 ± 0.03	78 ± 3
0.200	0.100	EC-PFP-deriv.	250 μg	0.158 ± 0.003	0.0792 ± 0.0015	79.2 ± 1.5
0.020	0.010	EC-PFP-deriv.	1.25mg	0.0126 ± 0.0004	0.0063 ± 0.0002	63 ± 2
0.000	0.000	EC-underiv.	5.0 mg	0.124 ± 0.038	0.06 ± 0.02	- -
		EC-PFP-deriv.	1.25mg	0.0026 ± 0.0018	0.0013 ± 0.0010	- -
		N/P-underiv.	5.0 mg	0.04 ± 0.02	0.02 ± 0.01	- -

[a]Per 2 g of chow.
[b]Means and standard error from triplicate assays; spiked samples are corrected for background of control chow.
Source: Ref. 40.

DiClBzd gives a good response to EC-GC and samples of chow and wastewater containing residues as low as 1.0 ppm and 20 ppb, respectively, may be accurately assayed by the procedure described. The sensitivity of DiClBzd via N/P-GC was about the same as EC-GC; however, the specificity of N/P-GC permitted injections of larger amounts of sample extractives, and assays of lower levels of residues could be achieved. Nevertheless, the limited sensitivities of DiClBzd with both detectors and the somewhat temperamental characteristics of the N/P system led us to investigate the possibility of derivatizing DiClBzd to enhance its electron-capturing properties. Typical EC gas chromatograms of PFP, TFA, and HFB derivatives of DiClBzd are presented in Figure 17 together with DiClBzd per se and a p,p'-DDT reference standard. The PFP and HFB derivatives gave about equal responses, and TFA-DiClBzd was about half as sensitive. The PFP derivative was therefore selected for use in the analytical procedure since it enhanced detector responses about 300-fold.

The spectrum of the PFP derivative of DiClBzd from a GC-mass spectrometer indicated the presence of two pentafluoropropionyl groups, probably one on each of the amino groups (see formula III, Fig. 16); this was consistent with the molecular weight of 544.

Tests with benzene solutions of DiClBzd and its PFP derivative stored at 5° and assayed periodically by EC-GC indicated that both compounds were stable for at least 22 days. The derivatization procedure as described yields excellent results, and essentially no PFP-DiClBzd is lost by washing the benzene reaction mixture with phosphate buffer (pH 6). The use of aqueous ammonia as a washing agent was discussed by Walle and Ehrsson [44] and it should be avoided. In tests where 3.0 and 0.75 N ammonium hydroxide were substituted for the phosphate buffer, recoveries of the PFP-DiClBzd were only 8 and 38%, respectively.

Results from triplicate samples of chow spiked with DiClBzd·2HCl at 0, 0.010, 0.10, 1.00, 10.0, 100, and 1000 ppm as determined by the three procedures are presented in Table 13. At levels of 1.0 ppm or more, recoveries and precision were good and the three procedures yielded comparable results. Therefore, for samples containing residues of this magnitude, analyses of underivatized extracts via EC-GC or N/P-GC are the procedures of choice. For levels below 1.0 ppm, analysis of the PFP-derivatized sample via EC-GC is recommended. Minimum levels of DiClBzd·2HCl detectable in chow (based on twice background) via EC-GC of DiClBzd and PFP-DiClBzd were 120 and 3 ppb, respectively; N/P-GC of either the free amine or the PFP derivative was about 40 ppb.

Data from samples of wastewater spiked with either the free amine or the salt at levels of 0, 0.1, 1.0, and 10.0 ppb and human urine spiked at 0, 1.0, and 20.0 ppb are presented in Table 14. Recoveries from wastewater spiked with 1.0 ppb or more were 75% or better and

Table 14 Gas Chromatographic Analysis of 3,3'-Dichlorobenzidine or Its Dihydrochloride Salt in Wastewater and Human Urine

Added[a]			Equivalents of sample/analysis	Recovered ($\bar{x} \pm SE$)[b]		
μg	ppb	Procedure	(mg)	μg	ppb	%
			Wastewater			
1.0	10.0	EC-underiv.	250	0.78 ± 0.02	7.8 ± 0.2	78 ± 2
		N/P-underiv.	250	0.82 ± 0.02	8.2 ± 0.2	82 ± 2
0.10	1.0	EC-PFP-deriv.	25	0.0749 ± 0.0054	0.749 ± 0.054	74.9 ± 5.4
0.10[c]	1.0	EC-PFP-deriv.	25	0.0785 ± 0.0016	0.785 ± 0.016	78.5 ± 1.6
0.01	0.1	EC-PFP-deriv.	125	0.0055 ± 0.0005	0.055 ± 0.005	55 ± 5
0	0	EC-underiv.	250	0.04 ± 0.00	0.4 ± 0.0	- -
		N/P-underiv.	250	0.03 ± 0.01	0.3 ± 0.1	- -
		EC-PFP-deriv.	125	0.0009 ± 0.0001	0.009 ± 0.001	- -
			Human Urine			
2.0[c]	20.0	EC-PFP-deriv.	2.5	0.776 ± 0.139	7.76 ± 1.39	38.8 ± 7
		N/P-underiv.	250	0.74 ± 0.16	7.4 ± 1.6	37 ± 8
0.10	1.0	EC-PFP-deriv.	25	0.047 ± 0.008	0.47 ± 0.08	47 ± 8
0	0	EC-PFP-deriv.	25	0.003 ± 0.000	0.03 ± 0.00	- -
		N/P-underiv.	250	0.09 ± 0.03	0.9 ± 0.3	- -

[a]Per 100 g of sample.
[b]Mean and standard error from triplicate assays; spiked samples are corrected for background of control samples.
[c]Spiked as DiClBzd·2HCl
Source: Ref. 40.

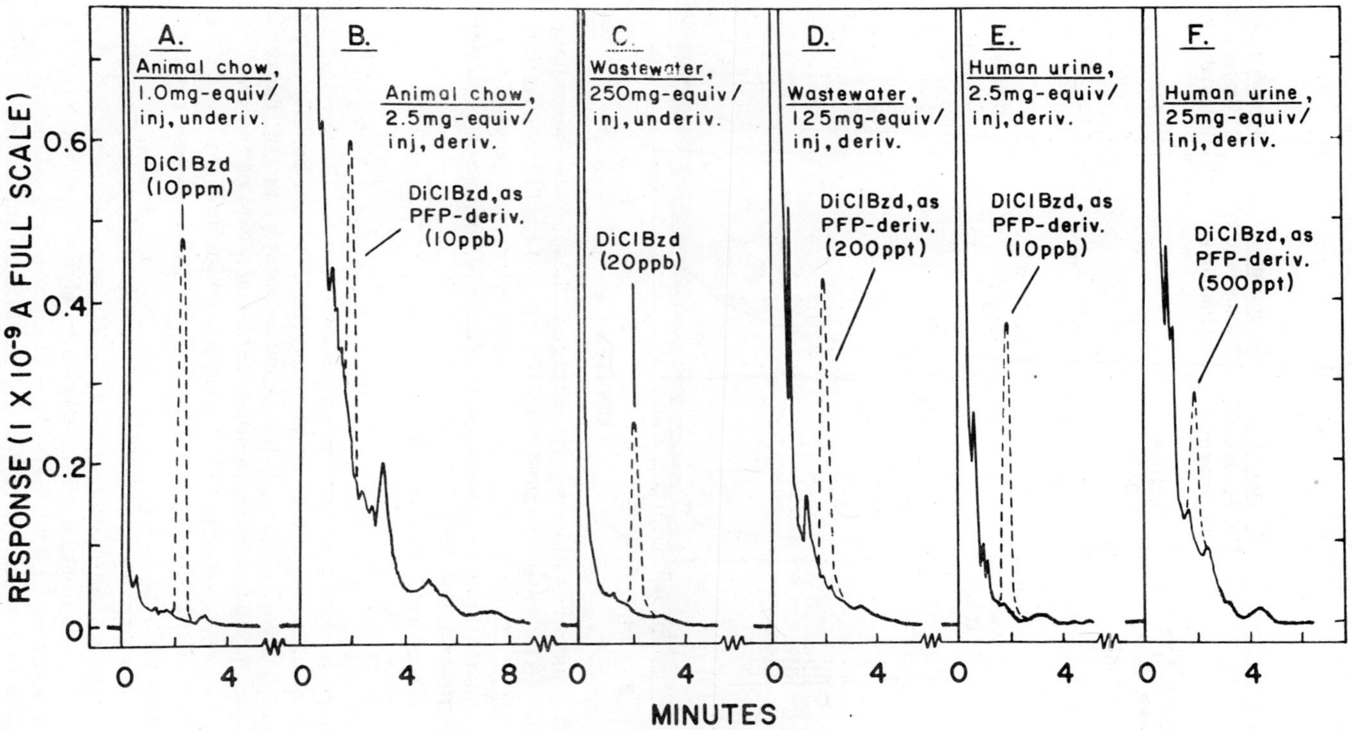

Figure 18 Electron capture gas chromatograms. Solid lines are untreated sample extracts; dashed lines (superimposed) illustrate responses of residues spiked into the extracts. In (A) and (C) neither the extract nor the DiClBzd was derivatized; all others were derivatized. All injections are in 5 μl of benzene. (From Ref. 40.)

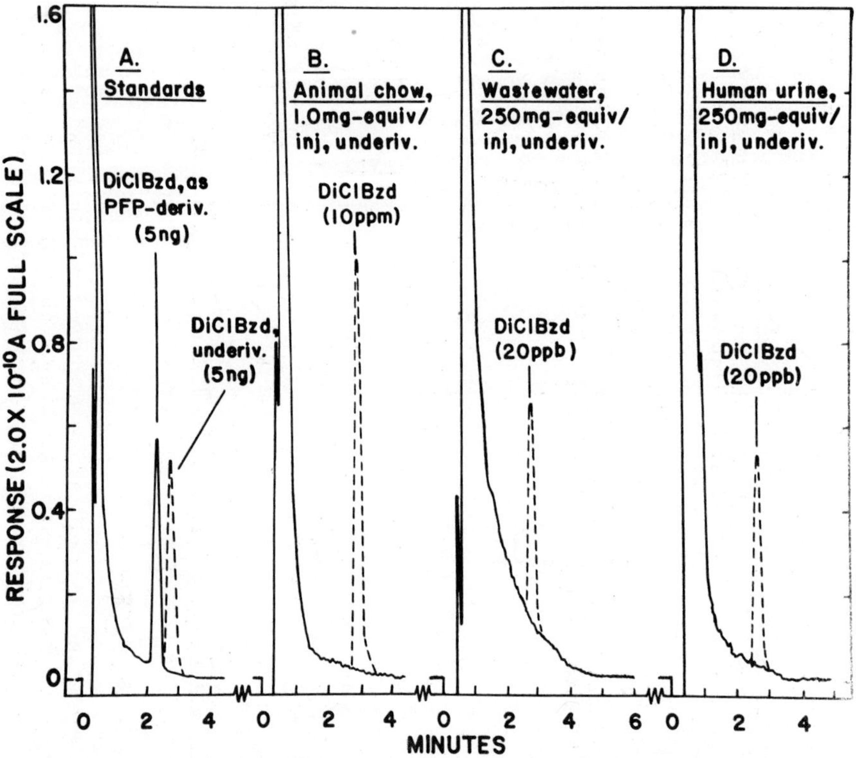

Figure 19 Gas chromatograms via nitrogen-phosphorus thermionic detection. (A) shows standards of DiClBzd and its PFP derivative; in (B), (C), and (D) solid lines are underivatized extracts of untreated samples; dashed lines (superimposed) illustrate responses of underivatized DiClBzd spiked into the extracts. All injections are in 5 μl of benzene. (From Ref. 40.)

those spiked at 0.10 ppb gave recoveries of 55 ± 5%. Wastewater containing as much as 10 ppb of residue may be analyzed by EC- or N/P-GC without derivatization. At levels below 10 ppb, EC-GC assays of the PFP derivative are recommended. Minimum levels of the free amine detectable in wastewater (based on twice background) by EC-GC of DiClBzd or PFP-DiClBzd were 0.80 and 0.018 ppb, respectively; N/P-GC was 0.60 ppb.

Recoveries from human urine spiked with 0, 1.0, and 20 ppb of the free amine or salt averaged 41 ± 8%. These losses occurred mostly during evaporation of the acidified acetone eluate from the XAD-2 column to a volume of 2 ml. The step is necessary to allow sufficient vaporization of volatile interferences from the sample to permit analysis

Table 15 Partition Values for 3,3'-Dichlorobenzidine

Solvent system	p Value
Hexane-acetonitrile	0.015
Hexane-80% acetone (20% water)	0.478
Chloroform-60% methanol (40% water)	0.974
Benzene-aqueous HCl (1 N)	0.093
Benzene-aqueous HCl (2 N)	0.0092
Benzene-aqueous HCl (4 N)	<0.0003
Benzene-aqueous NaOH (0.1 N)	0.98
Benzene-aqueous NaOH (1 N)	1.00
Chloroform-water	1.00
Chloroform-aqueous NaOH (0.1, 1, and 10 N)	1.00

Source: Ref. 40.

at the 1.0 ppb level; unfortunately, some of the residue is also lost in the process. Nevertheless, recoveries and sensitivity are sufficient to signal any accidental exposure of an employee to the chemical. Minimum amounts of DiClBzd detectable in human urine (based on twice background) were about 0.060 ppb via EC-GC of the PFP derivative and 1.8 ppb by N/P-GC.

Typical EC gas chromatograms of various untreated control extracts (derivatized or underivatized) before and after being spiked with DiClBzd or its PFP derivative are presented in Figure 18. Chromatograms of extracts (underivatized) spiked in a similar manner as determined by N/P-GC are presented in Figure 19 with standards of DiClBzd and PFP-DiClBzd. Sensitivities of equal amounts of Cl- and/or N-containing compounds were compared using the N/P detector and adjusting all responses (peak heights) in terms of the t_R of DiClBzd; the results were as follows:

Compound	Response (peak height relative to DiClBzd = 1.0)
3,3'-Dichlorobenzidine	1.0
3,3'-Dichlorobenzidine, PFP derivative	0.83
4,4'-Dichlorobiphenyl	0.028
Benzidine	0.59
p,p'-DDT	0.080

It is interesting to note that the response of DiClBzd is greater than would be expected from the chlorine response of 4,4'-dichlorobiphenyl plus the nitrogen response from benzidine; also the response from PFP-DiClBzd was not as great as DiClBzd. Appreciable responses were also obtained from the compounds that contained chlorine and no nitrogen.

Partition values (the fraction of solute partitioning into the non-polar phase of an equivolume immiscible binary solvent system) are useful in developing extraction and cleanup methods for confirmation of identity [15,18]. The values obtained for DiClBzd and some of which were used in developing the present methods are given in Table 15; they may also be useful to other investigators.

E. 4-Aminobiphenyl, 2-Naphthylamine, and Analogs [43]

General description of method

Procedures are described for monitoring trace levels of 4-aminobiphenyl, 2-naphthylamine, and their hydrochloride salts in wastewater, microbiological growth media, potable water, human urine, and mouse blood utilizing spectrophotofluorometry (SPF). The salient elements of the methods are extraction of the residues as the free amines with benzene, rapid cleanup on an alumina column, and quantification of the free amine in methanol via SPF. Potable water solutions of the salts are diluted with 0.01 N aqueous HCl and quantified directly by SPF. Ancillary analytical information concerning gas chromatography of the free amines, partitioning properties of the compounds between solvent pairs, their solubility and stability in water, and thin layer chromatographic data are presented. The compositions of various admixtures of 1- and 2-naphthylamine or their salts were determined by using SPF with calculations based on simultaneous equations.

Introduction

Studies of workers who were occupationally exposed have established 4-aminobiphenyl, 2-naphthylamine, and benzidine as human bladder carcinogens [1]. Of this group, 2-naphthylamine is generally considered to be one of the most dangerous environmental carcinogens to which humans have been exposed. Because of these and 11 other compounds known to cause, or suspected of causing cancer in humans by occupational exposure, the Standards Advisory Committee on Carcinogens to the U.S. Department of Labor have recommended their regulation.

Toxicological tests have been initiated at NCTR for some of these chemicals and are proposed for others; therefore, analytical methods were required. Several methods for aromatic amines were reported in the literature. Lugg [46] described optimum reaction conditions for the colorimetric determination of 24 phenols and aromatic amines by using commercially available stabilized diazonium salts. Bridges et al. [47] investigated the variation with pH of the excitation and fluorescence wavelengths and fluorescence intensity of several hydroxy- and aminobiphenyls with a view of using the data for determining hydroxybiphenyls in biological material; however, no actual substrates were assayed. Sawicki et al. [42] investigated column and thin layer chromatographic (TLC) and fluorometric behavior of 45 polynuclear aromatic amines and heterocyclic imines; Shimomura and Walton [48] studied the effects of zinc, cadmium, and nickel nitrates on the TLC separation of aromatic amines with silica gel and aluminum oxide. Masuda and Hoffmann [49] described a method for determining 1- and 2-naphthylamine in cigarette smoke. The compounds were derivatized by using pentafluoropropionic anhydride and the neutral fraction was cleaned up on Florisil; the N-pentafluoropropionamide was then assayed by electron capture (EC) gas chromatography (GC). Knight [50] assayed aminoaromatic compounds by GC with flame ionization detection (FID). Gupta and Srivastava [51] reacted acetic acid solutions of 48 substituted anilines and other aromatic amines with an aqueous peroxydisulfate solution to form colored products with differing absorption maxima in the visible range and El-Dib [35] reported a colorimetric procedure based on diazotization of primary aromatic amines and coupling with resorcinol or 1-naphthol. Recently, Jakovljevic et al. [52] described a method for assaying traces of 4-aminobiphenyl in 2-aminobiphenyl based on the separation of the free amines using TLC, extractions of the isolated materials from the plates, and fluorometric determination. However, none of these methods possess all of the qualities (specificity, sensitivity, accuracy, precision, versatility, and speed) required for our substrates; therefore, the following procedures for trace analysis were developed. The formulas of two of the carcinogens of current interest–4-aminobiphenyl and 2-naphthylamine–and four analogs are shown in Figure 20.

Experimental

Materials. 4-Aminobiphenyl (m.p. 52 to 54°; Aldrich Chemical Co., Milwaukee, Wisconsin), 1-naphthylamine (m.p. 49.1 to 50.3°; Fisher Scientific Co., Pittsburgh, Pennsylvania), and 2-naphthylamine (m.p. 111 to 113°; Sigma Chemical Co., St. Louis, Missouri) were used as received since they contained no extraneous GC peaks. The salts of the amines were prepared by bubbling an excess of anhydrous HCl through benzene solutions of each amine to precipitate its corresponding salt, then vacuum dried overnight at ambient temperature prior to use. Portions of the salts, after conversion back to the free amine, yielded the correct amount of product and were also void of extraneous GC peaks. The adsorbent (basic alumina, Brockman activity I; Fisher Scientific Co., No. A-941) was used as received. Sodium sulfate was anhydrous; all reagents were CP grade; and all solvents were pesticide grade. Ingredients for the microbiological culture media were purchased from Difco Laboratories, Detroit, Michigan, and the media were

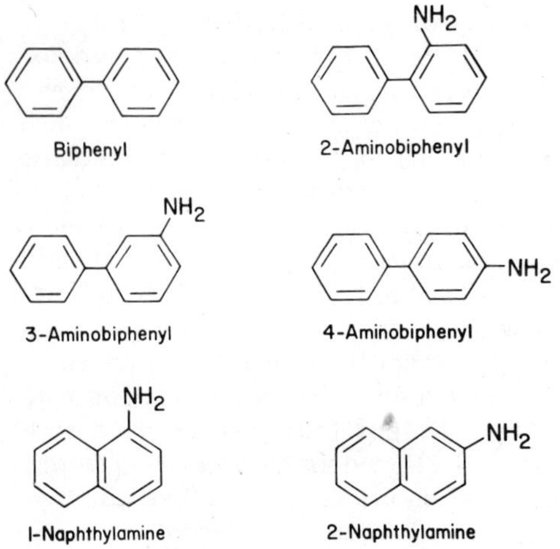

Figure 20 Formulas of the carcinogens 4-aminobiphenyl and 2-naphthylamine, and four analogs. (From Ref. 43.)

prepared in accordance with the instructions supplied by the manufacturer. All culture tubes were of borosilicate glass and equipped with Teflon-lined screw caps. The TLC plates (20 × 20 cm, Fisher No. 6-601A), precoated with silica gel GF (250 μm thick), were activated in an oven at 140° for 1 hr and allowed to cool in a desiccator prior to use.

Spectrophotofluorometric (SPF) Analysis. An Aminco-Bowman instrument equipped with a xenon lamp and a 1P28 detector was used with 1 cm^2 cells and a 2-2-2 mm slit program to measure fluorescence. All dilutions of free amine were freshly prepared in methanol and those of the salts were in 0.01 N HCl solution. Excitation (λ_{Ex}) and emission (λ_{Em}) wavelengths (nm) for maximum fluorescence and the corresponding relative intensities (RI) were given in Table 16. The instrument was frequently calibrated to produce an RI of 5.0 with a solution of 0.3 μg of quinine sulfate/ml of 0.1 N sulfuric acid (λ_{Ex} = 350, λ_{Em} = 450). Readings were corrected for solvent blanks and RI was plotted versus concentration of the six compounds on log-log paper to produce a standard curve. To ensure that the RI was within the linear range of the standard curve and thus unaffected by concentration quenching, samples were diluted with an equal volume of solvent to ascertain whether the RI was about half the undiluted solution. If it was not, dilution was continued until RI was halved. Preparation of samples for SPF analysis is fully described later in the experimental section. Extracts of wastewater, urine, medium, and blood for SPF analyses were first diluted to contain the equivalents of 10, 1, and 0.2 g sample/ml,

Table 16 Wavelengths for Maximum Fluorescence and Corresponding Relative Intensities

Compound	λ_{Ex} (nm)	λ_{Em} (nm)	RI (0.5 μg/ml)
Biphenyl	260	312	3.90
2-Aminobiphonyl	312	392	6.25
3-Aminobiphenyl	255	398	5.50
3-Aminobiphenyl·HCl	260	410	7.0
4-Aminobiphenyl	290	368	55.0
4-Aminobiphenyl·HCl	260	382	7.80
1-Naphthylamine	332	425	14.6
1-Naphthylamine·HCl	285	444	2.1
2-Naphthylamine	242	400	18.5
2-Naphthylamine·HCl	286	406	10.4

Source: Ref. 43.

respectively; further dilutions were made as required to be certain the RI was within the linear range of the standard curve. The RI of the untreated control sample was then subtracted from that of the unknown and the concentration (μg/ml) was determined from the standard curve. In the instances where the salts are assayed as the free amines, the analytical results were multiplied by the factors 1.22 for 4-aminobiphenyl and 1.25 for 2-naphthylamine to express them in terms of the salts.

Determinations of 1- and 2-naphthylamine or their salts in admixtures were performed by measuring the RI at the λ_{Ex} and λ_{Em} maxima for each compound and calculating the amount of each consistituent by using the simultaneous equations $I_a = F_{1a}C_a + F_{1b}C_b$ (1); $I_b = F_{2a}C_a + F_{2b}C_b$ (2), where I_a and I_b are the observed RI value at the λ_{Em} maxima of compounds a and b, respectively; C_a and C_b are the respective concentrations; and the F factors (1a, 2a, 1b, 2b) are proportionality constants for each constituent at each wavelength combination. The proportionality constants for each compound (0.1 μg/ml) were determined by measuring the RI at the wavelength maxima for both compounds.

Gas Chromatographic Analysis. A Hewlett-Packard model 5750 instrument equipped with an FID and a 100 cm glass column (4 mm i.d., 6 mm o.d.) containing 10% OV-101 (w/w) on Gas Chrom Q (80-100 mesh) was operated either isothermally or temperature programmed from 100 to 250° at the rate of 10°/min. The helium carrier flow was 100 ml/min and the injection port and detector temperatures were set at 275 and 295°, respectively. Temperature-programmed analyses, which were used to determine whether our standards contained extraneous GC

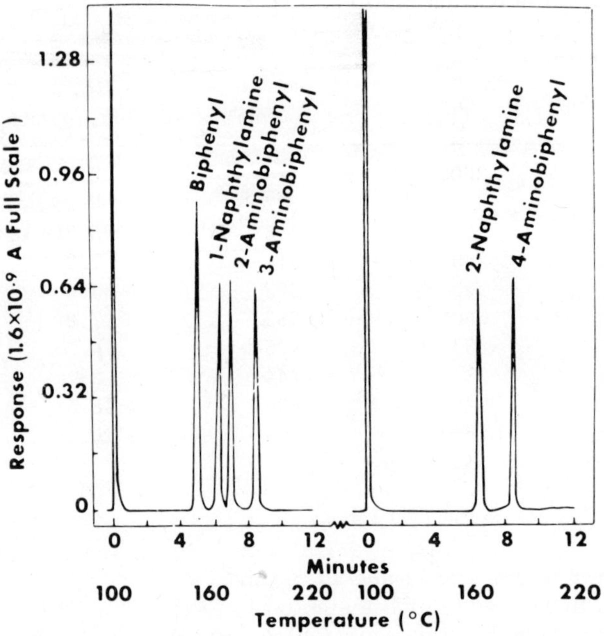

Figure 21 Typical temperature-programmed gas chromatograms (FID) of 500 ng amounts of each of the six aromatic compounds shown in Fig. 20 injected in 5 μl of chloroform. (From Ref. 43.)

peaks, yielded retention times (t_R) in minutes as follows: biphenyl, 5.30; 2-aminobiphenyl, 7.20; 3-aminobiphenyl, 8.50; 4-aminobiphenyl, 8.75; 1-naphthylamine, 6.50; and 2-naphthylamine, 6.65. Typical chromatograms are presented in Figure 21. For quantitative analysis of the individual free amines (e.g., for p-value determinations, the fraction of solute partitioning into the nonpolar phase of an equivolume immiscible binary solvent system), the column oven was operated isothermally at a temperature that resulted in a t_R of about 2 min. These temperatures were as follows: biphenyl, 140°; 2-aminobiphenyl, 165°; 3-aminobiphenyl, 180°; 4-aminobiphenyl, 185°; and 1- and 2-naphthylamine, 160°.

Solubility, p Values, and TLC Determinations. The solubilities of 4-aminobiphenyl, 2-naphthylamine, and their hydrochloride salts in water at 25 ± 2° were determined by SPF in a manner similar to that described by Bowman and King [6] for 2-acetylaminofluorene.

Extraction p values for the aromatic amines were determined in several solvent systems by GC in the manner described by Bowman and Beroza [16,18]. The TLC determinations were made by using a

Gelman model 51325-1 apparatus and glass plates precoated with silica gel GF. The plates were spotted with 5 μl methanol solutions (1 μg/μl) of the test compounds (biphenyl was used as a reference compound). After the developing solvent (Table 23) had ascended 13 cm above the spotting line (about 25 min), the plates were removed and the solvent allowed to evaporate. The spots were made visible by viewing them under ultraviolet (UV) light (254 nm) and the R_f values calculated.

Preparation of Samples for SPF Analysis

Microbiological growth media. Ten milliliters of the trypticase soy dextrose (TSD) or brain heart infusion (BHI) medium was added to a 30 ml culture tube containing 1 g of NaCl and 10 ml of benzene. After the addition of 0.2 ml of 10 N NaOH, the tube was sealed, shaken vigorously for 2 min, and centrifuged for 10 min at about 625 *g*. The benzene layer was carefully withdrawn by using a syringe and cannula and percolated through a plug of sodium sulfate (25 mm × 10 mm thick) in tandem with a glass column (12 mm i.d., Kontes No. 420,000) prepared by adding successively, a plug of glass wool, 5 g of sodium sulfate, 1 g of basic alumina, and 5 g of sodium sulfate. The medium was extracted with two additional 10 ml portions of benzene that were also percolated through the plug and column. Finally, the column was washed with 10 ml of dichloromethane-10% methanol to ensure complete elution of the free amine residue from the column. After the addition of 1 drop of diethylene glycol to serve as a keeper, the combined eluates were evaporated just to dryness by using water pump vacuum and a 60° water bath. The dry residue was dissolved in an appropriate amount of methanol for SPF analysis as the free amine.

Wastewater. One hundred milliliters of sample was added to a 160 ml culture tube containing 2 g of NaCl, then made alkaline with 0.5 ml of 10 N NaOH. The sample was then shaken for 2 min, centrifuged at about 50 *g* for 10 min, cleaned up, and prepared for analysis as described for media except that three 15 ml portions of benzene were used for extraction.

Blood. Procedures employing no hydrolysis as well as alkaline or acid hydrolysis of the sample prior to extraction were conducted as follows:

1. *No hydrolysis.* One milliliter of heparinized whole mouse blood was added to a 20 ml culture tube containing 6 ml of distilled water and 1 ml of 10 N NaOH. The contents were mixed, extracted three times with 10 ml portions of benzene, and prepared for SPF analysis as described for media.
2. *Alkaline hydrolysis.* Samples were analyzed as described under no hydrolysis except that the mixture in the sealed tube was held in an 80° heating block for 2 hr with gentle shaking at about 10 min intervals, then cooled to ambient temperature prior to extraction with benzene.

Potable water. Aqueous solutions of the hydrochloride salts, slated for use as the animals' drinking water, were assayed for proper concentration after sequential dilutions with 0.01 N HCl solution. The fluorescence of diluted sample (e.g., 0.1 ppm) was compared directly to that of a standard solution prepared in the same manner.

Human urine. Procedures utilizing alkaline, acid, or no hydrolysis prior to extraction were employed for urine as follows:

1. *No hydrolysis.* Analyses were performed exactly as described for wastewater.
2. *Alkaline hydrolysis.* Analyses were performed exactly as described for wastewater except that the alkaline solution in the sealed tube was heated in a water bath at 80° for 2 hr with gentle shaking at about 10 min intervals, then cooled to ambient temperature prior to extraction with benzene.
3. *Acid hydrolysis.* These analyses were also performed as described for wastewater except that 0.5 ml of 12 N HCl was substituted for the 10 N NaOH. This mixture was then heated at 80° for 2 hr, cooled, and made alkaline with 1 ml of 10 N NaOH prior to extraction with benzene.

Recovery Experiments. Triplicate samples of both biological media were separately spiked with 100 μl of methanol (or water) containing the appropriate amount of the free amine (or its salt) to produce concentrations at 0, 0.1, and 1.0 ppm. The samples were allowed to stand in the refrigerator (5°) overnight prior to extraction. Samples (1 ml) of heparinized mouse blood were spiked in the same manner at 0 and 2.0 ppm, held at 5° overnight, and analyzed as described. Wastewater and urine samples (100 ml) were spiked at 0 and 20 ppb by adding 1 ml of methanol (or water) containing the appropriate amount of compound, held at 5° overnight, and analyzed as described.

Stability Experiments. Aqueous 4-aminobiphenyl (about 1.0 and 100 ppm) dissolved in either deionized water or 0.01 N HCl (pH 2) was tested to determine the chemical stability of the compound and its acceptability to the animals under simulated test conditions. The animal drinking water dispenser for each cage (four mice per cage) consisted of a rubber stopper and a stainless steel "sipper tube" (8 mm o.d. × 90 mm long) containing a steel ball to serve as a valve. Triplicate dispensers, each containing 325 ml of the various levels of test solution, were placed in cages and exposed to ambient conditions (25 ± 2°) and continuous fluorescent lighting in the animal room. Samples (10 ml) were taken from each dispenser immediately and 1, 2, 4, 8, and 16 days later. The pH of each sample was determined and solutions of the salt were diluted and analyzed as described for potable water.

Results and discussion

The use of SPF as a means of assaying these compounds is indicated by their strong fluorescence intensities, which result in high sensitivity, and by the inherent specificity of the method. The RI values of the free amines in methanol are as much as seven times greater than those of the corresponding hydrochloride salts in 0.01 N HCl solutions. In these solvents the limit of detection, expressed as twice background, were about 1 to 2 and 2 to 5 μg/ml for the free amines and salts, respectively. As expected, the SPF response of the salts was highly dependent on pH, and assays of these compounds diluted with water alone were not reproducible. Excitation and emission spectra and standard curves for 4-aminobiphenyl, 1-naphthylamine, 2-naphthylamine, and their HCl salts are presented in Figures 22 to 24.

The choice of 0.01 N HCl as the solvent for administering 4-aminobiphenyl·HCl to the animals via their drinking water was based on results from stability studies presented in Table 17. Aqueous solutions containing 1.0 and 100 ppm of the salt diminished in concentration by about 72 and 43%, respectively, during the 16 day simulated test, whereas similar solutions in 0.01 N HCl diminished only 5% at the 1.0 ppm level and were essentially unchanged at 100 ppm. The high accuracy and precision of the results obtained with 0.01 N HCl solutions of 4-aminobiphenyl·HCl illustrate the utility of the method for obtaining rapid and reliable assays of the potable water formulations for use in animal experiments. Tests with other aqueous solutions [0.3% NaCl-HCl (0.5 N NaCl, 0.01 N HCl, pH 2) and 0.9% NaCl-HCl (0.15 N NaCl, 0.01 N HCl, pH 2)] of 4-aminobiphenyl salt yielded about the same stabilizing effects as 0.01 N HCl; however, they were not as palatable to the animals.

Results from assays of the two microbiological growth media are presented in Table 18. Recoveries from samples spiked with 0.10 and 1.0 ppm of 4-aminobiphenyl and its salt were 81 to 95%. However, low recoveries (44 to 85%) were obtained for 2-naphthylamine and its salt. The background fluorescence of unspiked media was 20 to 30 ppb. Data from wastewater collected from the decontamination of control animal cages (total solids content and pH were 217 ppm and 7.33, respectively) unspiked and spiked with 20 ppb of the two amines and their salts are presented in Table 19. Recoveries averaged 89%, precision was excellent, and the background of unspiked samples was 0.2 to 0.3 ppb. The method has been used successively for evaluating the performance of a laboratory-scale adsorber system similar to that described by Nony et al [53] that is required for the cleanup of 4-aminobiphenyl-containing wastewater prior to discharging it into the environment (see Section II.G).

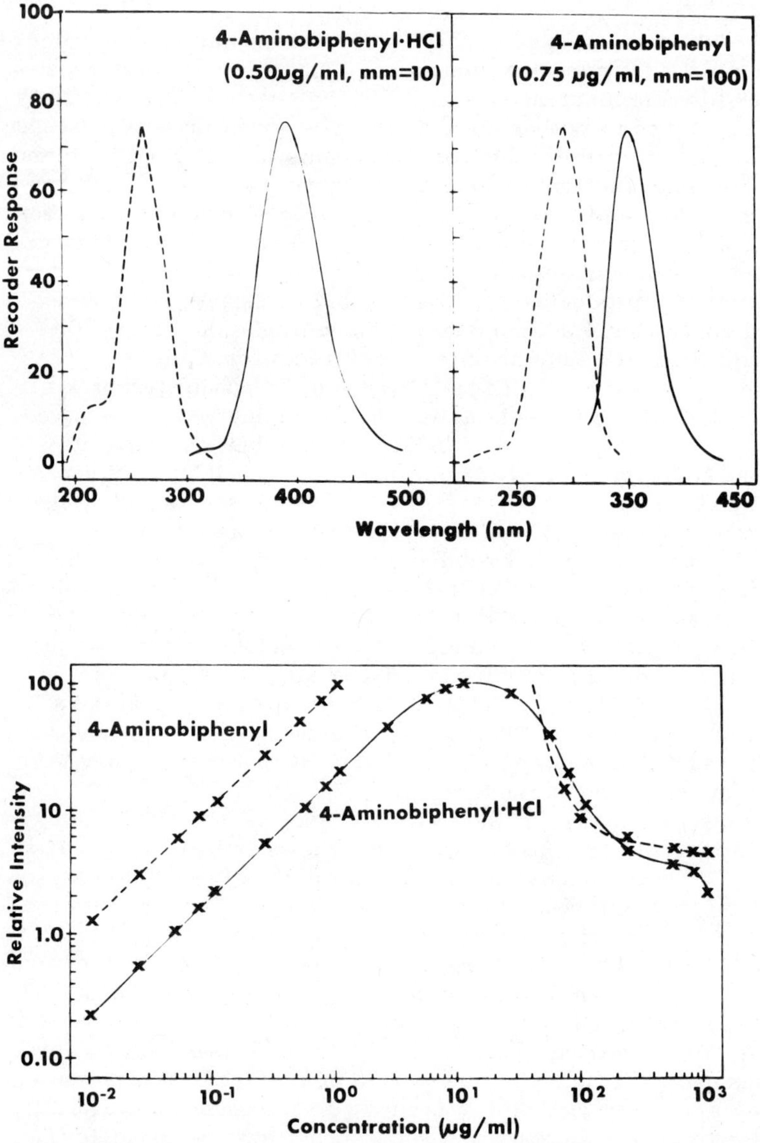

Figure 22 Top: Excitation (dashed line) and emission (solid line) spectra of 4-aminobiphenyl and its HCl salt. Bottom: Standard curves of 4-aminobiphenyl and its HCl salt in methanol and 0.01 N aqueous HCl, respectively. (From Ref. 43.)

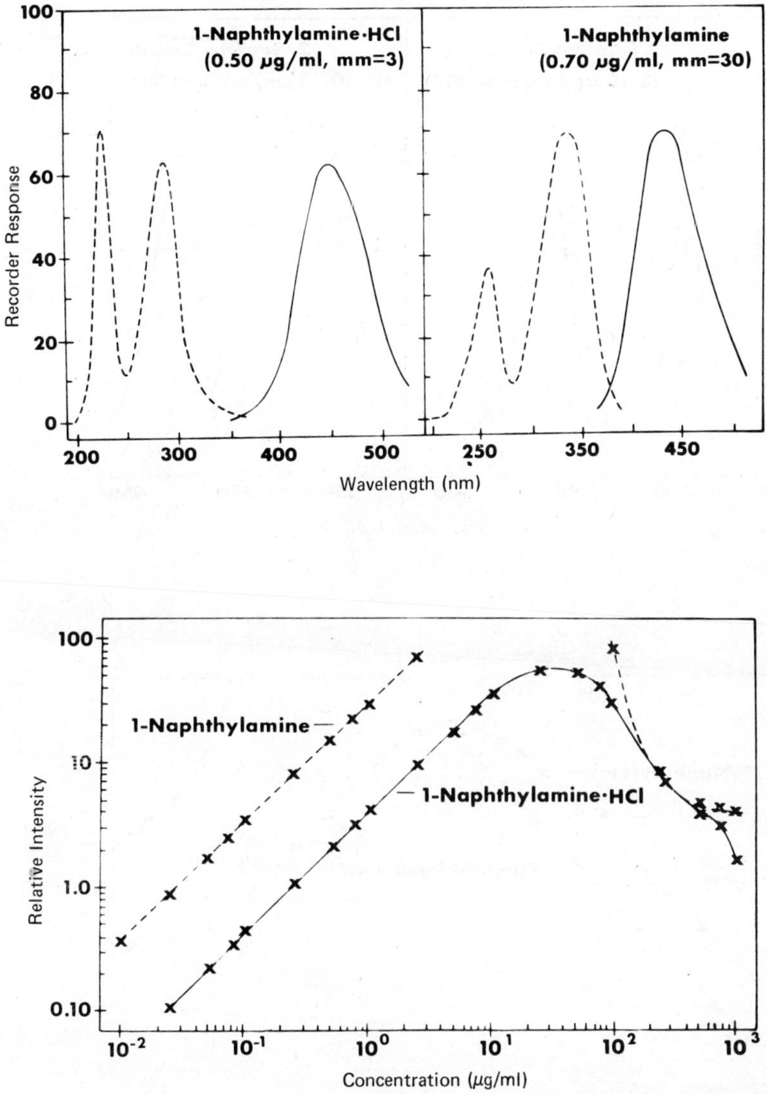

Figure 23 Top: Excitation (dashed line) and Emission (solid line) spectra of 1-naphthylamine and its HCl salt. Bottom: Standard curves of 1-naphthylamine and its HCl salt in methanol and 0.01 N aqueous HCl, respectively. (From Ref. 43.)

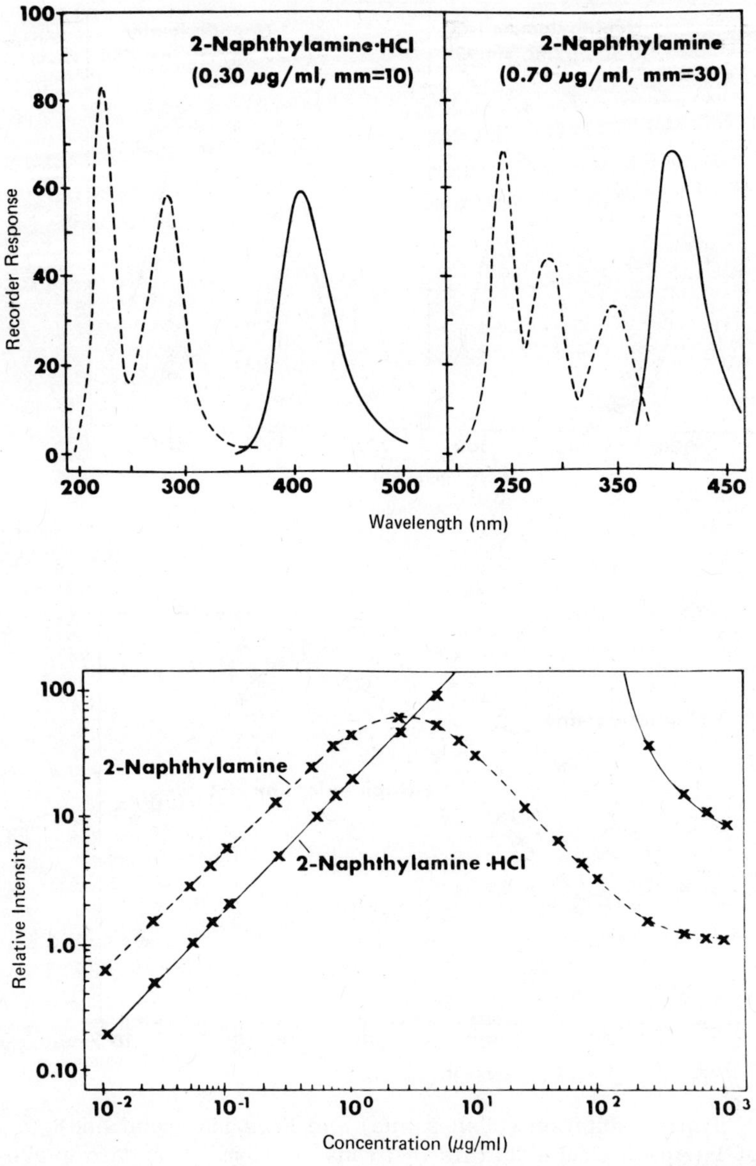

Figure 24 Top: Excitation (dashed line) and emission (solid line) spectra of 2-naphthylamine and its HCl salt. Bottom: Standard curves of 2-naphthylamine and its HCl salt in methanol and 0.01 N aqueous HCl, respectively. (From Ref. 43.)

Table 17 Stability of Aqueous Solutions of 4-Aminobiphenyl·HCl After Exposure to Stimulated Test Conditions for 16 Days

Sampling interval (days)	Concentration and pH of solutions indicated[a]							
	1.0 ppm solution[b]		100 ppm solution[b]		1.0 ppm solution[c]		100 ppm solution[c]	
	ppm	pH	ppm	pH	ppm	pH	ppm	pH
0	0.989 ± 0.003	2.03 ± 0.01	98.9 ± 0.35	2.02 ± 0.01	1.01 ± 0.001	7.47 ± 0.01	93.3 ± 0.001	4.17 ± 0.01
1	0.973 ± 0.012	2.07 ± 0.01	99.2 ± 0.42	2.03 ± 0.01	0.781 ± 0.001	7.03 ± 0.02	79.7 ± 0.06	4.08 ± 0.06
2	0.968 ± 0.005	2.04 ± 0.02	97.9 ± 0.90	2.06 ± 0.01	0.649 ± 0.019	6.70 ± 0.02	73.5 ± 0.17	3.95 ± 0.06
4	0.976 ± 0.021	2.05 ± 0.02	98.6 ± 1.0	2.02 ± 0.03	0.459 ± 0.020	6.63 ± 0.04	60.4 ± 2.3	4.01 ± 0.01
8	0.950 ± 0.001	2.04 ± 0.03	98.3 ± 0.31	2.00 ± 0.01	0.365 ± 0.023	6.81 ± 0.02	62.4 ± 0.66	3.94 ± 0.08
16	0.936 ± 0.002	2.06 ± 0.01	98.9 ± 0.50	2.05 ± 0.02	0.282 ± 0.011	6.45 ± 0.04	57.4 ± 1.1	3.91 ± 0.06

[a]Mean and standard error from triplicate assays.
[b]Aqueous HCl solution (0.01 N, pH 2); samples adjusted for control.
[c]Deionized water solution; samples adjusted for control.
Source: Ref. 43.

Table 18 Analysis of Two Biological Growth Media Spiked with 4-Aminobiphenyl, 2-Naphthylamine, and Their Hydrochloride Salts at 0, 0.10, and 1.0 ppm

Compound	Medium[a]	Added[b]		Recovered ($\bar{x} \pm$ SE)[c]	
		ppm	μg	ppm	%
4-Aminobiphenyl	BHI	0	0	0.031 ± 0.001	-
		0.10	1.0	0.086 ± 0.001	86 ± 1.0
		1.00	10.0	0.948 ± 0.033	94.8 ± 3.3
	TSD	0	0	0.024 ± 0.001	-
		0.10	1.0	0.081 ± 0.002	81 ± 2.0
		1.00	10.0	0.810 ± 0.006	81 ± 0.6
4-Aminobiphenyl·HCl	BHI	0	0	0.031 ± 0.001	-
		0.10	1.0	0.087 ± 0.001	87 ± 1.0
		1.00	10.0	0.855 ± 0.014	85.5 ± 1.4
	TSD	0	0	0.024 ± 0.001	-
		0.10	1.0	0.090 ± 0.003	90 ± 3.0
		1.00	10.0	0.908 ± 0.010	90.8 ± 1.0
2-Naphthylamine	BHI	0	0	0.015 ± 0.001	-
		0.10	1.0	0.070 ± 0.005	70 ± 5.0
		1.00	10.0	0.853 ± 0.030	85.3 ± 3.0
	TSD	0	0	0.018 ± 0.00	-
		0.10	1.0	0.051 ± 0.006	51 ± 6.0
		1.00	10.0	0.712 ± 0.035	71.2 ± 3.5
2-Naphthylamine.HCl	BHI	0	0	0.015 ± 0.001	-
		0.10	1.0	0.053 ± 0.001	53 ± 1.0
		1.00	10.0	0.701 ± 0.002	70.1 ± 0.2
	TSD	0	0	0.018 ± 0.00	-
		0.10	1.0	0.044 ± 0.007	44 ± 7.0
		1.00	10.0	0.646 ± 0.003	64.6 ± 0.3

[a]BHI, brain heart infusion; TSD, trypticase soy dextrose.
[b]Per 10 ml of sample.
[c]Mean and standard error from triplicate assays; spiked samples are corrected for controls. Methanol solutions from controls and 0.10 ppm samples for SPF readings contained an equivalent of 1.0 g of medium/ml; the 1.0 ppm samples contained 0.2 g.
Source: Ref. 43.

Table 19 Analysis of Wastewater Spiked with 4-Aminobiphenyl, 2-Naphthylamine, and Their Hydrochloride Salts at 0 and 20 ppb

	Added[a]		Recovered ($\bar{x}$ ± SE)[b]	
Compound	ppb	μg	ppb	%
4-Aminobiphenyl	0	0	0.3 ± 0.00	-
	20	2.0	19 ± 0.00	95
4-Aminobiphenyl·HCl	0	0	0.3 ± 0.00	-
	20	2.0	18 ± 0.00	90
2-Naphthylamine	0	0	0.2 ± 0.00	-
	20	2.0	18 ± 0.00	90
2-Naphthylamine·HCl	0	0	0.2 ± 0.00	-
	20	2.0	16 ± 0.00	80

[a]Per 100 ml of sample.
[b]Mean and standard error from triplicate assays; spiked samples are corrected for controls. Methanol solutions for SPF readings contained an equivalent of 10 g of water sample/ml.
Source: Ref. 43.

Whole mouse blood unspiked or spiked with 2.0 ppm of the two amines and their salts were assayed without hydrolysis or after alkaline or acid hydrolysis; results of these tests are presented in Table 20. Acid hydrolysis yielded the best recoveries (namely, 62 to 76%) and is therefore considered the method of choice; under these conditions the background fluorescence of unspiked samples was about 0.03 ppm.

Data from human urine unspiked and spiked with 20 ppb of the amines and salts are presented in Table 21. Better recoveries of the free amines were obtained without hydrolysis than by utilizing an alkaline hydrolysis step. On the other hand, alkaline hydrolysis enhanced recoveries of the salts; the reason for this behavior is not known. Acid hydrolysis of the urine was also performed; however, formation of a purple-colored product in both control and spiked samples prevented the assay by SPF.

Water solubilities of the two aromatic amines and their salts were required before analytical method development or formulation of spiked animal drinking water could be undertaken; however, these values could not be found in the literature. Results of our solubility tests, determined as described by Bowman and King [6] analyzed via SPF, were as given in Table 22.

Table 20 Analysis of Whole Mouse Blood (Heparinized) Spiked with 4-Aminobiphenyl, 2-Naphthylamine, and Their Hydrochloride Salts at 0 and 2.0 ppm

Compound	Hydrolysis	Added[a] ppm	Added[a] μg	Recovered ($\bar{x}$ ± SE)[b] ppm	Recovered ($\bar{x}$ ± SE)[b] %
4-Aminobiphenyl	None	0	0	0.022 ± 0.007	-
		2.0	2.0	0.206 ± 0.063	10 ± 3
	Alkaline	0	0	0.048 ± 0.001	-
		2.0	2.0	0.727 ± 0.081	36 ± 4
	Acid	0	0	0.034 ± 0.008	-
		2.0	2.0	1.51 ± 0.01	76 ± 0.5
4-Aminobiphenyl· HCl	None	0	0	0.022 ± 0.007	-
		2.0	2.0	0.115 ± 0.007	6 ± 0.4
	Alkaline	0	0	0.048 ± 0.001	-
		2.0	2.0	0.542 ± 0.020	27 ± 1
	Acid	0	0	0.034 ± 0.008	-
		2.0	2.0	1.23 ± 0.11	62 ± 6
2-Naphthylamine	None	0	0	0.021 ± 0.001	-
		2.0	2.0	0.088 ± 0.010	4.4 ± 0.5
	Alkaline	0	0	0.039 ± 0.004	-
		2.0	2.0	0.482 ± 0.046	24.1 ± 2.3
	Acid	0	0	0.027 ± 0.002	-
		2.0	2.0	1.37 ± 0.08	68.5 ± 4.2
2-Naphthylamine· HCl	None	0	0	0.021 ± 0.001	-
		2.0	2.0	0.160 ± 0.012	8 ± 0.6
	Alkaline	0	0	0.039 ± 0.004	-
		2.0	2.0	0.332 ± 0.034	16.6 ± 1.7
	Acid	0	0	0.027 ± 0.002	-
		2.0	2.0	1.51 ± 0.03	75.3 ± 1.3

[a]Per milliliter of sample.
[b]Mean and standard error from triplicate assays; methanol solutions of control and spiked samples for SPF readings contained an equivalent of 200 and 20 mg blood/ml, respectively. Spiked samples are corrected for controls.
Source: Ref. 43.

Table 21 Analysis of Human Urine Spiked with 4-Aminobiphenyl, 2-Naphthylamine, and Their Hydrochloride Salts at 0 and 20 ppb

		Added[a]		Recovered ($\bar{x}$ ± SE)[b]	
Compound	Hydrolysis	ppb	μg	ppb	%
4-Aminobiphenyl	None	0	0	0.008 ± 0.001	-
		20	2.0	0.019 ± 0.001	95 ± 1
	Alkaline	0	0	0.002 ± 0.000	-
		20	2.0	0.012 ± 0.000	60 ± 0
4-Aminobiphenyl·HCl	None	0	0	0.008 ± 0.001	-
		20	2.0	0.009 ± 0.001	45 ± 1
	Alkaline	0	0	0.002 ± 0.000	-
		20	2.0	0.011 ± 0.000	55 ± 0
2-Naphthylamine	None	0	0	0.003 ± 0.000	-
		20	2.0	0.016 ± 0.001	80 ± 1
	Alkaline	0	0	0.001 ± 0.000	-
		20	2.0	0.013 ± 0.001	65 ± 1
2-Naphthylamine·HCl	None	0	0	0.003 ± 0.000	-
		20	2.0	0.010 ± 0.001	50 ± 1
		0	0	0.001 ± 0.000	-
		20	2.0	0.015 ± 0.001	75 ± 1

[a]Per 100 ml of sample.
[b]Mean and standard error of triplicate assays; spiked samples are corrected for controls. Methanol solutions of control and spiked samples for SPF readings contained an equivalent of 10 g of urine/ml. Development of interferences upon acid hydrolysis of unspiked urine prevented the assay via SPF.
Source: Ref. 43.

Table 22 Solubility Test Results Analyzed by SPF

Compound	Solubility in water (mg/ml) at 25 ± 2°)
4-Aminobiphenyl	0.18
4-Aminobiphenyl·HCl	4.14
2-Naphthylamine	0.22
2-Naphthylamine·HCl	26.1

Source: Ref. 43.

Table 23 TLC R_f Values of the Carcinogens 4-Aminobiphenyl and 2-Naphthylamine, and Four Analogs in 10 Solvent Systems

Solvent system (v/v)	R_f values (× 100) of compound indicated					
	4-Amino-biphenyl	3-Amino-biphenyl	2-Amino biphenyl	Biphenyl	1-Naphthyl-amine	2-Naphthyl-amine
Chloroform	31	38	57	83	34	31
Chloroform-ethyl acetate (9:1)	58	61	79	94	61	57
Chloroform-diethyl ether (9:1)	58	62	83	97	62	57
Chloroform-acetone (9:1)	68	70	88	100	71	65
Chloroform-methanol (9:1)	90	90	96	100	90	85
Benzene	13	12	24	73	16	13
Benzene-ethyl acetate (9:1)	29	33	52	72	36	29
Benzene-diethyl ether (9:1)	30	33	56	77	36	29
Benzene-acetone (9:1)	43	46	65	75	47	41
Benzene-methanol (9:1)	62	63	73	78	63	58

Source: Ref. 43.

Table 24 Partition Values for the Carcinogens 4-Aminobiphenyl and 2-Naphthylamine, and Four Analogs in Seven Solvent Systems

	p Value[a]					
Solvent system	Biphenyl	2-Amino-biphenyl	3-Amino-biphenyl	4-Amino-biphenyl	1-Naphthyl-amine	2-Naphthyl-amine
Hexane-acetonitrile	0.38	0.11	0.03	0.24	0.08	0.03
Hexane-80% acetone (20% water)	0.90	0.73	0.53	0.51	0.48	0.44
Chloroform-water	0.98	1.0	1.0	1.0	1.0	1.0
Chloroform-60% methanol	1.0	1.0	0.98	0.99	0.95	0.94
Chloroform-aqueous NaOH						
(5.0 N)	-	1.0	1.0	1.0	1.0	1.0
(0.5 N)	-	1.0	1.0	1.0	1.0	1.0
(0.05 N)	-	1.0	1.0	1.0	1.0	1.0
Chloroform-aqueous HCl						
(5.0 N)	-	0.03	0.01	0.01	0.00	0.00
(0.5 N)	-	0.47	0.10	0.10	0.03	0.02
(0.05 N)	-	0.96	0.82	0.81	0.57	0.42
Hexane-dimethyl-formamide	0.21	0.04	-	0.01	-	-

[a]Fractional amount of solute partitioning into the nonpolar phase of an equivolume immiscible binary solvent system.
Source: Ref. 43.

Table 25 Analysis of 1- and 2-Naphthylamine and Their HCl Salts in Admixture by Using Simultaneous Equations

Added (μg/ml)		Found (calculated μg/ml)	
1-Naphthylamine	2-Naphthylamine	1-Naphthylamine	2-Naphthylamine
	Free Amines[a]		
0.50	0.50	0.49	0.50
0.50	0.10	0.49	0.11
1.00	0.10	1.00	0.09
2.00	0.10	1.90	0.08
0.50	0.01	0.48	0.02
	HCl Salts[b]		
1.00	1.00	1.00	0.97
0.50	0.10	0.48	0.11
1.00	0.10	1.00	0.09
2.00	0.10	1.90	0.08
5.00	0.10	4.70	0.06

[a]In methanol.
[b]In 0.01 N aqueous HCl.
Source: Ref. 43.

TLC Rf values for the aromatic amines (biphenyl was used as a reference compound) in 10 solvent systems are reported in Table 23. Anthracene may be substituted for biphenyl as the reference compound since their R_f values were identical in all of the systems tested. These data are useful in the development of cleanup procedures and for the separation and identification of the compounds in mixtures. Any two of the compounds tested may be separated from each other by choosing the appropriate solvent system. Aqueous solutions of the salts spotted and developed, as described, gave R_f values identical to those of the free amines.

Partition values are useful in developing extraction and cleanup methods and for confirmatory tests [16,18]. The p values for the compounds of interest were therefore determined via FID-GC, and the results are presented in Table 24. It is interesting to note that in the chloroform-aqueous NaOH systems, all normalities of NaOH tested (0.05 to 5.0 N) yielded p values of 1.0. On the other hand, with chloroform-aqueous HCl, 0.5 N HCl was not sufficient to partition the amines (as their HCl salts) completely into the aqueous phase; however, the use of 5.0 N HCl increased the partitioning efficiency and yielded p values no higher than 0.03.

Since 1-naphthylamine has been of commercial importance and it has been known to be contaminated with the carcinogen 2-naphthylamine, we investigated the possibility of assaying mixtures of the free amines or their salts via SPF using simultaneous equations. Results obtained for various mixtures of the compounds are presented in Table 25. At approximately equal concentrations, the results are quite good and are acceptable up to a ratio of 20:1 of the 1- and 2-substituted isomers; one part of 2-naphthylamine was detectable in 50 parts of 1-naphthylamine, but it could not be accurately quantified at that level.

F. 2,4-Diaminotoluene (2,4-TDA) and 2,6-Diaminotoluene (2,6-TDA) [54]

General description of method

A spectrophotofluorometric (SPF) method is described for the analysis of diaminotoluenes (TDA) in flexible polyurethane foams at the 1 ppm concentration level. Salient elements of the method are extraction of TDA with methanol, separation of the amines by thin layer chromatography (TLC), and SPF assay employing the Fluram reagent. Additional information is provided concerning structure verification of the Fluram adducts of 2,4-TDA by mass spectrometry and the use of this method for the assay of amines in urethane products derived from isocyanates other than the toluene diisocyanates (TDI).

Introduction

The inclusion of 2,4-diaminotoluene (2,4-TDA) in the list of potential carcinogens [55] published by the National Institute for Occupational Safety and Health (NIOSH) was the result of a number of toxicological studies [56-61] conducted during the past 40 years. In addition, the amine content of polyurethane foams is important in studies related to color stability, humid aging resistance, and other physical properties. Polyurethane foams are often used in warm, humid environments where loss of properties through hydrolysis is of concern. Since these foams are derived from the TDI, they would be expected to contain small quantities of the corresponding TDA compounds.

The most sensitive method for TDA in urethane foams involved mass spectrometric analysis of extracts with a detection level of 1000 ppm. Because severely degraded foams contained less than this amount, a more sensitive method was sought. Campbell et al. [62] used the relative NCO and NH infrared absorptions to follow hydrolysis of TDI ureas during development of humid age compression set. Tompa [63] used infrared spectroscopy to study cracking of solid urethanes caused by reaction of carbon dioxide with free isocyanate. Wilson [64] has improved the color stability of foams by derivatizing free amines. In *Analytical Chemistry of the Polyurethanes* [65], the only amine method cited by David and Staley was the colorimetric method of Guenchev and Atanasov [66]. There is a potentiometric method for amines in polyurethanes [67,68], and TDA methods using gas chromatography [69,70], paper and thin layer chromatography [71-74], and NMR [75]. However, none of these methods was sensitive enough for the authors' [54] purpose.

Recently, Rinde and Troll [76] reported a colorimetric amine assay in the nanomole range, based on the Fluram reagent introduced by Udenfriend [77]. Amines in water or body fluids were separated by thin layer chromatography (TLC) and assayed on the plate as stable, yellow derivatives. They did not study the TDA compounds; however, a TLC method was used by Kottemann [74] to identify these compounds and other aromatic amines at high concentrations in hair dyes. The following procedure combines TLC and SPF analysis for ppm levels of TDA in urethane foams.

Experimental

Test Chemicals and Reagents. The 2,4- and 2,6-TDA were obtained from Eastman and Aldrich, respectively, and were used without further purification. The Fluram reagent was purchased from the American Instrument Co., Silver Spring, Maryland. Methanol and acetone were Baker reagent grade solvents.

Extraction of Samples. A 1 to 2 g sample of a typical foam (1 to 250 ppm of TDA), weighed to the nearest milligram, is immersed in 75 ml of methanol contained in a 250 ml beaker and soaked for 5 min with occasional compression. The methanol extract is decanted and the foam is compressed to express as much methanol as possible. The extraction is repeated twice by using 75 ml portions of methanol. The combined extracts are concentrated, typically, to 25 ml for TLC; however, further dilution or concentration may be required if the TDA concentration is too high or too low.

Thin Layer Chromatography. Standard solutions of 2,4- and 2,6-TDA are prepared in methanol containing 2, 4, 8, 12, 16, and 20 μg/ml and 20 μl of each standard are spotted at six positions 3 cm from the bottom of the TLC plate. The foam extract is spotted at the seventh position. After drying, the plate is placed in a developing tank that contains 120 ml of chloroform, 33 ml of ethyl acetate, 20 ml of ethanol, and 7 ml of glacial acetic acid. Development is complete in about 1 hr when the solvent front has migrated 15 cm. The plate is dried in a horizontal position for 5 to 10 min and sprayed uniformly with a 0.015% solution of Fluram in acetone. The compounds are visualized by employing a long-wavelength, hand-held, UV light and the sides of the plate are marked in preparation for fluorescent scanning.

SPF Assay. The marked TLC plate is placed in a thin film chromatographic scanner (Model J4-8427), an accessory to an Aminco-Bowman Spectrophotofluorometer equipped with a photomultiplier microphotometer (Model J10-280) and a strip chart recorder with a 10 mv full-scale output. The plate position is adjusted so that the visible light spot produced when setting the excitation wavelength at 500 nm is in position to scan across the line of TDA spots. After closing the cover of the scanner and setting the excitation and emission wavelengths at 390 and 500 nm, respectively, the plate is scanned starting with the standard of highest concentration. Instability of the Fluram adducts places a time limit of 1 hr for scanning a plate after development.

Calculation of Data. A calibration curve is constructed on linear graph paper by plotting the peak heights of the standards versus concentration (μg/ml) and is used to determine the concentration of TDA in the foam sample extract. To express this value as ppm in the original foam sample, the following equation is used:

$$\text{TDA in foam (ppm)} = \frac{\text{TDA in extract } (\mu\text{g/ml}) \times \text{extract volume (ml)}}{\text{foam sample weight (g)}}$$

Results and discussion

Various techniques for the extraction of TDA from foams were evaluated, including Soxhlet extraction, extraction of foam cubes in the barrel of a 30 ml syringe using cold methanol and tetrahydrofuran; however, methanol was the solvent of choice used as described. In an extraction study using a hydrophilic polyether foam, extraction with water at 60° resulted in a 2,4-TDA concentration of 5.3 ppm; Soxhlet extraction with methanol for 1 hr gave 20 ± 6 ppm; manual extraction with cold methanol (as described) produced 20 ± 3 ppm; and tetroahydrofuran extraction resulted in 7 ppm for the manual method and 12 ppm for the syringe method. Since the TDA content may vary considerably in the same foam depending on the site of sampling, it would be premature to conclude that one type of foam inherently contains more TDA or a different isomer distribution than another. This nonuniform characteristic of foams was determined by assaying sample extracts in duplicate at the 10 to 15 ppm level. The precision, usually ±10% for a given extract, was ±30% for the six different samples of the same foam.

The identity of the TDA was established by comparison of R_f values versus TDA standards from the same TLC plate. The R_f values for 2,4-TDA and 2,6-TDA are about 0.25 and 0.40, respectively. An AEI model MS-12 mass spectrometer was used to confirm the identity of TDA sample extracts versus TDA standards. Scrapings from TLC plates were placed in the solids probe for analysis; identical mass spectra were obtained.

The method described was used to assay 11 commercial polyurethane foams of both hydrophilic and hydrophobic polyether and polyester types. The 2,4-TDA isomer content ranged from 6 to 442 ppm and the 2,6-TDA isomer, found only in 3 of the 11 foams, ranged from 8 to 80 ppm. The presence or absence of 2,6-TDA depends somewhat on mixing conditions and maximum foam temperature during the manufacturing process.

This method has also been used to assay the following amines in urethane products derived from isocyanates other than the TDI: bis(4-aminophenyl)methane (MDA) and the aliphatic amines bis(4-aminocyclohexyl)methane (reduced MDA) and isophorone diamine. Since the intensity of fluorescence of reduced MDA precludes assay at less than 100 ppm by the method described, larger foam samples would be required. Occasional interferences are encountered by the presence of polymeric amines, diethylenetriamine, 4,4'-diaminodiphenylurea, and other amino contaminants; nevertheless, an experienced analyst can recognize these by their shape, intensity, and position on the TLC plate. Polymeric amines usually remain at the origin. Adjustments in the composition of the developing solvents can usually correct poor separations.

G. Removal of Test Substances from Wastewater [53]

Introduction

It has been reported that the national goal for the control of water pollution is the elimination of pollutant discharge into navigable waters by the year 1985 [78]. In complying with the Federal Water Pollution Control Act amendments of 1972 (Public Law 92-500), industry often finds that it is more economical to treat wastewater for reuse than for discharge into the environment. Of the various processes available for the treatment of wastewater, the most promising are chemical treatment, filtration, activated carbon, and microscreening [79]. Peacock [80] concluded that physical chemical processes consisting of chemical flocculation, filtration, and granular activated carbon could replace conventional biological processes, especially when upsets from toxic chemicals could be anticipated.

The NCTR is engaged in long-term, low-dose feeding studies of known carcinogens [2-acetylaminofluorene (2-AAF) was our first test substance] and of potential carcinogens in mice and other experimental animals. In such studies, residues of the carcinogens are introduced into our wastewater primarily through the cleaning procedures used for decontaminating the animal cages, feeders, and containers used to prepare and store the toxicant-treated diets. Therefore, the objective of our wastewater cleanup is the total removal of any deleterious residues, thereby rendering the water safe for recycle or direct discharge into the environment.

The size of the complex of laboratories and ancillary functions places the NCTR in the small-to-medium category with regard to the magnitude of its wastewater program. When all programs become operational, about 500,000 gal of wastewater will be discharged daily. Prior to the development of our present wastewater treatment at NCTR, carcinogen-containing wastewater was isolated from other water and held in tanks pending the development of an acceptable means of removing the residues (2-AAF). However, to evaluate the effectiveness of any proposed cleanup system for wastewater, it was first necessary to develop a highly sensitive chemical procedure for the analysis of traces of the contaminant in wastewater. Since sub-ppb (ng/g) sensitivity was sought, special emphasis was also placed on the confirmation of the identity of trace amounts of the carcinogen. The following experiments describe what ultimately led to a workable means of cleaning up wastewater contaminated with traces of carcinogens [53].

Experimental

Analysis of 2-Acetylaminofluorene (2-AAF) in Wastewater. The following method for determining traces of 2-AAF was developed for use in evaluating the behavior of such residues in several experiments proposed for cleaning up contaminated wastewater.

Residues of 2-AAF and/or its hydrolysis product, 2-aminofluorene (2-AF), were assayed by a modification of the procedure of Bowman and King [6]. The sample (250 ml) in a 500 ml separatory funnel containing 2 g of sodium chloride and 1 ml of 10 N sodium hydroxide was extracted twice with 25 ml portions of chloroform, which were successively percolated through a plug of sodium sulfate (15 mm diam × 10 mm thick) and collected in a 100 ml glass-stoppered flask containing a boiling bead and 1 drop of diethylene glycol as a keeper. The contents were evaporated to near dryness under water pump vacuum at 60° and quantitatively transferred to a culture tube (20 × 150 mm, sealed with a Teflon-lined cap) by using three 2 ml portions of chloroform. The contents were evaporated to near dryness with a jet of dry air and finally to dryness with water pump vacuum and a 60° water bath. Hydrolysis of 2-AAF to 2-AF was then accomplished by adding 4 ml of methanol and 2 ml of concentrated HCl to the dry residue and heating it in the sealed tube at 85° for 2 hr using a tube heater (Kontes No. 720,000). After the tube had cooled, 3 ml of distilled water was added and the contents extracted twice with 7 ml portions of benzene; each portion of benzene was carefully withdrawn and discarded by using a 10 ml syringe and cannula. Next, 4 ml of 10 N sodium hydroxide was added and the contents extracted three times with 7 ml portions of benzene. Each portion was successively percolated through a plug of sodium sulfate (15 mm diam × 10 mm thick) and collected in a 50 ml glass-stoppered flask containing a boiling bead and 1 drop of keeper. The contents were evaporated just to dryness under water pump vacuum at 60° as described and the residue dissolved in 10 ml of methanol for subsequent spectrophotofluorescent (SPF) analysis.

An Aminco-Bowman instrument (American Instrument Co., Silver Spring, Maryland) equipped with a xenon lamp and a 1P28 detector was used with 1 cm cells and a 2-2-2 mm slit program to measure the fluorescence of the 2-AF (λ_{Ex} = 297 nm; λ_{Em} = 366 nm). Samples of water known to be free of carcinogens were carried through the entire procedure and used for correcting the analytical results. Since residues of 2-AAF are analyzed as 2-AF, the analytical results are multiplied by a factor of 1.23 to express them as 2-AAF. Recoveries of 2-AAF from water spiked at the 10 ppb level averaged about 80%; the analytical data are corrected for both background and recovery. Based on twice the background fluorescence, the sensitivity of the method to 2-AAF (assayed as 2-AF) is 0.2 ppb. The identity of 2-AAF and/or 2-AF residues in wastewater at levels as low as 0.2 ppb may be easily confirmed by comparing the excitation and emission maxima of the unknown sample with those for 2-AF. The analytical method detects combined residues of 2-AF and 2-AAF; since no residues of 2-AF have been found in the wastewater, all results are expressed as 2-AAF. The individual residues may be analyzed as described by Bowman and King [6].

Evaluation of Cleanup Procedures for Wastewater. Several possible approaches to cleaning up the wastewater were investigated in the laboratory; they include Millipore filtration, distillation, organic solvent extraction, alkaline hydrolysis, and carbon and nonionic polymeric adsorption. In addition, information concerning the adsorption of 2-AAF from aqueous dispersions by the soil at NCTR was also sought.

Two distillation experiments were performed to investigate the effectiveness of the process as a cleanup procedure and to approximate the vapor pressure of 2-AAF. In the first experiment, 200 ml of distilled water containing 2 mg of solid 2-AAF (10 μg/ml) was distilled at 1 atm until 100 ml of distillate was collected; the distillate was assayed for 2-AAF content. The initial concentration of 2-AAF in the distilling flask (10 ppm) and subsequent levels were undoubtedly below the saturation level at 100°. Second, 100 ml of distilled water and 200 mg of solid 2-AAF were distilled until 80 ml of distillate was collected. The distillate was analyzed for 2-AAF and the equation of Rassow and Schultzky [81] was used to approximate the vapor pressure. The water in the distilling flask was observed to be supersaturated with 2-AAF during the entire distillation.

In laboratory evaluations of adsorbents for removing traces of 2-AAF from water, glass columns containing activated carbon (Witco Grade 718, 50 g, 20 mm diam × 280 mm thick) or a nonionic polymeric resin (Amberlite XAD-2, 70 g, 20 mm diam × 240 mm thick) supported by a plug of glass wool and topped by a plug of glass wool were each prewashed with 2 liters of distilled water. Fifteen liters of an aqueous dispersion of 2-AAF (5.0 ppm) was then separately percolated by gravity through each column; 1 liter fractions from the columns were analyzed for residues of 2-AAF.

A sample of alluvial silt soil of the type found in the oxidation and equalization ponds of the sewage treatment system at NCTR was used for laboratory tests to determine its ability to absorb 2-AAF residues from aqueous dispersion. Duplicate 250 ml beakers were prepared by adding the appropriate amount of soil to provide a layer 6.5 cm in diameter and about 1.7 cm thick in the bottom of each container. Deionized water (150 ml) was added to one container to serve as a control and aqueous 2-AAF (150 ml, 5.0 ppm) was added to the other. The aqueous layers over the soil were about 4.1 cm deep. Another beaker (soil absent) containing 150 ml of the aqueous 2-AAF was also prepared to monitor any change in concentration due to settling or adsorption of the 2-AAF by the container. Aliquots (10 ml) of the aqueous phases were withdrawn from the geometrical center of the supernatants after they had stood at 25° for 2 hr; then 3, 7, 14, 21, and 28 days later. The containers were tightly sealed with aluminum foil, except during the sampling process, to prevent evaporation of the water and possible "co-distillation" of the 2-AAF. Evaporation of the water could also cause the 2-AAF residue to precipitate. Each aliquot was assayed for 2-AAF content.

Evaluation of Pilot-Scale Wastewater Cleanup System. A pilot-scale cleanup system for removing 2-AAF residues was implemented by modifying an existing system of stainless steel tanks. A flow diagram of the system is presented in Figure 25 and the 15 components are designated by the letters A through O; reference to the individual components is made by using these designations. The carcinogen-containing wastewater, isolated from other wastewater, was stored in two 30,000-gal tanks (A and B). The tanks were piped in a manner to allow the wastewater to flow into one (A) and be withdrawn from the other (B). Liquid levels in each tank were equalized through interconnecting pipes. Wastewater was forced through the filtration and adsorption system by using a horizontal single-stage centrifugal pump (C) driven by a 3-hp motor; the pump was rated at 5 gal/min against a 72-ft head. The water was pumped through a series of coarse (D), medium (E), and fine (F) depth filtration filter elements (40, 25 and 5 μm, respectively) for clarification and then through the primary adsorber (G), which consisted of 25 lb of Witco Grade 718 granular carbon contained in a conventional water treatment tank. The

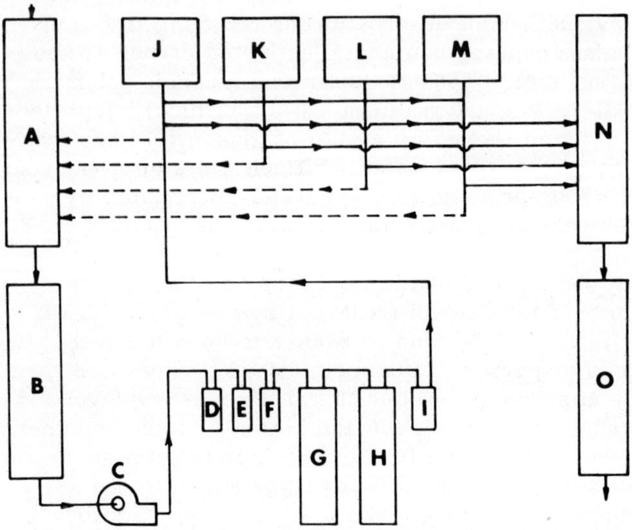

Figure 25 Flow diagram of pilot plant system for treating carcinogen-containing wastewater at NCTR, 1974. A and B, holding tanks for raw wastewater (30,000 gal each); C, centrifugal pump; D, E, and F, filters of 40, 25, and 5 μm, respectively; G, granular carbon (Witco Grade 718, 25 lb); H, polymeric resin (Amberlite XAD-2, 45 lb); I, membrane filter (99% retention of 0.45 μm particles); J, K, L, and M, holding tanks for cleaned-up wastewater (7,000 gal each); N and O, holding tanks for cleaned-up wastewater (30,000 gal each). (From Ref. 53.)

secondary adsorber (H) was located immediately downstream from the primary adsorber. It consisted of 45 lb of Amberlite XAD-2 nonionic polymer also contained in a conventional water treatment tank. This unit provided assurance that any 2-AAF residues penetrating the carbon adsorber would still be retained in the cleanup system. Finally, the water was passed through membrane filter (I). This filter (99% retention of 0.45 μm particles) was to retain any fine particles of the two adsorbents which might escape their respective tanks and carry adsorbed 2-AAF along with them. Treated water was stored in 5000-gal batches in the 7000-gal tanks (J, K, L, and M) pending the results of chemical analysis concerning the presence or absence of 2-AAF. These tanks were equipped with turbine mixers to allow representative sampling. Treated water found to contain 2-AAF is returned to tanks A and B for reprocessing. Water found to be free of 2-AAF is transferred to holding tanks (N and O) for reuse or discharge into the environment. The operation of the cleanup system was monitored by using a series of gauges and valves located in a manner that permitted the determination of pressure drop and 2-AAF concentration across any component of the system.

Results and discussion

Preliminary experiments with Millipore filtration (99% retention of particles 0.45 μm or larger) of actual wastewater (32.6 ppb of 2-AAF, pH 9.42) yielded a 40% cleanup, which presumably resulted from the removal of sludge which had sorbed a portion of the 2-AAF residue. Since the solubility of 2-AAF is about 7 ppm in water at 25° [6], filtration would not be expected to clean up the water effectively unless all of the residue had been irreversibly sorbed by the sludge. Moreover, the Millipore filtration concept proved unsatisfactory because the accumulation of sludge on the filter drastically reduced the rate of filtration. The experiment was repeated after the wastewater had been adjusted to a pH of 7.0 and essentially the same results were obtained.

The possibility of removing 2-AAF residues from the wastewater by organic solvent extraction was also investigated. After the wastewater was saturated with chloroform (about 1%, v/v), a single extraction of 100 ml of water by using 1 ml of chloroform removed 93% of the residue. The 1% solubility of chloroform in water is a decided disadvantage and makes this procedure impractical. A similar disadvantage would also be expected with other immiscible solvents of sufficient polarity to extract the 2-AAF from water.

Hydrolysis procedures such as 24-hr digestion (180°F) of wastewater previously adjusted to pH 11 with NaOH failed to destroy any of the 2-AAF. The compound is very difficult to hydrolyze, as is evidenced by the analytical procedure; such processes are not amenable to the decontamination of wastewater.

Results from distillation tests indicated that 2-AAF distills with water. Two hundred milliliters of water containing 10 ppm of 2-AAF (presumably in solution) yielded 1.3 μg (13 ppb) in the first 100 ml of distillate. In another test, 100 ml of water containing 2000 ppm of 2-AAF (supersaturated) contained 297 μg (3.71 ppm) in the first 80 ml of distillate. Results of this test were used to approximate the vapor pressure at 100° for 2-AAF at about 2.3×10^{-4} mm. Distillation, in addition to being inefficient, would be a slow process and its energy requirements are prohibitive.

In the laboratory tests, evaluating the effectiveness of adsorbents for removing 2-AAF residues from water by percolating 15 liters of aqueous 2-AAF (5.0 ppm) through them, residues (0.96 ppb) were found only in the 4 to 5 liter fraction from carbon. With XAD-2 resin, residues were detected only in the 3 to 5 and 12 to 14 liter fraction, which averaged 1.03 and 2.89 ppb, respectively. These few instances, where 2-AAF was found in the eluate, were believed to have resulted from small particles of the adsorbent being swept through channels in

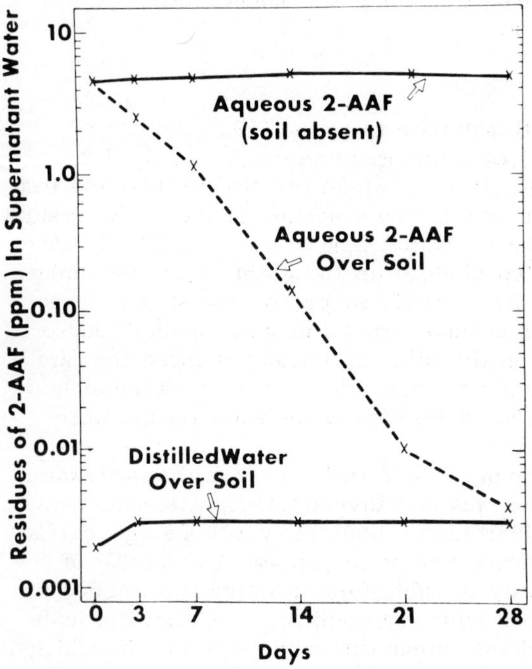

Figure 26 Adsorption of 2-AAF from an aqueous dispersion (5 ppm) by alluvial silt soil at NCTR. (From Ref. 53.)

the column; such difficulties could be overcome easily by using appropriate filters for the column effluent. There was no evidence that the adsorption capacity of either column for 2-AAF had been depleted, and both systems generally achieved a cleanup of 100,000-fold. Based on these data, a system consisting of filters and adsorption units was proposed for pilot-scale evaluation.

Results of tests to determine possible sorption of 2-AAF from aqueous dispersions by the alluvial silt soil at NCTR are illustrated in Figure 26. The concentration of the aqueous 2-AAF in the presence of soil declined from 5.0 to 0.004 ppm during the 28-day test period, while a portion of the same dispersion (soil absent) remained essentially unchanged. In the unlikely event that 2-AAF-containing wastewater accidentally escaped our cleanup and entered the sewage treatment process, none of the residues would be expected to be discharged from the NCTR. The 30 day journey through the sewage processing system would probably allow complete sorption of the residues by the soil.

Table 26 Residues of 2-AAF in Wastewater at Various Stages of the Pilot-Scale Cleanup Process

	Residues of 2-AAF (ppb)			
Wastewater processed (gal × 10^3)	Raw wastewater (untreated)[a]	After filtration	After filtration and carbon adsorption[b]	After filtration and carbon and resin adsorption[c]
0[d]	3.3	2.0	<0.2	<0.2
1	7.0	6.7	<0.2	<0.2
3	8.3	5.9	<0.2	<0.2
4	7.1	6.4	<0.2	<0.2
5	2.6	3.4	<0.2	<0.2
10	7.8	-	0.6	<0.2
18	8.5	-	1.2	<0.2
20	6.7	6.9	0.8	<0.2
30	7.5	-	<0.2	<0.2
35	3.2	-	<0.2	<0.2
40	3.8	-	<0.2	<0.2
45	3.0	-	<0.2	<0.2
50	4.3	-	1.1	<0.2
55	4.4	-	<0.2	<0.2
59	55.9	-	44.3	<0.2

[a]The pH ranged from 6.3 to 7.5; however, it was generally 7.0 ± 0.1.
[b]The carbon adsorber was replaced after 20,000, 30,000 and 50,000 gal were processed.
[c]No residues of 2-AAF were detected in any of the samples.
[d]Initial sample was taken after only a few gallons were processed.
Source: Ref. 53.

The pilot-scale cleanup system was evaluated by using 59,000 gal of 2-AAF-containing wastewater; results of the tests are presented in Table 26. Samples were collected across each major component of the system at 1000 gal intervals during the processing of the first 5000 gal. The depth filters were shown to have little or no effect on the residue levels of 2-AAF; therefore, routine monitoring of the water between the filters and the primary adsorber was discontinued. Nevertheless, the filters are considered necessary for the removal of suspended material that could accumulate in the adsorbers and cause a reduction of flow rate and/or deactivation of the adsorbents. No residues of 2-AAF penetrated either adsorber during the purification of the first 5000 gal. Slight penetration of 2-AAF residues through the carbon adsorber occurred during the processing of the next 5000 gal batch; nevertheless, only the depth filters were replaced at this point, and an additional 10,000 gal were processed in order to challenge the secondary adsorber. No residues penetrated the secondary adsorber during this treatment. The performance of the system indicated that the primary carbon adsorber should be changed after processing 10,000 gal of water, however, its longevity is undoubtedly related directly to the concentration of extraneous contaminants in the water. Therefore, after 20,000 gal of water had been processed, the carbon adsorber was replaced and another 10,000 gal processed. The effluents of both adsorbers were free of 2-AAF residues. At the 30,000 gal interval, the depth filters, carbon adsorber, and membrane filter were replaced and the water treatment process continued. No residues were detected in either adsorber effluent after 40,000 gal; the longevity of the carbon adsorber was again tested by subjecting it to an additional 10,000 gal of wastewater. At the 50,000 gal interval, 2-AAF residues had again penetrated the carbon but not the resin. The carbon adsorber was replaced and the treatment continued. As the holding tanks were being emptied (59,000 gal processed) residual sludge containing high levels of 2-AAF (e.g., 55 ppb) was inadvertently picked up from the bottom of the tank and introduced into the cleanup system. This caused high levels of 2-AAF (44 ppb) to penetrate the carbon adsorber; however, no residues passed the secondary adsorption unit. The pilot-scale evaluation was terminated when the supply of wastewater was essentially exhausted and sludge began to enter the system. Results of the evaluation are illustrated in Figure 27. No residues of 2-AAF (<0.2 ppb) were detected in the effluent of the secondary adsorber at any time during the tests. Flow rates of the wastewater through the cleanup system ranged from 0.8 to 1.7 gal/min with the pressure drop being greatest across the primary adsorber. The spent carbon adsorbent and filters removed from the system were destroyed by incineration at 900°. Contaminated XAD-2 resin may be incinerated or cleaned up by percolating acetone through it; the acetone effluent should be destroyed by incineration.

Future modifications of the cleanup system include the scaling up of the components to provide a higher capacity. This could be accomplished with several complete systems consisting of larger filters and adsorbers arranged in parallel. Each system would include two carbon adsorbers in tandem to protect the more costly polymeric resin. Once the upstream carbon unit becomes depleted, the second unit would be brought upstream and a new unit installed downstream. Fine-porosity depth filters should also be installed downstream from each adsorber to prevent particles of adsorbent from being carried from one unit to another and to protect the membrane filter.

Consideration was given to the recycling of the treated wastewater for use in the boilers and cooling tower at NCTR, and chemical analyses indicated that its quality was acceptable. However, microbiological assays of one of the treated samples revealed the presence

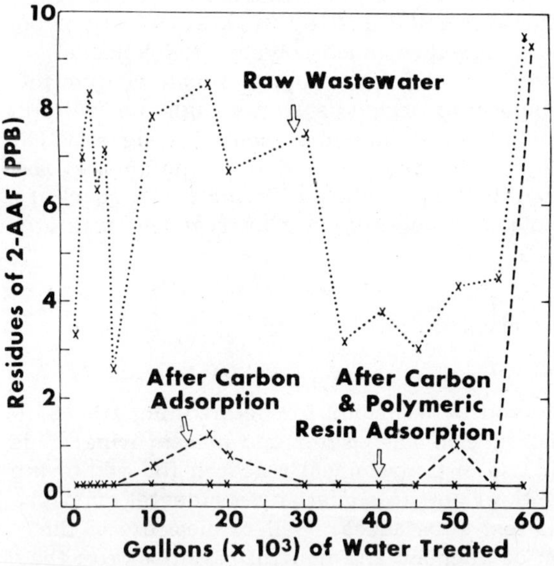

Figure 27 Residues of 2-AAF in raw wastewater (dotted line), after adsorption on activated carbon (dashed line), and finally on polymeric resin (solid line). Carbon adsorber was replaced after 20,000, 30,000, and 50,000 gal were treated. (From Ref. 53.)

of a variety of microorganisms that prevented its immediate reuse; chlorination would probably correct the deficiency.

In laboratory evaluations of the carbon and XAD-2 columns tested with wastewater as previously described, traces of all compounds tested thus far have been effectively removed by both adsorbents. These include 4-aminobiphenyl, benzidine, 3,3'-dimethylbenzidine, 3,3'-dimethoxybenzidine and 3,3'-dichlorobenzidine as free amines or HCl salts and 2-AAF, 2-AF, diethylstilbestrol, estradiol, lindane, and rotenone.

The pilot-scale cleanup system just described has functioned well for decontaminating relatively small volumes of wastewater, however, a system capable of processing much larger volumes of wastewater was required at the NCTR as toxicological testing was expanded. Such a high-capacity system, based on the principles of the pilot-scale cleanup, was designed and constructed; the total cost of the facility was about $1.5 million.

Other researchers [82] who face cleanup problems with relatively small volumes of contaminated wastewater are employing the basic principles described in our pilot-scale system.

It should be noted that any appreciable amounts of organic solvents present in the wastewater could destroy the adsorptivity of both the carbon and the XAD-2; therefore, such solvents are collected separately and destroyed by incineration. A possible alternative to separate collection and disposal of organic solvents might be found in the use of a new hydrophobic crystalline silica molecular sieve [83]. Although this product has not yet been evaluated by the author, the use of such a material is an attractive alternative for the removal of organic solvents of low molecular weights prior to treatment with other adsorbers.

H. Aromatic Amines in Admixture [84]

General description of method

A gas chromatographic method is described for determining traces of 11 aromatic amines in admixture in wastewater and human urine. This method was developed for use in toxicological research for monitoring the safe disposal of wastewater and to signal any accidental exposure of personnel to hazardous test substances. Salient elements of the procedure are: extraction of phenolic and neutral residues from the acidified sample, liquid-liquid partitioning cleanup and separation of neutral from phenolic residues at pH 14 and 10.2, acid hydrolysis of the neutral component, subsequent alkalinization of the sample and extraction of the basic residues as the free amines, conversion of selected residues to the corresponding pentafluoropropionyl (PFP) derivatives, and quantification by electron capture gas chromatography. Residues were detectable in wastewater and urine at the 0.1 and 1 ppb levels, respectively. Additional information is provided concerning partition values for all PFP derivatives in five solvent systems, structure verification of the derivatives by mass spectrometry, and the adaptation of this method to the monitoring of surfaces and air in potentially contaminated work areas.

Introduction

Two important factors relating to the control of test substances in nonclinical laboratory studies as proposed by the U.S. Department of Health and Human Services, Food and Drug Administration [85], are:

1. To provide assurance that personnel and work areas remain free of contamination by the substances.
2. To accomplish the safe disposal of contaminated experimental material.

Since long-term, low-dose toxicological studies with large numbers of mice at our laboratory include tests with several chemicals known to cause, or suspected of causing cancer in humans by occupational exposure [31,32,86], every effort must be made to ensure zero exposure of personnel to carcinogens by periodically monitoring samples of urine by using the most sensitive and specific analytical methods available [6,29,40,43]. In a similar manner, these methods are also used routinely to monitor wastewater that has been treated for the removal of test chemicals [53] prior to sewage treatment and eventual discharge into the environment. Methods based on spectrophotofluorescence (SPF), high-pressure liquid chromatography (HPLC), or electron capture gas chromatography (EC-GC) have served us well in determining traces [low or sub-ppb (ng/ml)] of a few chemicals analyzed separately. However, as the number of test compounds increases, such methods fail to detect, identify, and quantify all of the substrates when they are present in admixture [87]. It therefore became necessary to devise a procedure capable of simultaneously analyzing for traces of the substances of current interest at our laboratory. Formulas of these compounds, some of their analogs, and their abbreviations used in this presentation are described in Figure 28.

All of the compounds shown in Figure 28 may be classified according to their chemical properties as follows: (1) 10 primary amines (basic) and (2) one secondary amine (neutral). This provided the basis for separating them into groups via acidification, alkalinization, and solvent extraction. Because of the free hydrogen atoms present in all compounds, including the secondary amine (2-AAF) after acid hydrolysis and conversion to 2-AF, these compounds can be reacted with fluorinating agents [40,44] to produce derivatives that exhibit high sensitivity in assays using EC-GC.

The following procedure provides details for extraction, separation, detection, identification, and quantification of trace amounts of all 11 chemical carcinogens and analogs in admixture in wastewater and human urine by EC-GC of their pentafluoropropionyl (PFP) derivatives [84,88].

Experimental

Test Chemicals and Reagents. The chemicals shown in Figure 28 were obtained from several suppliers as previously reported by Bowman [6,29,40] and Holder et al. [43], who also described their properties and purity. (Note: See appropriate sections of this chapter concerning the individual compounds.)

All solvents were pesticide grade and all reagents were CP grade. Sodium sulfate and glass wool were extracted with benzene for 40 hr in a Soxhlet apparatus and dried in an oven overnight at 130° prior to use. All culture tubes were borosilicate glass and equipped with Teflon-lined screw caps. The 170 and 35 ml culture tubes were fabricated by Shamrock Scientific Glassware Co., Little Rock, Arkansas.

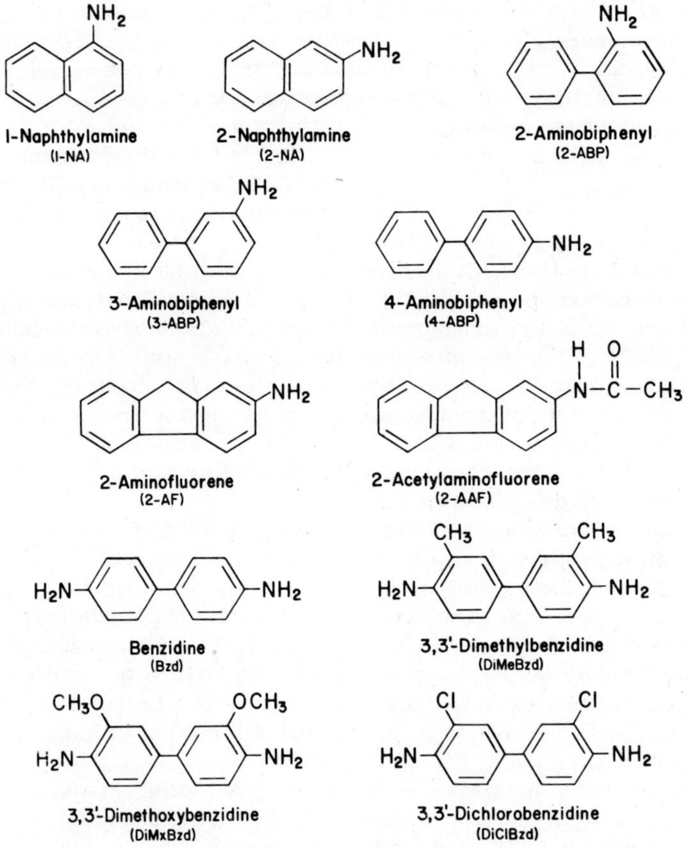

Figure 28 Formulas of 11 carcinogens and related compounds. (From Ref. 84.)

Pentafluoropropionic anhydride (PFPA) (No. 65193) and heptafluorobutyric anhydride (HFBA) (No. 27085) were obtained from Pierce Chemical Co., Rockford, Illinois, and Regis Chemical Co., Morton Grove, Illinois, respectively. A 100 μl Hamilton syringe, fitted with a Chaney adapter, was used to withdraw the derivatizing agent from the vial and deliver it into the reaction vessel. The trimethylamine (TMA) reagent (0.05 M in benzene), buffer solution (potassium monobasic phosphate, pH 6), and sodium hydroxide (1 N) were described by King et al. [89] and Bowman and Rushing [40]. The keeper solution was paraffin oil (20 mg/ml) in pentane.

Preparation of Samples for Gas Chromatographic Analysis

Wastewater. One hundred milliliters of the sample and 10 ml of concentrated HCL added to a 170-ml culture tube were shaken and allowed to stand for 5 min. Twenty milliliters of benzene was then added, the contents shaken for 1 min, then the tube was centrifuged at 550 rpm for 10 min. The benzene layer was carefully withdrawn by using a syringe and cannula, percolated through a plug of sodium sulfate (25 mm diam × 25 mm thick), and collected in a 100 ml round-bottom flask containing a glass bead and 0.5 ml of keeper solution. The extraction was repeated by using two additional 20 ml portions of benzene and the combined extracts, containing the neutral compound (2-AAF) and possibly some phenolic compounds (hormones) were evaporated just to dryness by using water pump vacuum and a 60° water bath. The acidified aqueous phase was then reserved for subsequent extraction of the basic compounds.

The flask containing the neutral and phenolic compounds was treated as described by Bowman and Nony [90]: 5 ml of benzene was used to transfer the residue to a 20 ml culture tube containing 4 ml of 1 N NaOH. The contents of the tube were shaken, centrifuged for 5 min at 1200 rpm, and the benzene layer transferred to a 35 ml culture tube also containing 4 ml of 1 N NaOH. The contents of the second tube was shaken and centrifuged as described and the benzene layer was carefully withdrawn and percolated through a plug of sodium sulfate (18 mm diam × 20 mm thick) and collected in a 50 ml round-bottom flask containing a glass bead and 0.5 ml of keeper solution. The flask and aqueous NaOH phases in both tubes were again sequentially washed and extracted in the same manner by using two additional 5 ml portions of benzene which were also percolated through a plug of sodium sulfate. The combined extracts containing the neutral fraction (2-AAF) were reserved for subsequent treatment. The contents of the 20 ml and 35 ml tubes were discarded.

The neutral fraction was evaporated to dryness as described and the residue transferred to a 20 ml culture tube by using three 1 ml portions of chloroform. The solvent in the tube was then evaporated to dryness in a tube heater (Kontes No. 720,000, Vineland, New Jersey) set at 40° by using a gentle stream of dry nitrogen. The dry residue was hydrolyzed as described by Bowman and King [6]: by heating the sealed tube containing 4 ml of methanol and 2 ml of concentrated HCl in a tube heater set at 85° for 2 hr. After the tube had cooled, 3 ml of water was added and the contents extracted three times with 7 ml portions of benzene. Each extract was carefully withdrawn and discarded by using a 10 ml syringe and cannula. Next, 4 ml of 10 N NaOH was added and the contents extracted three times with 7 ml portions of benzene. Each extract was successively percolated through a plug of sodium sulfate (18 mm diam × 20 mm thick) and collected in a 50 ml round-bottom flask containing a boiling bead and 0.5 ml of keeper solution.

The contents were evaporated just to dryness at 60° by using water pump vacuum as described; the residue was transferred to an 8 ml culture tube by using three 1 ml portions of benzene which were also evaporated to dryness in a tube heater at 50° by using a stream of dry nitrogen. The residue containing 2-AF was reserved for subsequent derivatization with PFPA and assay by EC-GC.

The acidified aqueous phase (basic fraction), previously reserved for later treatment, was made strongly alkaline by adding 15 ml of 10 N NaOH and extracted three times with 20 ml portions of benzene. Each extract was percolated successively through a plug of sodium sulfate (25 mm diam × 25 mm thick) and collected in a 100 ml round-bottom flask containing a boiling bead and 0.5 ml of keeper solution. The combined extracts were evaporated to dryness by using water pump vacuum and a 60° water bath. The residue was transferred to an 8 ml culture tube by using three 1 ml portions of benzene and evaporated to dryness in a tube heater at 50° with a stream of dry nitrogen. The residue was reserved for subsequent derivatization with PFPA and assay by EC-GC.

Human urine. Two 50 ml portions of the sample were separately added to 75 ml culture tubes, each containing 5 g of NaCl; 5 ml of concentrated HCl was added to one tube (neutral and phenolic fractions) and 5 ml of 10 N NaOH was added to the other tube (basic fraction). After the tubes were shaken and allowed to stand for 5 min the contents were extracted three times with 15 ml portions of benzene which were successively percolated through plugs of sodium sulfate (25 mm diam × 25 mm thick) and collected in 100 ml round-bottom flasks containing a boiling bead and 0.5 ml of keeper solution. Each of these combined extracts was then treated exactly as described for wastewater.

Recovery Experiments

Wastewater. Triplicate samples (100 g) of wastewater in 170 ml culture tubes were separately spiked with 1 ml of methanol containing the appropriate amount of eight selected carcinogens and analogs (i.e., 2-NA, 4-ABP, 2-AF, 2-AAF, Bzd, DiClBzd, DiMeBzd, and DiMxBzd) to produce residues of 0, 0.10, 1.0, and 10 ppb. The tubes were sealed, mixed, and allowed to stand overnight at 5° prior to analysis.

Human urine. Two sets of triplicate 50 g samples of urine in 75 ml culture tubes were separately spiked with 0.5 ml of methanol containing the appropriate amounts of the eight compounds used for wastewater to produce residues of 0, 2.0, and 20 ppb. The tubes were sealed, mixed, and allowed to stand overnight at 5° prior to analysis.

Preparation of Derivatives. Pentafluoropropionyl (PFP) derivatives and heptafluorobutyryl (HFB) derivatives of all compounds shown in Figure 28 (except 2-AAF) were prepared by our modification of the procedures reported by Walle and Ehrsson (44). For derivatization of amines, TMA solution (0.5 ml, 0.05 M) was added to an 8 ml culture tube containing the compounds (10 μg or less) dissolved in exactly 1.5 ml of benzene (total benzene = 2.0 ml) and followed by the addition of 50 μl of either PFPA or HFBA reagent. The tube was immediately sealed, shaken, heated in a 50° water bath for 20 min, cooled, and the reaction terminated by adding 2 ml of phosphate buffer (pH 6.0). The tube was shaken for 1 min, and after the phases had separated, the aqueous layer (bottom) was discarded. The extraction was repeated with an additional 2 ml portion of buffer; the tube was centrifuged for 1 min at 1000 rpm and the benzene layer (top) was either analyzed directly or appropriately diluted with benzene prior to analysis.

Final residues from the extraction and cleanup procedures of the basic and neutral fractions from wastewater or urine were dissolved in benzene (1.5 ml) and derivatized by using TMA solution and PFPA reagents as described. For assays of wastewater containing amine residues in the order of 0.10, 1.0, and 10 ppb, the entire extract (100 g equivalents) of the cleaned-up sample was derivatized and 5 μl injections containing 250, 25, and 2.5 mg equivalents, respectively, were assayed by EC-GC. Similarly, for assays of urine containing residues in the order of 2 or 20 ppb, the entire extract (50 g equivalents) was derivatized and 12.5 and 1.25 mg equivalents, respectively, were analyzed.

Gas Chromatographic Analysis. A Hewlett-Packard (Palo Alto, California) Model 5750B instrument equipped with a ^{63}Ni electron capture detector (Tracor, Inc., Austin, Texas) and 125 cm glass columns (4 mm i.d.) containing 5% Dexsil 300, 5% OV-101 or 5% OV-17, all on Gas Chrom Q (80-100 mesh) conditioned at 270° overnight prior to use, was operated isothermally at the various temperatures (Table 27) with a nitrogen carrier flow of 160 ml/min. The detector, operated in the dc mode, was 300° and the injection port was 20° higher than the column oven. Lindane and heptachlor epoxide were used as reference standards to monitor the performance of the EC-GC system; all injections were made in 5 μl of benzene. Assays of the three fractions from wastewater or urine were performed on a column of Dexsil 300. Because of the wide differences in t_R values for the various PFP derivatives, the basic fraction was first analyzed at 165° to quantify the 2-NA and 4-ABP, then at 220° for the other amines. The neutral fraction was also assayed at 220°. Derivatization samples of unknown residue content were quantified by relating their peak heights to known amounts of the corresponding PFP derivatives. Derivatized samples

Table 27 Retention Times of Two Electron-Capturing Derivatives of Carcinogens and Analogs on Three Chromatographic Columns

		Retention time (t_R, min) and oven temperature (°C) for column indicated[a]					
		Dexsil 300		OV-101		OV-17	
Compound	Derivative[b]	°C	t_R	°C	t_R	°C	t_R
2-Aminobiphenyl	PFP	165	1.65	155	2.20	165	1.90
(2-ABP)	HFB	165	1.70	155	2.40	165	1.90
1-Naphthylamine	PFP	165	1.80	155	2.00	165	2.00
(1-NA)	HFB	165	1.95	155	2.25	165	1.95
2-Naphthylamine	PFP	165	2.30	155	2.45	165	2.50
(2-NA)	HFB	165	2.50	155	2.75	165	2.50
3-Aminobiphenyl	PFP	165	4.50	155	4.80	165	4.90
(3-ABP)	HFB	165	4.85	155	5.50	165	4.90
4-Aminobiphenyl	PFP	165	5.05	155	5.40	165	6.10
(4-ABP)	HFB	165	5.55	155	6.30	165	6.10
2-Aminofluorene	PFP	220	1.70	210	1.60	220	1.75
(2-AF)	HFB	220	1.80	210	1.80	220	1.70
Benzidine	PFP	220	3.20	210	3.00	220	2.75
(Bzd)	HFB	220	3.55	210	3.60	220	2.65
3,3'-Dichlorobenzidine	Underiv.	220	6.60	210	4.80	220	11.85
(DiClBzd)	PFP	220	4.30	210	4.10	220	3.00
	HFB	220	4.70	210	5.20	220	2.90
3,3'-Dimethylbenzidine	PFP	220	4.90	210	4.10	220	3.75
(DiMeBzd)	HFB	220	5.50	210	5.20	220	3.60
3,3'-Dimethoxybenzidine	PFP	220	8.25	210	6.90	220	6.00
(DiMxBzd)	HFB	220	8.70	210	8.30	220	5.70
Lindane		165	4.15	155	3.70	165	6.40
(ref. std.)		220	0.85	210	0.85	220	1.00
Heptachlor epoxide		165	11.50	155	11.90	165	-
(ref. std.)		220	1.75	210	1.75	220	2.20

[a] All columns were 125 cm glass (4 mm i.d.), packed with 5% liquid phase on Gas Chrom Q (80-100 mesh); nitrogen carrier flowed at 160 ml/min.
[b] PFP and HFB are pentafluoropropionyl and heptafluorobutyryl derivative, respectively.
Source: Ref. 84.

of unknown 2-AAF content were quantified by relating the peak height of the resulting PFP-2-AF to a known amount of PFP-2-AF and then expressing the results as 2-AAF (2-AF × 1.23 = 2-AAF).

Results and discussion

A periodic analysis of the urine is one of the most convenient means of determining human exposure to test chemicals. Although partial metabolism of these substances is known to occur prior to excretion in the urine, the unaltered parent compound is also believed to be excreted in sufficient amounts to signal any appreciable exposure in the event that highly sensitive analytical procedures are employed. Therefore, in the absence of rapid and sensitive methods for a wide variety of metabolites of each of the test compounds shown in Figure 28, surveillance of personnel to detect accidental exposure to the test substances is based on periodic assays of the urine for traces of the parent compounds.

Recent development of methodology at our laboratory for assaying traces of DiClBzd [40] based on derivatization with fluorinated acid anhydrides led us to investigate the possibility of analyzing all the compounds in the same manner. Indeed, it was found that all these compounds, with the exception of 2-AAF, could be derivatized and analyzed with high sensitivity; 2-AAF, after hydrolysis to 2-AF [6] and subsequent derivatization, could also be analyzed.

Both PFP and HFB derivatives of all the compounds were prepared and subjected to GC analysis on columns of Dexsil 300, OV-101, and OV-17 by using a variety of isothermal operating conditions. Data concerning GC operations and retention times for all these compounds as well as underivatized DiClBzd and reference standards of lindane and heptachlor epoxide are presented in Table 27. DiClBzd was the only test substance that demonstrated appreciable electron-capturing properties without being subjected to derivatization; nevertheless, conversion of the compound to the PFP derivative enhanced its response about 300-fold, which agrees with the value reported by Bowman and Rushing [40]. Although the PFP and HFB derivatives of the various compounds yielded about the same response, the use of PFP derivatives was adopted because the reagent was easier to use and generally produced fewer interference peaks. Data concerning t_R values of the PFP derivatives (Table 27) indicate that Dexsil 300 is the column of choice for the analytical procedure because better separation was obtained. Although the present procedure for wastewater and urine employs PFP derivatives on a column of Dexsil 300, the data concerning both the PFP and HFB derivatives on all three column packings may be useful in confirmatory tests. Typical gas chromatograms of PFP derivatives of all the compounds, underivatized DiClBzd, and the reference standards assayed on the column of Dexsil 300 using various isothermal operating conditions are presented in Figures 29 and 30.

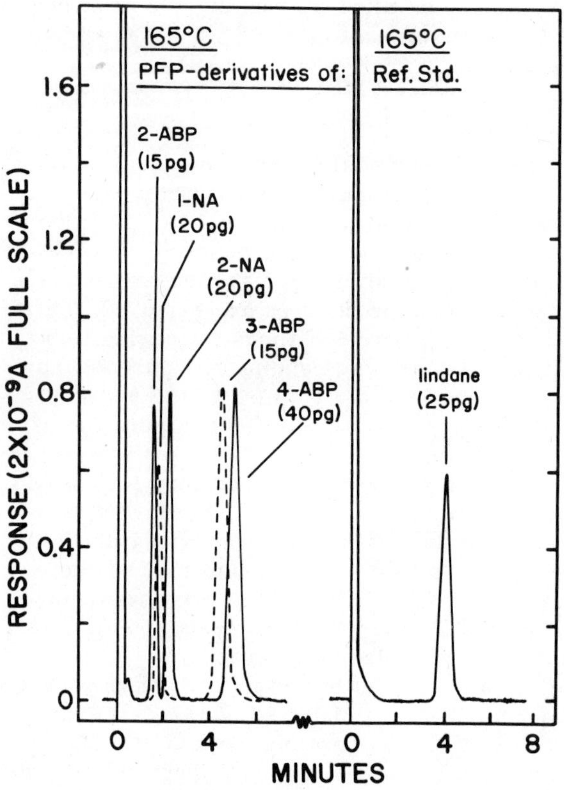

Figure 29 Electron capture gas chromatograms of standards of PFP derivatives of carcinogens, their analogs, and a reference standard of lindane. All injections were in 5 μl of benzene. (From Ref. 84.)

Excellent responses are obtained from injection of picogram amounts of the PFP derivatives.

The p values (fraction of solute partitioning into the nonpolar phase of an equivolume immiscible binary solvent system) are useful for confirming the identity of unknown GC peaks where insufficient amounts are available for test by other means. Therefore, such values for all of the PFP derivatives in five solvent systems, determined as described by Bowman and Beroza [15,18], are reported in Table 28. Additional p values were determined for all of the PFP derivatives in benzene versus the phosphate buffer (pH 6) used to terminate the derivatization reaction; all the values were found to be 1.0, which indicated that no loss of the derivative occurred during the process. Results from GC-mass spectrometric tests of the individual

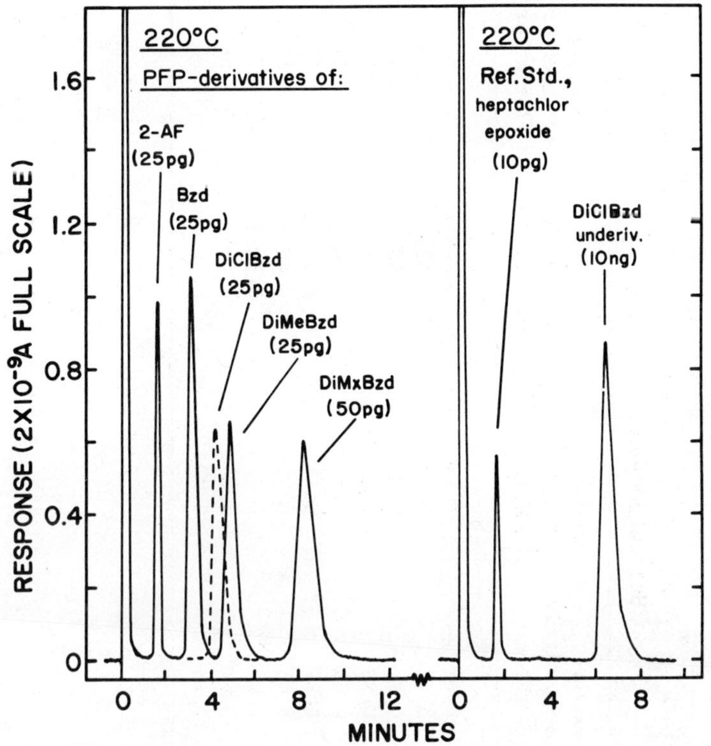

Figure 30 Electron capture gas chromatograms of standards of PFP derivatives of carcinogens, their analogs, a reference standard of heptachlor epoxide, and underivatized DiClBzd. All injections were in 5 μl of benzene. (From Ref. 84.)

derivatives to determine the number of PFP groups added to each compound during derivatization are also presented in Table 28. Bzd and its analogs each contained two PFP groups, while all the other compounds contained one PFP group.

Stability studies employing periodic assays of benzene solutions (5 ng/ml) of the PFP derivatives stored in sealed tubes at 5° indicated that all the compounds were essentially stable during a 10 month period.

The chemical properties of the test substances provided a convenient means of separating them into basic and neutral fractions. The analytical scheme used for the extraction, separation, and analysis of all 11 compounds in admixture in wastewater is illustrated in Figure 31. Salient elements of the procedure after separation of the sample into two fractions are hydrolysis of 2-AAF in the neutral fraction and

Table 28 Partition Values (p Values) and GC-Mass Spectrometric Verification of PFP Derivatives of Carcinogens and Analogs

Compound	PFP groups per molecule	Solvent system: Hexane-acetonitrile	Hexane-40% acetonitrile (60% water)	Heptane-90% ethanol (10% water)	Isooctane-90% acetone (10% water)	Isooctane-80% acetone (20% water)
1-NA	1	0.038	0.63	0.11	0.46	0.62
2-NA	1	0.052	0.77	0.12	0.45	0.70
2-ABP	1	0.090	0.91	0.27	0.42	0.70
3-ABP	1	0.050	0.88	0.13	0.48	0.76
4-ABP	1	0.044	0.85	0.13	0.44	0.74
2-AF	1	0.046	0.86	0.14	0.56	0.73
Bzd	2	0.016	0.45	0.020	0.48	0.66
DiClBzd	2	0.042	1.00	0.14	0.59	0.78
DiMeBzd	2	0.031	0.52	0.046	0.50	0.66
DiMxBzd	2	0.044	0.98	0.22	0.69	0.86

Source: Ref. 84.

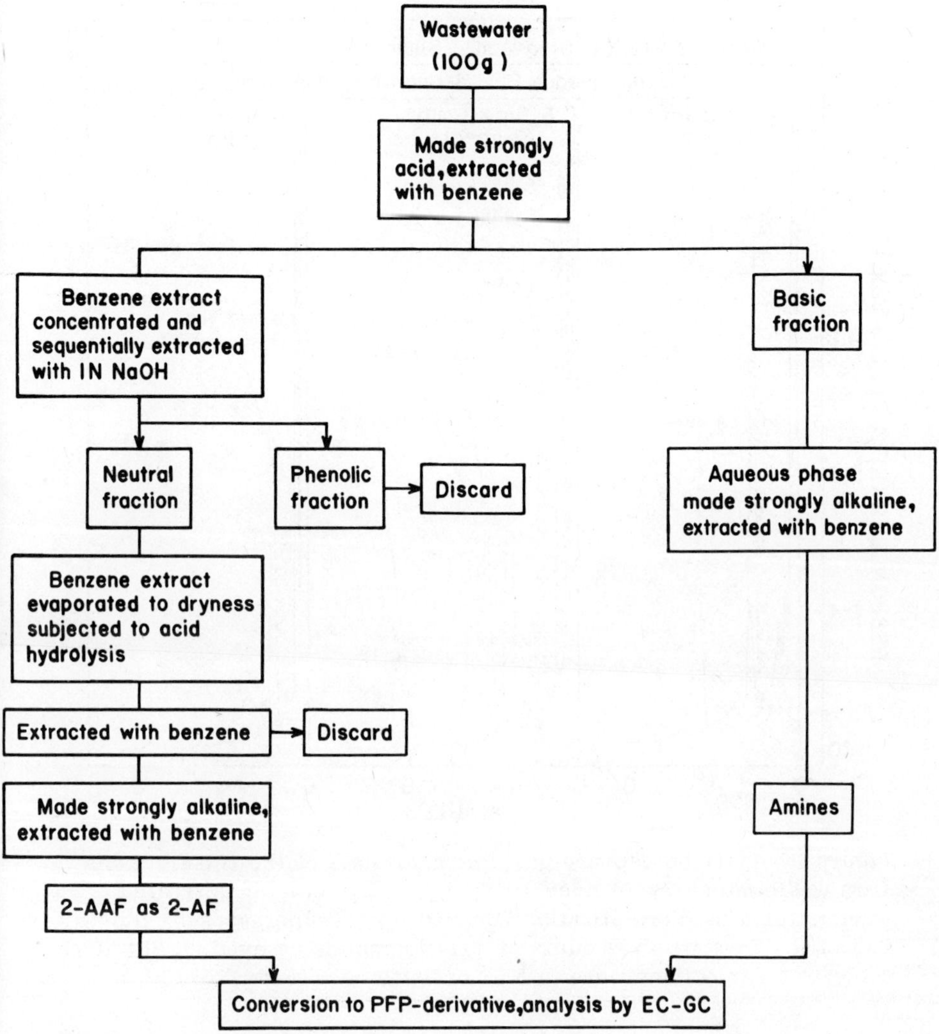

Figure 31 Scheme for extraction, separation, and analysis of 11 carcinogens and related compounds in admixture in wastewater. (From Ref. 84.)

extraction of the product (2-AF) as the free amine, extraction of the free amines from the basic fraction (pH 12), conversion of all residues to the PFP derivatives, and analysis via EC-GC by using two isothermal operating conditions.

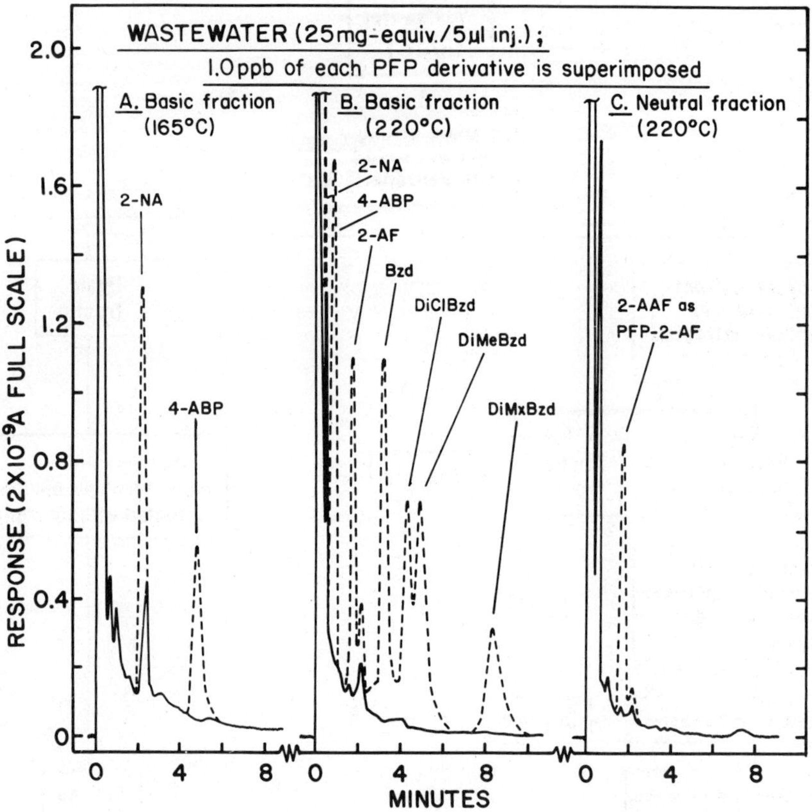

Figure 32 Electron capture gas chromatograms of the two fractions from wastewater. Solid lines are 25 mg equivalents of untreated wastewater after derivatization; dashed lines (superimposed) illustrate responses from 1 ppb amounts of the compounds assayed as PFP derivatives. All injections were in 5 µl of benzene. (From Ref. 84.)

Typical gas chromatograms of derivatized fractions from untreated wastewater together with 1 ppb amounts of eight of the compounds as PFP derivatives (superimposed) are presented in Figure 32. Resolution was excellent for six of the eight derivatives. Although baseline resolution was not achieved for DiClBzd and DiMeBzd, no problem was experienced in using peak height measurement to quantify residues as low as 0.1 ppb.

Results from triplicate assays of wastewater unspiked and spiked with 0.10, 1.0, and 10 ppb of eight of the compounds in admixture are presented in Table 29. Recoveries were generally good at the 10 ppb

Table 29 Analysis of Wastewater Unspiked and Spiked with 0.10, 1.0, and 10 ppb of Eight Carcinogens and Analogs in Admixture

	Recovery ($\bar{x}$ ± SE)[a]						
	Unspiked	Spiked with 0.10 ppb		Spiked with 1.0 ppb		Spiked with 10 ppb	
Compound	ppb	ppb	%	ppb	%	ppb	%
2-NA	0.123 ± 0.025	0.011 ± 0.004	11 ± 4	0.443 ± 0.039	44.3 ± 3.9	7.64 ± 0.60	76.4 ± 6.0
4-ABP	0.002 ± 0.001	0.040 ± 0.003	40 ± 3	0.657 ± 0.036	65.7 ± 3.6	8.52 ± 0.30	85.2 ± 3.0
2-AF	0.002 ± 0.000	0.022 ± 0.000	22 ± 0	0.555 ± 0.048	55.5 ± 4.8	8.17 ± 0.10	81.7 ± 1.0
2-AAF	0.002 ± 0.001	0.056 ± 0.006	56 ± 6	0.650 ± 0.042	65.0 ± 4.2	7.52 ± 0.06	75.2 ± 0.6
Bzd	0.002 ± 0.001	0.004 ± 0.003	4 ± 3	0.208 ± 0.009	20.8 ± 0.9	7.05 ± 0.33	70.5 ± 3.3
DiClBzd	0.003 ± 0.001	0.055 ± 0.004	55 ± 4	0.580 ± 0.064	58.0 ± 6.4	7.47 ± 0.08	74.7 ± 0.8
DiMeBzd	0.005 ± 0.002	0.028 ± 0.001	28 ± 1	0.583 ± 0.037	58.3 ± 3.7	8.39 ± 0.14	83.9 ± 1.4
DiMxBzd	0.003 ± 0.001	0.009 ± 0.001	9 ± 1	0.465 ± 0.048	46.5 ± 4.8	7.25 ± 0.10	72.5 ± 1.0

[a]Mean and standard error from triplicate assays; spiked samples are corrected for background of unspiked samples.

Source: Ref. 84.

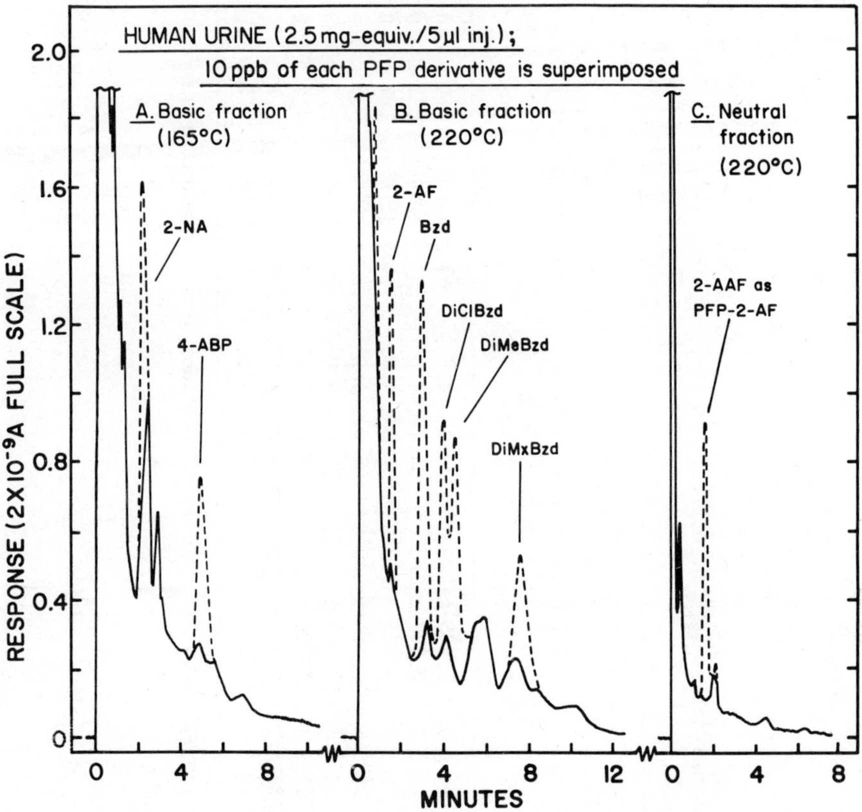

Figure 33 Electron capture gas chromatograms of the two fractions from human urine. Solid lines are 2.5 mg equivalents of untreated urine after derivatization; dashed lines (superimposed) illustrate responses of 10 ppb amounts of the compounds analyzed as PFP derivatives. All injections were in 5 µl of benzene. (From Ref. 84.)

level but tend to drop significantly at 1 ppb. At 0.10 ppb, recoveries of 2-NA, Bzd, and DiMxBzd were 11% or less; however, the fact that the compounds were detectable indicated that the procedure is useful even at this low level.

Urine is assayed by using the same scheme as for wastewater except that the sample is initially divided into two 50 ml portions. One of the portions is made strongly alkaline for extraction and analysis of the basic fraction (amines); the other is made strongly acid for extraction of phenolic and neutral (2-AAF) fractions and analysis of the neutral fraction after separation from the phenolic fraction. Typical

Table 30 Analysis of Human Urine Unspiked and Spiked with 2.0 and 20 ppb of Eight Carcinogens and Analogs in Admixture

	Recovered ($\bar{x}$ ± SE)[a]				
	Unspiked	Spiked with 2.0 ppb		Spiked with 20 ppb	
Compound	ppb	ppb	%	ppb	%
2-NA	0.788 ± 0.038	0.637 ± 0.172	31.9 ± 8.6	13.3 ± 0.7	66.6 ± 3.3
4-ABP	1.06 ± 0.08	1.03 ± 0.08	51.3 ± 4.0	17.3 ± 0.2	86.5 ± 1.1
2-AF	0.515 ± 0.031	0.480 ± 0.040	24.1 ± 2.0	14.9 ± 0.2	74.2 ± 1.0
2-AAF	0.023 ± 0.005	1.16 ± 0.12	57.7 ± 5.9	15.9 ± 0.8	79.2 ± 3.8
Bzd	0.213 ± 0.023	0.907 ± 0.023	45.1 ± 1.2	14.1 ± 0.2	70.4 ± 0.9
DiClBzd	0.830 ± 0.038	1.41 ± 0.06	70.7 ± 2.8	19.9 ± 0.3	99.3 ± 1.4
DiMeBzd	0.215 ± 0.037	0.973 ± 0.012	48.6 ± 0.4	17.3 ± 0.3	86.4 ± 1.3
DiMxBzd	2.13 ± 0.00	0.953 ± 0.021	47.5 ± 1.0	18.6 ± 0.3	92.6 ± 1.6

[a]Mean and standard error from triplicate assays; spiked samples are corrected for background of unspiked samples.

Source: Ref. 84.

electron capture gas chromatograms of the derivatized fractions from untreated urine together with 10 ppb amounts of eight of the compounds as PFP derivatives (superimposed) are presented in Figure 33. Results from triplicate assays of urine unspiked and spiked with 2.0 and 20 ppb of the eight compounds are presented in Table 30. Recoveries at the 20 ppb level were good; however, a marked decrease in recovery was found at the 2 ppb level. Also, background interferences from untreated urine as high as 2 ppb were observed in the case of DiMxBzd. Nevertheless, the procedure does serve as an excellent means of monitoring for residues of the compounds at levels of 1 to 2 ppb in the urine of our personnel.

Recent tests with the monoacetyl analog of benzidine (MoAcBzd), a metabolite of benzidine found in urine, have indicated that it also responds to the analytical procedure. The retention time (t_R) of PFP-MoAcBzd on the Dexsil 300 column operated at 220° was about 12.6 min. Quantitation of MoAcBzd, as the PFP derivative, is best accomplished with the Dexsil 300 column operated at 260° (t_R = 2.85 min). Under these conditions, a 5 μl injection of benzene containing 250 pg of PFP-MoAcBzd yields a response of about 6×10^{-10} A, which is about 10 times less than PFP-Bzd; nevertheless, this sensitivity is adequate for the measurement of MoAcBzd in urine at the low-ppb level.

It should be noted that no cleanup steps are used in the procedure for wastewater and urine; nevertheless, some cleanup was achieved by our method as a result of the extraction, separation, and derivatization steps. Bowen [91] was also able to assay for certain aromatic amines at ppb levels in aqueous waste streams via flame ionization GC without sample treatment in many cases. Although extensive studies of cleanup procedures were conducted at our laboratory employing XAD-2 resin and Sephadex LH-20 prior to derivatization and alumina and silica gel before and after derivatization, no system could be devised that allowed good recoveries of all compounds at the levels tested. Therefore, it appears that further refinement of the present procedure to improve sensitivity and recovery should be directed toward the individual compound and substrate.

This method may easily be adapted to the monitoring of work areas (animal cages, floors, apparatus, air filters, etc.) suspected of being contaminated with the test chemicals. The procedure currently used at our laboratory [29] for sampling surfaces employs a kit consisting of a cotton applicator and a 5 ml culture tube containing a known volume of a suitable solvent. The applicator is saturated with the solvent and used to swab a specific area, then the applicator is vigorously stirred in the solvent after each of several swabbings of the same area. In a similar manner fiberglass filters used to trap particulate matter from the air may be cut into small pieces and extracted with a suitable solvent. These extracts may then be screened for contaminants by slightly modifying the procedure described.

I. Triphenylmethane Dyes and Related Compounds [92]

General description of methods

Sensitive and specific high-pressure liquid chromatographic procedures are described for determining residues of gentian violet in animal feed, human urine, and wastewater down to levels of 10, 1, and 10 ppb, respectively. Animal feed is extracted with a solvent followed by cleanup on a column of Sephadex LH-20 prior to analysis. Human urine is extracted with dichloromethane followed by evaporation to dryness, and the residue is assayed directly without cleanup. Wastewater is processed through a C_{18} cartridge and after elution with a solvent, the eluate is assayed directly. Information is also reported concerning the stability of gentian violet in animal feed and its removal from industrial wastewater, and the application of these methods to the separation and analysis of six related triphenylmethane dyes.

Introduction

Gentian violet ([4-{bis(p-[dimethylamino]phenyl)methylene}-2,5-cyclohexadien-1-ylidine]dimethylammonium chloride; also known as hexamethylpararosaniline chloride and CI 42555) has been marketed since 1951 for a variety of uses. The compound (formula shown in Fig. 34) has been used to control fungi and intestinal parasites in humans, as an antimicrobial agent on burn victims, to treat umbilical cords of infants, as a vaginal cream, for various purposes in veterinary medicine, and as a pH indicator. It has also been used as a medicative feed additive in the poultry industry, even though it has never been approved by the Food and Drug Administration (FDA) for such use [93-95].

Fujita et al. [96] determined that gentian violet was mutagenic to *Bacillus subtilis, Escherichia coli,* and *Salmonella typhimurium,* and Norrby and Mobacken [97] found it cytotoxic to mammalian cells. Au et al. [98-99] demonstrated its genetic cytotoxicity to Chinese hamster ovary (CHO) cells and found it toxic to *Salmonella typhimurium* but not mutagenic. Wolfe [100] determined that gentian violet also inhibits DNA synthesis in *E. coli* B polymerase 1. Some triphenylmethane-classed dyes, of which gentian violet is a member, have been recognized as animal and human carcinogens. Case and Pearson [101] in 1954 noted the increased risk of bladder cancer in industrial workers engaged in the production of rosaniline ([2-methyl-4,4'-{(4-amino-2,5-cyclohexadiene-1-ylidene)methylene} dianiline]; CI 42510; a ring methylated primary amine analog of gentian violet). The leuco form of rosaniline induces renal, hepatic, and lung tumors in mice; hematopoietic tumors and mammary gland fibroadenomas also have been noted in rats [102]. Benzyl violet 4B(benzenemethanaminium,N-[4-{(4-[dimethylamino]phenyl)(4-[ethyl {(3-sulfophenyl)methyl}amino]phenyl)methylene}-2,5-cyclohexadien-1-

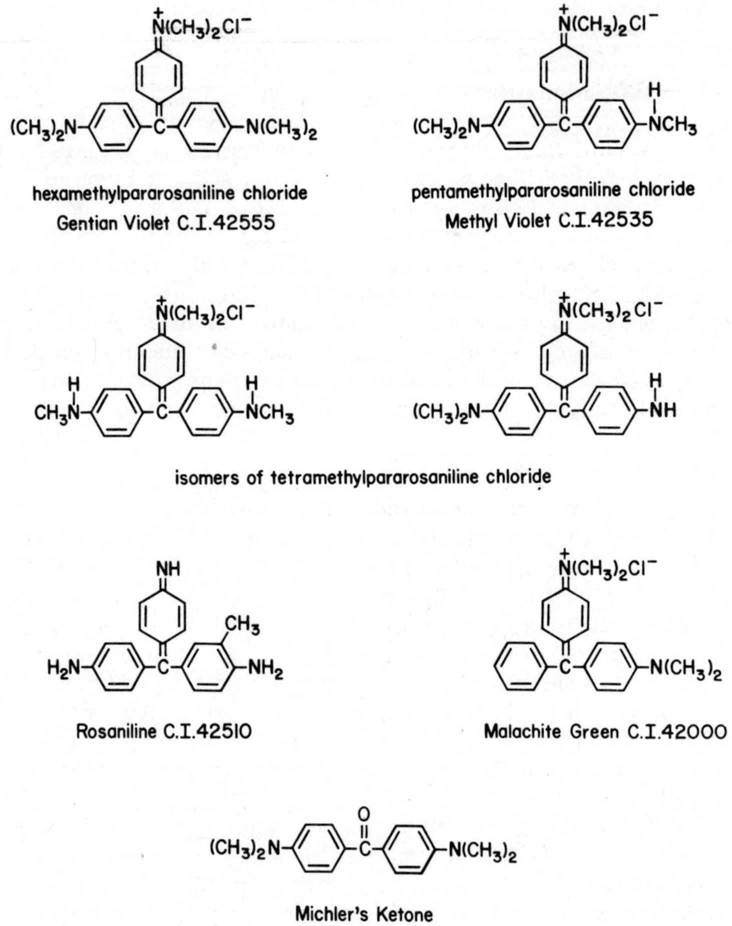

Figure 34 Formulas of gentian violet and six related compounds. (From Ref. 92.)

ylidine]-N-ethyl-3-sulfo-, hydroxide, inner salt, sodium salt; CI 42640; a benzyl sulfonate analog of gentian violet) was found to induce tumors in the ear ducts and mammary glands of female rats [103].

Studies were therefore proposed as part of the National Toxicology Program (NTP) to be carried out at the National Center for Toxicological Research (NCTR) to investigate any potential human hazard associated with the use of gentian violet in food-producing animals. Before such studies could be initiated, analytical chemical methodology was required to provide assurance that accurate doses of the substance are administered to the test animals via spiked feed and that the test agent is uniformly distributed and stable during preparation of the feed and during the feeding period of the animal study. Also, trace-level assays were required for urine of laboratory personnel to signal any accidental exposure to the test agent and for wastewater to provide assurance that the compound is not discharged into the environment.

Fisher [104] reported a paper chromatographic procedure for assaying mixtures of methyl violet (pentamethylpararosaniline chloride, CI 42535) and gentian violet. Marshall and Lewis [105] and Marshall [106] reported thin layer chromatographic (TLC) systems for the analysis of gentian violet and other commonly used histological stains. Van Mullem and MacGillavry [107] reported gravity-flow talcum column separations of triphenylmethane dye mixtures and correlated methyl substitution with their visible absorption maxima. Taylor [108,109] described methods for the analysis of gentian violet in chicken feed, tissue, and eggs; however, these procedures lacked specificity and data concerning precision and accuracy were not included. The procedure listed in the *United States Pharmacopeia* [110] requires that 400 mg of gentian violet be reacted with titanium trichloride and then titrated with ferric ammonium sulfate; the procedure is not specific because other triphenylmethane dyes also respond.

This work describes sensitive and specific procedures for the analysis of gentian violet in animal feed at levels within the range 1000 ppm to 10 ppb, 1 ppb in human urine, and 10 ppb in wastewater, as determined by high-pressure liquid chromatography (HPLC). Data concerning the stability of gentian violet in animal feed and ancillary analytical information pertaining to separation and analysis of several related compounds (structures shown in Fig. 34) are also included.

Experimental

Test Chemicals and Materials. Gentian violet was purchased from the Hilton-Davis Co. (Cincinnati, Ohio) and used as received. Their analysis of the product by the method described in the *United States Pharmacopeia* [110] was as follows: 98.5% gentian violet, 0.29% residue on ignition, 0.06% alcohol insolubles, <30 ppm lead content, and <10 ppm arsenic content. Additional purity and identification tests of the Hilton-Davis material were performed in our laboratories. Mass spectrometry (MS) positively identified the major constituent as gentian violet, a minor component as methyl violet, and a trace amount of a material believed to be tetramethylpararosaniline chloride; no other impurities were detected. HPLC employing a refractive index detector indicated only gentian violet. However, an ultraviolet (UV)-visible absorbance detector indicated a trace (0.02% of the total absorbance at 588 nm) of tetramethylpararosaniline chloride, 1% of methyl violet, and gentian violet; a trace of an unknown compound not detectable at 588 nm was also found at 254 nm. The sample was heated in a vacuum oven at 50° for 9 days at 23 mmHg and the volatiles (moisture) were found to be 2%; the oven temperature was limited since the compound is heat labile.

Four different samples of methyl violet were examined by HPLC for possible use as analytical standards. These included CI 680 and CI 42535 from Eastman Chemical Co. (Rochester, New York), CI 42535 from Aldrich Chemical Co. (Milwaukee, Wisconsin), and CI 42535B from Matheson, Coleman and Bell (Cincinnati, Ohio). All samples were found to be mixtures containing tetramethylpararosaniline chloride and methyl violet, with gentian violet as the major constituent. Since no pure standards of tetramethylpararosaniline chloride or methyl violet were commercially available, the material from the Aldrich Chemical Co. was selected for separation of its constituents by HPLC to obtain the standards sought. This sample was selected because of its relatively high content of tetramethylpararosaniline chloride and methyl violet. The standards, prepared as described in a subsequent section, were positively identified by MS.

Malachite green (ammonium, [4-{p-(dimethylamino)-α-phenylbenzylidene}-2,5-cyclohexadien-1-ylidene]dimethylchloride; CI 42000) and Michler's ketone (4,4'-bis[dimethylamino]benzophenone) were from Eastman; the rosaniline was from Aldrich.

Sulfan blue ([4-{α(p-[diethylamino]phenyl)-2,4-disulfobenzylidene}-2,5-cyclohexadien-1-ylidene]diethylammonium hydroxide inner salt, sodium salt, CI 42045) and isosulfan blue (the 2,5 isomer) were obtained from the Virginia Medical College (Richmond, Virginia).

The animal feed (Laboratory Chow, type 5010-C, Ralston Purina Co., St. Louis, Missouri) contained 6% fat, had a pH of 5.5, and 7.4% was volatile at 110° overnight.

The Sephadex LH-20 was from Pharmacia Fine Chemicals, Inc. (Piscataway, New Jersey); the C_{18} Sep Paks (No. 51910) were from Waters Associates, Inc. (Milford, Massachusetts).

The Amberlite XAD-2 resin was from the Mallinckrodt Chemical Co. (St. Louis, Missouri); the activated carbon was Witco grade 718 from the Continental Water Conditioning Co. (Little Rock, Arkansas).

Preparation of Columns. The Sephadex LH-20 columns (15 mm i.d., with a 250 ml reservoir, No. K-420280, Kontes Glass Co., Vineland, New Jersey) were prepared by adding 5 g of dry powdered Sephadex LH-20 to 60 ml of methanol in the column. The methanol was allowed to percolate through the bed, then the column was rinsed with 60 ml of 90% benzene-10% methanol and allowed to equilibrate with the solvent overnight before use. The column was regenerated after use by rinsing it with 60 ml of methanol followed by 60 ml of 90% benzene-10% methanol and allowed to equilibrate overnight as described.

The Sep Paks were rinsed with 10 ml of methanol followed by 10 ml of deionized water prior to use.

The column of activated carbon (30 mm i.d., with a 500 ml reservoir, Kontes No. K-420280) was prepared by adding a plug of glass wool, partially filling the column with deionized water, then adding 50 g of activated carbon followed by a second plug of glass wool. The column was rinsed with 3 liters of deionized water prior to use. A column of nonionic polymeric resin was prepared in a similar manner except that 70 g of Amberlite XAD-2 were substituted for the activated carbon.

High-Pressure Liquid Chromatography. The system for HPLC consisted of a Waters Associates (Milford, Massachusetts) Model 6000A solvent delivery system; a Rheodyne (Berkeley, California) Model 7120 septumless injector; an Altex (Berkeley, California) 10μ ODS guard column, 40 mm × 3.2 mm i.d.; a Waters μBondapak C_{18} reverse-phase column, No. 27324, 30 cm × 3.9 mm i.d.; a Tracor (Austin, Texas) Model 970 variable wavelength UV-visible absorbance detector; a Waters R-401 refractive index detector; and a Hewlett-Packard (Palo Alto, California) Model 7132A recorder. The mobile phase used for analysis of residues of gentian violet was 85% methanol-15% buffer (0.01 M potassium dihydrogen phosphate adjusted to pH 3 with phosphoric acid). This mobile phase, hereafter referred to as 85% methanol-15% buffer pH 3, flowed at a rate of 1 ml/min at a pressure of 900 psi. Under these conditions the retention times (t_R) for tetramethylpararosaniline chloride, methyl violet, and gentian violet were 4.9, 5.7, and 6.8 min, respectively. All residues of gentian violet were assayed at 588 nm and quantified by peak height. Mobile phases of 70% methanol-30% buffer pH 3 and 50% methanol-50% buffer pH 3 were used for ancillary assays of several analogs of gentian violet.

Separation of Constituents of Commercial Methyl Violet. The sample of commercial methyl violet from Aldrich, which contained 12% tetramethylpararosaniline chloride, 39% methyl violet, and 49% gentian violet, was separated into its constituents to provide standards of the first two components. The same HPLC system previously described was used except that the mobile phase was 70% methanol-30% buffer pH 3. Fifty microliters of methanol containing 50 μg of commercial methyl violet was injected into the chromatograph and the separated constituents collected as they eluted from the instrument. This process was repeated five times and assays of the separated fractions by HPLC indicated that each constituent was free of the others; MS analysis indicated that the constituents were correctly identified. Since MS did not distinguish between the two isomers of tetramethylpararosaniline chloride (Fig. 34) and their standards were not available, the isomeric nature of the single peak obtained by HPLC was not determined. Since assays of the constituents of commercial methyl violet by HPLC (based on percent of total absorption) and MS were in close agreement, the assumption was made that the molar absorptivities of tetramethylpararosaniline chloride, methyl violet, and gentian violet are essentially identical at their respective absorption maxima. Therefore, standard solutions of the tetramethylpararosaniline chloride and methyl violet were prepared by dilution to an absorbance value (at their maxima) corresponding to that of a 2.5 μg/ml standard of gentian violet at its maximum. A Perkin-Elmer (Norwalk, Connecticut) Model 550 UV-visible spectrophotometer was used to determine the absorption spectra for these solutions and for other compounds previously mentioned. The absorption maxima of tetramethylpararosaniline chloride, methyl violet, and gentian violet were found to be 573, 581, and 588 nm, respectively.

Extraction and Recovery Experiments. In preliminary tests to determine the solvents most efficient for extracting residues of gentian violet from animal feed, samples of the control animal feed (10 g) were spiked with 1 ml of 95% ethanol containing 100 μg (10 ppm) of the chemical. The open containers were allowed to stand at ambient temperature in the dark for 16 hr prior to extraction. The spiked samples were then shaken with various solvents on a reciprocating shaker for 1 hr unless otherwise specified. A 10 ml aliquot (1 g equivalent of feed) from each extract was cleaned up on a column of LH-20 and analyzed by HPLC.

After the appropriate extraction solvent was determined, triplicate 10 g samples were spiked to yield 0, 0.01, 0.1, 1, 10, 100, and 1000 ppm of gentian violet in animal feed by the addition of the appropriate amount of the chemical in 1 ml of 95% ethanol. The open flasks were allowed to stand in the dark for 16 hr, then the samples were extracted, cleaned up, and analyzed by HPLC to determine the accuracy and precision of the procedure.

Extraction and Cleanup of Animal Feed. A 10 g portion of the animal feed was weighed into a 250 ml conical flask, fitted with a glass stopper, and mechanically extracted for 1 hr with 100 ml of 99% methanol-1% 1 N HCl on a reciprocating shaker (No. 6000, Eberbach Corp., Ann Arbor, Michigan) at a rate of 200 excursions/min. Part of the extract was rapidly filtered through a small plug of glass wool in a funnel, collected in a 30 ml culture tube, and centrifuged at 1500 rpm for 5 min. (Note: All culture tubes were borosilicate glass equipped with Teflon-lined screw caps.) A 10 ml portion of the supernatant extract (1 g equivalent of animal feed) was transferred to a 100 ml round-bottom flask containing a glass bead and 1 drop of diethylene glycol to serve as a keeper and evaporated just to dryness in a 55° water bath by using water pump vacuum. (Note: A water bath temperature in excess of the value noted will degrade the gentian violet.) The residue was transferred to a Sephadex LH-20 cleanup column by using five successive 2 ml portions of 90% benzene-10% methanol followed by one 2 ml portion of 75% benzene-25% methanol, with each portion being allowed to percolate into the column bed. The column was washed with an additional 10 ml of 75% benzene-25% methanol and the eluate discarded. The gentian violet was then eluted with 10 ml of 75% benzene-25% methanol and collected in a 50 ml round-bottom flask containing a glass bead and 10 μl of diethylene glycol keeper. Samples containing more than 100 ppm of gentian violet require a larger elution volume (e.g., 17 ml are needed to quantitatively elute the residue at the 1000 ppm level). The eluate containing the gentian violet was evaporated as described and redissolved in an appropriate volume (1 ml or more) of methanol for analysis by HPLC.

Stability Experiments. Tests were performed to determine the stability of gentian violet in animal feed at the proposed dosage levels under simulated animal test conditions (i.e., 0 to 16 days, open container in the light) and storage conditions (i.e., 0 to 16 weeks, closed container in the dark). Batches of animal feed spiked with 0, 1, 10, 100, and 1000 ppm of gentian violet were prepared by adding the appropriate amount of the chemical in 50 ml of 95% ethanol to 1 kg of animal feed contained in a Patterson-Kelly (East Stroudsburg, Pennsylvania) Model LV Twin-Shell Lab Blender. The shell of the blender was operated at 20 rpm during the 25 min mixing process and the intensifier bar was operated at 3300 rpm during the first 5 min of mixing, then turned off. An additional 25 ml of 95% ethanol was added as a rinse during the intensifier bar operation. At the end of the blending process each batch was transferred to a stainless steel pan and dried in an autoclave at ambient temperature for 18 hr under reduced pressure (about 84 mmHg).

Each batch (1 kg) was divided into two 500 g portions for use in the short-term (simulated animal test conditions) and long-term (storage) stability tests. One 500 g portion of each batch was placed in an open glass crystallizing dish (10 cm × 19 cm diam) and allowed to stand in a fume hood at ambient temperature under incandescent lighting for 16 days. After gently remixing each batch by hand, duplicate 10 g samples were taken for analysis of gentian violet content at intervals of 0, 1, 2, 4, 8, 13, and 16 days after the initial blending. Duplicate 5 g portions were also taken at the same intervals and dried at 110° overnight to determine the dry matter content. The other 500 g portion of each batch was transferred to a glass amber bottle, sealed, and stored in the dark at ambient temperature. These were sampled for analysis of gentian violet and dry matter content at intervals of 0, 1, 2, 4, 8, 12, and 17 weeks after preparation.

Extraction of Human Urine. A 100 ml portion of human urine in a 165 ml culture tube was adjusted to pH 7.0 with 6 N NaOH. After the addition of 50 ml of dichloromethane, the tube was gently shaken by hand for 3 min with care taken to prevent emulsification of the contents. The tube was then centrifuged for 5 min at 500 rpm and the dichloromethane layer removed by syringe and cannula, percolated through 20 g of sodium sulfate in a glass funnel (3.0 cm diam), and collected in a 250 ml round-bottom flask. The extraction process was repeated with two additional 20 ml portions of dichloromethane, the sodium sulfate in the funnel washed with 5 ml of dichloromethane, and the combined extracts evaporated just to dryness on a 30° water bath by using water pump vacuum. The dry residue was transferred to a 50 ml round-bottom flask by using four successive 1 ml rinses of the dichloromethane, which were then evaporated to dryness as described. The residue was finally dissolved in 1 ml of methanol and 100 μl (10 g equivalents of urine) was injected for analysis by HPLC.

Extraction of Wastewater. A 100 ml portion of wastewater in a 100 ml syringe equipped with a Luer end fitting was forced through a C_{18} Sep Pak at a rate of about 15 ml/min. The gentian violet that concentrated from the wastewater at the top of the Sep Pak column was then eluted in 4 ml of 90% methanol-10% buffer pH 3; a 100 μl portion of the eluate (2.5 g equivalents of wastewater) was injected for analysis by HPLC.

Removal of Gentian Violet from Industrial Wastewater. An activated carbon column, prepared as described, was used to simulate a large-scale process used at the NCTR for the removal of hazardous residues from industrial wastewater prior to its discharge into the environment. Fifteen liters of aqueous gentian violet (1 ppm) was percolated through the column of activated carbon at a rate of about 100 ml/min. A 100 μl sample of each liter of effluent was injected directly for analysis by HPLC to determine the adsorption efficiency of the carbon for gentian violet. A column containing XAD-2 resin, prepared as described, was evaluated in the same manner.

Results and discussion

High-pressure liquid chromatography appeared to be a logical choice for the separation and quantitation of gentian violet because the compound has a high molar absorptivity and it is soluble in solvents such as methanol and water, which are commonly used as mobile phases. Although gentian violet was expected to have little retention on a reverse-phase column, it was thought that the molecule could possibly be paired with a counterion to produce a more hydrophobic species that would be retained. On the contrary, gentian violet was found to be retained by the reverse phase column and it could not be eluted with mobile phases of 100% methanol, acetonitrile, or dichloromethane. Upon further investigation of several paired-ion chromatographic systems, a mobile phase of 85% methanol-15% buffer pH 3 was selected

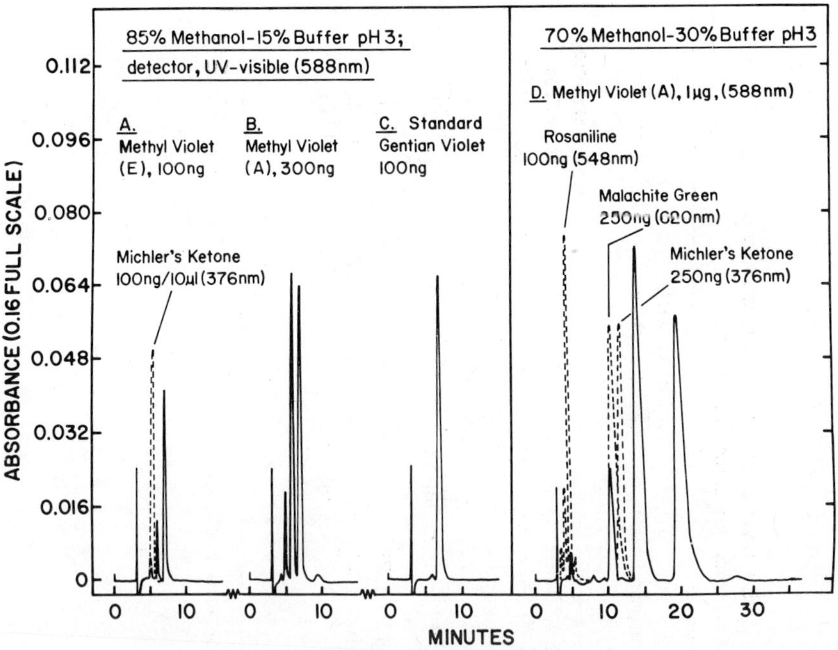

Figure 35 High-pressure liquid chromatograms of commercial methyl violet, gentian violet, and three related compounds. (A) and (B) illustrate two commercial samples of methyl violet; Michler's ketone measured at 376 nm is superimposed in (A) only for ancillary information. (C) is an analytical standard of gentian violet. In (D), chromatograms of a commercial sample of methyl violet, two triphenylmethane dyes, and Michler's ketone are superimposed. (E) and (A) denote products from Eastman and Aldrich, respectively. All injections are in 10 μl of methanol. (From Ref. 92.)

as the system for quantitative measurements of trace-level residues of gentian violet. Chromatograms A, B, and C of Figure 35 illustrate responses of commercial methyl violet and a standard of gentian violet obtained by using this system. It is interesting to note that the three major constituents of commercial methyl violet which are an analogous series differing by only one methyl group are essentially separated in less than 8 min. It was necessary to modify the mobile phase to 70% methanol-30% buffer pH 3 in semipreparative work to obtain standards of the tetramethylpararosaniline chloride and methyl violet. Chromatogram D of Figure 35 illustrates the separation of the three major constituents of commercial methyl violet; chromatograms of rosaniline, malachite green, and Michler's ketone are also superimposed.

Table 31 Retention Times and Responses of Several Dyes and a Dye Precursor at Their Respective Absorption Maxima and Their Relative Responses at the Maximum for Each Compound

Compound	Relative response at wavelength (nm) indicated							t_R (min) with mobile phase indicated			% Response/ng injected[a,b]
	635	620	588	581	573	548	376	b	c	d	
Malachite green	-	1.00	0.42	0.36	0.31	0.11	-	5.2	10.3	-	0.34
Gentian violet	-	0.29	1.00	0.93	0.86	0.71	-	6.8	19.5	-	0.41
Methyl violet	-	0.17	0.98	1.00	0.94	0.77	-	5.7	14.1	-	0.54
Tetramethylpararosaniline chloride	-	0.12	0.82	0.96	1.00	0.79	-	4.9	10.2	-	0.50
Rosaniline	-	0.04	0.13	0.23	0.46	1.00	-	3.5	4.4	12.8	0.72
Michler's ketone	-	0	0	0	0	0	1.00	5.2	11.7		0.31
Sulfan blue	1.00	-	-	-	-	-	-	-	-	11.1	-
Isosulfan blue	1.00	-	-	-	-	-	-	-	-	5.3	-

[a] 0.16 AUFS; determined at absorption maximum for compound indicated.
[b] 85% Methanol-15% buffer pH 3.
[c] 70% Methanol-30% buffer pH 3.
[d] 50% Methanol-50% buffer pH 3.
Source: Ref. 92.

It is suggested that this HPLC procedure may be useful for the identification, analysis, and quality control of triphenylmethane dyes used as biological stains and thus resolve some of the problems associated with the batch-to-batch variations in staining properties reported in the literature [106]. Michler's ketone is superimposed in Figure 35 as ancillary information because it is a precursor in one of the manufacturing processes for triphenylmethane dyes. The compound is not detected at 588 nm due to its low response at this wavelength; its adsorption maximum is 376 nm. Additionally, a mobile phase of 50% methanol-50% buffer pH 3 was evaluated to provide an adequate retention time for rosaniline in the event its analysis is sought; sulfan blue and isosulfan blue may also be analyzed by this system.

The t_R values, absorption maxima, and relative responses at various wavelengths for several triphenylmethane dyes and a dye precursor are presented in Table 31. The visible spectra of malachite

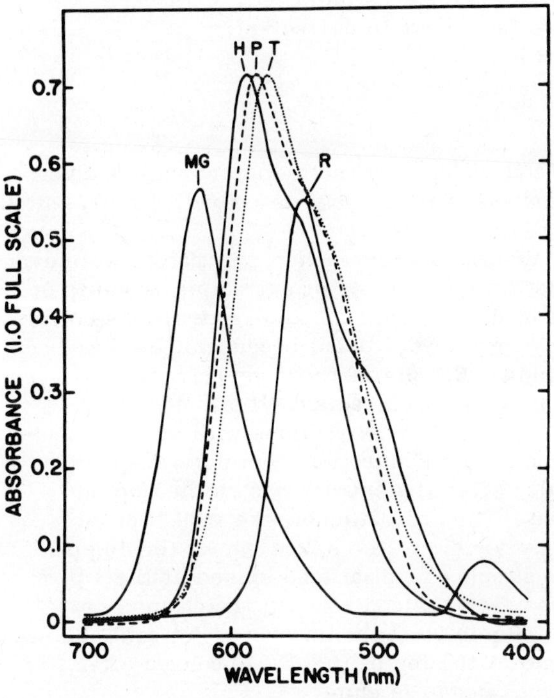

Figure 36 Visible absorption spectra of gentian violet (H) and four related compounds. MG, malachite green; P, methyl violet, T, tetramethylpararosaniline chloride; R, rosaniline. All concentrations are 2.5 μg/ml in 70% methanol-30% buffer pH 3 except R, which is 2 μg/ml. (From Ref. 92.)

Table 32 Residues Recovered from Animal Feed (10 g) Spiked with Gentian Violet (10 ppm) by Using Various Extraction Systems[a]

Solvent	Volume of solvent	Recovery (%)
Ethyl acetate	100	11
Tetrahydrofuran	100	15
Dichloromethane	100	29
Dichloromethane	100	59[b]
90% Dichloromethane-10% MeOH	100	73
91% Dichloromethane-9% MeOH	110	77[b]
Methanol	100	74
99% Methanol-1% 0.5 N HCl	100	78
99% Methanol-1% 1 N HCl	100	86
99% Methanol-1% 1 N HCl	100	86[c]
99% Methanol-1% 12 N HCl	100	81

[a]Mechanically shaken for 1 hr, except as indicated.
[b]HCl (15 ml, 1 N) added to feed prior to extraction.
[c]Mechanically shaken for 2 hr.
Source: Ref. 92.

green, gentian violet, methyl violet, tetramethylpararosaniline chloride, and rosaniline, determined as previously described, are presented in Figure 36.

A variety of solvent systems and extraction parameters were evaluated to determine the most efficient means of extracting residues of gentian violet from animal feed. However, Soxhlet extractions and the use of high-boiling solvents were avoided because of the heat labile nature of the compound. Results of these experiments are presented in Table 32. The highest extraction efficiencies (86%) were obtained from both 1 hr and 2 hr extractions with 99% methanol-1% 1 N HCl; the 1 hr extraction procedure was therefore adopted for the analysis of animal feed. After the extract was cleaned up on LH-20 and finally dissolved in 1 ml of methanol, the violet color of the gentian violet was easily visible to the naked eye at the 10 ppm level. Also, a cleaned-up sample of animal feed spiked at the 1 ppm level could be distinguished from the control. In the cleanup of animal feed spiked at the 100 ppb level the gentian violet could be seen as a very faint narrow band at the top of the LH-20 column after most of the yellowish coextractives began to elute.

Results from triplicate samples of animal feed spiked at levels of 0, 0.01, 0.1, 1, 10, 100, and 1000 ppm are presented in Table 33. Recoveries ranged from 72 to 90% and the standard error was generally less than 1%. Although it is possible to analyze samples containing residues of gentian violet in excess of 10 ppm by simply injecting

Table 33 HPLC Analysis of Animal Feed, Human Urine, and Wastewater Spiked at Various Levels with Gentian Violet

Gentian violet added		Gram equivalents of sample injected	Gentian violet recovered ($\bar{x}$ ± SE)[a]		
μg	ppm		μg	ppm	%
			Animal Feed[b]		
0	0	0.1	0.026 ± 0.003	0.0026 ± 0.0003	-
0.1	0.01	0.1	0.079 ± 0.002	0.0079 ± 0.0002	79 ± 2
1	0.1	0.1	0.725 ± 0.012	0.0725 ± 0.0012	72.5 ± 1.2
10	1	0.01	8.28 ± 0.05	0.828 ± 0.005	82.8 ± 0.5
100	10	0.01	86.3 ± 0.6	8.63 ± 0.06	86.3 ± 0.6
1000	100	0.001	889 ± 2	88.9 ± 0.2	88.9 ± 0.2
10,000	1,000	0.0001	8960 ± 40	896 ± 4	89.6 ± 0.4
			Human Urine[c]		
0	0	10	0.003 ± 0.001	0.00003 ± 0.00001	-
0.1	0.001	10	0.056 ± 0.005	0.00056 ± 0.00005	56 ± 5
1	0.01	10	0.580 ± 0.026	0.00580 ± 0.00026	58.0 ± 2.6
			Wastewater[c]		
0	0	2.5	0.012 ± 0.002	0.00012 ± 0.00002	-
1	0.01	2.5	0.605 ± 0.021	0.00605 ± 0.00021	60.5 ± 2.1

[a]Mean and standard error from triplicate assays; spiked samples are corrected for background of control samples

[b]Per 10 g of animal feed.

[c]Per 100 g of sample.

Source: Ref. 92.

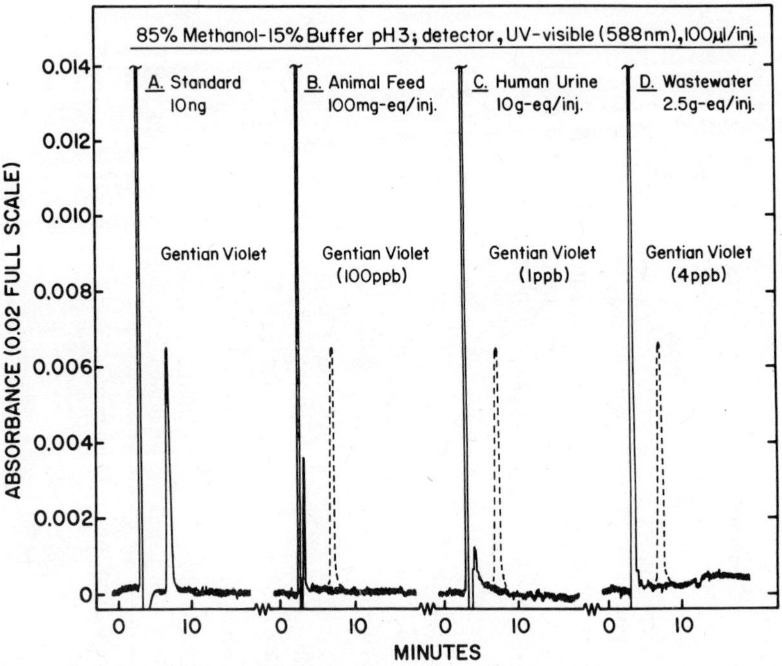

Figure 37 High-pressure liquid chromatograms of gentian violet alone and in extracts of animal feed, human urine, and wastewater. In (B), (C), and (D), solid lines represent cleaned-up extracts; dashed lines denote 10 ng of gentian violet spiked into the extracts. (From Ref. 92.)

the raw extract into the high-pressure liquid chromatograph, this procedure would undoubtedly reduce the life of the column. However, the analysis of trace levels in animal feed required cleanup on LH-20; therefore, the cleanup system was used for all analyses. Typical high-pressure liquid chromatograms of a standard of gentian violet and of a cleaned-up extract spiked with gentian violet (100 ppb) are presented in chromatograms A and B of Figure 37. The background response for gentian violet in the cleaned-up unspiked animal feed amounted to no more than the noise of the HPLC system, which was equivalent to 2.6 ppb of gentian violet.

Results from triplicate samples of human urine spiked with gentian violet at levels of 1 and 10 ppb and wastewater spiked at 10 ppb are also presented in Table 33. All recoveries were approximately 60% and the standard error was no more than 5%, even for the 1 ppb level in human urine. Typical chromatograms of cleaned-up unspiked extracts of human urine and wastewater with gentian violet superimposed at levels of 1 and 4 ppb are presented in Figure 37. As with cleaned-up unspiked animal feed, backgrounds for unspiked human urine and wastewater were attributed to the noise of the HPLC system, equivalent to about 30 and 120 parts per trillion of gentian violet, respectively. The procedure for human urine based on liquid-liquid partitioning, which was found to give excellent results, was developed before the analysis of wastewater was attempted. Later attempts to adapt this procedure to the analysis of wastewater yielded erratic and low recoveries of 6 to 30%. This was probably caused by the adsorption of the gentian violet onto particulate matter present in the wastewater, as evidenced by the light bluish particles that settled from the spiked wastewater that stood overnight. Consistent results were obtained only after the spiked wastewater was vigorously shaken to uniformly disperse the particles immediately prior to forcing the sample through the Sep Pak. The residues of gentian violet were then eluted from the Sep-Pak by using 90% methanol-10% buffer pH 3 and subjected to analysis.

Results from the experiments conducted to evaluate the efficiency of an activated carbon column to remove gentian violet from industrial wastewater indicated that no residue (<20 ppb) emerged from the column after the addition of 15 liters of aqueous gentian violet (1 ppm). It should be noted that 100 μl from each liter of effluent was taken for analysis, resulting in a minimum detectable level of 20 ppb, which was considered adequate to monitor the effluent of the column. On the other hand, if higher sensitivity is desired, the Sep-Pak procedure could yield an enhancement of about 25-fold. Nevertheless, these experiments indicated that activated carbon efficiently removes gentian violet from industrial wastewater, which is a prerequisite for release of the water into the environment. The column packed with XAD-2 resin, evaluated in a similar manner, failed to remove gentian violet from the wastewater.

Results from the stability studies of gentian violet in animal feed are presented in Table 34. These data clearly indicate that small amounts of gentian violet were unstable in feed during both short-term and long-term studies. The percentages of residues lost were more pronounced at the lower levels; for example, residues in animal feed spiked with 1 ppm of gentian violet declined by about 26% during both 16 days in simulated animal test conditions and 17 weeks in storage, whereas those spiked at the 1000 ppm level declined by about 11% under the same conditions; these losses were generally inversely related to the amount of gentian violet present in the feed. Therefore, the spiked animal feed must be prepared frequently to provide assurance that the requisite dosages are administered to the test animals.

Although the residue levels of gentian violet declined markedly during the stability test, no degradation products were observed during

Table 34 Results from Stability Studies of Gentian Violet in Animal Feed Spiked at Four Levels

Sampling interval	Gentian violet recovered (ppm)[a] Controls	1	10	100	1000
Days			Short-Term Study[b]		
0	0.003 ± 0.000	1.56 ± 0.08	10.4 ± 0.1	99.6 ± 0.5	1090 ± 10
1	0.003 ± 0.000	1.64 ± 0.05	10.8 ± 0.1	101 ± 0.0	1120 ± 10
2	0.003 ± 0.000	1.48 ± 0.03	10.4 ± 0.1	97.8 ± 0.8	1090 ± 10
4	0.003 ± 0.000	1.38 ± 0.02	10.5 ± 0.0	97.0 ± 0.1	1060 ± 0
8	0.004 ± 0.001	1.34 ± 0.05	9.48 ± 0.50	96.4 ± 0.1	1050 ± 10
13	0.003 ± 0.000	1.18 ± 0.01	8.02 ± 0.55	86.5 ± 1.1	1020 ± 0
16	0.004 ± 0.000	1.14 ± 0.04	8.42 ± 0.13	80.5 ± 0.3	980 ± 0
Weeks			Long-Term Study[c]		
0	0.003 ± 0.000	1.56 ± 0.08	10.4 ± 0.1	99.6 ± 0.5	1090 ± 10
1	0.004 ± 0.001	1.58 ± 0.01	9.72 ± 0.31	98.3 ± 0.3	1100 ± 10
2	0.003 ± 0.000	1.50 ± 0.03	10.7 ± 0.1	94.0 ± 0.8	1080 ± 10
4	0.003 ± 0.000	1.45 ± 0.00	10.2 ± 0.2	90.7 ± 1.7	1030 ± 10
8	0.003 ± 0.000	1.37 ± 0.04	9.38 ± 0.09	88.0 ± 2.1	1020 ± 10
12	0.004 ± 0.001	1.37 ± 0.01	8.25 ± 0.02	83.1 ± 0.0	971 ± 16
17	0.003 ± 0.000	1.16 ± 0.02	7.68 ± 0.28	75.2 ± 3.3	962 ± 22

[a]Mean and standard error from duplicate assays; corrected for background of control samples, recovery, and dry matter content.
[b]Open container, incandescent lighting, and ambient temperature.
[c]Sealed container, light-tight cabinet, and ambient temperature.
Source: Ref. 92.

the analysis of the samples. However, an evaluation of the data in Table 34 indicates that the decline in residues may be due, at least in part, to photodegradation and/or oxidation. The following ancillary experiment was performed to investigate this possibly. Fifty micrograms of gentian violet in 0.5 ml of methanol was left to evaporate in the bottom of a 50 ml round-bottom flask, covered with a beaker and placed under incandescent light for 19 days. The residue was then dissolved in methanol and the pink-colored solution analyzed by HPLC. No gentian violet was detected in this sample; however, several degradation products with t_R values less than that of gentian violet were observed. At present, no statement about the identity of the degradation products can be made. It should be emphasized that without the specificity of analysis by HPLC (Table 31), the degraded sample in the presence of the yellowish animal feed extract could be mistaken to contain gentian violet if analyzed by conventional spectrophotometry [108,109].

The procedures reported in this work provide the analyst with specific and sensitive means not previously available for the separation and determination of triphenylmethane dyes and related compounds.

This work was conducted under the auspices of the National Toxicology Program.

III. AZO COMPOUNDS

A. Analysis, Purification, and Stability of Azo Dyes and Pigments [111]

General description of methods

Impurities of aromatic amines in the azo dye and pigment, Direct Black 38 and Pigment Yellow 12, and in vitro stability of the dye were determined. These factors can affect the results of studies designed to ascertain whether the two compounds are metabolized to potential carcinogens in hamsters. Procedures for removing impurities from the two compounds are presented and may be applied to other water-soluble azo dyes and water-insoluble pigments. Electron capture gas chromatography of the heptafluorobutyryl derivatives of the impurities and degradation products was used to satisfy all the analytical requirements of the experiments. Because of the extremely insoluble nature of some azo compounds, especially pigments, the use of electron capture gas chromatography and the high sensitivity associated with the technique provides one of the few inexpensive means available for analyzing picogram amounts of impurities extracted from solutions containing milligram amounts of sample. Methods for stability studies of purified Direct Black 38 in water and in urine from hamsters and humans are described.

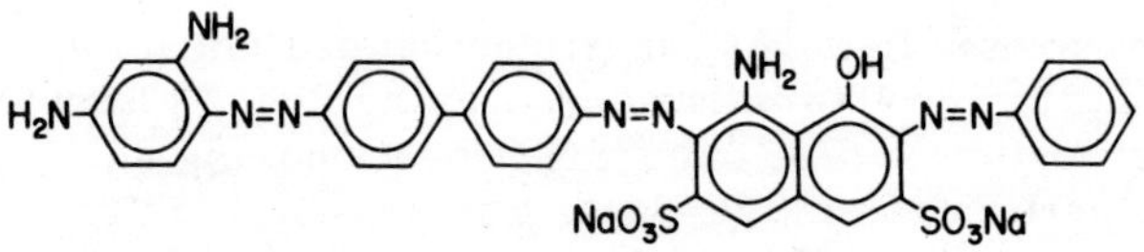

C.I. Direct Black 38

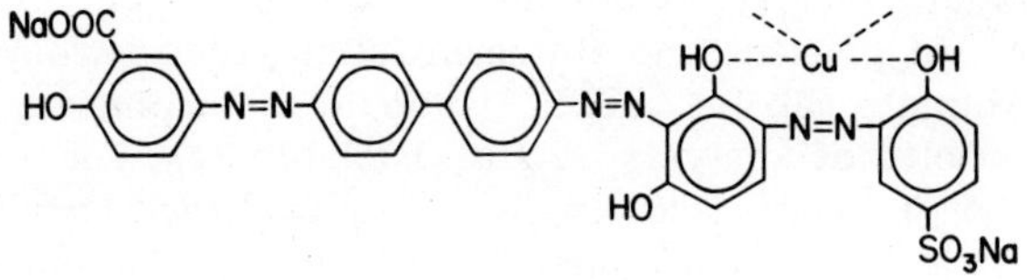

C.I. Direct Brown 95

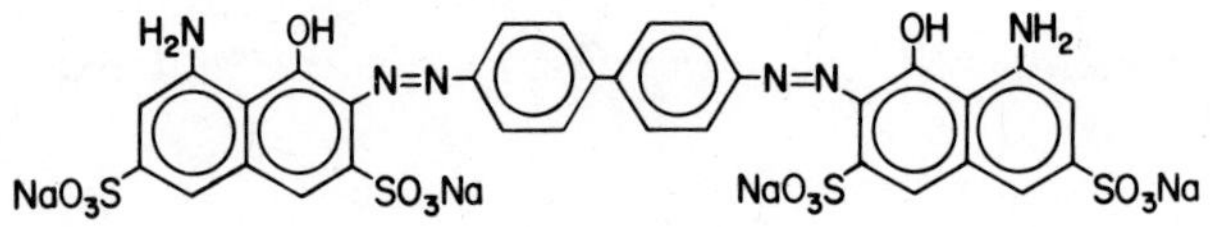

C.I. Direct Blue 6

Figure 38 Formulas of Direct Black 38, Direct Brown 95, and Direct Blue 6.

Introduction

Experiments that determine the toxicological effect of a test chemical require that the compound be examined for the presence of extraneous substances prior to the initiation of animal tests. The presence of excessive amounts of one or more impurities indicates that the compound must be purified to minimize or eliminate the effects of substances that might bias the experimental results [88]. Also, in cases where traces of the test compound are to be determined in substrates such as diet, tissues, and body fluids, there must be assurance that such residues are stable during the period required to perform the assays. Recent cooperative research between the National Center for Toxicological Research (NCTR) and the National Institute for Occupational Safety and Health (NIOSH) demonstrated the importance of determining the purity and stability of the test substance to validate toxicological experiments. Hamsters were to be given a single dose of Direct Black 38 (a benzidine-based, water-soluble dye) or Pigment

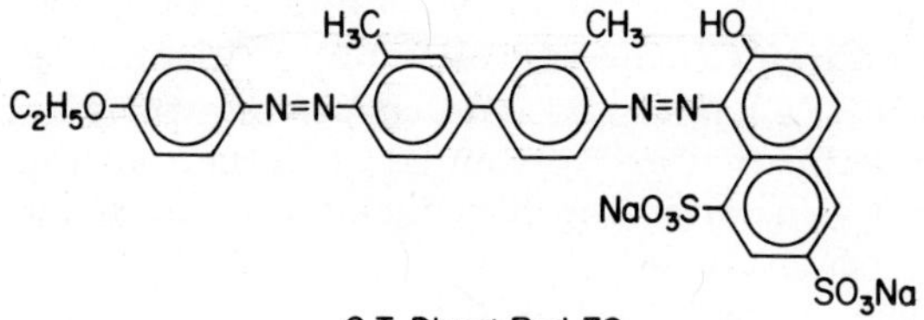

C.I. Direct Red 39

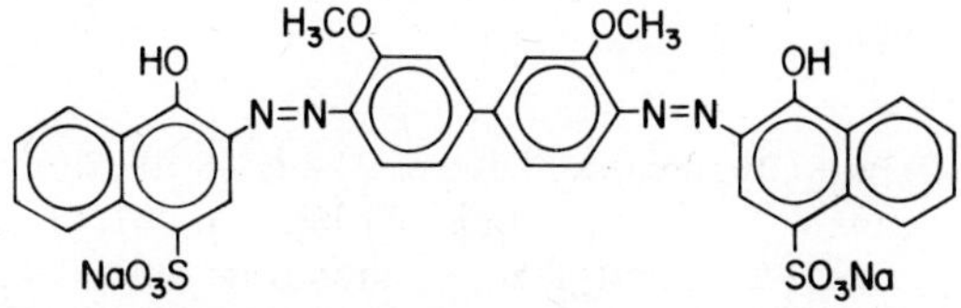

C.I. Direct Blue 8

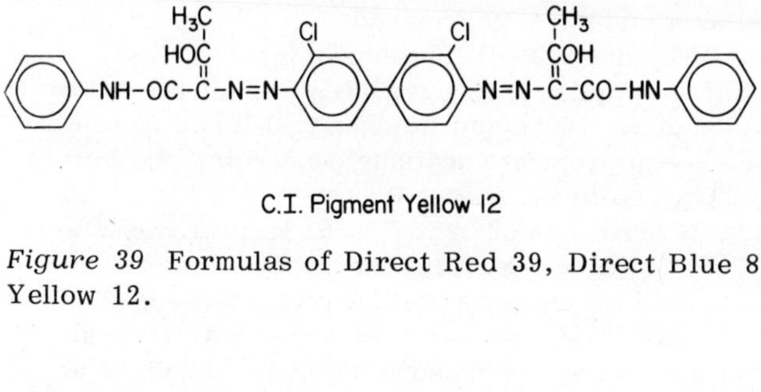

C.I. Pigment Yellow 12

Figure 39 Formulas of Direct Red 39, Direct Blue 8, and Pigment Yellow 12.

Yellow 12 (a 3,3'-dichlorobenzidine-based, water-insoluble pigment) followed by trace-level assays of the urine to measure any cleavage of the azo compounds to fragments that are known or suspected to cause cancer (e.g., benzidine, 3,3'-dichlorobenzidine). Formulas of Direct Black 38 and Pigment Yellow 12 are shown in Figures 38 and 39 together with other azo dyes that contain moieties of benzidine or its congeners.

Recently, sensitive and specific analytical procedures for determining trace levels of aromatic amines were developed at this laboratory [112]. These procedures, based on conversion of the free amines to heptafluorobutyryl (HFB) derivatives and subsequent quantification by electron capture gas chromatography (EC-GC), were employed to investigate and satisfy the purity and stability requirements of the metabolism studies. Procedures for the analysis and purification of Direct Black 38 and Pigment Yellow 12 and data concerning their purity before and after purification are presented, together with information regarding stability in water and hamster and human urine stored at three different temperatures.

Data obtained in these studies were used in the development of trace-level analytical methods for potentially carcinogenic metabolites of the dye and pigment in the urine of hamsters and humans [112] and were a prerequisite to metabolism studies based on the analysis of urine from hamsters dosed with the two compounds.

Experimental

Test Materials and Other Chemicals. Direct Black 38 (2,7-naphthalenedisulfonic acid, 4-amino-3-{[4'-[(2,4-diaminophenyl)azo] [1,1'-biphenyl]-4-yl]azo}-5-hydroxy-6-(phenylazo)-, disodium salt) was Lot No. 690 purchased from GAF Corp. (New York, New York). Pigment Yellow 12 (2,2'-[(3,3'-dichloro(1,1'-biphenyl)-4,4'-diyl)bis(azo)]bis(3-oxo-N-phenyl)butanamide) was purchased from the Dry Color Manufacturers' Association (Nutley, New Jersey). The 2,4-diaminoazobenzene (DiAmAzBz), also known as Basic Orange 2 or Chrysoidine Y, was purchased from Pfaltz and Bauer Co., Flushing, New York, and used as a standard as received. Benzidine (Bzd), 4-aminobiphenyl (4-ABP), and 3,3'-dichlorobenzidine (DiClBzd) were obtained from three suppliers, as previously reported by Bowman et al. [29], Holder et al. [43], and Bowman and Rushing [40], respectively. (Note: See appropriate sections concerning the individual compounds.) The azo dyes, Direct Brown 95 and Direct Blue 6, depicted in Figure 38 were Lots 237 and 45896, respectively, both obtained from GAF Corp. (New York, New York).

All solvents were distilled in glass and all reagents were CP grade. Sodium sulfate and glass wool were extracted with benzene for 40 hr in a Soxhlet apparatus and dried in an oven overnight at 130° prior to use. All culture tubes were borosilicate glass and equipped with Teflon-lined screw caps. The keeper solution was paraffin oil (20 mg/ml) in benzene.

Heptafluorobutyric anhydride (HFBA) (No. 63164) was obtained from Pierce Chemical Company, Rockford, Illinois. A 100 μl Hamilton syringe, fitted with a Chaney adapter, was used to withdraw the derivatizing agent from the vial and deliver it into the reaction vessel. A fresh vial (1 g) was used for each group of samples. The trimethylamine (TMA) reagent (0.05 M in benzene), phosphate buffer solution (pH 6), and sodium hydroxide (10 N) were described by Bowman and Rushing [40] and Nony and Bowman [84].

Extraction and Preparation of Sample for Analysis of Impurities

Direct Black 38. A 25 mg sample of Direct Black 38 contained in a 12 ml culture tube was dissolved in 5 ml of deionized water and extracted with a 5 ml portion of benzene by shaking the tube and contents vigorously for 1 min followed by centrifugation at 1000 rpm for 5 min. The benzene layer was carefully withdrawn by using a syringe and cannula, percolated through a plug of anhydrous sodium sulfate (18 mm diam × 20 mm thick) and collected in a 50 ml round-bottom flask containing a glass bead and 0.5 ml of keeper solution. The extraction was repeated by using two additional 5 ml portions of benzene, and the combined extracts, containing any free amine impurities, were evaporated just to dryness by using water pump (aspirator) vacuum and a 60° water bath. The residue was derivatized as described later. All water-soluble azo dyes can be analyzed for aromatic amine impurities as described. Slight adjustments in sample size or pH may be necessary to ensure complete dissolution of sample and that the impurities are in the free amine form. Some dyes may require dissolution in 0.01 N NaOH with warming and sonication to hasten the process.

Pigment Yellow 12. A 7.5 mg portion of Pigment Yellow 12 contained in a 170 ml culture tube was dissolved in 100 ml of chloroform and extracted with a 20 ml portion of 2 M HCl by shaking the tube and contents vigorously for 1 min. After the phases have separated, the upper layer (aqueous) was withdrawn by using a syringe and cannula, percolated through two pieces of filter paper (Whatman No. 42), and collected in another 170 ml culture tube. The extraction was repeated by using two additional 20 ml portions of 2 M HCl and the combined filtrates, containing any HCl salts of DiClBzd or other amines, were cooled to about 5°. An 18 ml portion of 10 N NaOH was added to the aqueous phase to convert the salts to their corresponding free amines, which were then extracted with three 20 ml portions of benzene. The combined extracts, collected in a 100 ml round-bottom flask, were treated as described for Direct Black 38. Other pigments may be analyzed as described or with minor adjustments in sample size to effect complete dissolution.

Preparation of Derivatives for Gas Chromatographic Analysis. The HFB derivatives of standards of the aromatic amine impurities in Direct Black 38 and Pigment Yellow 12 were prepared by the authors' modification [112] of the procedures reported by Walle and Ehrsson [44]. Briefly, the amines were derivatized in benzene by using HFBA reagent with TMA solution as a catalyst, as discussed in Section II.H.

Dry residues from the extraction of impurities from the dye or pigment were dissolved in benzene and converted to HFB derivatives as described. For assays of dye containing amine residues of no more than 400 ppm, the entire extract (25 mg equivalents of dye) was derivatized and 5 μl injections (62.5 μg equivalents of dye) were assayed by EC-GC. For assays of dye containing amine residues in excess of 400 ppm (e.g., DiAmAzBz), the final extract must be diluted with benzene and a suitable aliquot taken for derivatization to avoid depletion of the HFBA reagent.

For assays of pigment containing amine residues of no more than 1000 ppm, the entire extract (7.5 mg equivalents of pigment) was derivatized and 5 μl injections (18.75 μg equivalents of pigment) were assayed by EC-GC.

Gas Chromatographic Assays. A Hewlett-Packard (Palo Alto, California) Model 5750B instrument equipped with a ^{63}Ni electron capture detector (Tracor, Inc., Austin, Texas) was used as described by Nony and Bowman [112] and as presented in Section III.B. Impurities of Bzd, DiClBzd, and DiAmAzBz were analyzed on a column of 5% Dexsil 300 operated at 260°. Retention time (t_R) values for their HFB derivatives were 2.30, 2.95, and 1.85 min, respectively. The 4-ABP analyzed on the same column at 220° had a t_R value of 1.95 min. Heptachlor epoxide, used as a reference standard to monitor the performance of the EC-GC system, had t_R values at 260 and 220° of 1.65 and 3.95 min, respectively. All injections were made in 5 μl of benzene. All derivatized samples of unknown residue content were quantified by relating their peak heights to known amounts of the corresponding HFB derivatives.

Purification of Test Compounds

Direct Black 38. One liter portions of an aqueous solution of the dye (5 g/liter) were manually extracted 12 times in a separatory funnel with 1 liter portions of benzene which were subsequently discarded. The aqueous phase containing purified dye was then lyophilized and the dry material reassayed for impurities as previously described. Other water-soluble azo dyes may be purified in this manner.

Pigment Yellow 12. A dichloromethane solution (1500 ml) containing 150 mg of the pigment were extracted six times with 500 ml portions of 2 M HCl, which were discarded. The organic phase containing the purified pigment was then evaporated to dryness at 40° under water pump vacuum. The process was repeated 40 times to provide about 5 g of purified pigment which was reassayed for impurities as described. Other azo pigments may be purified in this manner or with modification to compensate for different solubilities in dichloromethane.

Stability Studies with Direct Black 38 in Water, Hamster, and Human Urine. Thirty milliliter amounts of water, hamster urine, and human urine were each spiked with 5000 ppm of purified Direct Black 38 and stored at 5, 25, and 37.5°; 5 ml samples were then withdrawn and analyzed immediately and 24, 48, 72, and 96 hr later. Each sample, contained in a 12 ml culture tube, was extracted and analyzed as described for impurities in Direct Black 38.

Results and discussion

Initial experiments with Direct Black 38, designed to determine the presence or absence of free aromatic amine impurities, indicated a large amount of an unknown compound perhaps generated during synthesis of the dye. Its presence prevented the assay of Bzd by an established electron capture gas chromatographic method [84]. Extracts of the dye, subjected to combined gas chromatography-mass spectrometry (GC-MS) and field desorption mass spectrometry (FD-MS), confirmed the identity of this compound as 2,4-diaminoazobenzene (DiAmAzBz), also known as Basic Orange 2. Further, an inspection of the structural formula of Direct Black (Fig. 38) reveals that DiAmAzBz is a moiety of the dye connected by a strong C—C bond. Nevertheless, a method to assay for small amounts of Bzd in the presence of large amounts of DiAmAzBz was accomplished by substituting the fluoroacylating reagent, heptafluorobutyric anhydride (HFBA), for pentafluoropropionic anhydride (PFPA), as reported by Nony and Bowman [112]. The resolution achieved as a result of using HFBA is depicted in Figure 40. The lower electron-capturing response obtained from HFB-DiAmAzBz as compared with HFB-Bzd is attributed to the number of HFB groups present in the derivatized molecule (i.e., one for DiAmAzBz and two for Bzd). Apparently, the amino group in the 2-position of DiAmAzBz is sterically hindered and does not derivatize under the conditions of this method; however, the sensitivity is still excellent. The known carcinogen, 4-ABP, is another impurity that was found to be present at a relatively high level in Direct Black 38; its presence was also confirmed by GC-MS and FD-MS. The presence of 4-ABP in the dye may be related to the synthesis of Bzd as an intermediate in the production process. As with Bzd and DiAmAzBz, 4-ABP is derivatized quantitatively with HFBA and is easily chromatographed at 220° with high sensitivity (Fig. 40).

Results of the EC-GC assays of the aromatic amine impurities in Direct Black 38 (GAF Lot No. 690) without and with purification were as follows:

Method of purification	Impurities (ppm)		
	Bzd	4-ABP	DiAmAzBz
None (as received)	< 0.1	150	9200
Soxhlet extraction	12	160	4800
Manual extraction	3.0	6.0	670

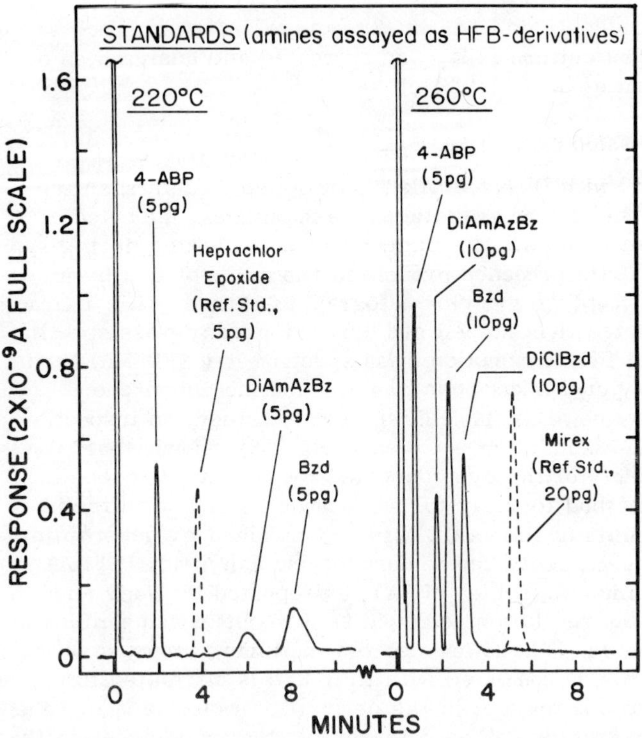

Figure 40 Electron capture gas chromatograms of HFB derivatives of impurities of Direct Black 38 and Pigment Yellow 12, and reference standards of heptachlor epoxide and mirex. All injections are in 5 μl of benzene. (From Ref. 111.)

The dye, as received, contained <0.1 ppm of Bzd, but because of the high levels of the carcinogen, 4-ABP, and DiAmAzBz, purification procedures were initiated. Initially, a 5 g sample of the dye was subjected to Soxhlet extraction with dichloromethane for 94 hr at a rate of 6 cycles/hr. The sample was dried, reassayed, and found to contain increased amounts of Bzd and 4-ABP and only a 50% reduction in DiAmAzBz. These data strongly indicated that the impurities might be occluded in the dye matrix and not be readily extracted by the Soxhlet procedure. As a consequence, the Soxhlet and the continuous liquid-liquid extraction procedures were abandoned since no satisfactory reduction of impurities was achieved. Finally, an aqueous solution of the dye was extracted manually with 12 portions of benzene (previously described), lyophilized, and the product assayed. Even though this procedure generated a 3 ppm level of Bzd, residues of 4-ABP and DiAmAzBz were diminished 25- and 14-fold, respectively; therefore, the process was adopted and the product used in animal studies since the purity vastly exceeded that obtained by other procedures.

The supply of Pigment Yellow 12, assayed by EC-GC as described, was found to contain 90 ppm of DiClBzd. No other aromatic amines were detected. As with Direct Black 38, the inefficient Soxhlet and continuous liquid-liquid extraction techniques were abandoned and the liquid-liquid extraction method using dichloromethane as previously described was used. An EC-GC assay of the pigment purified by the liquid-liquid extraction technique indicated a DiClBzd content of 0.3 ppm. This level, which was a 100-fold improvement over the Soxhlet procedures, was considered acceptable for the metabolic studies in animals. Because of the low solubility of Pigment Yellow 12 in both water and organic solvents, it was necessary to repeat the procedure 40 times to provide a sufficient quantity (about 5 g) of purified material for use in animal tests. Although the purification procedure is tedious, we know of no other method that will yield the desired purity.

Samples of Direct Brown 95 and Direct Blue 6 were also assayed for major aromatic amine impurities by using the methods described for Direct Black 38. The dyes, as received, contained 15 and 23 ppm of Bzd, respectively.

The stability tests with Direct Black 38 in water and in urine from hamsters were performed to validate the analytical procedure and the proposed conditions for collection and storage of animal samples, thus providing assurance that no in vitro degradation of the dye occurred. The dye was found to be essentially stable in water at both 5 and 25° during the 48-hr period. Also, the dye was stable at both temperatures in hamster urine up to 24 hr; however, after 48 hr at 25° the levels of Bzd and 4-ABP were appreciably higher. The results of a more comprehensive experiment with spiked hamster urine, conducted as previously described, are reported in Table 35. Again the dye was found to be stable up to 24 hr at all temperatures; then increasing amounts of Bzd and 4-ABP were found in subsequent samples held at 25 and 37.5°. These data indicate that essentially no degradation occurs in the analytical procedure; however, samples of urine from animal experiments should be collected under dry ice, then stored at -20° prior to analysis to prevent possible degradation of any dye that might be present in the urine. A similar experiment with Bzd and 4-ABP each spiked at 100 ppm into hamster urine showed that the residues were stable up to 96 hr.

The in vitro instability of the dye in hamster urine at temperatures near 25° led us to conduct a similar experiment with human urine;

Table 35 Stability of Purified Direct Black 38 in Hamster Urine

Sampling interval (hr)	Concentration of degradation product (μg/ml) at temperature (°C) indicated								
	Benzidine			4-Aminobiphenyl			2,4-Diaminoazo-benzene		
	5°	25°	37.5°	5°	25°	37.5°	5°	25°	37.5°
0	0.015	0.015	0.015	0.010	0.010	0.010	2.90	2.90	2.90
24	0.014	0.018	0.018	0.010	0.027	0.100	2.70	2.40	1.70
48	0.014	0.800	0.100	0.012	2.70	0.380	2.70	5.00	1.30
72	0.016	5.50	1.70	0.009	4.90	2.80	2.90	5.40	2.40
96	0.015	7.00	2.60	0.009	6.00	3.70	2.90	2.90	4.90

Source: Ref. 111.

the results are presented in Table 36. The dye was found to be stable up to 24 hr at all temperatures; then increasing amounts of Bzd and 4-ABP were found in subsequent samples held at 25 and 37.5°. The pattern of degradation in human urine was similar to that in hamster urine; however, the extent of degradation was considerably lower in the human urine. For example, after 96 hr at 25°, human urine contained only 0.13 ppm of Bzd compared with 7.00 ppm in hamster urine. These results can probably be explained by differences in urine dilutions, pH, and the presence of bacteria. Nevertheless, it is

Table 36 Stability of Purified Direct Black 38 in Human Urine

Sampling interval (hr)	Concentration of degradation product (μg/ml) at temperature (°C) indicated								
	Benzidine			4-Aminobiphenyl			2,4-Diaminoazo-benzene		
	5°	25°	37.5°	5°	25°	37.5°	5°	25°	37.5°
0	0.010	0.010	0.010	0.010	0.010	0.010	2.90	2.90	2.90
24	0.010	0.010	0.010	0.010	0.011	0.086	2.00	3.60	1.30
48	0.010	0.040	0.030	0.010	0.205	0.280	1.90	3.85	1.70
72	0.010	0.045	0.135	0.013	0.255	0.735	2.35	2.80	2.20
96	0.010	0.130	0.115	0.013	0.445	1.30	1.70	1.60	1.20

Source: Ref. 111.

definite that degradation of the dye does occur after 24 hr at 25 and 37.5° in both hamster and human urine. Consequently, since the inadvertent contamination of human urine with dye could occur at an industrial site, surveillance samples should be immediately frozen and transported under dry ice, and then stored at -20° prior to analysis. This procedure would also prevent cleavage of dyes by microorganisms.

The demonstrated instability of Direct Black 38 in vitro in hamster and human urine also signals the possibility that industrial discharge of the dye could ultimately contaminate the environment with breakdown products such as Bzd and 4-ABP. A similar phenomenon was reported by Games and Hites [86] as a result of their evaluation of dye manufacturing plant effluents. They observed an increased concentration of two chemicals *after* passing through the treatment plant and they concluded that chemical or biological degradation of dye molecules through reduction of azo linkages was the probably cause. Therefore, since enhanced toxicity of industrial wastewaters may occur during waste treatment, suitable cleanup precautions must be observed at the manufacturing site.

The chemical methods that the authors have described and referenced [29,40,43,84,112] are adequate for use as monitoring procedures to measure the degradation products of Direct Black 38 and similar compounds in both the urine from industrial workers and the effluent from manufacturing plants.

Stability tests with Pigment Yellow 12 were not conducted because of its extremely hydrophobic nature; however, effluents from manufacturing sites should be monitored for DlClBzd.

This work was conducted by the National Center for Toxicological Research under an interagency agreement No. 224-78-0004 for the National Institute for Occupational Safety and Health.

B. Trace Analysis of Potentially Carcinogenic Metabolites of Direct Black 38 and Pigment Yellow 12 [112]

General description of methods

Analytical chemical procedures are described for determining traces of possible metabolites of two azo compounds, Direct Black 38 and Pigment Yellow 12, in hamster urine and to monitor the urine from workers who may be occupationally exposed during the manufacture or use of the dye and pigment. These methods are used for metabolism studies designed to assess the hazards that may occur if the two compounds are converted by in vivo mechanisms to potential carcinogens. Salient elements of the procedure are: extraction of the free aromatic amines and neutral compounds, alkaline hydrolysis of the aqueous phase and extraction of any hydrolyzed conjugates as free amines, and the analysis of the free amines and acetylated metabolites directly by high pressure-liquid chromatography or by electron capture gas chromatography after conversion of the amines to heptafluorobutyryl derivatives. Residues of metabolites in hamster and human urine were determined at levels as low as 1 ppb. Ancillary data concerning hydrolysis of diacetylated metabolites and partition values for possible metabolites in various solvent systems are also presented.

Introduction

Recent epidemiological studies of workers in the dye industry showed an increased incidence of bladder tumors above that of the general population. Early attempts toward solving this problem indicated that many of the azo dyes and pigments used in large quantities contain benzidine or certain congeners, such as dichlorobenzidine, dimethylbenzidine, and dimethoxybenzidine. Although benzidine is known to be a carcinogen in humans [1], no similar evidence exists for the three congeners; however, they are known to be mutagenic [2] and to produce tumors in experimental animals. Akiyama [37] reported the release of dichlorobenzidine (DiClBzd) into the urine of exposed workers at a pigment manufacturing plant. Recent work at the National Cancer Institute (NCI) showed that the benzidine dyes Direct Black 38, Direct Brown 95, and Direct Blue 6 are carcinogenic in rats and hepatotoxic in mice [113]. In another study, Rinde and Troll [3] demonstrated the presence of free benzidine (Bzd) and monoacetylbenzidine (MoAcBzd) in the urine of rhesus monkeys fed four benzidine dyes. The colorimetric method they used was based on the reaction of trinitrobenzene sulfonic acid (TNBS) with compounds containing free amino groups, but no provision was made for the assay of diacetylbenzidine (DiAcBzd) and conjugated metabolites. An improvement of this method employing the reagent fluorescamine [76] increased the sensitivity of aromatic amines into the nanomole range; however, as with the TNBS method, only compounds with free amino groups were detected. Therefore, sensitive and specific analytical chemical methods were required to evaluate properly the results of metabolic studies in animals. Further assays for trace levels of these metabolites were necessary to monitor the urine from workers in the dye and pigment industries.

Methods for the analysis of free aromatic amines, including Bzd and DiClBzd, in human urine [29,40,84,88] are among the most sensitive and specific methods reported in the literature. Although Riggin and Howard [114] had difficulty derivatizing Bzd with fluoroacylating agents, no problem was experienced in this work when a catalyst of trimethylamine was used. The electron capture gas chromatographic (EC-GC) methods for DiClBzd [40] and Bzd [84] have minimum detectable levels in urine of about 60 ppt (pg/ml) and 1 ppb, respectively, analyzed as their pentafluoropropionyl derivatives. On the other hand, the procedure of Riggin and Howard [114] employing electrochemical

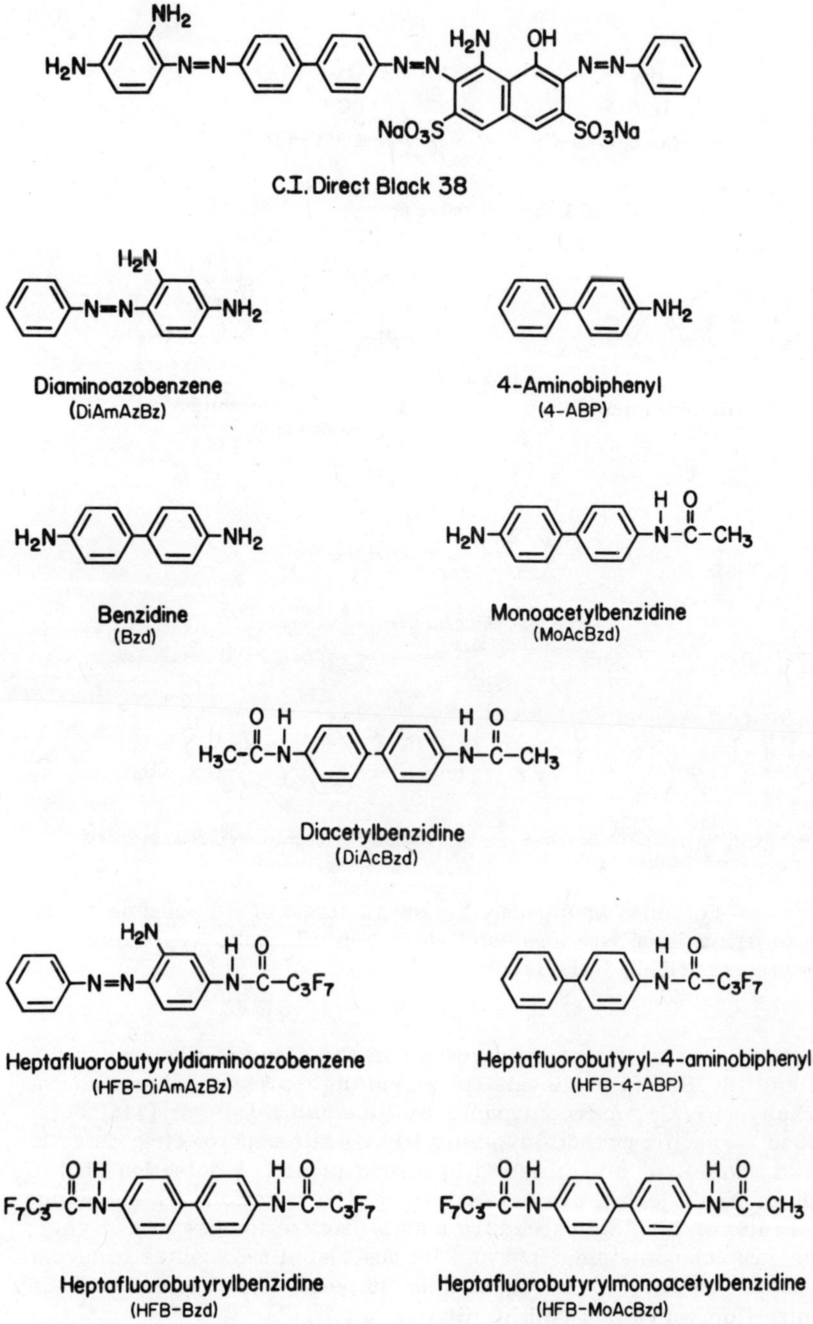

Figure 41 Formulas of Direct Black 38, its metabolites in urine from hamsters, and their heptafluorobutyryl (HFB) derivatives. (From Ref. 112.)

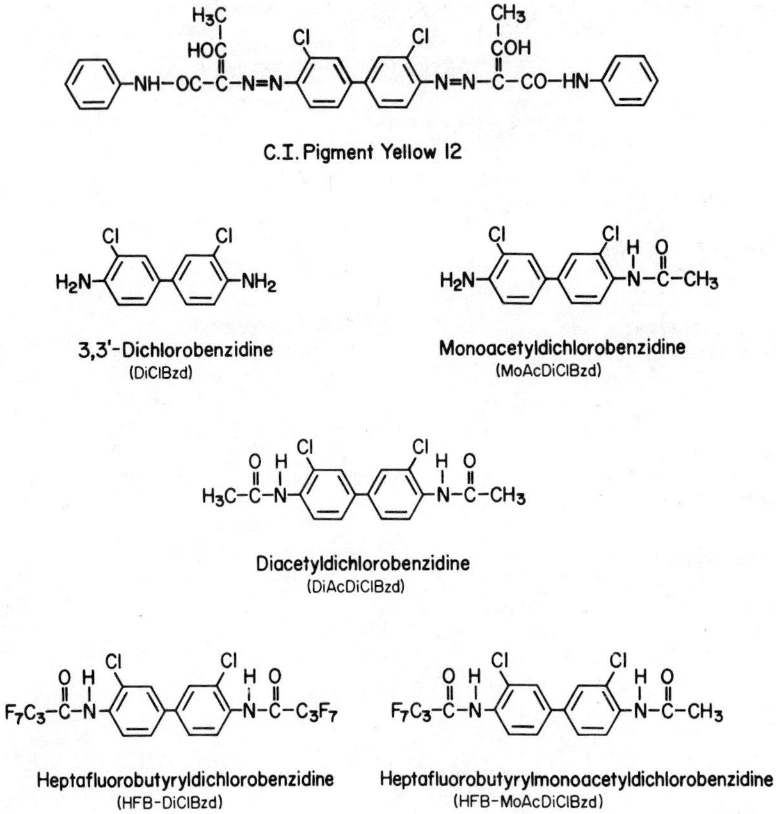

Figure 42 Formulas of Pigment Yellow 12, some of its possible metabolites in urine from hamsters, and their heptafluorobutyryl (HFB) derivatives. (From Ref. 112.)

detection is a significant improvement in the assay of wastewater for Bzd and DiClBzd at low levels (ppb) via high-pressure liquid chromatography (HPLC). A recent paper by Rice and Kissinger [115] described a specific method involving HPLC with amperometric detection of Bzd, MoAcBzd, and DiAcBzd in human urine. A detection limit of 10 pg of Bzd injected was determined by the criterion of a signal-to-noise ratio of 2. This procedure shows promise for use in assaying urine samples containing Bzd and its acetylated metabolites to levels as low as 10 ppb. Quantitation of levels below 10 ppb would probably require fluoroacylation and EC-GC.

Since methodology sufficiently sensitive and specific for determining possible metabolites of Direct Black 38 and Pigment Yellow 12

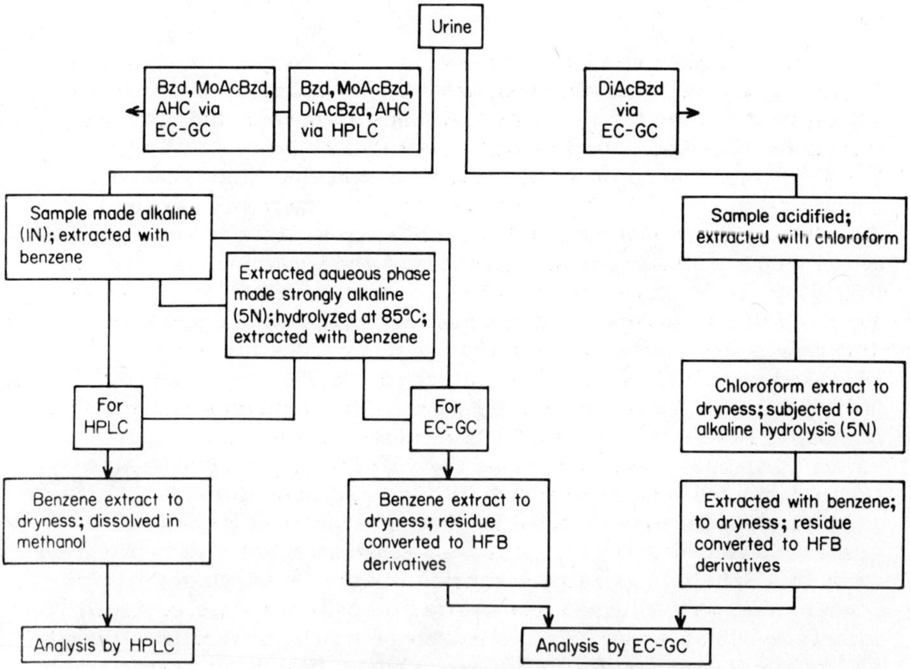

Figure 43 Scheme for extraction, separation, and analysis of benzidine (Bzd), monoacetylbenzidine (MoAcBzd), diacetylbenzidine (DiAcBzd), and alkaline hydrolyzable conjugates in urine. (From Ref. 112.)

in urine could not be found, methods were developed for use in cooperative research between the National Center forToxicological Research (NCTR) and the National Institute for Occupational Safety and Health (NIOSH).

The structural formulas of the dye and pigment, their possible metabolites in urine from hamsters and humans, and their heptafluorobutyryl (HFB) derivatives are presented in Figures 41 and 42. The abbreviations listed for the compounds in both figures are used throughout the text for the purpose of simplification. The scheme for the extraction, separation, and analysis of Bzd, MoAcBzd, and alkaline hydrolyzable conjugates in urine is depicted in Figure 43. Salient elements of the procedure are (1) extraction of the free aromatic amines and neutral compounds; (2) alkaline hydrolysis of the aqueous phase and extraction of any hydrolyzed conjugates as free amines; and (3) analysis of the free amines and acetylated metabolites directly by HPLC or by EC-GC after conversion to the HFB derivatives.

Experimental

Test Materials and Other Chemicals. The compounds shown in Figures 41 and 42 were obtained from various sources. Direct Black 38, Pigment Yellow 12, and DiAmAzBz were described and obtained from three suppliers, as previously reported by Nony and Bowman [111]. [Note: see appropriate sections concerning individual compounds (e.g., 4-ABP, Bzd, and DiClBzd).] The monoacetyl and diacetyl derivatives of Bzd and DiClBzd were synthesized and purified at the NCTR. The chemical structures of these compounds were confirmed by the electron impact (70 EV) spectra obtained via direct insertion using a Finnigan Instruments (Sunnyvale, California) Model 1015 mass spectrometer. Assays of the derivatives for purity by HPLC indicated MoAcBzd, 97.3%; DiAcBzd, 98.9%; MoAcDiClBzd, 90%; and DiAcDiClBzd, essentially pure. The impurities remaining in MoAcBzd, DiAcBzd, and DiAcDiClBzd were primarily the respective parent compounds and extraneous acetyl derivatives. The MoAcDiClBzd contained about 5% each of DiClBzd and DiAcDiClBzd.

All solvents were distilled in glass and all reagents were CP grade. Sodium sulfate and glass wool were extracted with benzene for 40 hr in a Soxhlet apparatus and dried in an oven overnight at 130° prior to use. All culture tubes were of borosilicate glass equipped with Teflon-lined screw caps. The keeper solutions were paraffin oil (20 mg/ml) in benzene for EC-GC assays and diethylene glycol for HPLC assays. (Note: The appropriate keeper solution must be used for each assay! Paraffin oil in benzene is not compatible with the HPLC procedure; also, the presence of diethylene glycol in the derivatization procedure for EC-GC depletes the reagents and produces interferences.)

Heptafluorobutyric anhydride (HFBA) (No. 63164) was obtained from Pierce Chemical Company (Rockford, Illinois). A 100 μl Hamilton syringe fitted with a Chaney adapter was used to withdraw the derivatizing agent from the vial and deliver it into the reaction vessel. A fresh vial (1 g) was used for each group of samples. The trimethylamine (TMA) reagent (0.05 M in benzene), buffer solution (potassium monobasic phosphate, pH 6), and sodium hydroxide (10 N) were described by Bowman and Rushing [40] and Nony and Bowman [84].

Preparation of Derivatives for Gas Chromatographic Assays. The heptafluorobutyryl (HFB) derivatives of the metabolites of Direct Black 38 and Pigment Yellow 12 shown in Figures 41 and 42 (except DiAcBzd and DiAcDiClBzd) were prepared by modification of the procedures reported by Walle and Ehrsson [44]. Briefly, the amines were derivatized in benzene by using HFBA reagent with TMA solution as a catalyst as discussed in Section II.H.

Final residues from the extraction procedures of the basic (free amine) fractions from hamster or human urine were dissolved in benzene (1.5 ml) and derivatized by using TMA solution and HFBA reagent as described. For assays of hamster urine containing amine residues in the order of 0.01, 0.1, 1.0, and not >10 ppm, the entire extract (1 g equivalent) of the sample was derivatized, and 5 μl injections containing 2500, 250, 25, and 2.5 μg equivalents, respectively, were assayed by EC-GC. For assays of hamster urine containing amine residues in excess of 10 ppm (e.g., MoAcBzd) the final extract must be diluted with benzene to a known volume in a calibrated tube or flask and a suitable aliquot taken for derivatization. For assays of human urine potentially containing amine residues in the order of 0.001, 0.01, 0.1, and 1.0 ppm, the entire extract (10 g equivalents) of the treated sample was derivatized and 5 μl injections containing 25,000, 2500, 250, and 25 μg equivalents, respectively, were assayed by EC-GC.

Gas Chromatographic Assays. A Hewlett-Packard (Palo Alto, California) Model 5750 B instrument equipped with a ^{63}Ni electron capture detector (Tracor, Inc., Austin, Texas) and a 6 ft glass column (4 mm i.d.) containing 5% Dexsil 300 on Anakrom Q (90/100 mesh) conditioned at 300° for 72 hr prior to use, was operated isothermally at 220, 260, and 280° with nitrogen as the carrier gas flowing at 160 ml/min. The detector operated in the dc mode was set at 330° and the injection port temperature was 20° higher than the column oven. Heptachlor epoxide and mirex were used as reference standards to monitor the performance of the EC-GC system; all injections were made in 5 μl of benzene. Because of the wide differences in retention time (t_R) values for the various HFB derivatives (Table 37), MoAcBzd and MoAcDiClBzd were analyzed at 280°; then Bzd, DiClBzd, and DiAmAzBz were analyzed at 260° and 4-ABP at 220°. DiAcBzd and DiAcDiClBzd must be hydrolyzed and converted to their corresponding free amines prior to derivatization with HFBA; these compounds are then analyzed at 260° as HFB-Bzd and HFB-DiClBzd. Hydrolyzed samples of unknown DiAcBzd and DiAcDiClBzd content that had been derivatized were quantified by relating the peak height of the HFB derivatives to known amounts of HFB-Bzd or HFB-DiClBzd, and the results were expressed as DiAcBzd (Bzd × 1.456 = DiAcBzd) or DiAcDiClBzd (DiClBzd × 1.332 = DiAcDiClBzd). All other derivatized samples of unknown residue content were quantified by relating their peak heights to known amounts of the corresponding HFB derivatives.

High-Pressure Liquid Chromatographic Assays. A Waters Associates, Inc. (Milford, Massachusetts) liquid chromatograph equipped with a Model 6000A solvent delivery system, a Model U6K septumless injector, a Tracor Model 970A variable-wavelength detector operated at 295 nm, and a 3.9 mm i.d. × 30 cm μBondapak C_{18} (reverse phase) column (Waters No. 27324) was used. The mobile phase, 50% methanol-50% potassium phosphate (0.01 M, pH 6.0), flowed at the rate of

Table 37 Retention Times of Possible Metabolites of Direct Black 38 and Pigment Yellow 12 (HPLC) and Their Heptafluorobutyryl Derivatives (EC-GC)

	Retention time (t_R, min) by method indicated			
	EC-GC at temperature (°C) indicated			
Compound	220°	260°	280°	HPLC
Benzidine (Bzd)	8.15	2.30	1.15	4.40
Monoacetylbenzidine (MoAcBzd)	a	10.6	3.95	5.50
Diacetylbenzidine (DiAcBzd)				7.65
2,4-Diaminoazobenzene (DiAmAzBz)	5.95	1.85	0.95	13.6
4-Aminobiphenyl (4-ABP)	1.95	0.85	0.55	14.4
3,3-Dichlorobenzidine (DiClBzd)	10.7	2.95	1.45	9.10
Monoacetyldichlorobenzidine (MoAcDiClBzd)	a	10.0	3.75	7.70
Diacetyldichlorobenzidine (DiAcDiClBzd)				6.30
Heptachlor epoxide (ref. std.)	3.95	1.65	1.00	-
Mirex (ref. std.)	15.0	5.20	2.75	-

[a]Low response precluded determination.
Source: Ref. 112.

1 ml/min with a pressure of 1600 psi. These conditions were used for assays of the metabolites of Direct Black 38, and their t_R values are reported in Table 37.

For assays of possible metabolites of Pigment Yellow 12, the mobile phase was adjusted to 60% methanol-40% potassium phosphate (0.01 M, pH 6.0) with a flow rate of 1 ml/min and a pressure of 1500 psi; the detector was operated at 292 nm. The t_R values for possible metabolites of Pigment Yellow 12 obtained under these conditions are also reported in Table 37. All injections were made in 5 μl of methanol.

For samples of unknown residue content, the residue was dissolved in 1 ml of methanol for analysis as described. Quantification was achieved by relating the peak height to known amounts of the corresponding metabolites.

Hydrolysis Studies of Diacetyl Compounds. Five microgram amounts of the diacetyl derivatives of Bzd and DiClBzd in 1 ml of methanol contained in 20 ml culture tubes were subjected to various concentrations of NaOH for 2 hr at 85° in a tube heater (Kontes No. 720,000, Vineland, New Jersey) to determine the optimum alkalinity required for complete cleavage of the compounds and recovery of the free amines. One milliliter portions of NaOH (0.5, 1.0, 2,0, 4.0, 6.0, 8.0, or 10 N) were added just prior to heating the compounds. After cooling to room temperature, 6 ml of deionized water was added, and the aqueous phase was extracted with three 8 ml portions of benzene which were successively percolated through a plug of anhydrous sodium sulfate (18 mm diam × 20 mm thick) and collected in a 100 ml round-bottom flask containing a boiling bead and 1 drop of keeper. The contents were evaporated just to dryness at 60° by using water pump (aspirator) vacuum; then 2 ml of methanol was added and again evaporated to dryness to remove any traces of benzene that could interfere with the HPLC assay. Finally, the dry residue was dissolved in 1 ml of methanol and 5 μl was injected for assay by HPLC.

Extraction and Preparation of Hamster Urine for Analysis of Metabolites of Direct Black 38

Benzidine (Bzd), monoacetylbenzidine (MoAcBzd), and diacetylbenzidine (DiAcBzd). One milliliter of sample, 4 ml of deionized water, 0.5 ml of methanol, 0.5 g of NaCl, and 0.5 ml of 10 N NaOH were added to a 20 ml culture tube, shaken, and allowed to stand for 5 min. A 5 ml portion of benzene was added to the tube and the contents shaken gently for 1 min; the tube was centrifuged at 1500 rpm for 5 min. The benzene layer was carefully withdrawn by using a syringe and cannula and percolated through a plug of anhydrous sodium sulfate (about 18 mm diam × 20 mm thick) into a 50 ml graduated cylinder. The extraction was repeated with three additional 5 ml portions of benzene. The combined extracts were then brought to exactly 30 ml and divided into two equal fractions: one for assay by HPLC and the other for assay by EC-GC. (The extracted aqueous phase was reserved for determining alkaline hydrolyzable conjugates.) A glass bead and the respective keeper solutions were added to each fraction contained in 100 ml round-bottom flasks, and the contents evaporated to near dryness by using water pump vacuum and a 60° water bath.

The residue for HPLC assay was dissolved in 2 ml of methanol and again evaporated to dryness as described, to remove any traces of benzene that could interfere with the assay. The residue was either assayed immediately or stored at 5° for subsequent assay by HPLC.

The residue for EC-GC assay was transferred to an 8 ml culture tube by using three 1 ml portions of benzene and evaporated to dryness in a tube heater at 50° with a stream of dry nitrogen. The residue was reserved for subsequent derivatization with HFBA and assay by EC-GC. (Note: Any DiAcBzd that may be present in this residue must be alkaline hydrolyzed prior to derivatization and assay by EC-GC. This procedure is discussed under "Preparation of Sample for Analysis of Diacetylbenzidine via EC-GC.")

Alkaline hydrolyzable conjugates (AHC) of benzidine (Bzd). The extracted aqueous phase reserved for alkaline hydrolysis of conjugates of Bzd was made strongly alkaline (5 N) by carefully adding 2 g of NaOH to the contents of the tube. Five milliliters of methanol was then added and the sealed tube was heated in a tube heater at 85° for 2 hr with occasional shaking. After the tube had cooled, any Bzd or other aromatic amine freed from the conjugates by the hydrolysis was extracted by using three 8 ml portions of benzene. The extracts were combined and evaporated to dryness as previously described. The residue was reserved for analysis by HPLC or subsequent derivatization with HFBA and assay by EC-GC.

Preparation of sample for analysis of diacetylbenzidine (DiAcBzd) via EC-GC. One milliliter of sample, 4 ml of water, 0.5 ml of methanol, and 0.5 ml of 1.2 N HCl were added to a 15 ml culture tube, shaken, and allowed to stand for 5 min. A 5 ml portion of chloroform was then added, the contents shaken gently for 2 min, and the tube centrifuged at 1500 rpm for 5 min. The chloroform layer was carefully withdrawn by using a syringe and cannula, percolated through a plug of anhydrous sodium sulfate (18 mm diam × 20 mm thick), and collected in a 50 ml round-bottom flask containing a glass bead and 0.5 ml of keeper solution. The extraction was repeated by using two additional 5 ml portions of chloroform, and the combined extracts containing DiAcBzd were evaporated just to dryness by using water pump vacuum and a 50° water bath. The residue was transferred to a 20 ml culture tube using three 1 ml portions of chloroform, and the solvent in the tube was then evaporated to dryness in a tube heater set at 50° by using a gentle stream of dry nitrogen. The residue was hydrolyzed by heating the sealed tube containing 1 ml of methanol and 1 ml of 10 N NaOH in a tube heater set at 85° for 2 hr. After the tube had cooled, 6 ml of deionized water was added and the contents extracted three times with 8 ml portions of benzene. Each extract was successively percolated through a plug of sodium sulfate (18 mm diam × 20 mm thick) and collected in a 50 ml round-bottom flask containing a boiling bead and 0.5 ml of keeper solution. The contents were evaporated just to dryness in the usual manner; the residue was transferred to an 8 ml culture tube by using three 1 ml portions of benzene which were also evaporated to dryness in a tube heater at 50° by using a stream of dry nitrogen. The residue containing benzidine was reserved for subsequent derivatization with HFBA and assay by EC-GC.

Extraction and Preparation of Hamster Urine for Analysis of Possible Metabolites of Pigment Yellow 12

3,3'-Dichlorobenzidine (DiClBzd), monoacetyldichlorobenzidine (MoAcDiClBzd), and diacetyldichlorobenzidine (DiAcDiClBzd). One milliliter samples were treated exactly as described for Bzd, MoAcBzd, and DiAcBzd.

Alkaline hydrolyzable conjugates (AHC) of dichlorobenzidine (DiClBzd). The extracted aqueous phase reserved for alkaline hydrolysis of conjugates of DiClBzd was made strongly alkaline (3 N) by adding 1.1 g of NaOH to the contents of the tube and treated exactly as described under "Alkaline Hydrolyzable Conjugates of Benzidine."

Preparation of sample for analysis of diacetyldichlorobenzidine (DiAcDiClBzd) via EC-GC. One milliliter of the sample, 0.5 ml of water, 0.5 ml of methanol, 4.0 ml of concentrated HCl, and 5 ml of benzene were added to a 15 ml culture tube and gently shaken for 5 min. The tube was centrifuged at 1000 rpm for 5 min and the benzene layer was carefully withdrawn by using a syringe and cannula, percolated through a plug of anhydrous sodium sulfate (18 mm diam × 20 mm thick), and collected in a 50 ml round-bottom flask containing a glass bead and 0.5 ml of keeper solution. The extraction was repeated by using two additional 5 ml portions of benzene, and the combined extracts containing DiAcDiClBzd were evaporated just to dryness in the usual manner. The residue was transferred to a 20 ml culture tube by using three 1 ml portions of benzene, and the solvent in the tube was then evaporated to dryness in a tube heater set at 50° by using a gentle stream of dry nitrogen. The dry residue was hydrolyzed by heating the sealed tube containing 1 ml of methanol and 1 ml of 6 N NaOH in a tube heater set at 85° for 2 hr. The contents of the tube were treated exactly as described for DiAcBzd via EC-GC. The final residue containing DiClBzd was reserved for subsequent derivatization with HFBA and assay via EC-GC.

Extraction and Preparation of Human Urine for Analysis of Metabolites of Direct Black 38 via EC-GC

Benzidine (Bzd) and monoacetylbenzidine (MoAcBzd). Ten milliliters of sample, 1 ml of methanol, 1 g of NaCl, and 1.0 ml of 10 N NaOH were added to a 30 ml culture tube, shaken, and allowed to stand for 5 min. A 10 ml portion of benzene was added to the tube and the contents shaken gently for 1 min; the tube was centrifuged at 1500 rpm for 5 min. The benzene layer was carefully withdrawn by using a syringe and cannula and percolated through a plug of anhydrous sodium sulfate (about 25 mm diam × 20 mm thick) and collected in a 100 ml round-bottom flask containing a glass bead and 0.5 ml of keeper solution. The extraction was repeated with three additional 10 ml portions of benzene, and the combined extracts were evaporated just to dryness in the usual manner. (The extracted aqueous phase was reserved for determining alkaline hydrolyzable conjugates.) The residue in the flask was transferred to an 8 ml culture tube by using three 1 ml portions of benzene and evaporated to dryness in a tube heater at 50° with a stream of dry nitrogen. The residue was reserved for subsequent derivatization with HFBA and assay by EC-GC. (Note: Any DiAcBzd in this residue must be alkaline hydrolyzed prior to derivatization and assay by EC-GC. This procedure is discussed under "Diacetylbenzidine."

Alkaline hydrolyzable conjugates (AHC) of benzidine (Bzd). The extracted aqueous phase reserved for alkaline hydrolysis of conjugates of Bzd was made strongly alkaline (5 N) by carefully adding 4 g of NaOH to the contents of the tube. Ten milliliters of methanol was then added and the sealed tube heated in a water bath at 85° for 2 hr with occasional shaking. After the tube had cooled, any Bzd or other aromatic amine freed from the conjugates by the hydrolysis was extracted by using three 8 ml portions of benzene. The extracts were combined and evaporated to dryness as described previously. The residue was reserved for subsequent derivatization with HFBA and assay by EC-GC.

Diacetylbenzidine (DiAcBzd). Ten milliliters of sample, 1 ml of methanol, and 1 ml of 1.2 N HCl were added to a 30 ml culture tube, shaken, and allowed to stand for 5 min. A 10 ml portion of chloroform was then added, the contents shaken gently for 5 min, and the tube centrifuged at 1500 rpm for 5 min. The chloroform layer was carefully withdrawn by using a syringe and cannula, percolated through a plug of anhydrous sodium sulfate (18 mm diam × 20 mm thick), and collected in a 100 ml round-bottom flask containing a glass bead and 0.5 ml of keeper solution. The extraction was repeated by using two additional 10 ml portions of chloroform, and the combined extracts containing DiAcBzd were evaporated just to dryness by using water pump vacuum and a 50° water bath. The residue was treated exactly as described for hamster urine under "Preparation of Sample for Analysis of Diacetylbenzidine via EC-GC."

Recovery Experiments

Hamster urine. Control urine from hamsters (300 ml) was diluted with 1200 ml of deionized water and sonicated for 5 min to disrupt sedimentary particles so that a sufficient supply of representative samples would be available for the complete development of analytical methodology. The diluted urine composite was stored at -20° when not in use.

Triplicate 5 ml samples of diluted urine composite, each containing 1 g equivalent of urine, were placed in 12 ml culture tubes and separately spiked with 50 μl of methanol containing the appropriate amount of Bzd, MoAcBzd, DiAcBzd, and 4-ABP to produce residues of 0, 0.01, 0.1, 1.0, and 5.0 ppm. In addition, MoAcBzd was spiked at the 200 ppm level. The tubes were sealed, mixed, and allowed to stand overnight at -20° prior to extraction and analysis by EC-GC.

In a similar manner, triplicate 5 ml samples of diluted urine composite were separately spiked as descirbed with the appropriate amount of Bzd, MoAcBzd, DiAcBzd, and 4-ABP to produce residues of 0, 0.5, 1.0, and 5.0 ppm. In addition, MoAcBzd was spiked at the 200 ppm level. The tubes were sealed, mixed, and allowed to stand overnight at -20° prior to extraction and analysis by HPLC.

Quadruplicate 5 ml samples of the diluted urine composite were separately spiked with the appropriate amount of Bzd, MoAcBzd, DiAcBzd, and 4-ABP to prepare residues of 1.0 ppm. One control sample (unspiked) was prepared. The tubes were sealed, mixed, and allowed to stand overnight at -20° prior to extraction and analysis by HPLC. Two of the extracted aqueous phases were again spiked in an identical manner and hydrolyzed (5 N NaOH) together with the other two extracted aqueous phases, which had not been spiked a second time. After hydrolysis and extraction with benzene, all samples were analyzed by HPLC.

Triplicate 5 ml samples of the diluted urine composite were separately spiked with the appropriate amounts of DiClBzd, MoAcDiClBzd, and DiAcDiClBzd to produce residues of 0 and 1.0 ppm. The tubes were sealed, mixed, and allowed to stand overnight at -20° prior to extraction and analysis by EC-GC and HPLC. In addition, 5 ml samples of the diluted urine composite were spiked with the appropriate amount of DiAcDiClBzd to produce residues of 0.01 and 0.1 ppm for assay only by EC-GC.

Human urine. Control human urine was collected and stored at -20° for use in the development of trace analytical methodology based on EC-GC analysis. Triplicate 10 ml samples of urine were placed in 30 ml culture tubes and separately spiked with 100 μl of methanol containing the appropriate amount of Bzd, MoAcBzd, DiAcBzd, DiAmAzBz, and 4-ABP to produce residues of 0, 0.001, 0.01, and 0.1 ppm. In addition, MoAcBzd was spiked at the 1.0 ppm level. The tubes were sealed, mixed, and allowed to stand overnight at -20° prior to extraction and analysis by EC-GC as described.

Quadruplicate 2.5 ml samples of control human urine were separeately spiked with the appropriate amount of Bzd, MoAcBzd, DiAcBzd, and DiAmAzBz to prepare residues of 1.0 ppm. One control

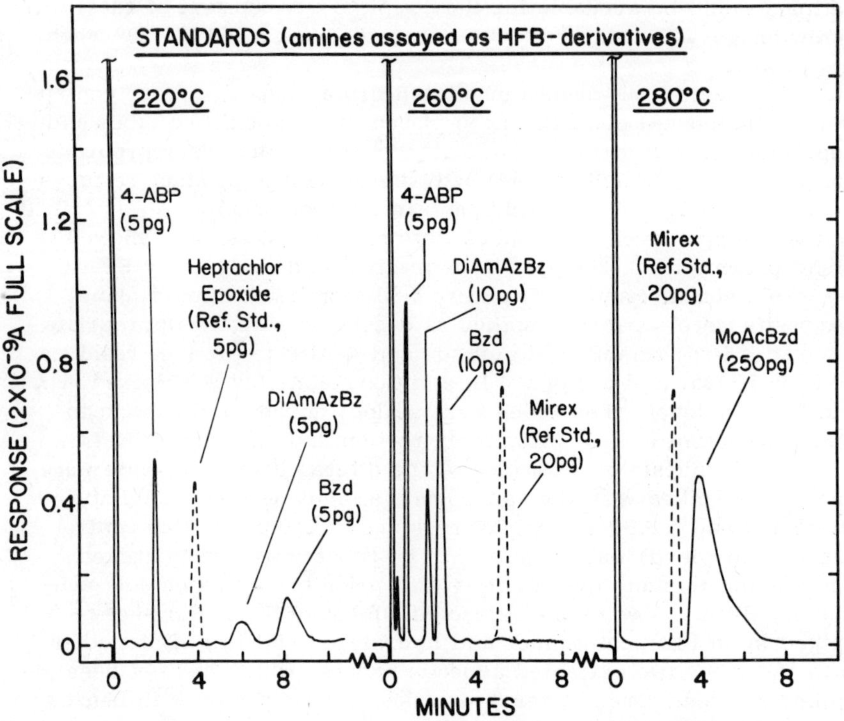

Figure 44 Electron capture gas chromatograms of HFB derivatives of metabolites of Direct Black 38, and reference standards of heptachlor epoxide and mirex. All injections are in 5 μl of benzene. (From Ref. 112.)

sample (unspiked) was prepared. The tubes were sealed, mixed, and allowed to stand overnight at -20° prior to extraction and analysis by HPLC as described. Two of the extracted aqueous phases were again spiked in an identical manner and hydrolyzed (5 N NaOH) together with the other two extracted aqueous phases, which had not been spiked a second time. After hydrolysis and extraction with benzene, all samples were analyzed by HPLC as described.

Results and discussion

EC gas chromatograms of derivatized standards of appropriate aromatic amines related to possible metabolites of Direct Black 38 (Fig. 41) and Pigment Yellow 12 (Fig. 42) are presented in Figures 44 and 45, respectively. Work reported previously [84] made use of pentafluoropropionic anhydride (PFPA) as the reagent of choice for derivatizing

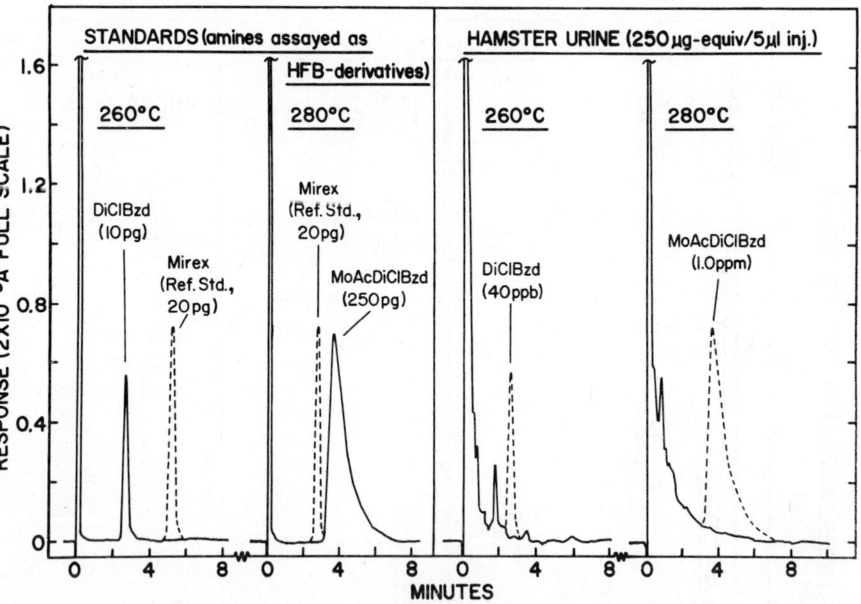

Figure 45 Electron capture gas chromatograms. Left: Solid lines are HFB-derivatives of possible metabolites of Pigment Yellow 12 in urine from hamsters; dashed lines are mirex reference standards. Right: Solid lines are derivatized extracts of urine from untreated hamsters; dashed lines (superimposed) illustrate responses from the possible metabolites analyzed as HFB derivatives. All injections are in 5 µl of benzene. (From Ref. 112.)

aromatic amines; however, the presence of a large amount of an impurity, 2,4-diaminoazobenzene (DiAmAzBz), also known as Basic Orange 2, in Direct Black 38 prevented the use of PFPA because of poor resolution between the PFP derivatives of DiAmAzBz and Bzd. Therefore, heptafluorobutyric anhydride (HFBA) was substituted for PFPA and since an acceptable degree of resolution was achieved (Fig. 44, 260°), HFBA was chosen for exclusive use in these methods where EC-GC was involved. The inclusion of 4-aminibiphenyl (4-ABP) in this project, as depicted in Figures 44 and 46, was necessary because of its presence as an impurity in Direct Black 38 and also its generation during metabolism of the dye as determined by preliminary feeding studies in hamsters. Although 4-ABP does not appear to be a metabolite of Direct Black 38 in humans, EC gas chromatograms of this compound in human urine (Fig. 47, 220°) have been included as guides in the event that it is detected as the free amine before or after alkaline hydrolysis of possible conjugates.

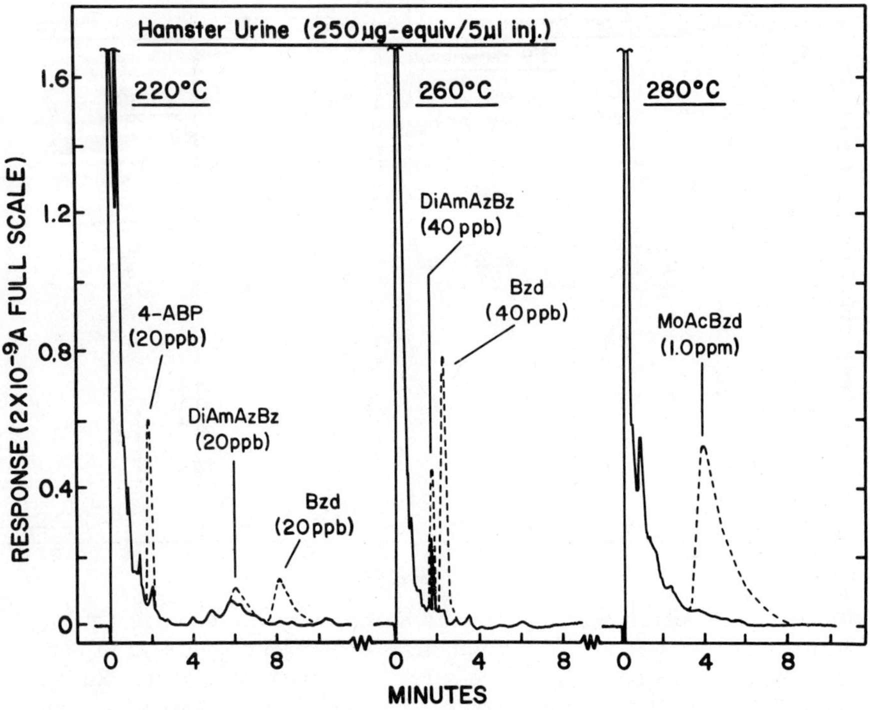

Figure 46 Electron capture gas chromatograms. Solid lines are derivatized extracts of urine from untreated hamsters. Dashed lines (superimposed) illustrate responses from metabolites of Direct Black 38 analyzed as HFB derivatives. All injections are in 5 μl of benzene. (From Ref. 112.)

Preliminary experiments with the HFB derivatives of MoAcBzd and MoAcDiClBzd indicated the need for GC column temperatures of 315° or higher to obtain chromatographic peaks with good symmetry. However, this condition, used with injector and detector temperatures of 340 and 360°, resulted in unpredictable responses, and early failure of the detector resulted. It therefore became necessary to lower the column temperature to 280° and the injector and detector temperatures to 300 and 330°, respectively. Under these conditions, the HFB derivatives of MoAcBzd and MoAcDiClBzd emerged from the GC column in a reasonably short time, but some tailing of the peaks was noted (Figs. 44 and 45). Also, with the column temperature at 280°, the t_R values increased as the amount of injected compound was decreased. Responses of unknown amounts of the two derivatives

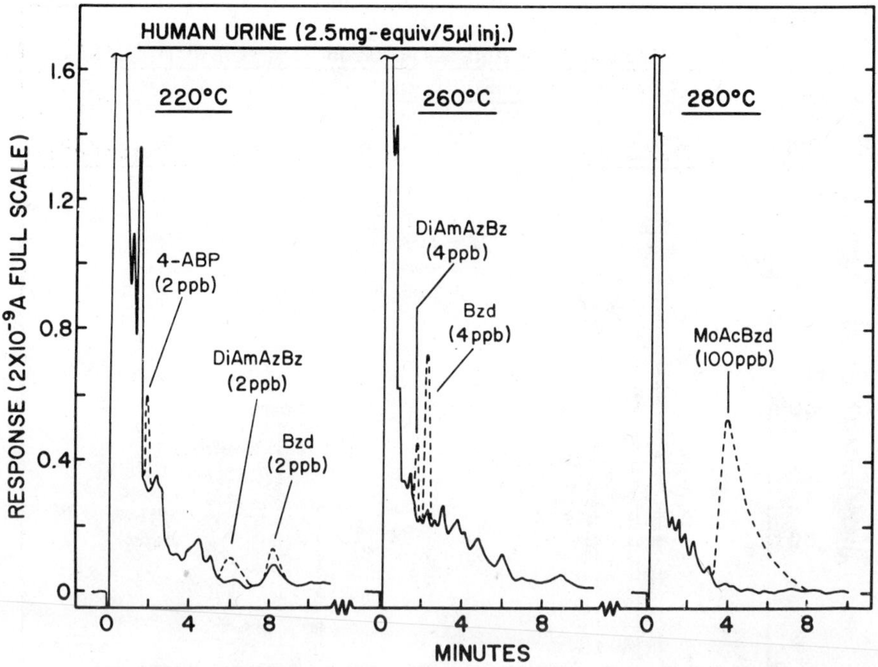

Figure 47 Electron capture gas chromatograms. Solid lines are derivatized extracts of control human urine. Dashed lines (superimposed) illustrate responses from metabolites of Direct Black 38 analyzed as HFB derivatives. All injections are in 5 µl of benzene. (From Ref. 112.)

were adjusted to compensate for changes in t_R values by using the ratio of their t_R values to those of a fixed amount of their respective standards. The validity of these corrections is evidenced by comparisons between parallel EC-GC and HPLC assays. Although considerable tailing of the peaks was obtained at 280°, no attempt was made to find an alternative column since the quantitative results were satisfactory and the thermal stability of Dexsil 300 is high. A summary of the EC-GC retention times of HFB derivatives of possible metabolites is presented in Table 37 with two reference standards, heptachlor epoxide and mirex. Since the t_R values of the MoAcBzd and MoAcDiClBzd depend on the amount injected, it should be noted that 250 pg amounts were used to obtain these values. The t_R values for the various metabolites as determined by HPLC are also presented in Table 37, and corresponding chromatograms are shown in Figures 48 and 49.

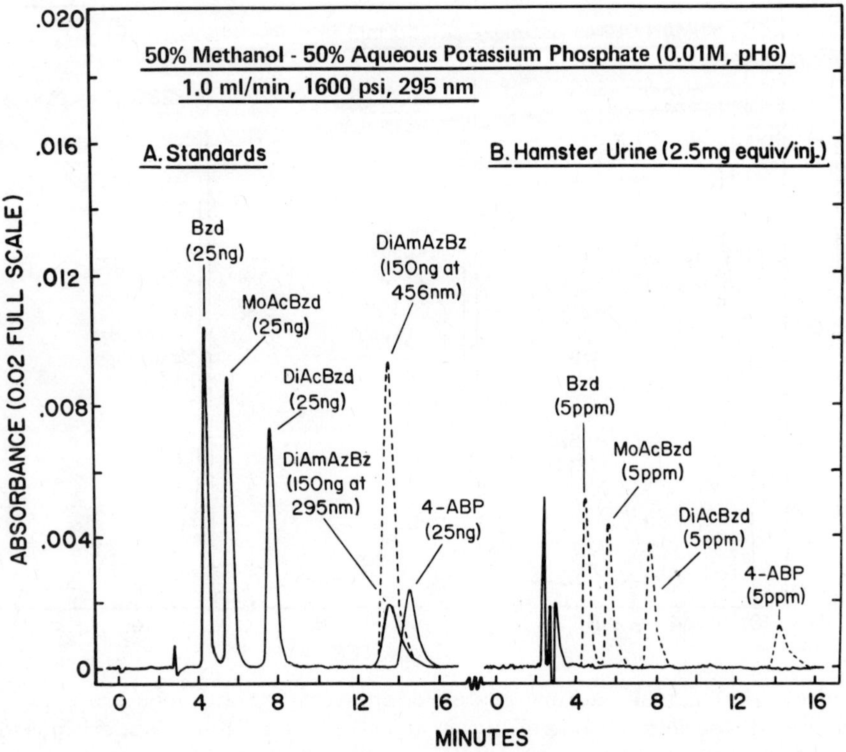

Figure 48 High-pressure liquid chromatograms. (A) Solid lines are standards of metabolites of Direct Black 38 assayed at 295 nm; dashed line illustrates the response of DiAmAzBz at its absorption maximum (456 nm). (B) Solid line is an extract of urine from untreated hamsters; dashed lines (superimposed) illustrate responses from the specified levels of metabolites in the urine extract. All injections are in 5 μl of methanol. (From Ref. 112.)

Before assays of hamster or human urine samples could be conducted, levels of background interference for each compound to be assayed were determined. Chromatograms of the various compounds are illustrated in Figures 44 to 47 (EC-GC) and Figures 48 and 49 (HPLC). The chromatograms depicted by solid lines are tracings of derivatized standards or derivatized extracts of urine from untreated hamsters or human controls. Dashed lines (superimposed) generally represent responses from derivatized standards spiked into extracts of urine from untreated hamsters and human controls. These data were used to calculate the minimum detectable levels for both methods, as reported in Table 38.

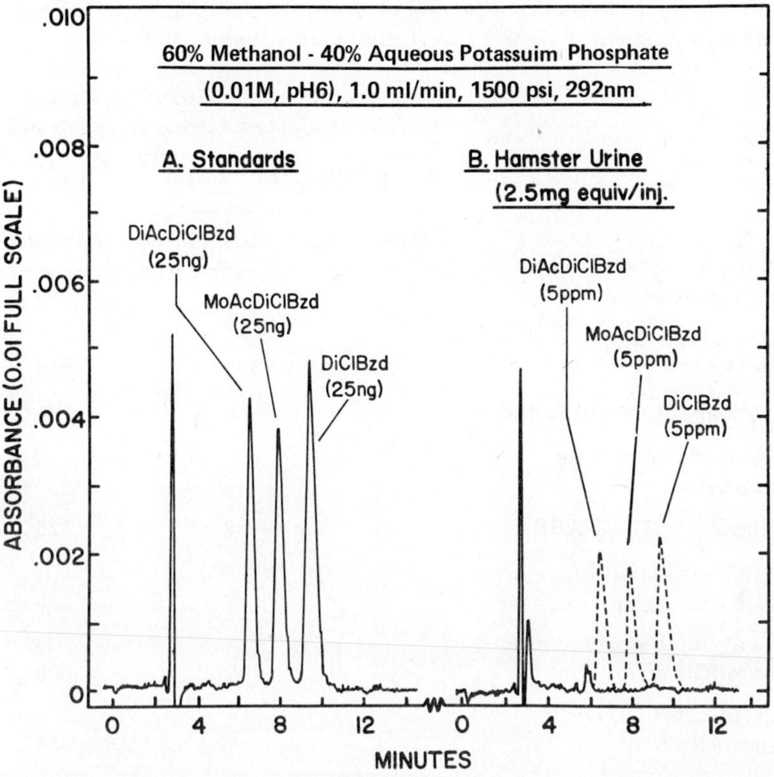

Figure 49 High-pressure liquid chromatograms. (A) Standards of proposed metabolites of Pigment Yellow 12. (B) Solid line is an extract of urine from untreated hamsters; dashed lines (superimposed) illustrate responses from the specified levels of proposed metabolites in the urine extract. All injections are in 5 μl of methanol. (From Ref. 112.)

The purity of the dye and pigment, as received, was determined by assaying for the presence of free aromatic amines by EC-GC [111]. Both compounds contained excessive amounts of impurities and each one was purified manually by a liquid-liquid extraction procedure [111].

The stability of the purified dye was tested in hamster and human urine at 5, 25, and 3.75° and found to be stable at 5° for at least 96 hr and at 25° for up to 24 hr. Based on these findings, essentially no degradation of the dye occurs in the analytical procedure. Nevertheless, it is recommended that samples of urine from hamsters

Table 38 Minimum Detectable Levels of Possible Metabolites of Direct Black 38 and Pigment Yellow 12 in Hamster and Human Urine

Compound	Minimum detectable level (ppb) by method indicated (twice background): EC-GC[a] Hamster	EC-GC[a] Human	HPLC Hamster
Benzidine (Bzd)	3	1	180
Monoacetylbenzidine (MoAcBzd)	70	2	210
Diacetylbenzidine (DiAcBzd)[b]	2	0.2	260
2,4-Diaminoazobenzene (DiAmAzBz)	5	1	850
4-Aminobiphenyl (4-ABP)	4	2	870
3,3'-Dichlorobenzidine (DiClBzd)	8	c	525
Monoacetyldichlorobenzidine (MoAcDiClBzd)	48	c	660
Diacetyldichlorobenzidine (DiAcDiClBzd)[b]	7	c	600

[a]Assayed as the HFB derivatives.
[b]Assayed as the HFB derivative after alkaline hydrolysis to the free amine.
[c]Not determined.
Source: Ref. 112.

or humans be collected and stored under dry ice initially, then at -20° prior to analysis to prevent possible degradation of any dye that might be present in the urine.

The assay of DiAcBzd and DiAcDiClBzd was straightforward when conducted by HPLC, as evidenced by the chromatograms shown in Figures 48 and 49. However, the presence of the two acetyl groups (Figs. 41 and 42) on each molecule and the absence of derivatizable functional groups prevented their assay by EC-GC. It therefore became necessary to develop a hydrolysis procedure to cleave the acetyl bonds and thereby release the free amines, Bzd and DiClBzd, for derivatization with HFBA. The results of the hydrolysis studies with DiAcBzd and DiAcDiClBzd are depicted in Figures 50

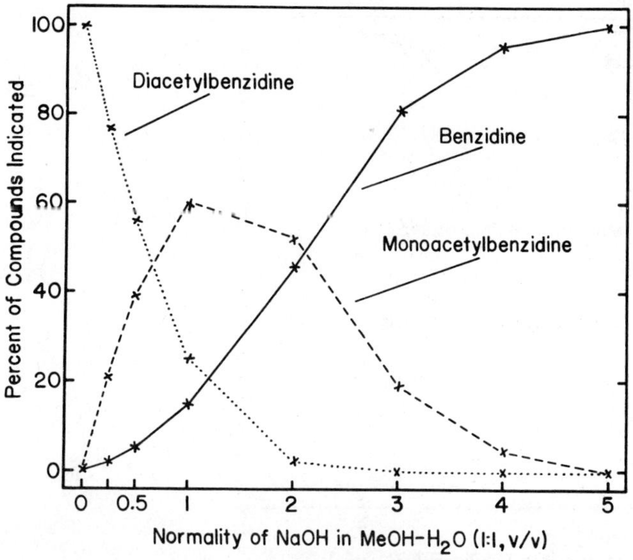

Figure 50 Alkaline hydrolysis of diacetylbenzidine. Dotted line illustrates the deacetylation of DiAcBzd; dashed line illustrates the generation of MoAcBzd from DiAcBzd and eventual deacetylation of MoAcBzd; solid line illustrates the gradual generation of Bzd from concurrent de-acetylations of DiAcBzd and MoAcBzd. Each data point represents a result from a 2 hr reaction at 85° at the indicated normality of NaOH. (From Ref. 112.)

and 51. The curves clearly indicate the progression of the hydrolysis reactions: the gradual decrease of the diacetyl (DiAc) compounds, the generation and eventual decrease of the monoacetyl (MoAc) compounds, and finally the complete conversion to Bzd or DiClBzd. Because 4 N NaOH appeared to be just sufficient for complete conversion to DiClBzd, 6 N NaOH was used for subsequent hydrolyses of DiAcDiClBzd to ensure that the reaction was complete.

Partition values (p values), which are defined as the fraction of solute partitioning into the nonpolar phase of an equivolume immiscible binary solvent system, are useful in developing extraction and cleanup methods and in confirming identity [15,18]. Hence such values, which were determined for Bzd, DiClBzd, and the respective MoAc and DiAc metabolites in several solvent systems by using HPLC, are reported in Tables 39 and 40. This information was then used to devise the scheme for extraction and separation shown in Figure 43. Salient elements of the procedures were as follows: extraction of free aromatic amines and neutral compounds with benzene (pH 14); dividing

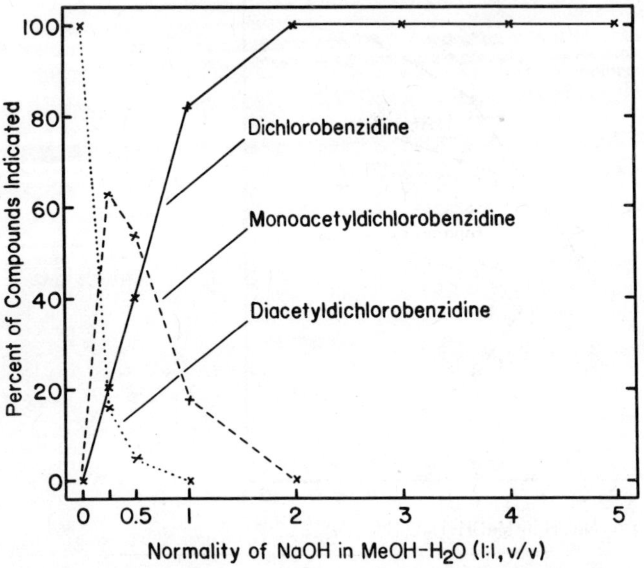

Figure 51 Alkaline hydrolysis of Diacetyldichlorobenzidine. Dotted line illustrates the deacetylation of DiAcDiClBzd; dashed line illustrates the generation of MoAcDiClBzd from DiAcDiClBzd and eventual deacetylation of MoAcDiClBzd; solid line illustrates the gradual generation of DiClBzd from the concurrent deacetylations of DiAcDiClBzd and MoAcDiClBzd. Each data point represents a result from a 2 hr reaction at 85° at the indicated normality of NaOH. (From Ref. 112.)

the extract into two known volumes; evaporating each to dryness and analyzing one residue dissolved in methanol by HPLC; and derivatizing the other residue with HFBA for analysis by EC-GC. The aqueous phase may still contain conjugated metabolites after this extraction; therefore, it is hydrolyzed under strongly alkaline conditions, extracted again with benzene, and any free amines are analyzed either directly by HPLC or after derivatization by EC-GC. For trace analysis of the neutral DiAc compounds via EC-GC, the residues must be separated from any free amines by extracting the highly acidified sample with chloroform. The residue from the chloroform extract is then subjected to hydrolysis, under strongly alkaline conditions, extracted with benzene, and the resulting free amine derivatized and analyzed by EC-GC. It should be noted that no laborious cleanup steps utilizing adsorbents such as silica gel or alumina are required even for trace analysis by EC-GC. Thus the method is greatly simplified and amenable to use with large numbers of samples. This scheme for the analysis of hamster urine, with slight modifications,

Table 39 Partition Values of Metabolites of Direct Black 38 as Determined by HPLC

Solvent system	p value		
	Bzd	MoAcBzd	DiAcBzd
Benzene-aqueous HCl (0.1 N)	0.00	0.00	0.24
Benzene-aqueous buffer (pH 7)	1.00	0.78	0.28
Benzene-aqueous NaOH (0.1 N)	0.95	0.69	0.25
Benzene-aqueous NaOH (1 N)	0.99	0.92	0.60
Chloroform-aqueous HCl (0.1 N)	0.00	0.031	1.00
Chloroform-aqueous buffer (pH 7)	1.00	1.00	1.00
Chloroform-aqueous NaOH (0.1 N)	1.00	0.98	0.93
Chloroform-aqueous NaOH (1 N)	1.00	1.00	0.97
Ethyl acetate-aqueous HCl (0.1 N)	0.00	0.045	1.00
Ethyl acetate-aqueous buffer (pH 7)	0.99	0.99	0.93
Ethyl acetate-aqueous NaOH (0.1 N)	1.00	0.99	0.94

Source: Ref. 112.

is also applicable to assays of samples containing possible metabolites of Pigment Yellow 12. Although other types of animal urine (e.g., rat or mouse) have not been tried, human urine is assayed by using this scheme with only slight adjustments of the volumes of sample and the amounts of reagents and solvents employed.

Results from triplicate assays of hamster urine unspiked and spiked with 0.01, 0.1, 0.5, 1.0, and 5.0 ppm of the metabolites of Direct Black 38 and also spiked only with MoAcBzd at the 200 ppm

Table 40 Partition Values of Possible Metabolites of Pigment Yellow 12 as Determined by HPLC

Solvent system	p value		
	DiClBzd	MoAcDiClBzd	DiAcDiClBzd
Benzene-aqueous HCl (8 N)	<0.003	<0.003	0.65
Benzene-aqueous HCl (6 N)	<0.003	0.01	0.92
Benzene-aqueous HCl (4 N)	<0.003	0.12	1.00
Benzene-aqueous buffer (pH 7)	1.00	1.00	1.00
Benzene-aqueous NaOH (1 N)	1.00	1.00	0.99

Source: Ref. 112.

Table 41 Analyses of Hamster Urine Unspiked and Spiked with 0.01, 0.1, 0.5, 1.0, 5.0, and 200 ppm of Metabolites of Direct Black 38

		Recovery of metabolites ($\bar{x} \pm SE$)[a]						
Metalites	Analytical method	Unspiked (ppm)	Spiked with 0.01 ppm (%)	Spiked with 0.1 ppm (%)	Spiked with 0.5 ppm (%)	Spiked with 1.0 ppm (%)	Spiked with 5.0 ppm (%)	Spiked with 200 ppm (%)
Bzd[b]	EC-GC	0.001 ± 0.000	c	10.8 ± 1.8	53.9 ± 10.1	71.9 ± 4.8	84.1 ± 1.5	d
Bzd	HPLC	0.090 ± 0.000	d	d	64.7 ± 0.5	73.8 ± 0.6	80.1 ± 2.2	d
MoAcBzd[b]	EC-GC	0.032 ± 0.002	c	61.9 ± 2.4	69.5 ± 6.1	85.8 ± 2.2	88.8 ± 4.7	72.6 ± 2.2
MoAcBzd	HPLC	0.100 ± 0.000	d	d	79.8 ± 1.4	89.5 ± 2.0	90.1 ± 1.2	95.2 ± 1.7
DiAcBzd[e]	EC-GC	0.001 ± 0.000	50.0 ± 0.0	53.0 ± 1.0	d	53.6 ± 0.3	55.2 ± 4.3	d
DiAcBzd	HPLC	0.130 ± 0.000	d	d	90.1 ± 1.8	87.8 ± 2.4	82.2 ± 0.7	d
4-ABP[b]	EC-GC	0.002 ± 0.001	37.8 ± 1.0	79.7 ± 2.6	78.3 ± 3.4	85.0 ± 2.1	93.2 ± 5.0	d
4-ABP	HPLC	0.430 ± 0.000	d	d	59.0 ± 8.0	82.4 ± 2.5	90.1 ± 3.0	d

[a] Mean and standard error from triplicate assays; corrected for background interference in the unspiked sample.
[b] Analyzed as the heptafluorobutyryl derivative.
[c] None detected above background.
[d] Not determined.
[e] Analyzed as the heptafluorobutyryl derivative after alkaline hydrolysis to Bzd.
Source: Ref. 112.

level are presented in Table 41. Recoveries determined by EC-GC and HPLC were generally good at levels of 0.1 ppm and above for all compounds except Bzd, which were 53.9 and 10.8% at the 0.5 and 0.1 ppm levels, respectively. Similar data were previously reported for Bzd in human urine [84]; however, the recovery did not decline appreciably until the 1 ppb level was assayed. It should be noted that hamster urine is markedly different from human urine in that it normally contains an unusually large amount of suspended solids that may have an adverse effect on the recovery of some compounds spiked at low levels. This phenomenon is evidenced in Table 41, where Bzd and MoAcBzd were not detected at the 0.01 ppm level, whereas recoveries of 50.0 and 37.8% were obtained at this level for DiAcBzd and 4-ABP, respectively.

The differences in recovery values between the EC-GC and HPLC methods are slight (Table 41); nevertheless, the generally lower recoveries obtained by EC-GC compared with HPLC are attributed to the larger number of manipulations in the EC-GC procedures. The most critical steps are probably those that involve evaporation to dryness and transfer of residues to other vessels.

No recovery experiments via HPLC were attempted at levels of 0.1 ppm or less since such levels are below the minimum detectable limits of the HPLC procedure. It should be emphasized that the HPLC procedure is an excellent choice for assays of metabolites in dosed animals where ppm amounts of the compounds are present. However, trace assays of metabolites in environmental samples containing sub-ppm levels of residues require the more sensitive EC-GC procedure.

The recovery experiment with hamster urine spiked with 1.0 ppm each of Bzd, MoAcBzd, DiAcBzd, and 4-ABP and extracted with benzene prior to respiking and alkaline hydrolysis resulted in recoveries of 70.0, 82.9, 79.6, and 79.7%, respectively, as determined by HPLC assay. These recoveries indicated efficient removal of the compounds from the urine. After respiking and alkaline hydrolysis, essentially 100% of the Bzd and 82.5% of the 4-ABP were recovered; thus the hydrolysis procedure did not interfere with recovery of these compounds.

In the experiment with hamster urine spiked with 1.0 ppm of each of the possible metabolites of Pigment Yellow 12, recoveries obtained via HPLC for DiClBzd, MoAcDiClBzd, and DiAcDiClBzd were 78.9, 83.7, and 80%, respectively, and the backgrounds were 0.240, 0,260, and 0.200 ppm, respectively. Assays by EC-GC of urine spiked at the 1.0 ppm level yielded recoveries for DiClBzd, MoAcDiClBzd, and DiAcDiClBzd of 89.0, 85.4, and 58.0%, respectively. At the 0.1 ppm level, recoveries of these compounds diminished to 53.6, 61.7, and 45.0%; the backgrounds from unspiked samples were 0.004, 0.024, and 0.004 ppm, respectively. None of these compounds could be detected in samples spiked at the 0.01 ppm level.

Table 42 Analysis of Human Urine Unspiked and Spiked with 0.001, 0.01, 0.1, and 1.0 ppm of Metabolites of Direct Black 38[a]

		Recovery of metabolites ($\bar{x}$ ± SE)[b]			
Metabolite	Unspiked (ppm)	Spiked with 0.001 ppm (%)	Spiked with 0.01 ppm (%)	Spiked with 0.1 ppm (%)	Spiked with 1.0 ppm (%)
Bzd	0.0002 ± 0.0001	c	53.4 ± 4.2	87.0 ± 5.2	d
MoAcBzd	0.0014 ± 0.0000	c	5.29 ± 0.36	61.1 ± 1.5	76.9 ± 2.5
DiAcBzd	0.0003 ± 0.0000	20.3 ± 4.0	65.5 ± 3.8	94.4 ± 2.3	d
DiAmAzBz	0.0008 ± 0.0003	c	37.6 ± 0.6	69.8 ± 1.7	d
4-ABP	0.0010 ± 0.0000	c	41.3 ± 1.9	76.5 ± 3.0	d

[a]Analyzed by EC-GC as the HFB derivatives. DiAcBzd analyzed after alkaline hydrolysis to Bzd.
[b]Mean and standard error from triplicate assays; corrected for background interference in the unspiked sample.
[c]None detected above background.
[d]Not determined.
Source: Ref. 112.

Results from triplicate EC-GC assays of human urine unspiked and spiked with 0.001, 0.01, and 0.1 ppm of the metabolites of Direct Black 38 and also spiked only with MoAcBzd at the 1.0 ppm level are presented in Table 42. All recoveries were excellent at the 0.1 ppm level; however, recoveries of all compounds decreased appreciably at the 0.01 ppm level. Only DiAcBzd (20.3%) was recovered at the 0.001 ppm level.

The recovery experiment with human urine spiked with 1.0 ppm each of Bzd, MoAcBzd, DiAcBzd, and DiAmAzBz and extracted with benzene prior to being respiked and subjected to alkaline hydrolysis resulted in recoveries of 76.8, 87.5, 85.7, and essentially 100%, respectively, as determined by HPLC assay. After the urine was respiked and subjected to alkaline hydrolysis, essentially 100% of all four compounds were recovered since the theoretical amounts of Bzd and DiAmAzBz were obtained.

Previously, assays for free aromatic amines in the urine has been the basis for monitoring humans who are potentially exposed [84]. However, the present procedure, which determines free amines, metabolites, and alkaline hydrolyzable conjugates, provides vastly improved sensitivity. In fact, the authors propose that in assays to monitor human urine, the samples be hydrolyzed at the outset to provide results that include both free and conjugated residues. Methods previously developed for monitoring urine that do not include a hydrolysis step will obviously fail to detect the conjugated amines.

For efficient monitoring of human urine it is suggested that equal portions of five samples be composited and analyzed by the hydrolysis procedure to determine if the composite is positive or negative for Bzd. If a given composite is negative, each sample in the composite may be considered negative. If a composite is positive, individual assays of the reserved samples (stored at -20°) are required to identify the positive sample(s). The benefits of this approach toward monitoring the urine of workers are evident since the method will also detect any other derivatizable aromatic amines and thus allow some judgment by the analyst concerning the identity or nature of the chemical(s), dye(s), or pigment(s) that could have caused a given occupational exposure.

This work was conducted by the National Center for Toxicological Research under an interagency agreement No. 224-78-0004 for the National Institute for Occupational Safety and Health.

C. 4-Dimethylaminoazobenzene (DiMeAmAzBz) [116]

General description of method

A facile method is described for the qualitative and quantitative determination of trace amounts of a regulated azo compound, DiMeAmAzBz, in dyestuff formulations by flame ionization gas chromatography and

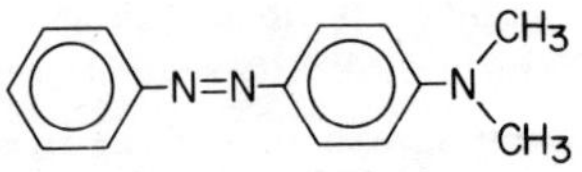

4-Dimethylaminoazobenzene

Figure 52 Formula of 4-dimethylaminoazobenzene.

thin layer chromatography. Four regulated aromatic amines that may be simultaneously determined by this method are benzidine, 1- and 2-naphthylamine, and 3,3'-dichlorobenzidine. The detection limit for the analysis was 100 μg/g, and recovery of aromatic amines from spiked dyestuffs was generally greater than 90% with a relative standard deviation of less than 10%.

Introduction

Exposure of workers to concentrations of DiMeAmAzBz in various matrices cannot exceed 0.1% according to guidelines published by the Occupational Safety and Health Administration [31]. Since this compound, as depicted in Figure 52, and the aromatic amines benzidine (Bzd), 1- and 2-naphthylamine (1- and 2-NA), and 3,3'-dichlorobenzidine (DiClBzd) are sometimes intermediates in the manufacturing of dyestuffs, it is possible that residual amounts may be present as contaminants in dyestuffs and dye intermediates. Thus, for both worker and user protection, accurate but reasonably simple analytical methods should be used to detect these compounds. The Environmental Protection Agency accepted the Chloramine-T complexation method as the official method for the analysis of Bzd in effluent [117], but because of interference, the method is not applicable to dyestuffs. Other chromatographic and spectrophotometric methods have been published describing the determination of one or more of these compounds in wastewater, air, urine, tissue, cigarette smoke, and food dyes [35,43,49,76,118-123]. Methods have also been described for the determination of Bzd and 2-NA in dyes by thin layer chromatography (TLC) [124,125] and for the determination of DiMeAmAzBz in dyes by paper chromatography [126]. The following work describes complementary TLC and gas chromatographic methods for the simultaneous determination of DiMeAmAzBz, Bzd, 1- and 2-NA, and DiClBzd in dyestuffs and dye intermediates. Although the detection limit of the analysis was established to comply with current governmental regulations [31], it can be lowered if needed.

Experimental

Reagents and Chemicals. Aromatic amine standards (reagent grade) were purchased from Pfaltz and Bauer, Inc. (Flushing, New

York) and used without further purification. Standard solutions in chloroform were prepared in a controlled area and stored at 4° in amber glassware. Organic solvents (spectrograde) were obtained from Matheson, Coleman and Bell. Photochemical degradation of labile amines was prevented by illuminating the laboratories with yellow light (devoid of UV components).

Preparation of Dyestuff Sample for Analysis. Three representative 1 g portions of dyestuff were added to each of three 15 ml centrifuge tubes fitted with ground glass stoppers. To one tube were added 400 μg each of the compounds under investigation. The dyestuff samples were dissolved or suspended in 4 ml of 0.5 N NaOH and 20 ml of chloroform was added. The mixtures were sonified for 6 min using a Heat Systems Ultrasonics Model W 185 Cell disruptor equipped with a microtip accessory and operated to provide a reading of about 50 W on the power meter. Then the mixtures were centrifuged at 1500 rpm for 15 min. Five milliliter aliquots of the resulting organic phases were transferred to 15 ml centrifuge tubes, washed with 5 ml of 6 N NaOH, and the washed organic phases were transferred to small screw-cap vials. Aliquots of the extracts were then analyzed by both gas chromatography and TLC.

Gas Chromatographic Analysis. A Tracor, Inc. (Austin, Texas) Model MT-220 instrument equipped with a flame ionization detector and a 6 ft glass column (3.5 mm i.d.) containing 3% OV-1 on Gas Chrom Q (100/200 mesh) was operated isothermally at 140° for the separation of 1- and 2-NA, or at 250° for the separation of Bzd, DiClBzd, and DiMeAmAzBz with helium as the carrier gas flowing at 60 ml/min. The detector and inlet temperatures were maintained at 270 and 250°, respectively. Aliquots (3 μl) of extracts were injected directly into the instrument.

Thin Layer Chromatography (TLC). TLC plates (20 × 20 cm) precoated with a 250 μm layer of silica gel G-F254 (EM Laboratories, Inc., Catalog No. 5767) were not activated prior to use. Aliquots (10 μl) of standard solutions or of the sample extracts were applied to the TLC plates by means of 5 μl capillary pipets (Microcaps, Drummond Scientific Co.). The plates were developed in the appropriate solvent system in tanks not saturated prior to use until the solvent migrated 15 cm upward from the bottom of the plate. Two solvent systems were used: system A was hexane-ethyl acetate-glacial acetic acid (80:20:5); system B was methylene chloride-acetone (90:10). The TLC plates were air dried for about 1 hr prior to scanning and measurement of fluorescence quenching. A Perkin-Elmer (Norwalk, Connecticut) Model MPF-2A fluorescence spectrophotometer equipped with a thin layer scanning accessory operated in the reflectance mode with an emission filter passing only the light above 430 nm was used for direct evaluation of thin layer chromatograms. Excitation and emission wavelengths were maintained at 264 and 524 nm, respectively.

Results and discussion

Complete separation of DiMeAmAzBz and the four aromatic amines was achieved by employing one or more combinations of TLC and flame ionization GC. TLC developing solvent system A was able to resolve all five compounds, as evidenced by the following R_f values:

Compound	TLC R_f values for solvent system indicated	
	A	B
Bzd	0.1	0.4
2-NA	0.4	0.7
DiClBzd	0.5	0.8
1-NA	0.6	0.8
DiMeAmAzBz	0.9	0.9

Benzidine, however, did not migrate much beyond the origin. To ensure accurate qualitative and quantitative TLC assays of Bzd, a second system of developing solvents was used (system B), which proved satisfactory for Bzd (R_f = 0.4); however, DiClBzd and 1-NA co-chromatographed. Therefore, system A was used to assay for 1- and 2-NA, DiClBzd, and DiMeAmAzBz, and system B was used solely for the assay of Bzd.

In a similar manner two GC column temperature conditions were required to completely separate all five compounds, as follows:

Compound	GC t_R values at temperatures indicated	
	Temperature (°C)	t_R (min)
1-NA	140	8.0
2-NA	140	8.6
Bzd	240	3.0
DiMeAmAzBz	240	3.8
DiClBzd	240	6.6

Temperature programming of the column oven would allow the separation of all five compounds in a single injection.

In the absence of interferences, the minimum detection limit by TLC was 100 ng of each amine (spotted in 10 μl of solvent), which is equivalent to 0.02% (220 ppm) with the quantities of dyestuff specified in the method. Similarly, the GLC detection limit was 15 ng (injected in 3 μl of solvent) or 0.01% (100 ppm). The detection limits can be decreased by concentrating the extracts. In the author's case [116],

Table 43 TLC and GC Analyses of a Dyestuff Spiked with 400 μg/g Each of DiMeAmAzBz and Four Aromatic Amines in Admixture

Compound	Assay	Recovery ($\bar{x}$ ± SE)[a] μg/g	%
DiMeAmAzBz	TLC	380 ± 10	95 ± 3
	GC	390 ± 60	97 ± 15
Bzd	TLC	410 ± 10	103 ± 3
	GC	391 ± 20	98 ± 5
DiClBzd	TLC	370 ± 10	93 ± 3
	GC	386 ± 40	96 ± 10
1-NA	TLC	410 ± 10	103 ± 3
	GC	420 ± 40	105 ± 10
2-NA	TLC	390 ± 10	98 ± 3
	GC	410 ± 30	103 ± 8

[a]Mean and standard error from quadruplicate assays; spiked samples were not corrected for background interference.
Source: Ref. 116.

a concentration step was avoided so that the analysis could be expedited.

Recovery data for a dyestuff spiked with DiMeAmAzBz and four aromatic amines determined by TLC and GC as described are presented in Table 43. Generally, the recoveries were greater than 90%, with standard errors for TLC of ±3% and for GC up to ±15%. Where recoveries were greater than 100%, this was attributed to interfering components present in some of the dyestuffs.

The relationship of peak height to compound concentration was linear via GC, but nonlinear via TLC [116]. The latter was probably caused by light scattering, since measurements were obtained in the reflectance mode [127]. No attempt was made to apply mathematical corrections to the TLC calibration data since the precision and accuracy obtained with the nonlinear standard curves were adequate for the purposes of the assay.

This method for five regulated compounds in dyestuffs is simple, fast, and capable of determining concentrations at least 10 times less than the minimum OSHA standard.

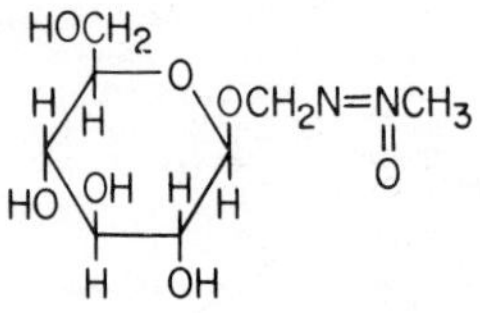

Figure 53 Formula of cycasin.

D. Cycasin [128]

General description of method

A quantitative method is described for the determination of cycasin in cycad flour by flame ionization gas chromatography. The flour is extracted with 70% ethanol and the residue from the dried extract is directly trimethylsilylated and assayed employing androsterone as an internal standard. The method is rapid, sensitive, and not hindered by contaminating compounds.

Introduction

Cycasin, β-D-glucosyloxyazoxymethane, depicted in Figure 53, is a toxin found in the seeds of the cycad plants [128]. Although widely distributed throughout the world about 200 million years ago, these plants are now limited to the tropical and subtropical zones, with occasional extension to temperature zone regions such as Florida, Japan, and Australia [5]. Cycads are used in many parts of the world as a source for medicines and for food. The size and depth of the roots of the plant probably account for the fact that they survive periods of drought as well as heavy storms, such as hurricanes and typhoons; thus they can provide food when other agricultural products are destroyed. The people who use cycads for food know that the seeds, stems, and tubers contain, besides an edible starch, poisonous substances that must be removed prior to use. Reported accidental poisonings may have occurred when cycad flour was hastily prepared at times of natural disasters. The appearance of clinical jaundice, observed after acute poisoning indicates that cycads are hepatotoxic for humans [5]. This is consistent with all observations in animals exposed to the toxin.

Cycasin has been analyzed previously by rigorous biological assay procedures via growth rates or liver lesions in rats [129] or by indirect chemical methods, some of which include acid treatment of the hydroxymethyl azoxymethane aglycone, liberating formaldehyde, which is determined colorimetrically by a chromotropic acid assay

[130] or a paper chromatographic modification [131]. In studies of the toxicity of cycasin, a rapid, specific, and sensitive method was needed to analyze extracts of cycad. The previous methods were not specific, owing to the many azoxyglycosides identified by Nagahama, designated neocycasins A-G [132]. The aglycone, methylazoxymethanol (MAM), considered to be the primary toxic agent [130,133], may also exist in extracts as a result of powerful endogenous β-glucosidase activity.

This method separates cycasin from other sugars by gas chromatography of the trimethylsilyl (TMS) derivative and permits its quantification in relation to androsterone as an internal standard.

Experimental

Materials. Cycasin, m.p. 145 to 146°, $[\alpha]_D$ - 46.5° (water), was obtained as a gift from A. Kobayashi, Kagoshima University (Japan). Androsterone, m.p. 182.5 to 183.5°, $[\alpha]_D$ + 89.5°, was purchased from Mann Research Laboratories, Inc. (New York, New York), and the β-glucosidase was obtained from Worthington Biochemical Corp. (Freehold, New Jersey).

Extraction of Cycasin from Cycad Flour. Ten 1 g samples of cycad flour, dried and powdered as described previously [129], were extracted by stirring in 3 ml of 70% ethanol for 1 min, followed by centrifuging at 2000 rpm for 10 min. The extraction was repeated four times; the extracts were combined and the volume adjusted to 25 ml with 70% ethanol. Recovery experiments were conducted by adding aliquots of a standard cycasin solution to portions of the extract.

Derivatization. Aliquots (1 to 2 ml) of the alcohol extract and 100 to 200 μg of the internal standard, androsterone, were placed in 12 ml glass-stoppered centrifuge tubes and evaporated to dryness under vacuum at 40°. Trimethylsilylation reagent (100 to 200 μl), consisting of a mixture of hexamethyldisilazane and trimethylchlorosilane in pyridine [134,135], was added to the dry residues and the reaction was allowed to go to completion at room temperature in 5 to 10 min.

Gas Chromatography. The TMS derivatives of the extracts were analyzed by two laboratories. One laboratory used a Hewlett-Packard (Palo Alto, California) Model 402 instrument equipped with a hydrogen flame ionization detector (FID) and a 6 ft glass column (1/8 in. i.d.) containing 3% OV-1 on Gas-Chrom Z (80-100 mesh) was operated isothermally at 230° with argon as the carrier gas. The other laboratory employed a Hewlett-Packard Model 810 instrument equipped with a FID and a 6 ft stainless steel column (1/8 in. i.d.) packed with HP Chromosorb W (100-120 mesh) coated with 3% OV-1 operated isothermally at 200° with helium as the carrier gas. All injections into the instruments were in 1 to 2 μl. Prior to assaying the samples, the response factor (RF) between the peak heights of the TMS derivatives corresponding to known quantities (1:1) of cycasin and the internal standard (IS), androsterone, was determined. The determination of the factor was repeated at the end of a series of analyses to verify the stability of the FID-GC system.

By predicting the range of the unknown concentrations of cycasin in a given extract, an exact amount of IS (approximately a 1:1 ratio) was added and the solvents removed by evaporation. Knowing the exact amount of IS added and the RF between the IS and cycasin standards, the amount of unknown cycasin can then be calculated by simple proportions. Also, the amount of the sample containing internal standard actually injected is not critical; thus injection variability is avoided. The amount of cycasin and internal standard is proportional to peak height.

Results and discussion

The retention time (t_R) values for cycasin and the IS (androsterone) were about 21.0 and 33.2 min, respectively, when determined at 230° using the Hewlett-Packard Model 402 instrument. Results of recovery experiments conducted in two laboratories by spiking aliquots of a standard solution of cycasin into 10 portions of the original extract were 94.7 ± 10.2 and 104.6 ± 13.4%, respectively. The cycasin content of cycad flour determined in these laboratories was 0.434 ± 0.014 and 0.423 ± 0.021 g/100 g, respectively. Reproducibility, recovery, actual visualization of the cycasin peak, high sensitivity of detection, and the convenience of direct analysis of the crude extract were obvious advantages of this GC method. TMS derivatization results in an ideally volatile derivative of the methylazoxymethoxyglycoside, as predicted from previous studies for carbohydrates and polyhydroxy compounds [134]. The stability of the derivative was improved by refrigerating at 5° when a storage time in excess of 24 hr was anticipated.

To strengthen the evidence that the peak in the chromatogram was cycasin alone, the extract was treated with β-glucosidase to degrade the β-glucoside. One gram of flour was incubated with 120 mg of β-glucosidase in 3 ml of water for 16 hr at 39°. After inactivating the enzyme by placing in a steam bath for 3 min, the mixture was extracted with 70% ethanol five times as described previously for the untreated samples. After TMS derivatization and injection into a GC, the absence of a peak at the t_R value of cycasin was a reasonably good indication that no other compound is co-chromatographed with cycasin.

A large unknown peak with a t_R value of 41 min observed in chromatograms of the TMS residue of crude extract of cycad flour was found to be susceptible to β-glucosidase activity. This indicated that it may be a disaccharide, and since one of the neocycasins, isolated by Nagahama [132], was thought to be a possible candidate for the unknown material, TMS derivatization of samples of neocycasins was conducted. However, no peaks corresponding to the t_R value of the unknown resulted.

REFERENCES

1. J. M. Price. *Benign and Malignant Tumors of the Urinary Bladder.* Medical Examination Publishing Co., Garden City, N.Y., 1971.
2. L. Fishbein. *Potential Industrial Carcinogens and Mutagens. EPA 560/5-77-005,* Office of Toxic Substances, U.S. Environmental Protection Agency, Washington, D.C., 1977.
3. E. Rinde and W. Troll. Metabolic reduction of benzidine azo dyes to benzidine in the Rhesus monkey. J. Natl. Cancer Soc. *55*(1), 181-182 (1975).
4. K. Venkataraman. *The Analytical Chemistry of Synthetic Dyes.* Wiley, New York, 1977.
5. G.L. Laqueur. Oncogenicity of cycads and its implications. In *Advances in Modern Toxicology*, Vol. 3 (H.F. Kraybill and M.A. Mehlman, Eds.). New York, 1977.
6. M. C. Bowman and J. R. King. Analysis of 2-acetylaminofluorene: residues in laboratory chow and microbiological media. Biochem. Med. *9*, 390-401 (1974).
7. E. K. Weisburger and J. H. Weisburger. Chemistry, carcinogenicity and metabolism of 2-fluorenamine and related compounds. Adv. Cancer Res. *5*, 331-431 (1958).
8. J. H. Weisburger and E. K. Weisburger. Biochemical formation and pharmacological, toxicological, pathological properties of hydroxylamines and hydroxamic acids. Pharmacol. Rev. *25*, 1-60 (1973).
9. B. B. Westfall. Estimation of 2-aminofluorene and related compounds in biological material. J. Natl. Cancer Inst. *6*, 23-29 (1945).
10. B. B. Westfall and H. P. Morris. Photometric estimation of N-acetyl-2-aminofluorene. J. Natl. Cancer Inst. *8*, 17-21 (1947).
11. R. B. Sandin, R. Melby, A. S. Hay, R. N. Jones, E. C. Miller, and J. H. Miller. Ultraviolet spectra and carcinogenic activities of some fluorene and biphenyl derivatives. J. Am. Chem. Soc. *74*, 5073-5075 (1952).
12. C. C. Irving. N-Hydroxylation of 2-acetylaminofluorene in the rabbit. Cancer Res. *22*, 867-873 (1962).
13. J. H. Weisburger, E. K. Weisburger, H. P. Morris, and H. A. Sober. Chromatographic separation of some metabolites of the carcinogen N-2-fluorenylacetamide. J. Natl. Cancer Inst. *17*, 363-374 (1956).

14. H. R. Gutmann and R. R. Erickson. The conversion of the carcinogen N-hydroxy-2-fluorenylacetamide to o-amidophenols by rat liver in vitro (an inducible enzymatic reaction). J. Biol. Chem. *244*, 1729-1740 (1969).
15. M. Beroza and M. C. Bowman. Identification of pesticides at nanogram level by extraction p-values. Anal. Chem. *37*, 291-292 (1965).
16. M. C. Bowman and M. Beroza. Extraction p-values of pesticides and related materials in six binary solvent systems. J. Assoc. Off. Anal. Chem. *48*, 943-952 (1965).
17. F. R. Fullerton. National Center for Toxicological Research, Jefferson, Ark. Personal communication.
18. M. C. Bowman and M. Beroza. Identification of compounds by extraction p-values using gas chromatography. Anal. Chem. *38*, 1544-1549 (1966).
19. M. Beroza, M. N. Inscoe, and M. C. Bowman. Distribution of pesticides in immiscible binary solvent systems for cleanup and identification and the extraction of pesticides from milk. Res. Rev. *30*, 1-61 (1969).
20. J. R. King and M. C. Bowman. 4-Ethylsulfonylnaphthalene-1-sulfonamide (ENS): analytical chemical behavior and trace analysis in five substrates. Biochem. Med. *12*, 313-330 (1975).
21. G. M. Bonser and D. B. Clayson. A sulphonamide derivative which induces urinary tract epithelial hyperplasia and carcinomas of the bladder epithelium in the mouse. Br. J. Urol. *36*, 26-34 (1964).
22. D. B. Clayson and G. M. Bonser. The induction of tumours of the mouse bladder epithelium by 4-ethylsulphonylnaphthalene-1-sulphonamide. Br. J. Cancer *19*, 311-315 (1965).
23. D. B. Clayson, J. A. Pringle, and G. M. Bonser. 4-Ethylsulphonylnaphthalene-1-sulphonamide: a new chemical for the study of bladder cancer in the mouse. Biochem. Pharmacol. *16*, 619-626 (1967).
24. P. F. Levi, J. C. Knowles, D. M. Cowen, M. Wood, and E. H. Cooper. Disorganization of mouse bladder epithelium induced by 2-acetylaminofluorene and 4-ethylsulfonylnaphthalene-1-sulfonamide. J. Natl. Cancer Inst. *46*, 337-343 (1971).
25. A. Flaks, J. M. Hamilton, and D. B. Clayson. Effect of ammonium chloride on incidence of bladder tumors induced by 4-ethylsulfonylnaphthalene-1-sulfonamide. J. Natl. Cancer Inst. *51*, 2007-2009 (1973).
26. W. J. Moore. *Physical Chemistry*, 4th ed. Prentice-Hall, Englewood Cliffs, N.J., 1972.
27. M. C. Bowman and M. Beroza. Gas chromatographic detector for simultaneous sensing of phosphorus- and sulfur-containing compounds by flame photometry. Anal. Chem. *40*, 1448-1452 (1968).
28. J. W. Stanley. National Center for Toxicological Research, Jefferson, Ark. Personal communication.

29. M. C. Bowman, J. R. King, and C. L. Holder. Benzidine and congeners: analytical chemical properties and trace analysis in five substrates. Int. J. Environ. Anal. Chem. *4*, 205-223 (1976).
30. L. Rehn. Blasingeschwulste bei Anilinarbeitern. Arch. Klin. Chir. *50*, 588-600 (1895).
31. Carcinogens. Occupational health and safety standards. *Fed. Reg. 39,* 3756-3797 (Jan. 29, 1974).
32. T. J. Haley. Benzidine revisited: a review of the literature and problems associated with the use of benzidine and its congeners. Clin. Toxicol. *8*, 13-42 (1975).
33. L. J. Sciarini and J. W. Meigs. Biotransformation of the benzidines. Arch. Environ. Health *2*, 108-112 (1961).
34. R. K. Baker and J. G. Deighton. The metabolism of benzidine in the rat. Cancer Res. *13*, 529-531 (1953).
35. M. A. El-Dib. Colorimetric determination of aniline derivatives in natural waters. J. Assoc. Off. Anal. Chem. *54*, 1383-1387 (1971).
36. J. M. Glassman and J. W. Meigs. Benzidine (4,4'-diaminobiphenyl) and substituted benzidines. A.M.A. Arch. Ind. Hyg. Occup. Med. *4*, 519-532 (1951).
37. T. Akiyama. The investigation of the manufacturing plant of organic pigment. Jikeikai Med. J. *17*, 1-9 (1970).
38. D. B. Clayson, E. Ward, and L. Ward. The fate of benzidine in various species. Acta Unio Int. Contra Cancerum. *15*, 581-586 (1959).
39. E. Rinde. A specific assay for the determination of trace amounts of the bladder carcinogen benzidine and other aromatic amines: Detection of benzidine liberated metabolically from benzidine azo dyes. Thesis, New York University, 1974.
40. M. C. Bowman and L. G. Rushing. Trace analysis of 3,3'-dichlorobenzidine in animal chow, wastewater and human urine by three gas chromatographic procedures. Arch. Environ. Contam. Toxicol. *6*, 471-482 (1977).
41. T. Gadian. Carcinogens in industry, with special reference to dichlorobenzidine. Chem. Ind. (Lond.) *19*, 821-831 (1975).
42. E. Sawicki, H. Johnson, and K. Kosinski. Chromatographic separation and spectral analysis of polynuclear aromatic amines and heterocyclic imines. Microchem. J. *10*, 72-102 (1966).
43. C. L. Holder, J. R. King, and M. C. Bowman. 4-Aminobiphenyl, 2-naphthylamine, and analogs: analytical properties and trace analysis in five substrates. J. Toxicol. Environ. Health *2*, 111-129 (1976).
44. T. Walle and H. Ehrsson. Quantitative gas chromatographic determination of picrogram quantities of amino and alcoholic compounds by electron capture detection: I. Preparation and properties of the heptafluorobutyryl derivatives. Acta Pharm. Suec. *7*, 389-406 (1970).

45. H. Ehrsson, T. Walle, and H. Brotell. Quantitative gas chromatographic determination of picogram qualities of phenols. Acta Pharm. Suec. *8*, 319-328 (1971).
46. G. A. Lugg. Stabilized diazonium salts as analytical reagents for the determinations of air-borne phenols and amines. Anal. Chem. *35*, 899-904 (1963).
47. J. W. Bridges, P. J. Creaven, and R. T. Williams. The fluorescence of some biphenyl derivatives. Biochem. J. *96*, 872-878 (1965).
48. K. Shimomura and H. F. Walton. Thin-layer chromatography of amines by ligand exchange. Sep. Sci. *3*, 493-499 (1968).
49. Y. Masuda and D. Hoffmann. Quantitative determination of 1-naphthylamine and 2-naphthylamine in cigarette smoke. Anal. Chem. *41*, 650-652 (1969).
50. J. A. Knight. Gas chromatographic analysis of γ-irradiated aniline for aminoaromatic products. J. Chromatogr. *56*, 201-208 (1971).
51. R. C. Gupta and S. P. Srivastava. Oxidation of aromatic amines by peroxodisulphate ion. Z. Anal. Chem. *257*, 275-277 (1971).
52. I. M. Jakovljevic, J. Zynger, and R. H. Bishara. Thin layer chromatographic separation and fluorometric determination of 4-aminobiphenyl in 2-aminobiphenyl. Anal. Chem. *47*, 2045-2046 (1975).
53. C. R. Nony, E. J. Treglown, and M. C. Bowman. Removal of trace levels of 2-acetylaminofluorene (2-AAF) from wastewater. Sci. Total Environ. *4*, 155-163 (1975).
54. J. L. Guthrie and R. W. McKinney. Determination of 2,4- and 2,6-diaminotoluene in flexible urethane foams. Anal. Chem. *49*, 1676-1680 (1977).
55. H. E. Christensen and T. T. Luginbyhl. Suspected carcinogens– a subfile of the NIOSH toxic substances list. (NIOSH) 75-190, 1975.
56. T. Yoshida, T. Shimauchi, and C. Kin. Experimentelle Studien ueber die Entwicklung des Harnblasentumors. Gann *35*, 272-274 (1941).
57. N. Ito, Y. Hiasa, Y. Konishi, and M. Marugami. Development of carcinoma in liver of rats treated with m-toluenediamine and the synergistic and antagonistic effects with other chemicals. Cancer Res. *29*, 1137-1145 (1969).
58. M. Umeda. Production of rat sarcoma by injection of propylene glycol solution of 2,4-diaminotoluene. Gann *46*, 597-604 (1955).
59. J. McCann, E. Choi, E. Yamasaki, and B. N. Ames. Detection of carcinogens as mutagens in the *Salmonella*/microsome test: assay of 300 chemicals. Proc. Natl. Acad. Sci. USA *72*, 5135-5139 (1975).
60. B. N. Ames, H. O. Kammen, and E. Yamasaki. Hair dyes are mutagenic. Identification of a variety of mutagenic ingredients. Proc. Natl. Acad. Sci. USA *72*, 2423, 2427 (1975).

61. C. Burnett, B. Lanman, R. Giovacchini, G. Wolcott, R. Scala, and M. Keplinger. Long-term toxicity studies on oxidation hair dyes. Food Cosmet. Toxicol. *13*, 353-357 (1975).
62. G. A. Campbell, T. J. Dearlove, and W. C. Meluch. Humid age compression set in high resilience polyurethane foam. J. Cell. Plast. *12*, 222-224 (1976).
63. A. S. Tompa. Infrared study in potassium bromide disks of the stability and hydrolysis of aromatic polyurethane foams. Anal. Chem. *44*, 1056-1058 (1972).
64. C. L. Wilson. Improving the color stability of polyurethane foams. U.S. Patent 2,921,866; January 19, 1960.
65. D. J. David and H. S. Staley. *Analytical Chemistry of the Polyurethanes*, Vol. 16. Wiley-Interscience, New York, 1969.
66. M. Guenchev and B. Atanasov. New color reactions of the aromatic amines. C. R. Acad. Bulgare Sci. *9*, 41-44 (1956).
67. E. A. Emelin and T. V. Lepina. Determination of end amino groups in polyamides and polyurethanes. USSR Patent 474,734; June 25, 1975.
68. E. A. Emelin. Direct potentiometric determination of end amino groups in polymers. Zh. Anal. Khim. *30*, 335-339 (1975).
69. F. Willeboordse, Q. Quick, and E. T. Bishop. Direct gas chromatographic analysis of isomeric diaminotoluenes. Anal. Chem. *40*, 1455-1458 (1968).
70. C. R. Boufford. Determination of isomeric diaminotoluenes by direct gas-liquid chromatography. J. Gas Chromatogr. *6*, 438-440 (1968).
71. S. Goldstein, A. A. Kopf, and R. Feinland. Analysis of oxidation dyes in hair colorants by thin-layer and gas chromatography. Proc. Joint Conf. Cosmet. Sci., 19-38 (1968).
72. I. Pinter, M. Kramer, and J. Kleeberg. Detection and determination of p-phenylenediamine in the presence of p-tolylenediamine in hair dyes. J. Parfuem. Kosmet. *46*, 61-64 (1965).
73. G. F. Macke. Tetracyanoethylene as a thin-layer chromatographic spray reagent. J. Chromatogr. *36*, 537-539 (1968).
74. C. M. Kottemann. Two-dimensional thin-layer chromatographic procedure for the identification of dye intermediates in arylamine oxidation hair dyes. J. Assoc. Off. Anal. Chem. *49*, 954-959 (1966).
75. A. Mathias. Analysis of diaminotoluene isomer mixtures by nuclear magnetic resonance spectrometry. Anal. Chem. *38*, 1931-1932 (1966).
76. E. Rinde and W. Troll. Colorimetric assay for aromatic amines. Anal. Chem. *48*, 542-544 (1976).
77. S. Udenfriend, S. Stein, P. Boehlen, W. Dairman, W. Leimgruber, and M. Weigele. Fluorescamine. Reagent for assay of amino acids, peptides, proteins and primary amines in the picomole range. Science *178*, 871-872 (1972).

78. H. M. Malin, Jr. Industry looks at wastewater reuse. Environ. Sci. Technol. 7, 500 (1973).
79. J. M. Cohen and I. J. Kugelman. Wastewater treatment: physical and chemical methods. J. Water Pollut. Control Fed. *45*, 1027-1038 (1973).
80. C. G. Peacock, Chem. Abstr. *74*, 67408K (1971).
81. B. Rassow and H. S. Schultzky. General pricniples of "codistillation." Z. Angew. Chem. *44*, 669-670 (1931).
82. J. N. Keith. How to design a building safe against hazards. Occup. Health Safety *47*, 46-48 (1977).
83. E. M. Flanigen, J. M. Bennett, R. W. Grose, J. P. Cohen, R. L. Patton, R. M. Kirchner, and J. V. Smith. Silicalite, a new hydrophobic crystalline silica molecular sieve. Nature (Lond.) *271*, 512-516 (1978).
84. C. R. Nony and M. C. Bowman. Carcinogens and analogs: trace analysis of thirteen compounds in admixture in wastewater and human urine. Int. J. Environ. Anal. Chem. 5, 203-220 (1978).
85. Nonclinical laboratory studies: proposed regulation for good laboratory practices. *Fed. Reg. 41,* 51206-51230 (Nov. 19, 1976).
86. L. M. Games and R. A. Hites. Composition, treatment efficiency and experimental significance of dye manufacturing plant effluents. Anal. Chem. *49*. 1433-1440 (1977).
87. M.C. Bowman. Control of test substances. Clin. Toxicol. *15*, 583-595 (1979).
88. M. C. Bowman. Trace analysis: a requirement for toxicological research with carcinogens and hazardous substances. J. Assoc. Off. Anal. Chem. *61*, 1253-1262 (1978).
89. J. R. King, C. R. Nony, and M. C. Bowman. Trace analysis of diethylstilbestrol (DES) in animal chow by parallel high-speed liquid chromatography, electron-capture gas chromatography and radioassays. J. Chromatogr. Sci. *15*, 14-21 (1977).
90. M. C. Bowman and C. R. Nony. Trace analysis of estradiol in animal chow by electron-capture gas chromatography. J. Chromatogr. Sci. *15*, 160-163 (1977).
91. B. E. Bowen. Determination of aromatic amines by an adsorption technique with flame ionization gas chromatography. Anal. Chem. *48*, 1584-1587 (1976).
92. L. G. Rushing and M. C. Bowman. Determination of gentian violet in animal feed, human urine and wastewater by high-pressure liquid chromatography. J. Chromatogr. Sci. *18*, 224-232 (1980).
93. J. E. Hoover (Ed.). *Remington's Pharmaceutical Sciences*. Mack Publishing Co., Easton, Pa., 1975, p. 1091.
94. N. A. Littlefield. National Center for Toxicological Research, Jefferson, Ark. Personal communication.
95. D. P. Ducharme. Bureau of Veterinary Medicine, Food and Drug Administration, Washington, D.C. Personal communication.

96. H. Fujita, A. Mizuo, and K. Hiraga. Mutagenicity of dyes in the microbial system. Tokyo Toritsu Eisei Kenkyusho Kenkyu Nempo *27*, 153-158 (1976).
97. K. Norrby and H. Mobacken. Effect of triphenylmethane dyes on proliferation in human normal fibroblast-like and established epithelial cell lines. Acta Dermato-Venereol. *52*, 476-483 (1972).
98. W. Au, S. Pathak, C. J. Collie, and T. C. Hsu. Cytogenetic toxicity of gentian violet and crystal violet on mammalian cells in vitro. Mutat. Res. *58*, 269-276 (1978).
99. W. Au, M. A. Butler, S. E. Bloom, and T. S. Matney. Further study of the genetic toxicity of gentian violet. Mutat. Res. *66*, 103-112 (1979).
100. A. D. Wolfe. Influence of cationic triphenylmethane dyes upon DNA polymerization and product hydrolysis by *Escherichia coli* polymerase, I. Biochemistry *16*, 30-33 (1977).
101. R. A. M. Case and J. T. Pearson. Tumors of the urinary bladder in workmen engaged in the manufacture and use of certain dyestuff intermediates in the British chemical industry: II. Further consideration of the role of aniline and the manufacture of auramine and magenta (fuchsine) as possible causative agents. Br. J. Ind. Med. *11*, 213 (1954).
102. O. G. Prokofeva and M. A. Zabezhinskii. Carcinogenicity of fuchsin derivatives. Vopr. Onkol. (Leningr.) *22*, 66-77 (1976).
103. Y. Ikeda, S. Horiuchi, A. Imoto, Y. O. Kadama, Y. Aida, and K. Kobayashi. Induction of mammary gland and skin tumors in female rats by feeding of benzyl violet 4B. Toxicology *2*, 275 (1974).
104. A. Fisher. Paper chromatographic analysis of a mixture of pentamethyl- and hexamethylpararosaniline chloride and hexamethylpararosaniline chloride. Chromatographia *11-12*, 481-482 (1968).
105. P. N. Marshall and S. M. Lewis. A rapid thin-layer chromatographic system for Romanowsky blood stains. Stain Technol. *49*, 235-240 (1974).
106. P. M. Marshall. Thin-layer chromatography of some cationic dyes commonly used in histology. J. Chromatogr. *129*, 277-285 (1976).
107. P. J. Van Mullem and F. MacGillavry. Chromatography of some triphenylmethane dye mixtures. K. Ned. Akad. Wet. Proc. *61*, 66-77 (1958).
108. G. W. Taylor. U.S. Patent 3,915,637; 1975.
109. G. W. Taylor. U.S. Patent 4,033,721; 1977.
110. United States Pharmacopeial Convention, Inc. *The United States Pharmacopeia,* 19th rev. ed. Mack Publishing Co., Easton, Pa., 1974, pp. 219-220, 617-620.

111. C. R. Nony and M. C. Bowman. Analysis, purification and stability: requirements for a metabolism study of an azo dye and pigment. J. Anal. Toxicol. *4*, 63-67 (1980).

112. C. R. Nony and M. C. Bowman. Trace analysis of potentially carcinogenic metabolites of an azo dye and pigment in hamster urine as determined by two chromatographic procedures. J. Chromatogr. Sci. *18*, 64-74 (1980).

113. *Thirteen Week Subchronic Toxicity Studies of Direct Blue 6, Direct Black 38, and Direct Brown 95 dyes. NIH 78-1358 (1978).* National Cancer Institute, Department of Health, Education and Welfare, Washington, D.C.

114. R. M. Riggin and C. C. Howard. Determination of benzidine, dichlorobenzidine, and diphenylhydrazine in aqueous media by high performance liquid chromatography. Anal. Chem. *51*, 210-214 (1979).

115. J. R. Rice and P. T. Kissinger. Determination of benzidine and its acetylated metabolites in urine by liquid chromatography. J. Anal. Toxicol. *3*, 64-66 (1979).

116. J. Schulze, C. Ganz, and D. Parkes. Determination of trace quantities of aromatic amines in dyestuffs. Anal. Chem. *50*, 171-174 (1978).

117. Toxic pollutant effluent standards. Standards for benzidine; final decision. *Fed. Reg. 42*, 2617-2618 (Jan. 12, 1977).

118. G. Ghetti, E. Bartalini, and A. Forni. Colorimetric method for the determination of benzidine for use in the evaluation of occupational exposure. Med. Lav. *59*, 176-179 (1968).

119. G. Ghetti, E. Bartalini, G. Armeli, and L. Pozzoli. Separation and determination of aromatic amines in various substances. Calibration of new analytical methods for use in industrial hygiene laboratories. Lav. Um. *20*, 389-400 (1968).

120. D. B. Parihar, S. P. Sharma, and K. K. Verma. Investigations of methemoglobinemic and carcinogenic poisons as π complexes with 2,4,6-trinitroanisole and picramide. Forensic Sci. Soc. J. *10*, 77-82 (1970).

121. S. Laham, J. Farant, and M. Potvin. Biochemical determination of urinary bladder carcinogens in human urine. Occup. Health Rev. *21*, 14-23 (1970).

122. R. L. Jenkins and R. B. Baird. The determination of benzidine in wastewaters. Bull. Environ. Contam. Toxicol. *13*, 436-442 (1975).

123. R. W. Weeks, B. J. Dean, and S. K. Yasuda. Detection limits of chemical spot tests toward certain carcinogens on metal, painted and concrete surfaces. Anal. Chem. *48*, 2227-2233 (1976).

124. A. Suzuki. Determination of benzidine in direct dyes by thin layer chromatography. Bunseki Kagaku *21*, 1025-1028 (1972).

125. E. J. Dixon and D. M. Groffman. The determination of unsulphonated primary aromatic amines in water-soluble food dyes and other food additives. Analyst (Lond.) *100*, 476-481 (1975).

126. I. Shimizu. Separation and identification of oil-soluble dyes by partition paper chromatography. Yukagaku *17*, 35-38 (1968).

127. V. Hezel. Direct quantitative photometry on thin-layer chromatograms. Angew. Chem. *12*, 298-306 (1973).

128. W. W. Wells, M. G. Yang, W. Bolzer, and O. Mickelsen. Gas-liquid chromatographic analysis of cycasin in cycad flour. Anal. Biochem. *25*, 325-329 (1968).

129. M. E. Campbell, O. Mickelsen, M. G. Yang, G. L. Laquer, and J. C. Keresztesy. Effects of strain, age and diet on the response of rats to the ingestion of *Cycas circinalis*. J. Nutr. *88*, 115-124 (1966).

130. H. Matsumoto and F. M. Strong. The occurrence of methylazoxymethanol in *Cycas circinalis* L. Arch. Biochem. Biophys. *101*, 299-310 (1963).

131. D. K. Dastur and R. S. Palekar. Effect of boiling and storing on cycasin content of *Cycas circinalis* L. Nature (Lond.) *210*, 841-843 (1966).

132. T. Nagahama. Studies on neocycasins, new glycosides of cycads. Bull. Fac. Agric. Kagoshima Univ. *14*, 1 (1964).

133. T. Nishida, A. Kobayashi, T. Nagahama, K. Kojima, and M. Jamane. Cycasin, a new toxic glycoside of *Cycas revoluta*: IV. Pharmacology of cycasin. Seikagaku *28*, 218 (1956).

134. C. C. Sweeley, R. Bentley, M. Makita, and W. W. Wells. Gas-liquid chromatography of trimethylsilyl derivatives of sugars and related substances. J. Am. Chem. Soc. *85*, 2497-2509 (1963).

135. C. C. Sweeley, W. W. Wells, and R. Bentley. Gas chromatography of carbohydrates. In *Methods in Enzymology*, Vol. 8 (E. F. Neufeld and V. Ginsburg, Eds.). Academic Press, New York, 1966, pp. 95-108.

4
Estrogens

EDWARD D. HELTON* National Center for Toxicological Research, U.S. Food and Drug Administration, Jefferson, Arkansas

MARY C. WILLIAMS and ROBERT H. PURDY Southwest Foundation for Research and Education, San Antonio, Texas

I. INTRODUCTION

In the last two decades, there has been an explosive increase in the use of estrogens for a variety of purposes, such as contraception and the therapy of the menopausal and postmenopausal state. In addition to these purely medical areas, agriculture has made increasingly extensive use of estrogenic hormones in the feeding of poultry and cattle. Concurrent with their clinical and industrial use, problems with regard to occupational exposure during their synthesis have resulted in numerous instances of endocrine toxicity [1]. Thus the potential exposure of humans to both small and large quantities of estrogen, on a chronic basis, has become a situation involving millions of people. Recently, estrogens have been reported to be present in drinking water, soil, and foliage [2].

In 1931, Lacassagne demonstrated that large doses of estrogen given continuously to a special strain of male mice were capable of inducing breast tumors. Since that time, the role of estrogenic hormones in tumorigenesis has come under increasingly intensive investigation. The results of such exposure, in the light of modern knowledge, have been inadequately explored. For instance, the metabolism of diethylstilbestrol, which has been used for over 40 years, is only now being resolved; knowledge of its pharmacokinetics is still minimal. The major plasma metabolite of ethynylestradiol, the chief estrogenic constituent of birth control pills, has yet to be unequivocally identified, in spite of the commercial introduction of this agent in 1961. In large

*Present affiliation: New Mexico State University, Holloman Air Force Base, New Mexico.

measure, this has been due to the lack of application of appropriate chemical technology which can adequately trace these hormones through the animal organism and identify the chemical transformations involved or the responses of the tissues to these chemicals or their derivatives at the cellular level. Recent advances in molecular biology and biochemical techniques have now made such investigations possible, and their intensive application to a problem with such wide ramifications is essential. Today, estrogens are involved not only with the question of breast cancer, but recent epidemiological studies have suggested a role in endometrial carcinoma, hepatic tumors, and in the case of prenatal exposure, subsequent development of permanent oligospermia, vaginal adenosis, and adenocarcinoma of the cervix. Thus the scope of potential hazards related to estrogen use has widened, and well-publicized concern over these issues has demonstrated the need for specific and quantitative methods for the determination of relatively low concentrations of estrogens and estrogen metabolites in body tissues and fluids.

A further factor adding to the general concern in this area is the present realization that certain other types of aromatic hydrocarbons are converted to cytotoxic, mutagenic, or carcinogenic substances by normal enzymatic mechanisms previously thought to be involved merely with metabolic detoxification. The principal reactive intermediates formed during the metabolic activation of estrogens are currently believed either to result from the superoxide oxidation of estrogen catechols, or to be arene oxide intermediates. The formation of catechol estrogens is now recognized to be a major pathway in the oxidative metabolism of estrogenic hormones [3]. These catechols are further oxidized to intermediates which irreversibly bind cellular components, including DNA [4-6]. This covalent linkage is analogous to that which occurs upon activation of other types of polycyclic aromatic hydrocarbons that are precarcinogens. Thus, in this respect, catechol estrogen oxidation and reactivity may be regarded as a potentially carcinogenic process. From such studies it may be possible to distinguish between a direct action of estrogen metabolites on tumor formation in experimental animals or an effect of estrogens as tumor promoters which is not directly related to their metabolism.

Catechol formation through phenolic oxides could proceed via the dienol epoxides (2 and 4, Fig. 1) and their keto tautomers (1 and 3, Fig. 1). Three of these isomeric enones (1 and 3) have recently been synthesized by LeQuesne et al. [7] as the 17β-acetoxy derivatives. The Δ^1 isomeric epoxides (1) of known configuration and one of the Δ^4 isomeric epoxides (3) of unestablished configuration were assayed for their effect on the chemical transformation of mouse fibroblast cells [8]. The preliminary data showed that Δ^1-4α,5β-epoxide was approximately as active as 3-methycholanthrene, and apparently at least two orders of magnitude more active than estradiol-17β in causing the formation of typical transformed foci. These epoxides are

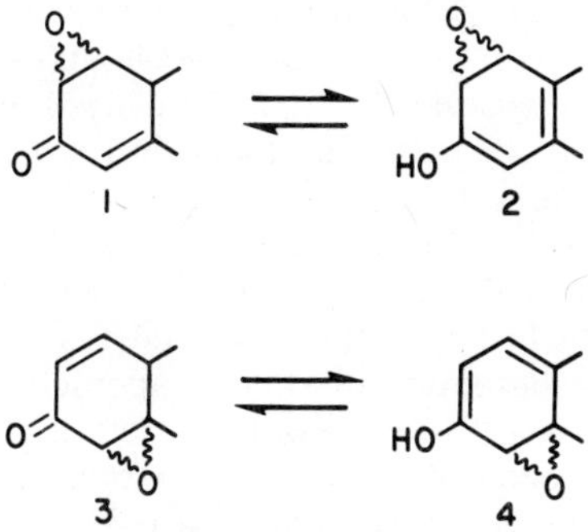

Figure 1 Structures of synthetic isomeric epoxides: 1 and 3, of 17β-acetoxyestrenes, and their dienol epoxide tautomers, 2 and 4.

relatively stable to base in alcoholic solution but are rapidly tautomerized to catechols under acidic conditions. It remains to be determined if these epoxides can be isolated as transient intermediates of estrogen metabolism in mammalian systems, and further, if there is an enzyme-catalyzed formation of catechol estrogens from a particular configuration of these epoxides. The latter circumstances is now relatively simple to measure using HPLC, but a radiolabeled intermediate might be enzyme bound and not capable of detectable exchange under the usual in vitro conditions of catechol formation.

Estrogen metabolism involves primarily, if not exclusively, oxidation of the molecule, as opposed to pregnane- and androstane-type steroids, which undergo mostly reductive metabolism. Although oxidative metabolism of estrogens alters their polarity and binding interactions with cellular receptors, we do not truly understand in any greater detail the significance of the conversion of estradiol-17β to estrone or estrone's subsequent oxidation and reduction to the weaker estrogen estriol. Furthermore, evidence has been accumulating to suggest that oxidation to the catechol estrogens may have profound significance. Investigators have reported that catechol estrogens (particularly 2-hydroxyestradiol-17β) may serve as uterine antiestrogens and/or modulators of hypothalamopituitary function as a result of their competitive binding to both uterine and pituitary estrogen receptors [9,10]. This capacity for receptor binding, coupled with the ability of the brain to produce catechol estrogens [11], suggests an interesting and attractive mechanism of estrogen control.

The nonsteroidal estrogen diethylstilbestrol (DES), a stilbene, has been suspected of being a chemical carcinogen [12]. Possibly it is bioactivated through epoxidation of the aliphatic double bonds. There is evidence that DES may bioactivate by two other mechanisms. One would be the oxidation of DES to a p-quinone, which would no doubt be reactive; the other mechanism would be an oxidation of the terminal aliphatic methyl group, which could conceivably become bioactive through acylation and subsequent cleavage. Although binding of DES to DNA is known [13,14], the nature of the adducts and the mechanisms of bioactivation are still unclear.

DES has been shown to cause a significant number of chromosomal aberrations and polyploid cell formation in Chinese hamster ovarian cells [15]. Although numerous attempts to apply the bacterial tester strains of the Ames assay system to the detection of the mutagenic activity of estrogens have been unsuccessful, DES has been found to cause mutation at the thymidine kinase locus of L5178Y mouse lymphoma cells [16]. Rüdiger et al. [17] have also reported that DES is capable of inducing sister chromatid exchange in cultured human fibroblasts. The DES metabolites DES-epoxide (E-DES-2',3'-oxide) and Z,Z-dienestrol were found to be 10-fold and 70-fold more active, respectively, than DES. However, Purdy et al. [8] found that neither of these metabolites was active in causing the malignant transformation of Balb/c 3T3 mouse fibroblast cells at a concentration (50 nM) where DES was an effective transforming agent.

Thus the need for a better understanding of estrogens and their metabolism is obvious, and our shortcomings with regard to obtaining answers relate closely to our bioanalytical technology. In this chapter we review the current analytical procedures for the analysis of steroidal, nonsteroidal, and ethynylated estrogens. Diethylstilbestrol and zearalanol are used as representative of nonsteroidal estrogens; estradiol-17β and 17α-ethynylestradiol are used as examples of steroidal estrogens. Trenbolone acetate is also discussed because of its probable use in the future as a significant anabolic agent in the food-animal industry.

A. Steroidal Estrogens

The natural estrogen estradiol-17β (E_2) and the synthetic estrogen 17α-ethynylestradiol (EE_2) serve here as the representatives for this class of female hormones (Fig. 2). Metabolism E_2 usually begins with oxidative conversion to estrone [18], followed by subsequent sulfation to estrone-3-sulfate, which is the principal circulating estrogen [19]. The sulfate is in turn cleaved, and estrone (or estradiol) can then be oxidized at C-2 to form the catechol, which may be subsequently methylated. Alternatively, hydroxylation at C-6 can occur; however, more commonly estrone is oxidized to the 16α- or 16β-hydroxy products, which after C-17 ketone reduction become estriol or epiestriol, respectively. Although more exotic oxidations of estradiol or estrone do occur, the described events are the most common, based on quantitative identification of metabolic products. The 3- and/or 17-glucuronide conjugates of the steroid oxidative metabolites, as well as the 3-sulfo-16-glucuronides of estriol, are formed prior to excretion.

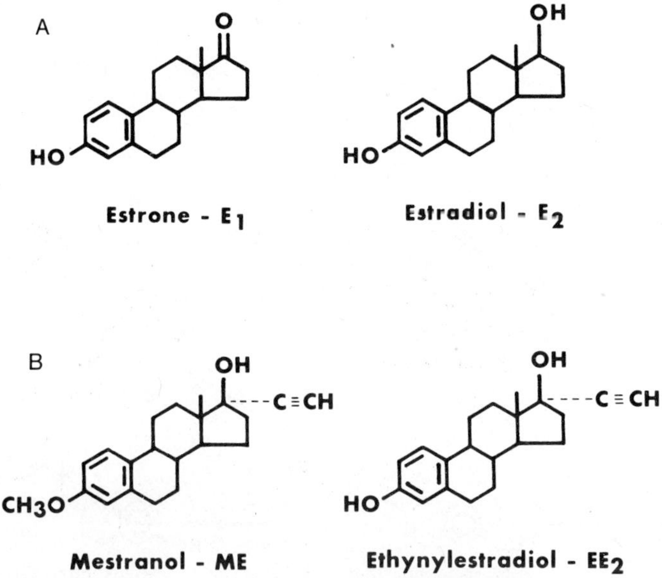

Figure 2 Structures of (A) natural and (B) synthetic estrogens.

The synthetic estrogen EE_2 undergoes A-ring oxidation and methylation, as does estradiol [18]; however, the 17α-ethynyl or propargylic alcohol group imparts special metabolic reactivity to these oral contraceptive estrogens (Fig. 3). Early investigations [20] demonstrated the ethynyl group to be reactive by the identification of D-homoannulated compounds, providing evidence that one of the acetylenic carbons was incorporated into the cyclohexyl D ring. Later investigations [21,22] have also demonstrated the ethynyl group to be metabolically cleaved, which thus results in one other unique reaction. The recent work of Ortiz de Montellano and coworkers [23] has now provided convincing evidence that ethynyl steroids are bound covalently to the prosthetic heme of cytochrome P-450 in liver microsomes. The 16β-hydroxy product of EE_2 has also been identified [21] and demonstrates that a 17-keto function is not always a prerequisite to 16β-hydroxylation. At this time, evidence suggests that the ethynylated estrogen metabolites undergo the same series of glucuronidations and sulfations prior to excretion that occur with estradiol.

B. Nonsteroidal Estrogens

Nonsteroidal estrogens such as diethylstilbestrol, dienestrol, zearalenone, and zearalanol are of special interest not only because of their

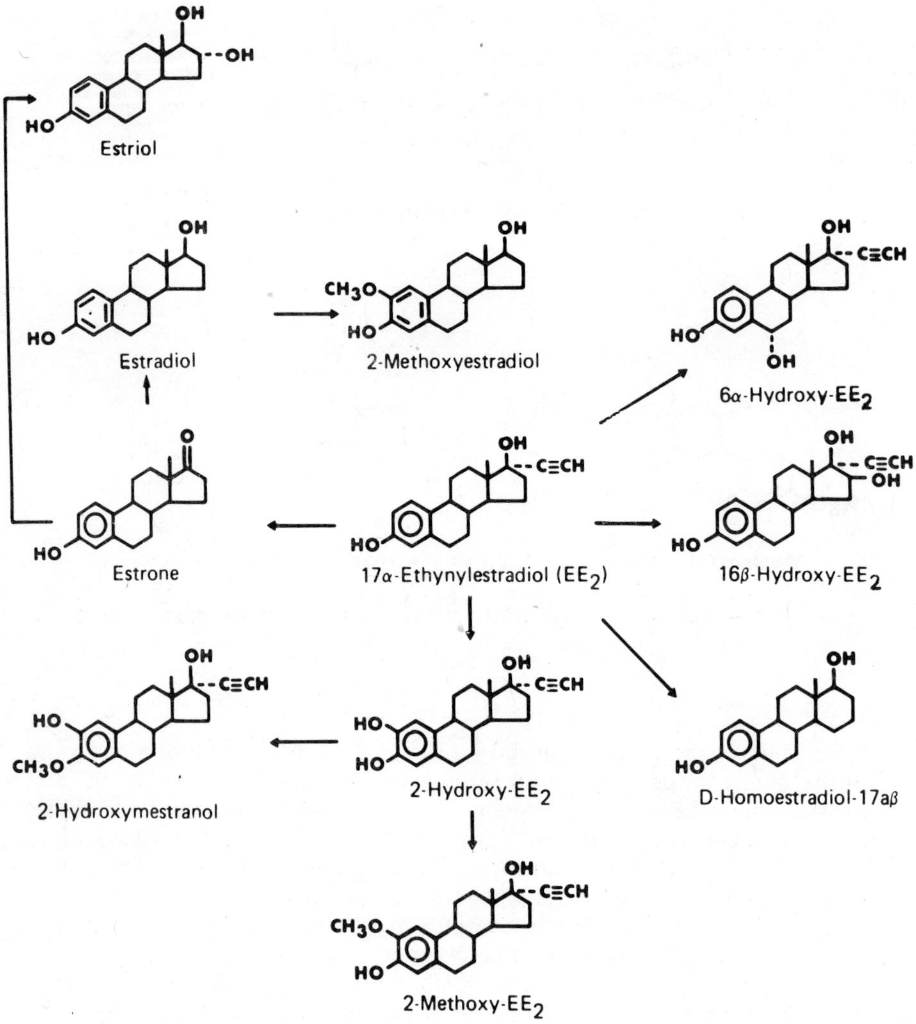

Figure 3 Pathways of metabolism of ethynylestradiol (EE_2) in the primate.

clinical and commercial use but because they demonstrate the diversity of chemical structure that can be potent hormonally (Figs. 4 and 5). Compared to the steroidal estrogens, they each have hydroxylated benzene ring(s) and oxygen functions at opposing ends of the molecule, with a distance between these oxygen functions of 11 to 12 Å. These molecular features are usually present in substances found to be estrogenic.

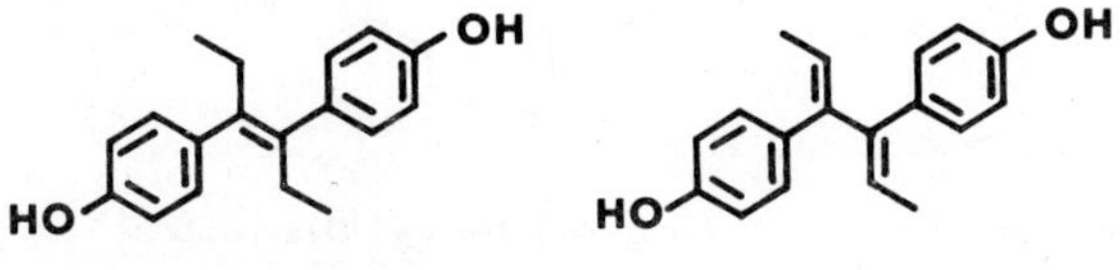

Diethylstilbestrol - DES **Dienestrol**

Figure 4 Structures of the nonsteroidal estrogens diethylstilbestrol (DES) and E,E-dienestrol.

The metabolism of DES is complex, and a great deal remains to be clarified. Tentative identifications have demonstrated [18,24] the stilbene to undergo ring oxidation and methylation, as do the steroidal estrogens (Fig. 6). DES metabolism diverges from steroidal metabolism when oxidation of the aliphatic portions of the molecule is considered. Definitive proof [25] for both oxidation of the terminal methyl groups to form the ω-hydroxylation products and oxidation of the aliphatic chain to dienestrol has demonstrated DES to undergo unique oxidative steps dissimilar to steroidal metabolism. The identification of a catechol derived from dienestrol has recently been made [26]. All of these products chiefly undergo glucuronidation prior to excretion. DES also undergoes carbon-carbon cleavage reactions [27] that yield p-hydroxypropiophenone and p-hydroxy-2-hexene-4-one (Fig. 7). Here again, these reactions are unique to the stilbene since ring cleavage is not common for steroids.

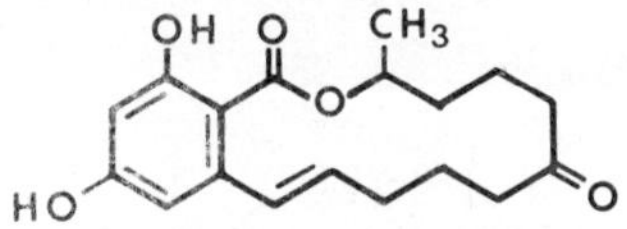

(S)-zearalenone

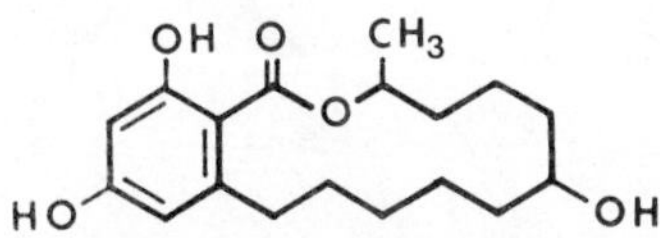

(S)-zearalanol (Ralgro®)

Figure 5 Structures of the phytoestrogens (S)-zearalenone and (S)-zearalanol.

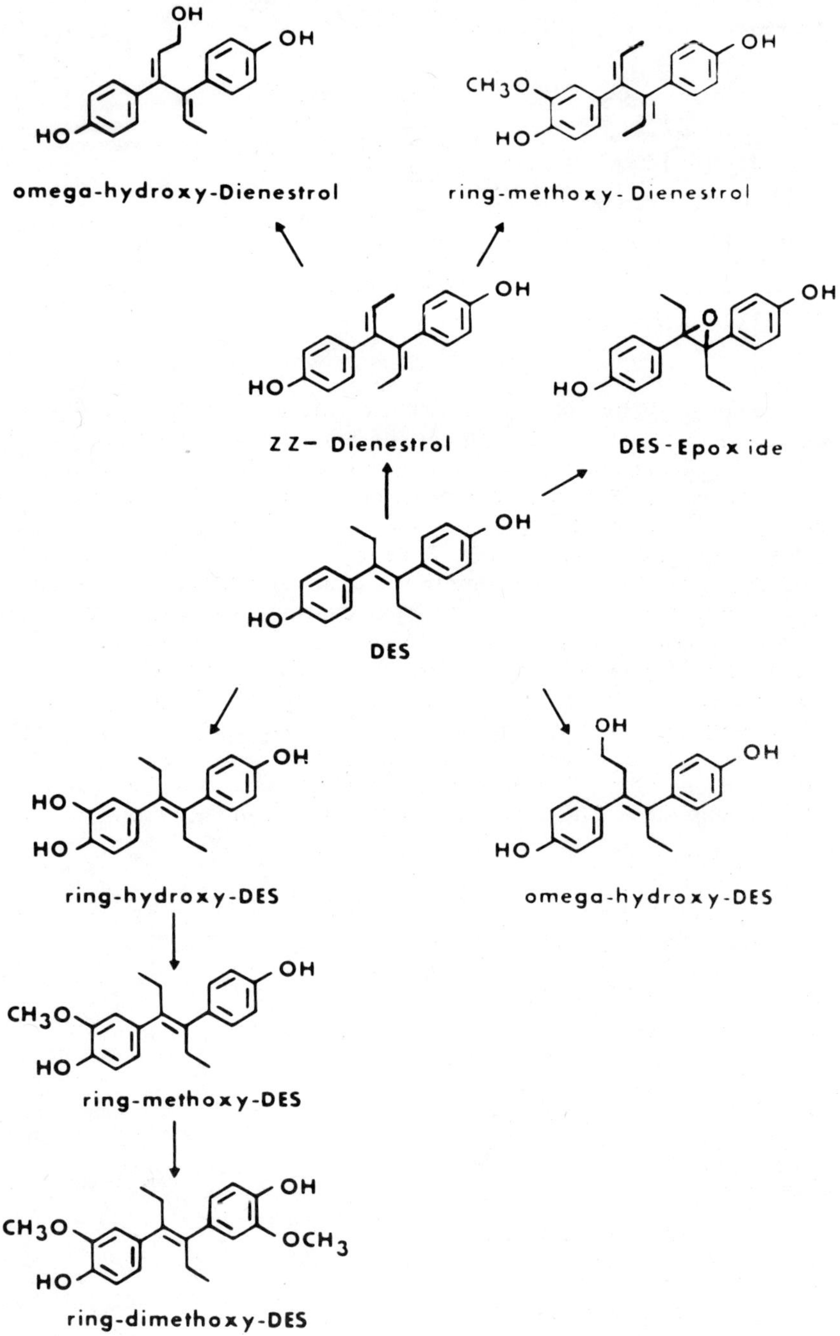

Figure 6 Pathways of metabolism of diethylstilbestrol (DES) in mammalian systems.

p - hydroxypropiophenone

3 - (p-hydroxyphenyl)-
2-hexene-4-one

Figure 7 Structures of cleavage products derived from diethylstilbestrol.

The study of DES metabolism is also complicated by the fact that the molecule exists in equilibrium between the cis (25%) and trans (75%) isomers. The rate of isomerization is controlled by the polarity of the solvent, in that the isomer interconversion is thought to be a second-order reaction that requires transfer of a phenolic proton of one molecule to the aliphatic double bond of another [28]. The greater potential the solvent has for trapping the proton, the slower the isomerization proceeds. In the radiosynthesis of DES, two by-products commonly appear. One is pseudo-DES, which is the $\Delta^{2,3}$-hexane rather than the $\Delta^{3,4}$-hexene of DES; the other is hexestrol, which has hexane as the aliphatic portion of the molecule. It is of interest to note, however, that the pseudo-DES ω-hydroxy product has been found as a metabolic product in mice after the administration of apparently pure DES. If, in fact, pseudo-DES and/or its ω-hydroxy product are true metabolites of DES, the double-bond shifts would be unique to stilbene estrogens.

Zearalenone is a phytoestrogen produced by the fugus *Fusarium* (Fig. 5). This mycotoxin is used commercially as a growth promotion agent in livestock in a reduced form called zearalanol (Ralgo). Zearalenone is distinguished from diethylstilbestrol not only structurally but by the fact that it occurs as a natural product in the food chain. Physiologically, it serves in the control of the reproductive process of *Fusarium roseum* [29], which has a wide variety of hosts, including tomatoes, bananas, barley, oats, and corn. Although zearalenone was not fully characterized chemically until 1966 [29], the products of *Fusarium* were associated with hyperestrogenism in swine as early as 1928 [29]. Its estrogenic effects with regard to reproductive capacity in livestock have been the essential impetus for the study of this mycotoxin.

The metabolism of zearalenone in laboratory animals is not well defined, although preliminary studies [30] have reported the compound to be excreted by the rat as the parent compound and its glucuronide conjugates [29]. Apparently, no significant studies of zearalanol metabolism in animals have been performed. The most definitive research with regard to zearalenone metabolism has been performed in

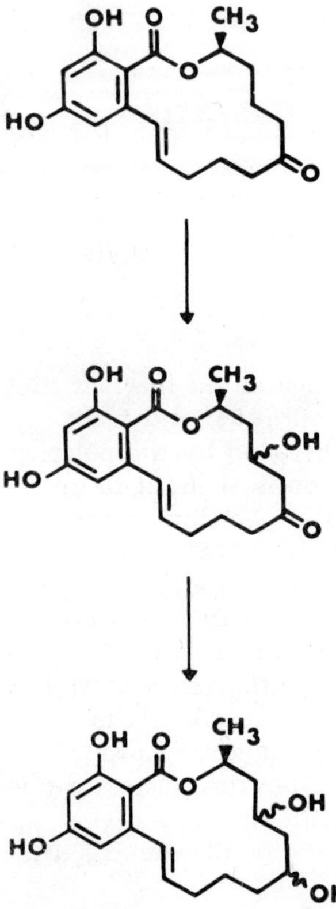

Zearalenone

8'-Hydroxy-Zearalenone

8'-Hydroxy-Zearalenol

Figure 8 Metabolism of zearalenone in the fungal species *Fusarium roseum* Graminearum. (From Ref. 29.)

the fungal species *Fusarium roseum* Graminearum; [29] the principal metabolism included hydroxylated products of zearalenone on the lactone ring at positions 6 and 8 and ring cleavage to produce derivatives of phenylacetic acid (Fig. 8). The cleavage of the lactone ring sets zearalenone apart from the steroidal estrogens. Zearalanol, which remains unstudied, differs significantly from diethylstilbestrol in that it has one three-thousandth of DES's oral activity [29]. It has also reportedly a very low tissue distribution [29]. Whether these molecular and hormonal traits reduce the interest for the study of zearalenone's metabolism remains to be seen.

II. EXTRACTION PROCEDURES

A. Urine and Bile

Efficient extraction of estrogens from urine or other aqueous media is very dependent on the chemical nature of the estrogen. Most unconjugated (aglycone) steroidal or nonsteroidal estrogens can be efficiently extracted from aqueous solutions (containing both the conjugated forms and the aglycones) with any number of organic solvents, such as chloroform, benzene, ethyl acetate, and ethers. When the extracts are from tissue that contains lipids and estrogen glycosides, this simple partition may not be advisable. In a recent study E_2-17β-D-glycoside was found in the ether phase [31]. The simplicity and efficiency of these liquid-liquid phase extractions have long prompted steroid chemists either to acid hydrolyze, solvolyze, or enzymatically hydrolyze urine samples prior to extraction, thus cleaving the water-soluble steroid conjugates and freeing the lipophilic estrogen aglycone. There are, however, estrogen metabolites (tetrols) of both steroidal and nonsteroidal estrogens which are water soluble and generally unextractable with most organic solvents. The desire to study these very polar metabolites and the ever present steroid conjugates found in urine and to a lesser extent in the fecal material has resulted in the development of varied technology to remove the compounds from an aqueous phase for both concentration and purification of these products. The earliest and most effective procedures [32] were to saturate the urine with ammonium sulfate or sodium chloride, which resulted in a simple case of competitive hydration between the salt and the estrogen conjugates. Due to the residual lipophilic nature of the estrogen conjugate and the fact that the salt effectively dehydrated the conjugate, extraction of the milieu with a somewhat polar yet hydrophobic solvent such as tertiary butyl alcohol or diethyl ether-ethanol (3:1) then removed the estrogen conjugates.

Nonionic polymeric adsorbents (XAD-2)

The advent and use of the neutral resin Amberlite XAD-2 (Rohm and Haas) has made extraction of estrogen conjugates simple and efficient. Kushinsky and Tang [33] were the first to introduce this technology for these estrogen conjugates. The routine procedure as developed by Bradlow for numerous steroid conjugates [34] has been widely utilized. The urine is thoroughly mixed with the polymer or passed through a prepared column of the resin. Subsequent water washes of the polymer remove considerable amounts of the endogenous salts and pigments. This washing is then generally followed by elution with either ethanol, methanol, or aqueous alcohol to strip the estrogen conjugates from the adsorbent. A product that is similar to XAD-2 and has been used successfully in the study of DES conjugates is Porapak Q (Waters Associates). This product is used in an identical manner to XAD-2. It is important to point out, however, that the XAD-2 presently on the market differs from the earlier commercial products. To restore its quantitative extraction capacity, Bradlow [35] recommended making the triethylamine salt of the estrogen conjugates prior to XAD-2 extraction.

Detailed Procedure for Extraction of Urinary Estrogen Conjugates Using Amberlite XAD-2 [34,35]

1. Place XAD-2 in an all-glass gravity-flow chromatographic column and wash the polymer with 2 volumes of methanol and then acetone. Follow this by a thorough wash with distilled water and a reverse-flow wash with water to remove the fines.
2. Urine is applied to the column and allowed to pass from the column. The estrogen is adsorbed to the polymer.
3. An equal volume of 0.5 M, pH 7.2 triethylamine sulfate is then passed through the column to convert the conjugates to the triethylamine salt.
4. The residual water on the column is displaced by 200 to 300 ml of petroleum ether.
5. The estrogen conjugates are then washed off the resin with the methanol or ethanol.

B. Feces, Tissues, and Feeds

Extraction of estrogens or their metabolic products from feces, tissues, and feeds is complicated by the fact that the compounds are trapped in a solid phase and are often composed of both polar and nonpolar products. Consequently, most if not all of the analytical extraction procedures begin with a homogenization or liquefaction step to allow effectively extraction. However, blood cells require only the addition of water or a polar organic solvent for cellular disruption. In the case of feces, some investigators lyophilize or heat dry the feces to remove the water present prior to extraction.

Solvent extraction is initiated by the addition of organic solvent, usually a polar alcohol, to solubilize both polar and nonpolar estrogens. This extract is then partitioned between an organic and an aqueous phase to separate water-soluble from nonpolar products. In certain instances, the initial alcohol extract is applied to a preparative column so as to elute by solvent selection the polar from the nonpolar fraction.

In practically every instance following the homogenization and extraction of a solid phase, there is an insoluble residue. When radiolabeled estrogens are used, the amount of residual radioactivity is determined by burning a representative sample of the residue in a commercial oxidizer or by chemically hydrolyzing and solubilizing the sample with strong alkali or a commercial solubilizer. The net effect, of course, is to liquefy the residue and thereby allow an accurate count by liquid scintillation spectrometry.

Extraction of diethylstilbestrol metabolic products from feces and tissues [36]

1. Either dried feces or ground tissue is placed into a Soxhlet extractor and refluxed for 24 hr with absolute ethanol and finally extracted for 48 to 72 hr with diethyl ether.
2. In the case of tissue, the alcohol extracts are extracted five times with an equal volume of ether. The ether-insoluble material is mixed with 2 volumes of water and acidified with 10 ml of 10% phosphoric acid and filtered. The acid filtrate is extracted again three times with ether.
3. The Soxhlet ether extracts and those resulting from the extraction of the acidified ethanol extract are combined and partitioned against a pH 9 to 10 bicarbonate solution to remove glucuronide conjugates.
4. The remaining ether phase is then extracted with 1 N NaOH to extract the phenolic aglycones. Following neutralization of the aqueous phase, the phenolic products are extracted from the aqueous fraction by chloroform.
5. The conjugates are removed from the bicarbonate by adjustment to pH 3.0, saturation with sodium sulfate, and extraction with diethyl ether.
6. In the case of the feces, the ethanol and ether Soxhlet extracts can be combined immediately because the feces were dehydrated prior to extraction.

Alternative procedure for extraction of diethylstilbestrol metabolic products from feces and tissues [37]

1. The feces or tissue is homogenized with methanol and shaken for 48 hr at 2°.
2. The extract is taken to dryness and dissolved in distilled water and the residue applied to a Porapak Q (Waters Associates) column.
3. A 100 to 200 ml step gradient of water-methanol is applied (0, 30, 50, 80, and 100% methanol). The polar or conjugated products are eluted between 50 and 80% methanol, whereas the free or aglycone metabolites are eluted by 100% methanol.

Extraction of estradiol metabolites from feces [38]

1. The feces are homogenized in ethanol and centrifuged.
2. The supernatant is evaporated to dryness in vacuo and the residue is dissolved in 20% (v/v) aqueous methanol and left for 48 hr at -20°.*

---

*All temperature data are in degrees Celsius.

3. The soluble estrogen metabolites are then passed through an Amberlyst-15 column, followed by solvent extraction.
4. Addition of hexane-dichloromethane elutes the nonpolar products from the column; the subsequent addition of n-butanol removes the polar tetrol products from the column.
5. It is of importance to point out that initial extraction of this procedure succeeds in removing only approximately 50% of the total estrogen present in the feces. If this is due to the extreme polarity of the products, a more exhaustive extraction in a Soxhlet extractor or use of methylal-methanol (4:1, v/v) as the solvent may provide a more efficient procedure.

Extraction of ethynylestradiol metabolites from hepatocyte cells [39]

1. The cells are homogenized in methylal-methanol (4:1) and the resulting homogenate allowed to set 18 hr at 2°.
2. The homogenate is centrifuged and the supernatant removed. The pellet is washed and centrifuged three times with a 2 to 3 volume excess of the methylal-methanol solvent. Each wash is added to the original extract.
3. The combined extracts are reduced in vacuo to near dryness and the residue is partitioned between benzene and water. The water contains the estrogen conjugates, whereas the benzene phase contains the aglycones.

Extraction of estradiol, diethylstilbestrol, and zearalenone or zearalanol from animal chow [40-42]

1. Twenty grams of animal chow is placed into a 250 ml flask and extracted mechanically with 100 ml of methanol for 2 hr.
2. The extract is filtered through a plug of glass wool and a 50 ml aliquot of the original 100 ml extract is placed in a screw-cap culture tube containing 100 ml of H_2O and 6 g of sodium chloride.
3. The mixture is extracted three to five times with 20 ml of benzene and each successive benzene extract is filtered through anhydrous sodium sulfate. The benzene extracts are combined and evaporated to dryness in vacuo.
4. The E_2 and DES residues are successively washed with benzene-methanol (9:1) (2 ml) and each wash allowed to percolate into a small Sephadex LH-20 column and, following placement of the sample, the column is eluted with additional solvent (20 ml of E_2 and 30 ml of DES). Zearalenone (Z) or Zearalanol is treated similarly but is placed on the column with benzene. The column is further eluted for each of these

compounds with benzene. The final wash from the column for E_2, DES, and zearalenone and its derivative is accomplished with 20, 25, 50, and 60 ml of benzene-methanol (9:1), respectively.

5. The final column eluate is taken to dryness in vacuo, dissolved in benzene, and transferred to a solution of 1 N NaOH (4 ml of E_2, 8 ml of DES, 10 ml of Z). Following centrifugation, the benzene layer is removed and the aqueous phase extracted twice more with benzene. For E_2 and DES, the alkaline solution is neutralized with 10 ml of 1 M sodium bicarbonate, then the aqueous phase extracted three times with benzene, each phase being filtered through anhydrous sodium sulfate. The zearalenone or zearalanol method is identical except that neutralization is carried out with pH 4.0 boric acid buffer.
6. The benzene extracts are taken to dryness and transferred to a silica gel column (3% water) by sequential transfer with benzene. For E_2 and DES, they are eluted from the column with 30 and 20 ml of benzene-4% acetone, respectively. For zearalenone and zearalanol, the compounds are eluted from the column with 49:1 and 47:3 benzene-acetone, respectively, with volumes of 50 and 60 ml.

III. ISOLATION AND PURIFICATION TECHNIQUES

Current methods, such as gas chromatography-mass spectrometry (GC-MS) and radioimmunossay (RIA) for identification and quantitation of estrogens and estrogen metabolites in biological materials, require extensive purification of the samples prior to final analysis. Isolation of individual compounds or groups of related compounds is most effectively and efficiently accomplished by employing one or more chromatographic fractionation procedures. A variety of such techniques are available, and selection of the appropriate one is based on the requirements of the final analytical procedure.

A. Conjugates

Valuable physiological information is lost in both chemical and enzymatic hydrolysis of the water-soluble conjugates; thus there is interest in chromatographic systems for profiling and defining the types of conjugation present in body fluids and tissues. A number of chromatographic media have been employed for fractionating the hydrophilic estrogen conjugates. The ionic character of these conjugates enabled Hahnel [43-45], Hobkirk et al. [46,47], and Musey et al. [48] to separate the major ones on DEAE Sephadex in the presence of NaCl. Taking advantage of the cation exchange properties of the lipophilic gel, Sephadex LH-20, in the presence of electrolytes, Tikkanen and Adlercreutz [49] separated all of the estriol conjugates known to occur in pregnancy urine. With this stationary phase and similar solvent system, profiles of urinary ethynyl estrogen conjugates have also been obtained [22]. This technique permits study of interspecies [22] and intraspecies [50] differences in estrogen metabolism. Alteration of the solvent system permits profiling of the conjugates of DES [51].

Separation of conjugated estrogens by high-pressure liquid chromatography is accomplished rapidly (e.g., 30 min versus 4 to 18 hr on Sephadex), with greater resolution and considerably smaller volumes of solvent. Van der Wal and Huber [52] demonstrated separations of estrogen conjugates on ion exchange columns and optimized the systems with respect to 30 compounds [53]. Determination of the level of urinary estriol-16-glucuronide in pregnant women was accomplished by this technique in 2 hr. Faster separations of similar compounds have been achieved on columns with stationary phases chemically bonded to microparticulate support materials [54-57]. The variety of these commercially available columns, either ion exchange or bonded phase, permits optimization of the chromatographic system for specific conjugate classes.

Gas chromatography with on-line mass spectrometric detection has been investigated as a tool for profiling estrogen conjugates in body fluids. Permethyl [58], propyl [59], and methylsilyl [60] derivatives have been employed. However, the greatest value of GC-MS techniques in estrogen conjugate studies has been elucidation of conjugate structure, specifically the position of glucuronide attachment to the aglycone moiety.

B. Aglycones

In all but a few cases, paper chromatography, the classical technique for steroids, has been replaced by the relatively inexpensive and rapid technique of thin layer chromatography (TLC). Heftmann [61], using silica gel G, has summarized R_f values for the major natural estrogens in 17 solvent systems and has reviewed many of the numerous estrogen TLC techniques that have been developed. Recently, TLC was used as the isolation procedure for ethynylestradiol and trenbolone acetate in feed [62] prior to GC analysis, and for 17α-estradiol and trenbolone acetate in urine [63] prior to fluorometric analysis. The use of high-performance TLC improves separations and detection of DES, zearalanol, and many of the natural estrogens [64]. For the catechol estrogens, which readily undergo oxidative decomposition, impregnation of the stationary phase with ascorbic acid is required [65-67].

Sephadex LH-20 column chromatography has had a considerable impact on steroid methodology. It has provided a quantitative and reproducible means of purifying substances without contributing impurities that interfere with sensitive identification techniques. Rinsing residual radioactivity and polar pigments from the column after each use allows columns to be used almost indefinitely. Although LH-20 has been the medium used for purifying plasma extracts for radioimmunoassay (RIA) procedures, the only systematic study of a wide variety of estrogens was done by Lisboa and Strassner [68] for 23 estrogens in six solvent systems. For epimeric and closely related compounds which are not resolved, this type of column may not be the most suitable. However, it is extremely useful for the analysis of complex extracts from large volumes of urine that at times are necessary in identification studies of unknown metabolies [21]. If reused, it becomes relatively inexpensive and gives the analyst information as to the kind and polarity range of radiolabeled metabolites present. Some derivatives of LH-20 have also proved to be useful in isolation techniques. Alkylated C_{11}-C_{14} LH-20 and alkylated C_{15}-C_{18} LH-20 columns used in a reverse-phase solvent system effectively remove contaminating pigments from metabolites isolated by LH-20 separation of urinary ethynyl estrogens [21]. Sulfoethyl (SE) LH-20 and triethylaminohydroxylpropyl hydroxyalkyl (TEAPHA) LH-20 appear to be potentially useful; Axelson and Sjovall [69] separated the estrogens from interfering steroids present in plasma extracts, thereby permitting GC-MS evaluation. However, TEAPHA is a strong base, necessitating caution if the steroids to be studied are alkali labile.

The use of 17α-ethynyl steroids in contraceptive formulations stimulated interest in specific and sensitive methods for isolating ethynylated steroids from biological fluids. The binding affinity of the olefin to the silver ion has been utilized in these techniques. Columns [70,71] and thin layer plates [72,72] impregnated with silver nitrate capture small quantities of ethynylated steroids from large amounts of foreign materials. With some of these methods, investigators have noted low recoveries and deethynylation. The silver-sulfoethyl cellulose column [71] eliminated some of these deficiencies and has been successfully employed in isolating ethynyl compounds for GC-MS identification studies [21,71].

Over the past decade high-pressure liquid chromatography (HPLC) has played an increasing role as a separative analytical technique. Development of sensitive detectors, continually improving stationary phases for columns, and sophisticated elution systems have encouraged investigators to apply this technique to the analysis of estrogens. A high degree of separation efficiency has been demonstrated with a variety of columns and elution systems for natural estrogens [74-81], ethynyl estrogens [82-84], equine estrogens [73,85,86], and DES

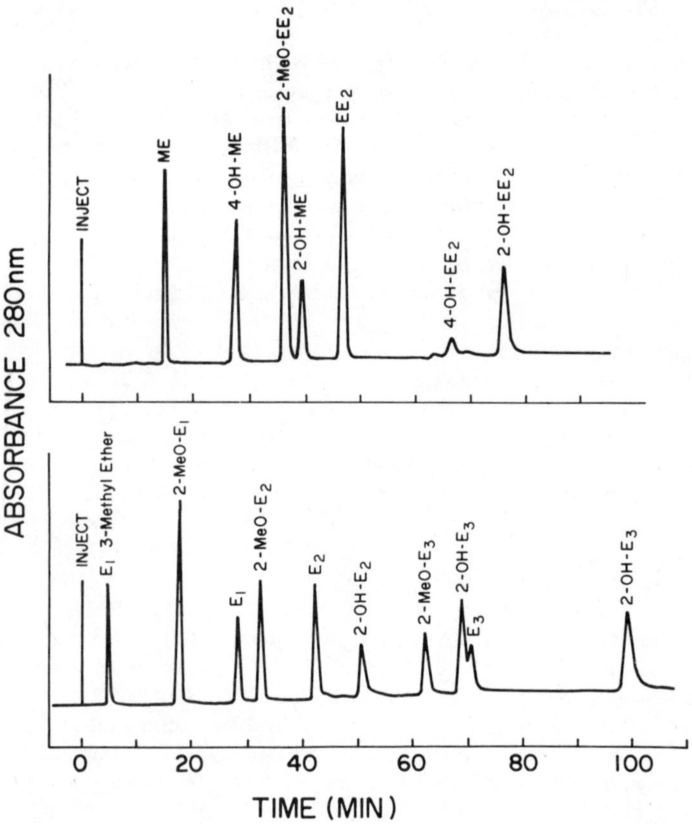

Figure 9 Separation of metabolites of ethynylestradiol (EE_2) and mestranol (ME), upper curve, and estrone (E_1), estradiol-17β (E_2), and estriol (E_3), lower curve, by HPLC on a 0.46 × 50 cm Chromegabond Diol column using a gradient of isopropanol in heptane.

[87-90]. A normal-phase separation by HPLC of some oxidized metabolites of estradiol and ethynylestradiol is shown in Figure 9. A similar chromtogram of some DES metabolites is illustrated in Figure 10.

When biological extracts are applied to adsorption HPLC columns, some irreversible adsorption occurs. The resultant degradation of stationary phase requires column replacement after a time. Precolumns eliminate some of the damage but can lead to loss in efficiency. By chemically binding the stationary phase to the solid support, stable and reproducible columns have been produced which avoid the problems of irreversible adsorption. Some of these columns were designed

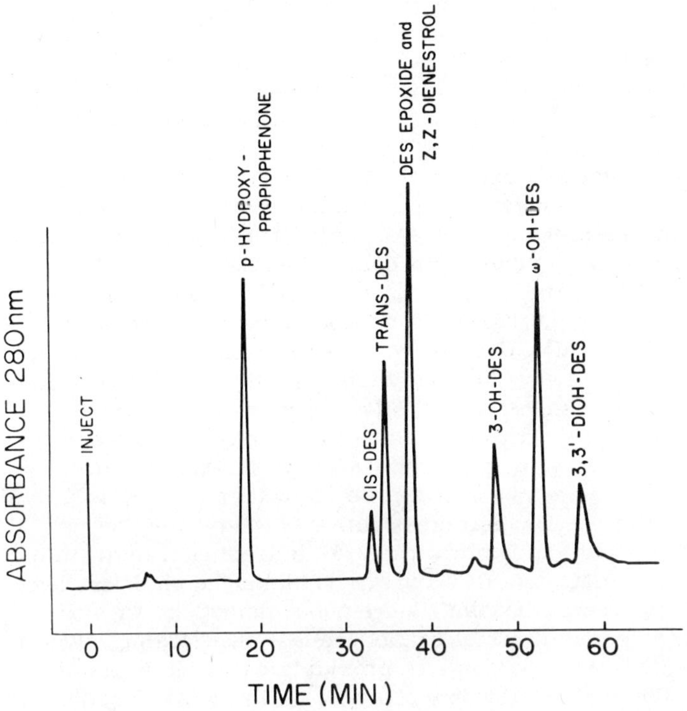

Figure 10 Separation of the metabolites of diethylstilbestrol (DES) by HPLC on a 0.46 × 60 cm Chromegabond Diol column using a gradient of ethanol in heptane.

for either reverse- or normal-phase operation and can be rinsed with a polar solvent between runs to remove residual pigments or radioactivity without loss of resolving capacity. Reverse-phase separations for estrogens have been demonstrated on columns of C_{18} alkyls chemically bonded to a microparticulate support [80, 87]. However, some of the best separations for a wide variety of estrogens have been obtained with a normal-phase solvent system of isopropanol in heptane on microparticulate columns with one of the following chemically bonded functional groups: ether [85, 85], NH_2 [79], and diol (Figs. 9 and 10; Refs. 8, 83, 84). Roos [86], using an ether-bonded ETH Permaphase column for aglycone separations, identified and measured eight of the conjugated and esterified estrogens in pharmaceutical tablets. Six estrogens in pregnancy urine were rapidly isolated by Fantl et al. [79] and the level of estriol determined using an NH_2 Bondapak column. Williams and Goldzieher [84] have obtained chromatographic profiles of as many as 20 ethynyl and nonethynyl metabolites of 23, 17α-ethynylestradiol on the weakly polar Chromegaprep Diol column. By gradually increasing the percent of isopropanol in heptane in a linear gradient, better resolution with symmetrical peaks was achieved in less time than with the chromatographic separation of similar compojnds on LH-20.

The type of detector used in the HPLC system determines the level of sensitivity. The refractive index detector has only limited use in work with estrogens because of its low sensitivity. For estrogens and DES the fixed-wavelength detector at 280 nm with detection limites of 20 ng [76] is the most commonly used. In practice, the most sensitive setting (0.005 AUFS on most detectors) produces considerable noise level. With the variable-wavelength detector, which permits monitoring to below 200 nm, the sensitivity is doubled using 230 nm, and trebled using 217 nm [79]. Flame ionization detection can monitor milligram quantities of estrogens of pharmaceutical interest for microgram quantities of impurities [82]. In the absence of a sensitive universal detector, chemical derivatization is used to provide additional sensitivity. For estrogens with a carbonyl function at C-17 (estrone, equilin, and equilenin), the 2,4-dinitrophenyl hydrazine derivatives can be detected at 365 nm [86]. Dansylation of estrogens [78] provides the means of using fluorescence detection; with this technique the detection limits of estriol are less than 400 pg. Electrochemical detection [81] is capable of providing detection limits of 1 to 5 ng per injection of the catechol estrogens, with identical responses for their methyl ethers. Considerable improvement in the means of detection will be necessary before HPLC becomes the quantitative method of choice for samples containing extremely low levels of estrogens.

Although continuous radioactivity detection has not been demonstrated in conjunction with HPLC of estrogens, on-line scintillation counters are commercially available and the technique has been used in metabolism studies [91-93]. HPLC with on-line mass spectrometry would permit positive identification and rapid quantitation.

Isolation and profiling of urinary metabolites of ethynylestradiol by HPLC [84]

1. Urine is collected for 72 hr following the ingestion of radiolabeled ethynylestradiol (usually 25 μCi), then extracted with XAD-2 Amberlite (Rohm and Haas). (No unconjugated metabolites are to be found in urine properly collected.)
2. Hydrolyze an aliquot, 50,000 to 100,000 dpm ^{3}H and/or ^{14}C, with *Helix pomatia* phenol sulfatase which contains β-glucuronidase (Sigma Type H-1.)
3. Extract released aglycones with 3 volumes of diethyl ether.

4. Evaporate ether extract to dryness using reduced pressure at 40°.
5. Dissolve extract in 200 to 300 μl of isopropanol (Burdick and Jackson, UV grade).
6. Inject the sample on a Chromegaprep diol column (ES Industries), 9.6 mm × 50 cm, having a flow of 7.5 ml/min and a pressure of 1000 psi.
7. Use linear gradient programming (Waters Solvent Programmer) to achieve an effective change of 2.25 to 15.00% isopropanol in heptane during a 158 min interval; pump A, heptane (Burdick and Jackson, UV grade); pump B, 15% isopropanol in heptane; gradient 6, 15 to 100% B in 158 min.
8. Upon completion of program, rinse column with MeOH to remove pigments and residual radioactivity.
9. During program, collect 1 min fractions directly into scintillation vials (Gilson-Mini Escargot); dry and count with appropriate scintillation fluid.
10. Plot radioactivity versus time to provide a profile of the radiolabeled metabolites.
11. After matching relative retention times of unknowns to the positions of reference compounds using the same gradient, the percent of total radioactivity under each peak can be calculated. (Some of the reference ethynyl estrogen metabolites are not commercially available.)
12. Using this same technique with fraction collection into tubes provides material for identification of unknown peaks using GC-MS or reverse-isotope recrystallization.

Urinary metabolites of diethylstilbestrol using Sephadex LH-20 and HPLC [51,94]

1. Remove unconjugated metabolites by extracting urine with benzene.
2. After processing the radiolabeled urine conjugates through XAD-2 (see Section II.a), dry and extract in vacuo. (Some samples require additional chromatography on Sephadex G-25).
3. Chromatograph conjugates on a Sephadex LH-20 (Pharmacia) column, 340 × 25 mm, using methanol-ethanol (50:50, v/v) as the mobile phase. Counting of a suitable aliquot (usually one-tenth or one-fifth of each fraction) provides information for the plotting of radioactivity versus fraction number. Four of these peaks are hydrolyzable with β-glucuronidase.
4. Hydrolyze the glucuronide fractions with beef liver β-glucuronidase (Sigma, Type B-10) in 0.1 N sodium acetate buffer, pH 5.0.
5. Extract deconjugated DES metabolites by partitioning three times with benzene.

6. Chromatograph by HPLC each fraction on a μPorasil column, 4 mm × 30 cm, using a mobile phase of hexane-$CHCl_3$-MeOH (70:27.5:2.5, v/v/v). Set flow at 1.0 ml/min, 600 psi. Count each fraction in a liquid scintillation counter.
7. Plot radioactivity versus fraction number. The parent compound (cis-trans isomers) will elute from the HPLC column at approximately 20 and 13 min, respectively.
8. Subject these radioactive fractions and others to trimethylsilylation and GC-MS analysis as described in Section IV.

Urinary metabolites of diethylstilbestrol using TLC and radio-GLC [24,25,95]

1. Collect urine for 4 days (at 24 hr intervals) following the ingestion of radiolabeled DES.
2. Saturate urine with ammonium sulfate and extract with mixture of ether-ethanol (3:1, v/v). Concentrate the extracts using a rotary evaporator.
3. Prepare 36 g of alumina column (neutral, Brockmann activity I, suspended in 96% ethanol). Apply sample to column.
4. Elute each fraction with 100 ml of the following solvents:
   a. 96% ethanol for unconjugated compounds
   b. Water for the sulfates and mercapturic acids
   c. Phosphate/citrate buffer, pH 6, for the glucuronides
   d. 20% aqueous formic acid for the polar and unidentified metabolites
5. Hydrolyze glucuronides with bacterial β-glucuronidase and sulfates with *Helix pomatia* aryl sulfatase (Serva). Extract released aglycones with ethyl ether.
6. Obtain a radio-thin layer chromatographic profile of metabolites by applying sample to a 250 mm silica gel HF_{254} glass plate (E. Merck), developing with benzene-ethyl acetate (1:1, v/v) and scanning in a flow counter. The counting efficiency is much higher for ^{14}C than for ^{3}H.
7. Perform radio-GLC [95], allowing one portion of the effluent to detect mass and the other portion to detect the radiolabeled peaks.
   a. For GLC use a 6 ft × 2 mm glass column packed with 3% OV-225 on Gas Chrom Q (100-200 mesh). Prepare trimethylsilylated derivatives using bis(trimethylsilyl)acetamide (BSA). Inject samples using an injector temperature of 250°, a detector temperature of 280°, and a column temperature of 160 to 200° with an increase of 4°/min. Retention times (min) for the following compounds have been determined:

DES*	12.4-14.6
Ring-methoxy-DES*	15.2-17.9
Dienestrol	18.8
Ring-methoxydienestrol	2.4
Δ-Hydroxy-DES*	16.7-18.0
Δ-Hydroxydienestrol	22.4

Run electron impact mass spectra at 70 eV using a Varian 2700 chromatograph-Varian CH 7 mass spectrometer.

b. The radiolabeled peaks can be detected by appropriate counting of the effluent after oxidative conversion.

IV. QUANTITATIVE ANALYSIS AND IDENTIFICATION

A. Gas Chromatography

Gas chromatography (GC), with its high resolution and sensitivity, has been used effectively as a quantitative technique for estrogens. Adlercreutz [96] and Heftmann [97] have reviewed its use in estrogen determinations. Methods using packed columns [98] have low efficiency, and some losses occur due to adsorption to the support particles and column walls. Some of the recent methods using open tubular columns [69, 99] eliminate this defect. GC suffers from the necessity of derivatizing the estrogens to make them volatile and from the exposure of the derivatives to high temperature, with the risk of degradation.

The level of sensitivity for GC methods is determined by the means of detection. Flame ionization detection limits are in the range of 10 ng. Using derivatives suitable for electron capture, the sensitivity of detection can be as low as 1 ng. Using the trifluoroacetate (TFA) and heptafluorobutyrate (HFB) derivatives of DES [100], as little as 2 ng/g in beef liver can be detected. Recently, electrolytic conductivity and electron capture detection for GC have been compared for derivatives of DES [101]: Electron capture is 10- to 100-fold more sensitive. The use of GC with detection of radioactivity in the effluent has been shown to be useful for the demonstration of DES metabolites [24, 25, 95].

Procedure for electron capture-gas chromatographic determination of estradiol, diethylstilbestrol, and zearalenone/zearalanol [40-42]

1. Add exactly 0.5 ml of benzene to a 50 ml round-bottom flask containing a DES, E_2, or zearalenone sample (dry residue).

---

*Cis-trans isomers.

To this flask are added 0.1 M trimethylamine (TMA) and pentafluoropropionic anhydride (PFPA). (For DES, 0.1 ml + 0.01 ml PFPA; for E_2, 0.2 ml TMA + 0.02 ml PFPA). These reagent quantities are used for a sample containing 500 ng or less.

2. The flask is sealed immediately with a glass stopper and swirled gently at room temperature for 20 min. The reaction is terminated by adding 1 ml of 1 M phosphate buffer (pH 4.2) and mixed by shaking 30 sec.
3. To the DES or zearalenone/zearalanol reaction mixtures exactly 1.4 ml or 0.5 ml of benzene is added, respectively. Exactly 1.3 ml of benzene is added to the estradiol reaction mixture. The appropriate reaction mixture is transferred to an 8 ml culture tube.
4. Allow phase separation and remove the lower aqueous phase. Wash the organic layer again with 0.1 ml of 1 M phosphate buffer. Transfer benzene phase to a clean 8 ml culture tube containing 1 g of anhydrous Na_2SO_4 and shake for 30 sec.
5. Remove the benzene phase and store in a clean, dry tube for subsequent electron capture-gas chromatographic analysis.
6. Gas chromatographic conditions for DES analysis: 5% OV-101 on Gas Chrom Q (80-100 mesh) in a 100 cm × 4 mm glass column is conditioned overnight prior to use at 275°. It is operated isothermally at 185° in the dc mode with nitrogen as the carrier gas (160 ml/min). The injection port temperature is 20° greater than the column and the detector is at 300°. With these conditions, the PFPA deriviative of cis and trans DES have retention times of 1.70 and 2.65 min, respectively. All injections are made in 5 μl of benzene.
7. Gas chromatographic condition for the analysis of *zearalenone-zearalanol*: 5% Dexsil on 80-100 mesh Gas Chrom Q is conditioned in a 100 cm × 4 mm glass column at 275° overnight prior to use. Nitrogen is the carrier gas (160 ml/min), with the injection port temperature at 240°, the detection at 270°, and the column at 220°. All injections are made in 5 μl of benzene. Zearalenone and zearalanol have retention times of 2.05 and 4.05 min, respectively.
8. Gas chromatographic conditions for the analysis of *estradiol*: 5% OV-25 (a phenyl-methyl silicone, 75% phenyl) on Gas Chrom Q (80-100 mesh) in a 300 cm × 4 mm glass column is conditioned overnight at 270° prior to use. During analysis, the column is operated isothermally at 235° in the dc mode with a nitrogen flow rate of 160 ml/min. The detector temperature is 275° and the injection port temperature is 255°. A 5 μl benzene sample yields a retention time of 2.95 min for estradiol-17β.

B. Spectrophotometry

The utilization of ultraviolet spectroscopy for the identification and quantitation of estrogens suffers from a lack of both specificity and sensitivity. Its use in biochemical or bioanalytical studies is therefore limited when dealing with samples of relatively low purity and mass. Excitation spectroscopy or fluorometry has greater specificity and sensitivity and, in the case of diethylstilbestrol analysis, it is as sensitive as gas-liquid chromatography in the electron capture or flame ionization mode. Infrared spectroscopy is also a technique for estrogen identification, and although it is definitive, the purity and mass of sample required for analysis make it generally impractical.

Fluorescent procedure for the quantitation of DES [102]

1. Prepare a stock solution of DES (0.4 mg/ml) in pure ethanol. Place this stock solution in four quartz tubes and irradiate for different intervals with ultraviolet light to determine the length for time of maximum fluorescence.
2. A dried tissue extract or chromatographic preparation of diethylstilbestrol is dissolved in 5 ml of pure ethanol; 2.5 ml is transferred to a quartz tube, with the remainder to be used in a cuvette for fluorescent intensity measurement.
3. Determine the fluorescent intensity of the cuvette sample without irradiation to establish a preirradiation reading. Irradiate the quartz sample and transfer the contents to a cuvette to measure the fluorescence intensity at 410 nm.
4. Make all samples alkaline by the addition of 0.5 ml of 1 N potassium hydroxide. Mix thoroughly and allow to stand 10 min, then measure the fluorescence intensity. The addition of the basic solution in the presence of ultraviolet energy results in the photocyclization of DES to phenanthrenedione, which has a maximum of 410 nm.
5. The difference in fluorescence between the base-treated, nonirradiated sample and the irradiated samples represent the DES present.

Fluorometric analysis of trenbolone acetate [103]

1. A tissue extract of urinary preparation of trenbolone acetate is purified on a silica gel thin layer chromatographic plate using chloroform-ethyl acetate (2:1).
2. The R_f value for trenbolone acetate is 0.68. The eluted zone is dissolved in 75% 6 M HCl in methanol and excited at 365 nm. A reversible fluorescence occurs at 498 nm and the sensitivity of the assay is about 1 ng.

C. Mass Spectroscopy

The ultimate technique for analysis and quantitation of estrogenic hormones is the use of mass spectroscopy. It can not only quantitate the compound but can simultaneously provide an authenticating mass spectrum. Analysis of estrogens by mass spectroscopy is generally preceded by gas chromatographic purification. Separation of the estrogen from the biological milieu prior to mass spectroscopy simplifies the analysis. There are instances where, with good extractive and chromatographic purification, a sample can be directly analyzed by probe insertion. Derivatization of the sample prior to probe insertion does enhance the estrogens' volatility. It is required when gas-liquid chromatography is used prior to either electron impact or chemical ionization analysis. In most instances, obtaining a chromatographic blank is advisable so that its spectrum can be computer-subtracted from the experimental sample. The use of a chromatographic blank can be particularly helpful in electron impact spectra, which generate a far more complex spectrum than chemical ionization. Other modes of mass spectral analysis that can be used for estrogen quantitation are atmospheric ionization (AI) and field desorption (FD). AI provides a simplistic spectrum that is usable in instances requiring high sensitivity and is particularly useful in conjunction with a deuterium standard for $^{12}C/^{13}C$ analysis. FD is not well suited for the analysis of aglycones, owing to their excessive volatility. However, FD can be very useful in the analysis of estrogen glucuronides in the free acid state because of the technique's ability to ionize a polar compound without excess thermal energy. When, in fact, estrogen glucuronides are presented for analysis as a sodium or potassium salt, usually the salts must be complexed in fructose or Crown ether to reduce their masking effect on FD analysis. Estrogen glucuronides are volatilized by simple methylation of the carboxyl function and subsequent trimethylsilylation of available hydroxyls. The volatile product is then separated by gas chromatography and analyzed by electron impact (EI) [59,60]. EI mass spectrometry of the TFA and HFB derivatives of DES [100] lends itself well to confirmation of DES metabolites. The mass spectra of DES, dienestrol, and hexestrol, and their diacetates, dimethyl ethers, and bis-trimethylsilyl ethers have been reported by Engel and colleagues [104].

Quantitation and identification by mass spectroscopy is limited by one underlying principle: the authentic compound must be available for spectral confirmation. Although this is true for chromatographic and photospectral analysis as well, it has long been acknowledged that both similar and completely dissimilar compounds can cochromatograph or have very similar descriptive spectra. In contrast, in the case of mass spectroscopy, the likelihood that two similar or dissimilar compounds have both identical molecular weights and spectra is far lower. Thus, in pursuing the analysis of an estrogen compound with mass spectrometry, comparison with the original compound is imperative.

Using mass fragmentography or selected ion monitoring for ultrasensitive analysis, in conjunction with modern computer technology, the investigator can focus the entire analysis on the quantitative and qualitative presence of an estrogenic hormone dominant spectral peak. By ignoring all other extraneous peaks and performing repetitive scanning for only the molecular ion and other dominant ions, the sensitivity for the desired compound is increased. Monitoring only certain ions allows partial integration of the ion currents and thus enhances sensitivity. This technology is becoming particularly effective when used in conjunction with an authentic deuterated compound [105]. Similarly, computer comparison of the $^{12}C/^{13}C$ ratio in the molecular ion can allow a very accurate estimation of the endogenous estrogen present. Using mass fragmentography (MF) Adlercreutz et al. [106] demonstrated increased sensitivity with a toleration for larger amounts of impurities. Even the extremely low levels of estrogens in circulating fluids can be detected using this technique [107-109[. The trimethylsilyl ether derivatives of the catechol estrogens show highly characteristic fragmentation patterns [110], thereby aiding in their identification.

Mass fragmentography determination of estradiol-17β in serum [106]

1. About 50 ng of [2,4,16,16-^{2}H]-estradiol is added to a 2 to 5 ml sample of serum and the serum sample is extracted three times with an equal volume of anhydrous diethyl ether. A standard curve is also prepared using 50, 100, and 200 pg of estradiol-17β, assayed together with the unknown(s).
2. The extract is purified on a small Sephadex LH-20 column (0.6 × 8 cm) using chloroform-heptane-methanol-water (500:500:75:3, v/v/v/v) as the mobile phase. Estradiol is eluted from the column in 7 to 11 ml of eluent.
3. The sample is dried and derivatized to a trimethylsilyl derivative by reacting the residue with 100 µl of N,O-bis (trimethylsilyl)trifluoracetamide-pyridine (1:1, v/v) for 30 min at 60°.
4. The sample in hexane is injected into a gas chromatograph-mass spectrometer [1% OV-1 on Supelcoport, (80-100 mesh), 2 m × 3 mm i.d., 230°, He 25 ml/min, retention time 3 min, molecular separator 250°].
5. The protium/deuterium ratio for the molecular ions at 416 and 420 nm is calculated by computer analysis and compared mathematically to the $^{1}H/^{2}H$ ratio of the original deuterated estradiol standard.

6. With the injection of 10 ng of deuterated estradiol per gas chromatographic-mass spectrometric analysis, the shift in the $^1H/^2H$ ratio resulting from the presence of endogenous estradiol will allow accurate determination of 10 pg.

Procedures for the characterization of steroidal estrogen glucuronides by GC-MS [59]

1. The sodium salts of the glucuronides in aqueous solution are processed through a column of Amberlite CG-120 H-type resin. The methanol eluate is taken to dryness in vacuo.
2. The residue is derivatized to give the n-propyl esters by adding a solution of hydrogen chloride-n-propanol and allowing the reaction mixture to stand at room temperature for 30 min.
3. The reaction mixture is then evaporated to dryness and treated with trimethylsilyl imidazol or trimethylsilyl-d_9 imidazole for 30 min at room temperature.
4. The derivative sample is injected into a 3 m × 2.5 mm glass column with 1% Dexsil 300 g.c. on Gas Chrom Q (80-100 mesh). Column oven temperature is kept at 265° for 20 min and then programmed to 310° at a rate of 1°/min. The carrier gas flow rate (helium) is 30 ml/min. The temperature for the injection port, separator, and ion source is 330°. The accelerating voltage, ionization energy, and the trap current are 3.5 kV, 70 eV, and 60 μA, respectively.
5. Molecular ions from the electron impact analysis will not always be observed, but frequently a $[M - 15]^+$ ion representing the loss of a methyl group is found. The use of the deuterated TMS derivative is helpful in structural elucidation by comparing the mass unit shifts of fragments thought to contain the TMS derivative to similar fragments from unlabeled glucuronides.
6. The aglycone moiety provides considerable interpretation for glucuronide characterization. Those, for instance, with an aliphatic acetal linkage (estriol and 16-epiestriol glucuronides) give fragment ions of m/e 231, 325, 415, and 431. In the case of the 3-glucuronide of estriol, an interesting fragment of the parent compound forms with an m/e of 504. It was found to represent the tri-TMS derivative of estriol which forms during the simultaneous cleavage of the ether linkage between estrogen and glucuronic acid.

Conditions for GC-MS identification of diethylstilbestrol metabolic products [94]

1. Chromatographically purified samples of diethylstilbestrol metabolic products are evaporated under nitrogen to dryness

and derivatized with a 5:1 mixture of bis(trimethysilyl)-acetamide and trimethylchlorosilane. The reaction mixture is heated at 85° for 14 min.
2. A 3 μl aliquot is injected into a gas chromatograph using a 5 ft × 2 mm i.d. glass column packed with 3% OV-225.
3. The injection port and interface oven temperature was 225° and the column oven temperature was programmed at 10°/min for 190 to 235°. The manifold temperature was 60°.
4. The mass spectrometer is operated in the electron impact mode using repetitive scanning. The ionizing voltage is 70 eV and the carrier helium gas flow is 30 μl/min.
5. This system will separate the cis/trans isomers of DES and each will give a molecular ion of m/e 412. The isomers of dienestrol, which are also separable, will each give molecular ions of m/e 410.

D. Radioassays

The utilization of radiolabeled estrogens for the quantitation of endogenous estrogenic hormones has revolutionized the efficiency and sensitivity of their analysis. One of the earliest uses of radiolabeled hormones was to perform the experiment with the tritium-labeled estrogen or its metabolic precursor and then add a known amount of authentic [^{14}C]estrogen product to serve as both a chromatographic marker and an internal standard for losses during purification. The double-isotope derivative assay is another form of radioassay that utilizes two-isotope technology; however, it allows the quantitative estimation of unlabeled estrogen hormone. Here, authentic radio-labeled product is added to the analysis mixture as an internal standard and, following purification, the product is derivatized with a differently labeled reagent of known specific activity. The amount of derivatizing reagent consumed in the derivatization reaction is the quantitating factor. The higher the specific activity of the reagent, the greater the sensitivity of the assay. It is important to point out, however, that these assays are time consuming and tedious.

The most noted and no doubt most widely used radioassay for estrogen quantitative analysis is the radioimmunoassay. The underlying phenomenon of the assay is the chemical specificity of an antibody for an antigen and the quantitation of that reaction by allowing an authentic radiolabeled estrogen to compete with unlabeled hormone for interaction with the antibody. The numerical quantiation results from a standard curve generated from reacting various levels of unlabeled compound with the radiolabeled estrogen and the antibody. The assay's sensitivity is based on the specific activity of the radiolabeled hormone used and its specificity is predicated on the antibody's steric specificity for the antigen. Both of these factors have improved through the years with the advent of mulitlabeled tritiated estrogens with very high specific activity (>100 ci/mmol) and the improvement of antigen synthesis that allows better steric exposure of the estrogen hormone. The resultant problem of high cross reactivity that can occur when the antigen has low steric specificity can be one of the assay's greatest shortcomings. For instance, if an estradiol antibody has a 3% cross reactivity with estrone, this phenomenon can become quite important when an experimental sample has present 100 times more estrone that estradiol. Chromatographic separation prior to the assay is normally used to solve this problem. The occurrence of a high experimental blank is still another problem the radioimmunoassay may give for the investigator. Often, the blank sample can generate a very high value that leaves the scientist in a quandary with regard to its validity and the advisability of subtracting the value from all experimental samples. Normally, however, a high blank value can be reduced by improving either the required bioanalytical technology or quality of the reagents used.

Other radioassays, such as the competitive protein binding assay, have been developed. Usually, the estrogen cellular receptor or testosterone estradiol binding globulin is used as the agent of specificity in assays where the endogenous product to be measured competes against authentic radiolabeled hormone. Because these natural proteins also have considerable cross reactivity, the specificity of the assay can be questionable. Other major problems of the use of this type of assay are the stability of the receptor or blood proteins and the presence of contaminating proteins in the preparation, which can result in high-capacity, nonspecific binding of the estrogen hormone. A standard curve is generated for mathematical quantitation, as in the case of the radioimunoassay.

Radioenzymic assays have been envisioned for quite some time, but in fact their practicability has been limited by the inability to obtain a specific enzyme preparation. An elegant assay for determining the concentration of catechol estrogens through the use of an enzyme preparation of catechol O-methyltransferase and a tritiated methyl donor is one of the first radioenzymic assays for estrogens [111]. No doubt, as the sophistication of enzyme purification continues to develop, such assays will develop greater utility. Since, in fact, estrogen metabolism proceeds primarily by ring oxidation, the controlled and specific incorporation of radiolabeled oxygen could serve as a quantitating method. The problems that radioenzyme assays will face in the future will probably be those of enzyme purity, optimization of the reaction kinetics, presentation of a pure substrate, and subsequent purification of the product.

Procedure for receptor protein assay for estradiol [112]

1. The uteri of immature rabbits are homogenized in a blender at 4° in three volumes of buffer (0.01 M Tris-HCl, pH 8.0, 0.001 M EDTA, 0.25 M sucrose) using four 30 sec pulses at 2 min intervals. Cellular debris is removed by centrifugation at 100 *g* for 15 min and the resulting supernatant is centrifuged at 105,000 *g* for 1 hr to obtain the cytosol. The cytosol is stored in liquid nitrogen.
2. Twenty microliter aliquots of the cytosol are incubated with tritiated 17β-estradiol (10,000 cpm) plus either standards of unlabeled E_2 or the experimental samples. The volume is taken to 0.5 ml with 0.01 MTris buffer, pH 8.0, 1 mM EDTA. The samples are incubated at 4° overnight or at 23° for 1 hr. Standards are run in triplicate and experimental samples are run in duplicate.
3. At the end of the incubation period, a 0.5 ml suspension of 0.01 M Tris, pH 8.0, containing 0.5% activated charcoal (Norit A) and 0.5% Mann D-grade dextran, is added to each incubation sample. After a 15 min incubation in an ice bath, the samples are centrifuged 15 min at 4°.
4. The supernatant is decanted into a scintillation vial and counted. A standard curve is plotted and the concentration of estradiol in the unknown samples is determined from the curve.

Double-isotope derivative procedure for the determination of estrogens in milk [113]

1. To detect estrone, estradiol-17β, or estradiol-17α, the appropriate tritiated estrogen is added as a marker. The aqueous phase is then extracted with diethyl ether and cooled to -20°. The extraction mixture is placed in a -50° bath and the ether layer removed and taken to dryness under nitrogen.
2. The residue is redissolved in ether and treated with 70% methanol to precipitate the lipids with cooling and centrifugation.
3. The supernatant which contains the estrogen is reacted with p-iodophenylsulfonyl-^{35}S chloride (pipsyl chloride) and the carbon-3 pipsylates of the estrogen(s) are formed. A liquid scintillation counter is then used to determine the amount of ^{35}S consumed in the derivatization reaction.
4. This procedure would obviously allow simultaneous determination of a number of estrogens in solution. However, a chromatographic separation of each carbon-3 pipsylate of the desired estrogen to be quantitated would be required.

Table 1 Physical Constants of Estrogen Hormones

	IUPAC Name	Molecular weight	Empirical formula	Melting point	Maximum UV	ε
Dienestrol	4,4'-(1,2-Diethylidene-1,2-ethylene)bisphenol	266.32	$C_{18}H_{18}O_2$	227-228	228	29,100
Diethylstilbestrol	(E)-4,4"-(1,2-Diethyl-1,2-ethylene)bisphenol	268.34	$C_{18}H_{20}O_2$	169-172	236	22,000
Estradiol-17β	Estra-1,3,5(10)-triene-3,17β-diol	272.37	$C_{18}H_{24}O_2$	173-119	280	2,000
Estriol	Estra-1,3,5(10)-triene-3,16α,17β-triol	288.37	$C_{18}H_{24}O_3$	282	280	2,300
Estrone	3-Hydroxyestra-1,3,5(10)-trien-17-one	270.36	$C_{18}H_{22}O_2$	254.5-256	280	2,300
17*a*-Ethynylestradiol	17α-Ethynyl-1,3,5(10)-estratriene-3,17β-diol	296.39	$C_{20}H_{24}O_2$	141-146	281	2,040

Mestranol	17α-Ethynyl-3-methoxy-1,3,5(10)-estratrien-17β-ol	310.42	$C_{21}H_{26}O_2$	150-151	280	2,280
Trenbolone	17β-hydroxyestra-4,9,11-trien-3-one	270.38	$C_{18}H_{22}O_2$	186	239 340.5	5,260 28,000
Zearalanol	3,4,5,6,7,8,9,10,11,12-Decahydro-7,14,16-trihydroxy-3-methyl-1-H-benzoxacylotetradecin-1-one	322.41	$C_{18}H_{26}O_5$	146-148 178-180	218 265 304	
Zearalenone	3,4,5,6,9,10-Hexahydro-14,16-dihydroxy-3-methyl-1H-2-benzoxacyclotetradecin-1,7(8H)-dione	318.36	$C_{18}H_{22}O_5$	164-165	264 274 316	29,700 13,909 6,020

Source: Refs. 115 and 116.

Procedure for the radioenzymatic determination of catechol estrogens in tissue [111]

1. Catechol O-methyltransferase is isolated from rat liver by first homogenizing the liver in 4 volumes (w/v) of isotonic KCl, filtering through cheesecloth, and centrifuging at 14,000 *g* for 30 min. The supernatant is then centrifuged for 60 min at 105,000 *g*, the supernatant removed and filtered through glass wool to remove any particulate material, and the pH adjusted to 5.3 with 1.0 M acetic acid. The resulting suspension is centrifuged at 14,000 *g*, the supernatant adjusted to pH 7.0, and an ammonium sulfate precipitation carried out according to Nikodejevic et al. [114]. The precipitate containing the catechol O-methyltransferase is solubilized in 0.001 M phosphate buffer (pH 7.0) and then dialyzed three times overnight against 0.01 M phosphate (pH 7.0) containing 0.001 M dithiothreitol. The dialysate is centrifuged for 2 hr at 105,000 *g* to remove a yellow-brown precipitate. The supernatant is removed, divided, and used in the subsequent assay.
2. Tissue is homogenized at 0 to 2°C in 25 to 40 volumes of 0.1 N HCl and then extracted with 3 to 4 volumes of diethyl ether by vortexing for 30 sec. The ether supernatant is collected by centrifugation at 10,000 *g* for 10 min and is transferred to a glass-stoppered tube for evaporation under nitrogen. Following evaporation the sample is immediately stored on ice (0 to 2°).
3. The sample is dissolved in 0.15 ml of 0.1 Tris-HCl buffer (pH 7.6), and the enzymatic assay is initiated by the addition of 0.05 ml of the following mixture: (1) 0.025 ml of 0.1 Tris-HCl buffer (pH 7.6), (2) 0.01 ml of 1 M $MgCl_2$, (3) 0.01 ml of catechol O-methyltransferase, (4) 0.005 ml (2.5 mCi) of ^{3}H-S-adenosylmethionine (specific activity ca. 11.2 Ci/mmol). The incubation is carried out at 37° for 60 min and the reaction is terminated by the addition of 0.5 ml of 0.5 M borate buffer, pH 10.0.
4. Blanks for the assay consist of (1) an equal volume of 0.1 N HCl and (2) tissue oxidized with 2 to 4 mg of $NaIO_4$/ml of homogenate (37° for 15 min) to destroy the catechol estrogen present. Each blank is treated identically to the experimental sample. Standards are made up from authentic 2-OH estrone and 2-OH estradiol dissolved in ethanol and then diluted to appropriate volume with 0.1 N HCl.
5. The incubation mixture, following termination of the reaction, is extracted with 6 ml of heptane. An aliquot of the organic phase which contains the methylated catechol estrogens is

counted to determine total radioactivity. Subtraction of the blank value is performed to provide the actual value of total catechol.

6. Individual values for each methylated catechol can be obtained by thin layer chromatographic separation of the heptane extract using silica gel plates and a mobile phase of $CHCl_3$-MeOH-HOAc (95:3:1) or by HPLC (Fig. 4-9). Chromatographic standards are prerequisite to this separation. See Table 1.

ACKNOWLEDGMENT

This investigation was supported in part by Grant 5R01-CA24629-01, awarded by the National Cancer Institute, Department of Health and Human Services.

REFERENCES

1. J. M. Harrington, R. O. Rivera, and L. K. Lowry. Occupational exposure to synthetic estrogens–the need to establish safety standards. Am. Ind. Hyg. Assoc. J. *39*, 139-143 (1978).
2. I. Okuno and W. H. Higgins. Method for determining residues of mestranol and ethynylestradiol in foliage, soil, and water samples. Bull. Environ. Contam. Toxicol. *18*, 428-435 (1977).
3. H. P. Gelbke, P. Ball, and R. Knuppen. 2-Hydroxyoestrogens–chemistry, biogenesis, metabolism and physiological significance. Adv. Steroid Biochem. Pharmacol. *6*, 81-154 (1977).
4. E. Hecker and F. Marks. Zum Stoffwechsel und Wirkungsmechanismus der Oestrogene: VII. Die o-Hydroxylierung von Oestron in Rattenleber und ihre Beziehung zur Proteinbindung sowie zur p-Hydroxylierung und zu Hydroxylierungen in aliphatischen Positionen. Biochem. Z. *343*, 211-226 (1965).
5. E. C. Horning, J.-P. Thenot, and E. D. Helton. Toxic agents resulting from the oxidative metabolism of steroid hormones and drugs. J. Toxicol. Environ. Health *4*, 341-361 (1978).
6. W. Jaggi, W. K. Lutz, and C. Schlatter. Covalent binding of ethinylestradiol and estrone to rat liver DNA in vivo. Chem. Biol. Interact. *23*, 13-18 (1978).
7. P. W. LeQuesne, A. D. Durga, V. Subramayam, A. H. Soloway, R. W. Hart, and R. H. Purdy. Biomimetic synthesis of catechol estrogens: potentially mutagenic arene oxide intermediates in estrogen metabolism. J. Med. Chem. *22*, 239-240 (1980).
8. R. H. Purdy, M. L. Meltz, J. W. Goldzieher, T. J. Goodwin, and M. J. Williams. Chemical transformation by estrogens in mammalian cell culture system. Proceedings of the 62nd Annual Meeting of the Endocrine Society, Washington, D.C., 1980, Abstr. #787, p. 277.

9. I. J. Davies, F. Naftolin, K. J. Ryan, J. Fishman, and J. Siu. The affinity of catechol estrogens for estrogen receptors in the pituitary and anterior hypothalamus of the rat. Endocrinology *97*, 554-557 (1975).
10. C. Martucci and J. Fishman. Direction of estradiol metabolism as a control of its hormonal action–uterotrophic activity of estradiol metabolites. Endocrinology *101*, 1709-1715 (1977).
11. J. Fishman, F. Naftolin, I. J. Davies, K. J. Ryan, and Z. Petro. Catechol estrogen formation by the human fetal brain and pituitary. J. Clin. Endocrinol. Metab. *42*, 177-180 (1976).
12. A. L. Herbst, P. Cole, T. Colton, S. J. Robboy, and R. E. Scully. Age-incidence and risk of diethylstilbestrol-related clear cell adenocarcinoma of the vagina and cervix. Am. J. Obstet. Gynecol. *128*, 43-50 (1977).
13. A. B. Okey and D. W. Nebert. Covalent binding of diethylstilbestrol to DNA catalyzed by hepatic and uterine microsomes. Proc. Am. Assoc. Cancer Res. *20*, 205 (828) (1979).
14. M. Metzler and J. A. McLachlan. Peroxidase-mediated binding of diethylstilbestrol and catechol estrogens to DNA: a potential factor for their carcinogenicity. Cancer Treat. Rep. *63*, 1181 (188) (1979).
15. M. Ishidate, Jr., and S. Odashima. Chromosome tests with 134 compounds on Chinese hamster cells in vitro–a screening for chemical carcinogens. Mutat. Res. *48*, 337-353 (1977).
16. D. Clive, K. O. Johnson, J. F. S. Spector, A. G. Batson, and M. M. M. Brown. Validation and characterization of the L5178Y/$TK^{+/-}$ mouse lymphoma mutagen assay system. Mutat. Res. *59*, 61-108 (1979).
17. H. W. Rüdiger, F. Haenisch, M. Metzler, F. Oesch, and H. R. Glatt. Metabolites of diethylstilbestrol induce sister chromatid exchange in human cultured fibroblasts. Nature (Lond.) *281*, 392-394 (1979).
18. H. M. Bolt. Metabolism of estrogens–natural and synthetic. Pharmacol. Ther. *4*, 155-181 (1979).
19. R. H. Purdy, L. L. Engel, and J. L. Oncley. The characterization of estrone sulfate from human plasma. J. Biol. Chem. *236*, 1043-1050 (1961).
20. M. T. Badel-Aziz and K. I. H. Williams. Metabolism of 17α-ethynylestradiol and its 3-methyl ether by the rabbit: an in vivo D-homoannulation. Steroids *13*, 809-820 (1969).
21. M. C. Williams, E. D. Helton, and J. W. Goldzieher. The urinary metabolites of 17α-ethynylestradiol-9α,11ξ-^{3}H in women. Chromatographic profiling and identification of ethynyl and non-ethynyl compounds. Steroids *25*, 229-246 (1975).
22. E. D. Helton, M. C. Williams, and J. W. Goldzieher. Oxidative metabolism and de-ethynylation of 17α-ethynylestradiol by baboon liver microsomes. Steroids *30*, 71-83 (1977).

23. P. R. Ortiz de Montellano, K. L. Kunze, G. S. Yost, and B. A. Mico. Self-catalyzed destruction of cytochrome P-450: covalent binding of ethynyl sterols to prosthetic heme. Proc. Natl. Acad. Sci. USA *76*, 746-749 (1979).
24. M. Metzler and J. A. McLachlan. Peroxidase-mediated oxidation, a possible pathway for metabolic activation of diethylstilbestrol. Biochem. Biophys. Res. Commun. *85*, 874-884 (1978).
25. M. Metzler, W. Muller, and W. C. Hobson. Biotransformation of diethylstilbestrol in the rhesus monkey and the chimpanzee. J. Toxicol. Environ. Health *3*, 439-450 (1977).
26. J. Weidenfeld, P. Carter, V. N. Reinhold, S. B. Tannier IV, and L. L. Engel. Metabolism of diethylstilbestrol: identification of a catechol derived from dienestrol. Biomed. Mass. Spectrom. *5*, 587-590 (1978).
27. M. Metzler and J. McLachlan. Oxidative metabolites of diethylstilbestrol in the fetal, neonatal and adult mouse. Biochem. Pharmacol. *27*, 1087-1094 (1978).
28. V. W. Winkler, M. A. Nyman, and R. S. Egan. Diethylstilbestrol cis-trans isomerization and estrogen activity of diethylstilbestrol isomers. Steroids *17*, 197-207 (1971).
29. C. J. Mirocha, S. V. Pathre, and C. M. Christensen. Zearalenone, In *Mycotoxins in Human and Animal Health* (J. V. Rodricks, C. W. Hesseltine, and M. A. Mehlman, Eds.). Pathotox Publishers, Park Forest South, Ill., 1977, p. 341.
30. C. J. Mirocha, S. V. Pathre, and C. M. Christensen. Zearalenone. In *Mycotoxins in Human and Animal Health* (J. V. Rodricks, C. W. Hesseltine, and M. A. Mehlman, Eds.). Pathotox Publishers, Park Forest South, Ill. 1977, p. 345.
31. P. N. Rao, R. H. Purdy, M. C. Williams, P. H. Moore, Jr., J. W. Goldzieher, and D. S. Layne. Metabolites of estradiol-17β in bovine liver: identification of the 17β-D-glucopyranoside of estradiol-17α. J. Steroid Biochem. *10*, 179-185 (1979).
32. F. Foggitt and A. E. Kellie. The isolation of urinary 17-oxo steroid and corticosteroid glucuronides. Biochem. J. *91*, 209-217 (1964).
33. S. Kushinsky and J. (Wu) Tang. Conjugated oestrogens: I. Liquid-liquid extraction of conjugated oestrogens in urine by means of liquid anion exchanger. Acta Endocrinol. *43*, 345-360 (1963).
34. H. L. Bradlow. Extraction of steroid conjugates with a neutral resin. Steroids *11*, 265-272 (1968).
35. H. L. Bradlow. Modified technique for the elution of polar steroid conjugates from Amberlite-XAD-2. Steroids *30*, 581-582 (1977).
36. G. E. Mitchell, Jr., A. L. Neumann, and H. H. Draper. Metabolism of tritium labeled diethylstilbestrol by steers. J. Agric. Food Chem. *7*, 509-512 (1959).

37. P. W. Aschbacher and E. J. Thacker. Metabolic fate of oral diethylstilbestrol in steers. J. Anim. Sci. *39*, 1185-1192 (1974).
38. J. S. Elce and P. P.-C. Lai. Water-soluble metabolites of the estrogens. Quantitation of C-18 tetrols in rat feces. Steroids *27*, 335-352 (1976).
39. E. D. Helton, D. A. Casciano, Z. R. Althaus, and H. D. Plant. Metabolism of 17α-ethynylestradiol by intact liver parenchymal cells isolated from mouse and rat. J. Toxicol. Environ. Health *3*, 953-963 (1977).
40. M. C. Bowman and C. R. Nony. Trace analysis of estradiol in animal chow by electron-capture gas chromatography. J. Chromatogr. Sci. *15*, 160-163 (1977).
41. J. R. King, C. R. Nony, and M. C. Bowman. Trace analysis of diethylstilbestrol (DES) in animal chow by parallel high-speed liquid chromatography, electron-capture gas chromatography, and radioassays. J. Chromatogr. Sci. *15*, 14-21 (1977).
42. C. L. Holder, C. R. Nony, and M. C. Bowman. Trace analysis of zearalenone and/or zearalanol in animal chow by high pressure liquid chromatography and gas-liquid chromatography. J. Assoc. Off. Anal. Chem. *60*, 272-278 (1977).
43. R. Hahnel. Use of Sephadex ion exchanger for the separation of conjugated urinary estrogens. Anal. Biochem. *10*, 184-192 (1965).
44. R. Hahnel and M. Ghazali bin Abdul Rahman. Improved gradient elution for the separation of urinary steroid conjugates on DEAE-Sephadex columns. Clin Chim. Acta *13*, 797-799 (1966).
45. R. Hahnel and M. Ghazali bin Abdum Rahman. Separation of urinary oestrogen sulphates from oestrogen glucosiduronates on diethylaminoethyl-Sephadex columns. Biochem. J. *105*, 1047-1053 (1967).
46. R. Hobkirk, P. Musey, and M. Nilsen. Chromatographic separation of estrone and 17β-estradiol conjugates on DEAE-Sephadex. Steroids *14*, 191-206 (1969).
47. R. Hobkirk and M. Nilsen. Separation of monoglucosiduronate conjugates of estrone and 17β-estradiol by DEAE-Sephadex chromatography. Anal. Biochem. *37*, 337-344 (1970).
48. P. I. Musey, D. C. Collins, and J. R. K. Preedy. Isocratic separation of estrogen conjugates on DEAE Sephadex. Steroids *29*, 657-668 (1977).
49. M. J. Tikkanen and H. Adlercreutz. Separation of estriol conjugates on Sephadex. Acta Chem. Scand. *24*, 3755-3757 (1970).
50. M. C. Williams, A. de la Pena, and J. W. Goldzieher. Geographic differences in the pharmacokinetics of ethynyl estrogens. J. Toxicol. Environ. Health *4*, 499 (1978).
51. E. D. Helton, B. J. Gough, J. W. King, Jr., J. P. Theont, and E. C. Horning. Metabolism of diethylstilbestrol in the C3H

mouse: chromatographic systems for the quantitative analysis of DES metabolic products. Steroids *31*, 471-484 (1978).

52. Sj. Van der Wal and J. F. K. Huber. High-pressure liquid chromatography with ion-exchange celluloses and its application to the separation of estrogen glucuronides. J. Chromatogr. *102*, 353-374 (1974).
53. Sj. Van der Wal and J. F. K. Huber. Separation of estrogen glucuronides, sulfates and phosphates on ion-exchange cellulose by high-pressure liquid chromatography. J. Chromatogr. *135*, 305-321 (1977).
54. J. Hermansson. Reversed-phase liquid chromatography of steroid glucuronides. J. Chromatogr. *152*, 437-445 (1978).
55. Sj. Van der Wal and J. F. K. Huber. Comparative study of several phase systems for the separation of estrogen conjugates by high-pressure liquid chromatography. J. Chromatogr. *149*, 431-453 (1978).
56. P. I. Musey, D. C. Collins, and J. R. K. Preedy. Separation of estrogen conjugates by high pressure liquid chromatography. Steroids *31*, 583-592 (1978).
57. B. Fransson, K.-G. Wahlund, I. M. Johansson, and G. Schill. Ion-pair chromatography of acidic drug metabolites and endogenic compounds. J. Chromatogr. *125*, 327-344 (1976).
58. R. M. Thompson. Gas chromatographic and mass spectrometric analysis of permethylated estrogen glucuronides. J. Steroid Biochem. *7*, 845-852 (1976).
59. H. Miyazaki, M. Ishibashi, M. Itoh, N. Morishita, M. Sudo, and T. Nambara. Analysis of estrogen glucuronides: I. Characterization of estrogen glucuronides by gas chromatography mass spectrometry. Biomed. Mass Spectrom. *3*, 55-59 (1976).
60. E. D. Helton, H. E. Hadd, M. C. Williams, P. N. Rao, and J. W. Goldzieher. Synthesis of 17β-D-glucupyranosiduronic acid of 17α-ethynylestradiol. J. Steroid Biochem. *9*, 237-238 (1978).
61. E. Heftmann. *Chromatography of Steroids* (Journal of Chromatography Library, Vol. 8). Elsevier, Amsterdam, 1976, p. 81.
62. J. M. Wal, J. C. Peleran, and G. Bories. Mise au point du dosage simultané de l'éthynyl-oestradiol et de l'acétate de Trenbolone dans les aliments composés au moyen du couplage chromatographie sur couche mince–chromatographie en phase gazeuse. J. Chromatogr. *136*, 165-169 (1977).
63. K. Vogt. Thin-layer chromatographic-fluorometric determination of trenbolone and 17α-estradiol in urine of fattening male calves after subcutaneous injection of Revalor, Trenbolone acetate or 17β-estradiol. Chem. Abstr. *88*, 85561y (1978).
64. H. Jarc, O. Ruttner, and W. Krocza. Der quantitative Nachweis von Oestrogenen und thyreostatika mittels Dunnschichtchromatographie und Hochleistungsdunnschicht-chromatographie in tierischen Substraten. J. Chromatogr. *134*, 351-358 (1977).

65. H. P. Gelbke and R. Knuppen. A new method for preventing oxidative decomposition of catechol estrogens during chromatography. J. Chromatogr. *71*, 465-471 (1972).
66. C. E. Morreal and T. L. Dao. Protection of estrogenic hormones by ascorbin acid during chromatography. Steroids *25*, 421-426 (1975).
67. H. P. Gelbke and G. Stubenrauch. The detection of A-ring-hydroxylated estrogens and their methyl ethers on ascorbic acid-impregnated paper and thin-layer chromatograms. J. Chromatogr. *120*, 239-242 (1976).
68. B. P. Lisboa and M. Strassner. Gel chromatography of steroid oestrogens on Sephadex LH-20. J. Chromatogr. *111*, 159-164 (1975).
69. M. Axelson and J. Sjovall. Analysis of unconjugated steroids in plasma by liquid-gel chromatography and glass capillary gas chromatography-mass spectrometry. J. Steroid Biochem. *8*, 683-692 (1977).
70. B. D. Kulkarni and J. W. Goldzieher. Isolation of 17α-ethynyl steroids by column chromatography on silver impregnated florisil. Steroids *13*, 467-475 (1969).
71. E. D. Pellizzari, J. Liu, M. E. Twine, and C. E. Cook. A novel silver-sulfoethyl cellulose column for purification of ethynyl steroids from biological fluids. Anal. Biochem. *56*, 178-190 (1973).
72. M. T. A. Aziz and K. I. H. Williams. Decomposition of 17α-ethynylestradiol and its ethers on silver nitrate impregnated silica gel thin layer plates. Steroids *12*, 167-170 (1968).
73. A. Ercoli, R. Vitali, and R. Gardi. Adsorbents for detection, isolation and evaluation of ethynyl steroids. Steroids *3*, 479-485 (1964).
74. S. Siggia and R. A. Dishman. Analysis of steroid hormones using high resolution liquid chromatography. Anal. Chem. *42*, 1223-1229 (1970).
75. J. F. K. Huber, J. A. R. J. Hulsman, and C. A. M. Meijers. Wuantitative analysis of trace amounts of estrogenic steroids in pregnancy urine by column liquid-liquid chromatography with ultraviolet detection. J. Chromatogr. *62*, 79-91 (1971).
76. R. J. Dolphin. The analysis of estrogenic steroids in urine by high-speed liquid chromatography. J. Chromatogr. *83*, 421-430 (1973).
77. R. J. Dolphin and P. J. Pergande. Improved method for the analysis of estrogenic steroids in pregnancy urine by high-performance liquid chromatography. J. Chromatogr. *143*, 267-274 (1977).
78. G. J. Schmidt, F. L. Vandemark, and W. Slavin. Estrogen determination using liquid chromatography with pre-column fluorescent labelling. Pittsburgh Conference on Analytical Chemistry and Applied Spectroscopy, Cleveland, Ohio, 1978, Paper no. 240 (Chromatogr. Rep. No. 17).

79. V. Fantl, C. K. Lim, and C. H. Gray. Separation of oestrogens and determination of oestriol in human pregnancy urine. In *High Pressure Liquid Chromatography in Clinical Chemistry* (P. F. Dixon, C. H. Gray, C. K. Lim, and M. S. Stoll, Eds.). Academic Press, New York, 1976, pp. 51-57.
80. P. G. Satyaswaroop, E. Lopez de la Osa, and E. Gurpide. High pressure liquid chromatographic separation of C_{18} and C_{19} steroids. Steroids, *30*, 139-145 (1977).
81. K. Shimada, T. Tanaka, and T. Nambara. CL. Separation of catechol estrogens by high-performance liquid chromatography with electrochemical detection. J. Chromatogr. *178*, 350-354 (1979).
82. G. Cavina, G. Moretti, A. Mollica, and R. Antonini. Analysis of steroid mixtures by column chromatography with continuous monitoring of the eluate by a flame ionization detector. J. Chromatogr. *60*, 179-184 (1971).
83. M. C. Williams and J. W. Goldzieher. High-pressure liquid chromatography profiling of the urinary metabolites of 17-ethynylestradiol and mestranol. J. Toxicol. Environ. Health *4*, 498-499 (1978).
84. M. C. Williams and J. W. Goldzieher. Metabolism of the ethynyl estrogens. Preparative HPLC profiling of radiolabeled urinary estrogens. In *Biological/Biomedical Applications of Liquid Chromatography II* (G. L. Hawk, ed.) (Chromatographic Science Series, Vol. 12). Marcel Dekker, New York, 1979, p. 395.
85. A. G. Butterfield, B. A. Lodge, and N. J. Pound. High-speed liquid chromatographic separation of equine estrogens. J. Chromatogr. Sci. *11*, 401-405 (1973).
86. R. W. Roos. Determination of conjugated and esterified estrogens in pharmaceutical tablet dosage forms by high-pressure, normal-phase partition chromatography. J. Chromatogr. Sci. *14*, 505-512 (1976).
87. R. W. Roos. Identification and determination of synthetic estrogens in pharmaceuticals by high-speed, reversed-phase partition chromatography. J. Pharm. Sci. *63*, 594-599 (1974).
88. C. Hesse, K. Pietrzik, and D. Hoetzel. Identification and quantitative determination of diethylstilbestrol and dienestrol by high-speed liquid chromatography. Chem. Abstr. *87*, 18342u (1977).
89. D. Maysinger, C. S. Marcus, W. Wolf, M. Tarle, and J. Casanova. Preparation and high-performance liquid chromatography of iodinated diethylstilbestrols and some related steroids. J. Chromatogr. *130*, 129-138 (1977).
90. A. R. Lea, W. J. Kayaba, and D. M. Hailey. Analysis of diethylstilbestrol and its impurities in tablets using reversed-phase high-performance liquid chromatography. J. Chromatogr. *177*, 61-68 (1979).

91. D. R. Reeve and A. Crozier. Radioactivity monitor for high-performance liquid chromatography. J. Chromatogr. *137*, 271-282 (1977).
92. V. K.-O. Vollmer, A. v. Hodenberg, A. Poisson, R. Bode, and E. Schauerte. Metabolismus und Pharmakokinetik von Piprozolin bei Ratte, Hund und Mensch: I. Mittleilung: Untersuchungen mit radioaktiv markierter Substanz. Arzneim. Forsch. *27*, 502-508 (1977).
93. A. V. Hdenberg, W. Klemisch, and K.-O. Vollmer. Metabolismus und Pharmakokinetik von Piprozolin bei Ratte, Hund und Mensch: II. Mitteilung: Erstellung von Metabolitenprofilen mit Hilfe der Kopplung HPLC-Radioaktivitatsdetektor nach direkter Injektion von Urin und Galle auf eine Reversed-Phase-Saule. Arzneim. Forsh. *27*, 508-511 (1977).
94. E. D. Helton, D. E. Hill, G. W. Lipe, T. J. Sziszak, and J. W. King, Jr. The metabolism of diethylstilbestrol in the rhesus monkey and chimpanzee. J. Environ. Pathol. Toxicol. *2*, 521-537 (1978).
95. H.-G. Neumann and J. Schenk. Radio gas chromatography of drug metabolites in tissue extract. Xenobiotica *3*, 435-450 (1973).
96. H. Adlercreutz. Determination of several estrogens in various biological fluids by gas-liquid chromatography. In *Methods of Hormone Analysis* (H. Breuer, D. Hamel, and H. L. Kruskemper, Eds.). Georg Thieme Verlag, Stuttgart, 1976, pp. 480-499.
97. E. Heftmann. *Chromatography of Steroids* (Journal of Chromatography Library, Vol. 8). Elsevier, Amsterdam, 1976, p. 83.
98. M. Axelson. Deactivation of gas chromatographic systems for quantitative analysis of MO-TMS derivatives of steroids at the picogram level. J. Steroid Biochem. *8*, 693-698 (1977).
99. J. P. Fels, L. Dehennin, and R. Scholler. Determination of estrogens by gas-liquid chromatography with an open tubular column, J. Steroid Biochem. *6*, 1201-1203 (1975).
100. J. J. Ryan and W. F. Miles. Derivatives of diethylstilbestrol (DES), mass spectral properties and their use in biological analysis. Int. J. Environ. Anal. Chem. *5*, 133-141 (1978).
101. J. F. Lawrence, J. J. Ryan, and R. Leduc. Comparison of electron capture and electrolytic conductivity for the gas chromatographic detection of some perchloro derivatives of diethylstilbestrol. J. Chromatogr. *147*, 398-400 (1978).
102. J. M. Goodyear and N. R. Jenkinson. Irradiation fluorometric method for estimation of diethylstilbestrol in beef liver tissue. Anal. Chem. *33*, 853-856 (1961).
103. K.-L. Oehrle, K. Vogt, and B. Hoffmann. Determination of trenbolone and trenbolone acetate by thin-layer chromatography

in combination with a fluorescence colour reaction. J. Chromatogr. *114*, 244-246 (1975).

104. L. L. Engel, P. J. Marshall, J. C. Orr, V. N. Reinhold, and P. Carter. The mass spectra of diethylstilbestrol and related compounds. Biomed. Mass Spectrom. 5, 582-586 (1978).

105. J. Zamecnik, D. T. Armstrong, and K. Green. Serum estradiol-17β as determined by mass fragmentography and by radioimmunoassay. Clin. Chem. *24*, 627 630 (1978).

106. H. Adlercreutz, M. J. Tikkanen, and D. H. Hunneman. Mass fragmentographic determination of eleven estrogens in the body fluids of pregnant and nonpregnant subjects. J. Steroid Biochem. 5, 211-217 (1974).

107. H. Adlercreutz, F. Martin, O. Wahlroos, and E. Soini. Mass spectrometric and mass fragmentographic determination of natural and synthetic steroids in biological fluids. J. Steroid Biochem. *6*, 247-259 (1975).

108. D. S. Millington. Determination of hormonal steroid concentrations in biological extracts by high resolution mass fragmentography. J. Steroid Biochem. *6*, 239-245 (1975).

109. H. Breuer and L. Siekmann. Mass fragmentography as reference method in clinical steroid assay. J. Steroid Biochem. *6*, 685-688 (1975).

110. H. O. Hoppen and L. Siekmann. Gas chromatography–mass spectrometry of catechol estrogens. Steroids *23*, 17-34 (1974).

111. S. M. Paul and J. Axelrod. A rapid and sensitive radioenzymatic assay for catechol estrogens in tissues. Life Sci. *21*, 493-502 (1977).

112. S. Korenman. Use of receptor proteins for steroid-hormone assays. Methods Enzymol. *36*, 49-58 (1975).

113. M. Mondain-Monval-Gerondeau, M. Castanier, and R. Scholler. Determination of estrogens in cow milk. C. R. Acad. Sci., Ser. D. *271*, 2381-2384 (1970).

114. B. Nikodejevic, S. Senoh, J. W. Daly, and C. R. Creveling. Catechol-O-methyltransferase: II. A new class of inhibitors of catechol-O-methyltransferase; 3,5-dihydroxy-4-methoxybenzoic acid and related compounds. J. Pharmacol. Exp. Ther. *174*, 83-93 (1970).

115. *The Merck Index*, 9th ed. Merck & Co., Rahway, N.J. 1976.

116. J. P. Dusza, M. Heller, and S. Bernstein. Ultraviolet absorption. In *Physical Properties of the Steroid Hormones* (L. L. Engel, Ed.). MacMillan, New York, 1963, pp. 69-287.

5
Mycotoxins

ALBERT E. POHLAND and CHARLES W. THORPE Bureau of Foods, U.S. Food and Drug Administration, Washington, D.C.

I. INTRODUCTION

A. Historical Background

A fascinating, challenging area of scientific research has been the study of fungal metabolism. Of particular interest are the secondary metabolites produced by the fungi, that is, those metabolites serving no known physiological function. Many of these secondary metabolites have been isolated and identified, and many have been found to be toxic to other living organisms. The *toxic* secondary fungal metabolites have been termed "mycotoxins" from the Greek word "mykes", meaning fungus, and the Latin word "toxicum", meaning poison; diseases caused by exposure to mycotoxins are termed "mycotoxicoses." This review concentrates on mycotoxins that may pose a hazard to human health from their presence, known or suspect, in foods and feeds, and for which analytical methods have been developed. Particular attention is paid to the following mycotoxins: aflatoxins, ochratoxin, patulin, penicillic acid, roquefortine, sterigmatocystin, T-2 toxin, and diacetoxyscirpenol (structures are shown in Fig. 1). Zearalenone could well be included in this list; however, it is discussed in Chapter 4.

The problem of mycotoxicoses of humans and animals has been with us throughout recorded history. On the one hand, it represents a sad tale of ignorance, disease, death, and economic loss; on the other hand, it presents an exciting story of research, discovery, development of new drugs (e.g., penicillin), and the development of

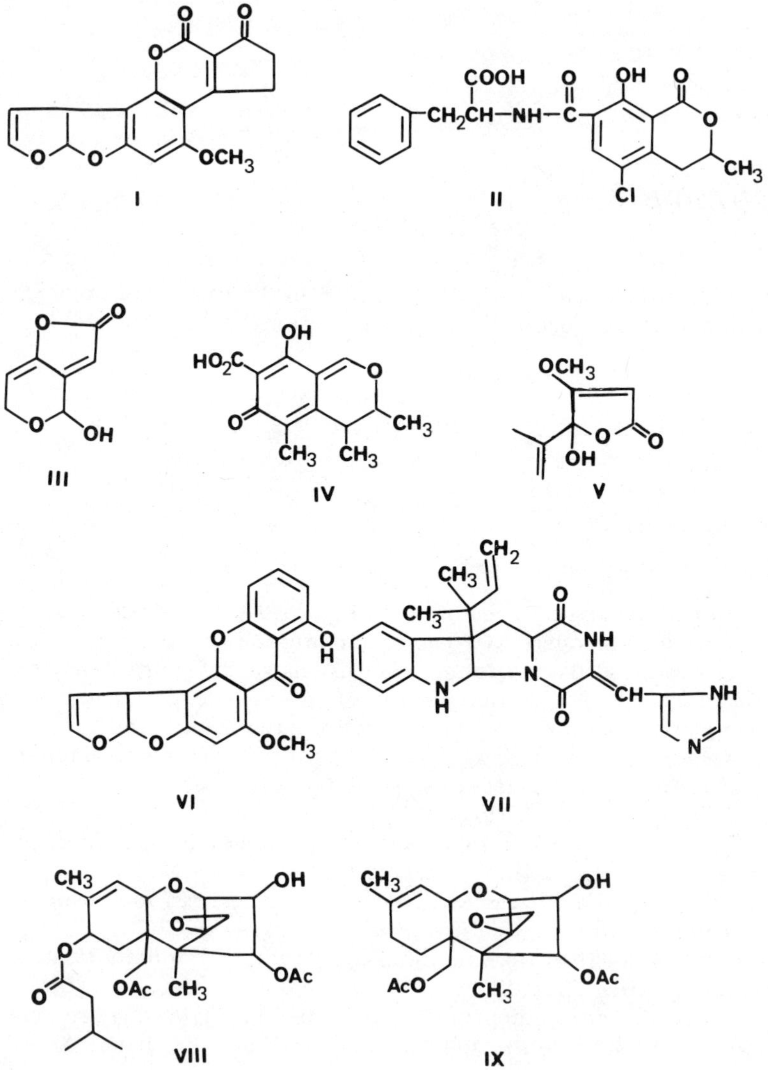

Figure 1 Structures of some common mycotoxins: (I) aflatoxin B_1, (II) ochratoxin A, (III) patulin, (IV) citrinin, (V) penicillic acid, (VI) sterigmatocystin, (VII) roquefortine, (VIII) T-2 toxin, (IX) diacetoxyscirpenol.

ways to control unwanted exposure through education, industry/ government regulation, and detoxification.

A summary of known or suspect human mycotoxicoses is found in Table 1 [1]. The earliest well-documented mycotoxicosis, ergotism, was caused by the ingestion of the sclerotium of *Claviceps purpurea*, a fungus that parasitizes principally rye and barley. The growing fungus produces, as secondary metabolites, lysergic acid and a wide variety of derivatives of lysergic acid (including LSD); these metabolites are responsible for the mycotoxicoses, the principal symptoms of which are gangrene resulting from constriction of the blood vessels, and a wide variety of effects on the central nervous system, including painful convulsions, epileptic fits, and hallucinations. In the Middle Ages the disease was known as "Saint Anthony's Fire," presumably because those afflicted might be cured by going to the church of Saint Anthony, where they apparently received bread prepared from uncontaminated rye or wheat and so recovered. In France in 994 an epidemic of ergotism resulted in the deaths of about 40,000 people. With the shift from rye to wheat in Europe in the 1700-1800s, ergotism was encountered less frequently. Today, because of processing technology, the sclerotia are largely removed before conversion into flour, and the disease is rarely encountered. Furthermore, today some of the ergot "mycotoxins" are offered as useful drugs.

Table 1 Occurrence of Human Mycotoxicoses

Mycotoxicoses	Years	Fungus (Mycotoxin)	Syndrome
Ergotism	994	*Claviceps purpurea* (lysergic acid der.)	Gangrene, CNS effects
Cardiac beriberi	1890	*P. citreoviride* (?) (citreoviridin?)	CNS effects
Alimentary toxic aleukia	1913 1945	*F. sporotrichioides* (a trichothecene)	Hemorrhage, leukopenia
Stachybotryotoxicosis	1930	*S. atra* (a trichothecene)	Dermatitis, hemorrhage
Balkan endemic nephropathy	1952	*A. ochraceus?* (ochratoxin?)	Nephritis
Aflatoxicosis	1963	*A. flavus* (aflatoxin)	Hepatitis

Other cases of human mycotoxicosis are less readily documented. The epidemiological evidence (cause-and-effect relationships are not firmly established) is strong that each of the human toxicoses listed in Table 1 was due to exposure to mycotoxins. Unfortunately, research is hindered either because the mycotoxicosis is no longer prevalent, or because food samples and/or tissue samples are no longer available for analysis. A brief review follows.

In rural Japan in the last half of the nineteenth century an acute heart disease, termed "cardiac beriberi," was prevalent and was said to be associated with consumption of polished rice, which, apparently, was frequently moldy. As better control was exerted and the quality of the rice improved, the disease became less common and finally disappeared. Many years later it was proposed that the principal mold present was probably *Penicillium citreo-viride*, which was found to produce an extremely potent mycotoxin, citreoviridin; this toxin was later shown to cause neurotoxic effects in experimental animals similar to those observed earlier in cases of cardiac beriberi in humans.

In Russia and Eastern Europe during World Wars I and II, a severe outbreak of a disease affecting the hematopoietic system occurred. Many thousands of people were affected, and the mortality rate approached 60%. The symptoms included extreme leukopenia, severe hemorrhage, and exhaustion of the bone marrow; the disease was therefore called alimentary toxic aleukia (ATA). A large number of studies related to the disease have led to the conclusion that the toxicosis resulted from ingestion of bread and other foods containing flour milled from overwintered grains that had become moldy; the molds implicated were of the *Fusarium* genus. We now know that many of the *Fusarium* species produce a group of toxic metabolites known as trichothecenes; based on current knowledge of the toxic effects of these compounds, it has been proposed that the trichothecenes, in particular T-2 toxin, were causative agents in ATA. In fact, a number of retained mold isolates from the last Russian incident [2] have demonstrated the ability to produce T-2 toxin.

Stachybotryotoxicosis, although not a severe human problem, has been observed particularly among farmers handling hay and straw, and is apparently due to toxins produced by *Stachybotrys atra*, a saprophyte frequently found on cellulose-rich substrates. The mycotoxicosis is characterized by a severe dermatitis, hemorrhage, and rhinitis, symptoms not unlike those observed with ATA. It is now believed that the mycotoxins involved are trichothecenes.

In the early 1950s a disease known as Balkan endemic nephropathy became evident in rural areas of Bulgaria, Rumania, and Yugoslavia [3]. Mortality rates of up to 40% were common in certain areas of Bulgaria. The major symptoms were severe nephropathy, often accompanied by urinary tract tumors. In 1974, Krogh [4] proposed that ochratoxin might be the causal agent, based upon the similarity of symptoms to renal changes observed in pigs exposed to ochratoxin A.

Recent surveys of foods in Yugoslavia show a much higher contamination frequency and level of ochratoxin in cereals produced in endemic areas than those grown in nonendemic areas [5]. Further studies are needed to establish a cause-and-effect relationship.

With the discovery of aflatoxin in the early 1960s the study of human mycotoxicoses underwent a complete metamorphosis. Up to this point, the acute effects of mycotoxins were responsible for the observed mycotoxicoses. To be sure, there have been 16 cases in which aflatoxin involvement was claimed, postulated, or suspected, the most severe of which occurred in 1974 in India [6, 7]. In this disaster about 25% of the exposed population (320 people) died of eating aflatoxin-contaminated corn (estimated level of contamination, about 15 ppm). However, contamination levels of such magnitude are not frequently encountered. In 1962 aflatoxin was shown to be a potent hepatocarcinogen; in every species of animal studied it was observed to be carcinogenic. This development quickly led to extensive studies of the possible relationship between aflatoxin exposure and human liver cancer, the development of sensitive analytical methods for detecting aflatoxin, and the survey of foods and feeds for the presence of aflatoxins. The result of this intensive activity is that in some minds the aflatoxins "are now considered to have acquired the doubtful distinction of being human carcinogens" [8]. However, it must be recognized that, for many reasons, even with the great deal of effort already expended, only a debatable association and not a direct cause-and-effect relationship has been established [9].

With the advent of the aflatoxins and the realization that mycotoxins may also exhibit subacute toxicity (i.e., mutagenic, teratogenic, carcinogenic), the study of mycotoxicoses took on a new perspective. We now know that many of the mold metabolites show carcinogenic activity. It is consequently important that sensitive analytical methods be developed to measure human exposure to such compounds at very low levels so that health risks associated with such exposure can be estimated.

It is also appropriate at this point to emphasize that there are many ideopathic diseases which may involve a mycotoxicosis: "farmer's lung," "mushroom worker's lung," "coffee worker's lung," "bird breeder's lung," to name a few. It is also important to realize that mycotoxicoses are undoubtedly much more common in livestock than in humans [10]. A great deal of effort and research has been expended to evaluate the effects of mycotoxins on food-producing animals. Certainly, the economic losses are immense; some of the more common animal mycotoxicoses are listed in Table 2. To obtain a better understanding of the factors leading to such mycotoxicoses and to learn how to control the problem, we need better analytical methods for detecting the mycotoxins in animal feeds and in the meat, milk, and eggs produced from animals exposed to mycotoxins.

Table 2 Occurrence of Animal Mycotoxicoses

Mycotoxicosis	Mycotoxin	Species affected	Symptom
Aflatoxicosis	Aflatoxin	All	Liver tumors, death
Dendrodochiotoxicosis	Trichothecenes	Horses	Dermatitis
Diplodiasis	Diplodiatoxin	Cattle	Ataxia, paralysis
Facial eczema	Sporidesmins	Sheep, cattle	Photosensitivity
Fescue foot	Butenolide	Cattle	Gangrene
Ochratoxicosis	Ochratoxin	Cattle, pigs	Nephritis
Rubratoxicosis	Rubratoxin	Cattle, pigs	
Slobber factor	Slaframine	Cattle, sheep	Excessive salivation
Stachybotryotoxicosis	Trichothecenes	Cattle, horses	Hemorrhage
Fusariotoxicosis	Zearalenone	Pigs	Vulvovaginitis

B. Occurrence of Mycotoxins in Foods and Feeds

With the advent of aflatoxin and the realization that mold growth on foods could lead to contamination of the food by mycotoxins, some of which exhibited carcinogenic activity, a great deal of effort was applied to the development of sensitive analytical methods for the detection of the mycotoxins in foods and feeds. These methods have been extensively utilized in recent years to survey foods and feeds for mycotoxins. These studies are important to the estimation of exposure (incidence and level) and calculation of risk. Several excellent reviews have been published relating some of these studies [11-13].

In summary, these studies indicate a measurable occurrence of the following mycotoxins in foods (Table 3): aflatoxin, citrinin, ochratoxin, patulin, penicillic acid, roquefortine. There has been some concern about sterigmatocystin because of its high carcinogenicity and structural similarity to aflatoxin B_1; however, extensive surveys have not revealed a significant contamination problem (although it was found in some badly molded samples of wheat and green coffee and in the moldy rind of aged cheese).

Table 3 Occurrence of Mycotoxins in Foods

Mycotoxin	Susceptible foods	Levels observed (range ng/g)
Aflatoxin	Peanuts	1-100
	Tree nuts	2-172
	Corn (grits)	1-15,000
	Copra meal	1-200
	Other grains	
	Rice, figs, lentils	
	Soybeans	1-10
	Sorghum	13-50
	Meat, milk, eggs	
Ochratoxin [11]	Corn	15-200
	Wheat	15-115
	Barley	10-189
	Coffee beans	20-360
Patulin	Apple juice	1-1,000
	Apple cider	20,000-45,000
Penicillic acid	Beans	11-179
	Cheese	
Roquefortine	Blue cheese	68,000
Sterigmatocystin	Cheese (intentionally molded)	5-600

Source: Refs. 11-13.

Animal feeds are generally compounded from lower-quality ingredients than human foods and are often stored in such a manner as to become moldy. Such feeds have frequently been implicated in animal mycotoxicoses. Table 4 summarizes some of the available information on the occurrence of mycotoxins in feeds. The presence of mycotoxins in feeds used for food-producing animals is of public health concern because of the possible transmission of the toxin or toxic metabolites into the meat, milk, or eggs [14].

The occurrence data found in Tables 3 and 4 must be considered only as an indication of what might be expected in terms of mycotoxin contamination of foods and feeds. Contamination is highly dependent on environmental conditions that lead to mold growth and toxin production. Data on incidence and level are, of course, limited by many factors, including the accuracy and sensitivity of the analytical method,

Table 4 Occurrence of Mycotoxins in Feeds

Mycotoxin	Susceptible commodities	Levels observed (range ng/g)
Aflatoxin	Cottonseed, cottonseed meal	1-100
	Corn	1-15,000
	Peanut meal	
	Copra meal	
Citrinin	Feeds	700-80,000
	Barley	160-2,000
	Corn, rice, wheat	
Ochratoxin	Wheat, oats, rye, barley	16-27,500
	Corn	45-5,125
Penicillic acid	Corn	5-230
Trichothecenes		
T-2	Mixed feed	76-300
DAS	Mixed feed	380-500
DON	Corn	100-1,800
	Mixed feed	40-1,000
Zearalenone	Barley, sorghum	10
	Corn	10-6,400
	Mixed feed	210-3,600
	Sesame meal	1,500

the sampling procedures, the capabilities of the analyst, and most important, the resources available to conduct the necessarily extensive surveys.

C. Toxicology

Several excellent reviews of the toxicological properties of the various known mycotoxins have been published [15-18]. It is not the intent of the authors to evaluate this information critically, but rather to discuss briefly the toxicological properties of those major mycotoxins (from the standpoint of possible effects on human health) singled out in the introduction for discussion, and to identify the toxicological properties of other mycotoxins that might reasonably be anticipated as contaminants of foods and feeds. A summary of the principal toxicological properties of these mycotoxins is found in Table 5.

Table 5 Toxicological Properties of Mycotoxins

Name	LD_{50} (mg/kg) oral/mouse	Subacute toxicity[a]	Principal effect	Susceptible commodities
Aflatoxin B_1	9	A, B, C	Hepatocarcinogen	See Tables 3 and 4
Brevianamide A				Corn, grains
Citreoviridin	29		Neurotoxin	Rice
Citrinin	50	B	Nephrotoxin	See Table 4
Cyclochlorotine	6.5		Hepatotoxin	Rice, grains
Cyclopiazonic acid	36		Neurotoxin	Grains
Diacetoxyscirpenol				
Ergot alkaloids	7.3		Neurotoxin	Grains
Luteoskyrin	220	A, B(?)	Hepatotoxin	Rice, grains
Ochratoxin A	20 (rat)	A(?), C	Nephrotoxin	See Tables 3 and 4
Patulin	25	A(?), B, C		See Table 3
Penicillic acid	530	A(?), B, C		See Tables 3 and 4
Penitrem A	10	C	Neurotoxin	Corn, grains
PR toxin	760		Neurotoxin	Cheese, grains, rice
Roquefortine	15-20 (i.p.)		Neurotoxin	See Table 3
Rubratoxin B	400	C	Nephrotoxin	Corn, grains
Rugulosin	83 (i.p.)	A, B	Hepatotoxin	Grains, rice
Sterigmatocystin	800	A, B	Hepatotoxin	Grains, coffee
T-2 toxin	7	A(?), C	Dermal toxin	See Table 4
Vomitoxin (deoxynivalenol)	70 (i.p.)		Dermal toxin	See Table 4
Zearalenone	>10 g/kg	B	Estrogen	See Table 4

[a] A, carcinogenic; B, mutagenic; C, teratogenic.

Aflatoxin

A number of excellent reviews have described the acute and chronic effects of the aflatoxins [19-21]; for an in-depth analysis of the toxicological properties of the aflatoxins, these authoritative reviews should be consulted.

Because of the fact that feeds are controlled for quality less rigorously than foods, and consequently are more likely to be contaminated with aflatoxin, animals are exposed to higher levels of aflatoxins more frequently than are humans. The result has been the occasional occurrence of acute aflatoxicosis in animals, and a probable huge economic loss, accrued as a result of reduced weight gain and egg and milk production due to subacute exposure of farm animals to aflatoxin through the feed. It has been observed in experimental animals that chronic exposure to aflatoxin results initially in loss of appetite, loss of weight, and general unthriftiness accompanied by generalized jaundice and cirrhosis of the liver. Acute aflatoxicosis results in widespread hemorrhage, fatty accumulation in the liver, and death. The severity of the acute effect is species dependent, with rabbits, ducklings, pigs, trout, and rats being moderately susceptible, whereas mice, hamsters, and chicks are relatively resistant. As was indicated previously, humans have also succumbed to the acute effects of aflatoxins [6, 7]. In all these studies aflatoxin B_1 was found to be the most acutely toxic.

Of course, it is its hepatocarcinogenicity that has been primarily responsible for the intense research activity revolving around aflatoxin over the past 20 years. The Shasta strain of trout and Fisher strain of rat appear to be the most sensitive species tested; as little as 1 μg/kg aflatoxin B_1 in the diet results in the development of liver carcinoma, making aflatoxin B_1 one of the most potent hepatocarcinogens known (in these species).

Direct experimentation on the effects of aflatoxin in humans obviously is not possible; however, a great deal of circumstantial and epidemiological evidence has been developed which tends to incriminate the aflatoxins in human carcinogenesis [8, 9]. This evidence may be summarized as follows:

1. In every animal species studied, including the nonhuman primate, the aflatoxins produce liver cancer in a dose-related manner.
2. Low-level, extensive exposure through foods has been documented, with peanuts and corn being the major commodities contaminated.
3. Epidemiological studies indicate a significant correlation between levels of aflatoxin in foods, levels ingested, and liver cancer in certain areas of the world.

4. The aflatoxins are heat stable and survive normal food preparation.
5. There is no contrary evidence.

It has been pointed out that, based on current knowledge of incidence and levels of aflatoxin in foods and LD_{50} values for nonhuman primates, it is unlikely that an adult would receive a high enough dose in a short enough period of time to cause death; however, infants and children might be at risk [9]. This line of reasoning has led to tho postulation that aflatoxin might be involved in some way in other human disease syndromes, including Indian infantile cirrhosis, Reye's syndrome, and labrea hepatitis; in each of these cases the syndrome is characterized in part by a similar liver pathology (acute encephalopathy and fatty degeneration of the liver). More recently it has been proposed, at least in the case of Reye's syndrome, that initial viral infection coupled with exposure to aflatoxin was the cause [22, 23]. A great deal of effort is currently being applied to the study of these diseases of unknown etiology.

Citrinin

In an extensive study of the metabolites produced by molds, Raistrick and his coworkers in 1931 isolated and identified citrinin from cultures of *P. citrinum* [24]. Ten years later it was shown to possess strong antibiotic activity against gram-positive bacteria [25]; however, its toxic properties prevented its use for therapeutic purposes. In particular, citrinin was found to be a potent nephrotoxin in experimental animals (rats, dogs, poultry, guinea pigs, etc.; in rabbits it was found to be hepatotoxic) [26].

The widespread occurrence of a severe renal disorder in pigs (porcine nephropathy) in Denmark, which was associated with ingestion of moldy feed, led to the finding that citrinin was present in such feeds, usually in conjunction with another nephrotoxin, ochratoxin A; the contaminating mold was predominantly *P. viridicatum* [27]. In humans, a fatal type of human nephritis, called Balkan endemic nephropathy, is observed extensively in certain areas of the Balkan countries, in which the renal pathology is similar to that of ochratoxin-induced porcine nephropathy. In 1974, Krogh [4] suggested that the two diseases have a common etiology, and that a possible cause may be exposure to ochratoxin A, with citrinin exerting a strong synergistic effect [28]. Citrinin shows synergistic activity toward both ochratoxin A and penicillic acid [15].

Although citrinin has been found to be mutagenic (*B. subtilis*) and embryotoxic, it has not been identified to date as having carcinogenic activity [29]; however, Roberts and Mora have reported [30] the presence of anaplastic areas in the pancreas and kidneys of chickens fed citrinin, and suggested that their findings may indicate that, at least in the chicken, citrinin may be a carcinogen. Because of the association of citrinin-producing mold species with many moldy feed toxicoses, the investigation of citrinin as the causative agent must be encouraged.

Ochratoxin [31]

Ochratoxin A is known to be produced by at least 14 *Penicillium* and *Aspergillus* species; it is sometimes accompanied by small amounts of the corresponding dechloro derivative, ochratoxin B. It is a dihydroisocoumarin containing, in the 7-position, a carboxylic acid function which is linked to L-β-phenylalanine. The amide function is relatively easily hydrolyzed to yield the nontoxic ochratoxin α (this readily occurs in the gut or rumen). Several excellent reviews of the toxicological properties of the ochratoxins have been published (31, 32).

Ochratoxin A has been shown to be a potent nephrotoxin in all species of animals in which it has been studied to date, including birds, fish, and mammals. It has been observed frequently in feeds contaminated by *P. viridicatum*. These feeds have been associated with several incidences of spontaneous ochratoxicoses (chickens, turkeys, swine). The most severe of these in terms of numbers of animals involved and economic loss was in Denmark, where ochratoxin A was observed as the major disease determinant of porcine nephropathy. Residues of ochratoxin A were also found in the tissues of nephrotic animals, and in those animals affected, the highest levels of ochratoxin A were found in the kidneys. Analysis of kidneys for ochratoxin A is the basis for the current control program in Denmark to prevent the occurrence of ochratoxin A residues in Danish hams.

Human renal disease is not uncommon; many cases are encountered with unknown etiology. Krogh's suggestion that ochratoxin A might be a disease determinant in BEN, mentioned above, was later supported by the finding, in limited surveys, that the incidence and levels of ochratoxin A in foods were higher in the endemic areas. These observations must be confirmed and expanded before a causal relationship can be definitely established.

Concern over the presence of ochratoxin A in foods and feeds arises for several additional reasons:

1. It has been found to be teratogenic in mice, rats, hamsters, and the chicken embryo.
2. It has been found that a high incidence of urinary tract tumors occurs in areas of high incidence of BEN.
3. Kanisawa et al. [33, 34] recently reported the occurrence of renal tumors in mice fed 40 ppm ochratoxin A for 45 weeks.

Consequently, although ochratoxin A has been implicated as a carcinogen, the experimental proof is tenuous and must be pursued further.

Patulin

Several detailed reviews covering the toxicological properties of patulin have been published [13, 35]. Patulin was originally identified as a potent antibiotic against both gram-positive and gram-negative bacteria since its discovery in 1942; it was tested extensively at one time for use as an antibiotic against the common cold. The idea was discarded when some of its undesirable side effects (dermal irritation, stomach irritation, nausea, vomition) became better known. These data indicated that humans could tolerate exposure to fairly heavy doses of patulin without acute effects; however, the question of cumulative effects and/or subacute toxicity is still open.

There is some circumstantial data implicating patulin in a mycotoxicosis of cattle in Japan and in Europe. However, no definitive studies have been conducted to confirm the involvement of patulin.

Of more concern from the standpoint of human health has been the report by Dickens and Jones [36] of tumor formation at the site of injection in six of eight male rats given 0.2 mg of patulin in arachis oil twice a week for 61 to 64 weeks. There is no evidence at this time, however, that patulin is an oral carcinogen, and a chronic study of patulin administered to rats by intubation revealed the absence of observable tumors.

Penicillic acid

Another mycotoxin produced in good yields in culture by molds frequently found growing on foods and feeds is penicillic acid. It was one of the first mycotoxins involved in a toxicosis to be isolated and identified (1913). As with patulin, its antibiotic properties were quickly noted. It is only moderately toxic (see Table 5); however, like patulin, it was found to form transplantable tumors at the point of injection in rats and mice; the dosage was 0.1 to 2.0 mg/kg penicillic acid injected subcutaneously twice a week for 52 to 65 weeks [37, 38]. There is no new evidence implicating penicillic acid as an oral carcinogen, although it has been reported to be mutagenic toward *B. subtilis* but not toward other bacterial test strains. Recent studies have indicated a facile reaction between penicillic acid (and patulin) and bond-SH-containing compounds; this probably accounts for the lack of toxicity of feeds containing this mycotoxin.

Roquefortine [39]

Roquefortine is one member of an unusual class of alkaloidal metabolites apparently derived from tryptophan. These compounds are capable of exerting a devastating effect on the central nervous system, resulting in tremors, seizure, and death in experimental animals. The LD_{50} (i.p.) in male mice is a low 15 to 20 mg/kg. No information is currently available relative to the subacute toxicity of roquefortine. The fact that it is produced by the mold commonly used in the commercial preparation of blue cheese, together with the general interest in the tremorgens as a class of toxic mold metabolites, led to the development of analytical methods for its detection in foods.

Sterigmatocystin

Sterigmatocystin was discovered during a systematic study of fungal metabolites [40]; it represented the first of a long list of metabolites containing the unusual dihydrofurofuran moiety. The elegant structural analysis studies leading to its structural determination were invaluable later in establishing the structures of the aflatoxins, versicolorins, austocystins, and related compounds and derivatives.

Although sterigmatocystin was found to have relatively low acute toxicity in the mouse (800 mg/kg), it was found to exhibit much greater toxicity in the Wistar rat (120 mg/kg, female) [41]. In 1966, Dickens et al. showed it to be carcinogenic by subcutaneous injection; this finding was complemented in 1970 by Purchase, who showed it to be a potent hepatocarcinogen in the rat [41]. Later studies showed it to be capable of producing tumors in the lungs as well as in the liver in mice.

The finding of carcinogenic activity, its close structural relationship to aflatoxin B_1, the common occurrence of molds (particularly *A. versicolor*) capable of producing sterigmatocystin on foods and feeds, and the ability of certain species to produce extremely large quantities (up to 12 g/kg) of sterigmatocystin in culture has encouraged the development of suitable analytical methods for the analysis of foods and feeds for this mycotoxin.

Trichothecenes [42, 43]

As previously noted, strong circumstantial evidence exists that one or more of the approximately 40 trichothecene metabolites were involved in the severe outbreaks of alimentary toxic aleukia and stachybotryotoxicoses in humans in Eastern Europe, and in the severe problem of fusariotoxicoses of farm animals which occurs frequently in many areas of the world. With an oral LD_{50} of 4.8 mg/kg in the mouse, the trichothecene T-2 toxin exhibits an acute toxicity equivalent to that of aflatoxin.

At the present time, only four of the known trichothecenes (T-2 toxin, deoxynivalenol, diacetoxyscirpenol, and nivalenol) have been identified as occurring naturally in grains. These compounds, singly or in combination, exhibit a wide range of toxic effects in experimental animals, including (1) feed refusal, vomition, diarrhea; (2) severe hemorrhage; edema, and necrosis of skin, mucous membranes, and brain tissue; (3) destruction of hematopoietic tissue; and (4) a variety of nervous disorders. In addition, these compounds are severely teratogenic and apparently interfere with antibody synthesis, predisposing animals to disease by affecting the immune response mechanism.

Although the trichothecenes studied have not been found to be mutagenic, there is tenuous evidence for carcinogenic activity. Schoental et al. [44-46] have reported the formation of tumors (benign and malignant) of the pituitary, brain, pancreas, and mammary gland, adenocarcinoma of the stomach and duodenum, and cardiovascular lesions in rats exposed to T-2 toxin. These observations have led to the suggestion that the *Fusarium* mycotoxins, probably trichothecenes, may play a role in development of tumors of the digestive tract and possibly are involved in some way in the close association between corn cultivation and esophageal cancer in some parts of Africa [47].

Other mycotoxins

A large number of mycotoxins are, of course, suspected of being contaminants of foods and feeds based upon the common occurrence in these commodities of the fungi that elaborate them. Many have been implicated in animal mycotoxicoses; some exhibit subacute toxicity. The toxicological properties of some of these mycotoxins are tabulated in Table 5 [13, 15-17].

D. Regulation and Control

The finding that aflatoxin, a common food contaminant, might be a potent hepatocarcinogen required control of exposure through foods and feeds, even though an estimate of risk could not be made. Most decisions in the face of uncertainty were made on the side of safety. However, it must be appreciated that "control" in an underdeveloped country involves balancing the certain risk of starvation against the uncertain risk of cancer, whereas in an industrialized country, where the standard of living is high, "control" takes on the attributes of a *defensive* mechanism. The result has been a wide variation in the type of control mechanisms and regulatory levels set by various countries [8, 19, 48] for mycotoxins in foods and feeds, with particular differences between producing and consuming countries.

There are many different facets to control, including (1) educational activities designed to make people aware of the problem and its consequences; (2) research activities aimed at developing crops resistant to invasion by the fungi, harvesting and storage techniques that protect the crops from fungal invasions, methods and techniques for identifying/quantitating the mycotoxin in foods and feeds, and decontamination techniques; and (3) the development and implementation of regulations controlling the amounts reaching the consumer.

In the United States regulatory control is exerted only in the case of aflatoxin. The need for control of other mycotoxins is being considered; however, insufficient evidence is currently available to require regulatory control activity. The legal basis for regulatory control in the United States is Section 402a (1) of the Federal Food, Drug, and Cosmetic Act, which prohibits from interstate commerce any adulterated food (i.e., any food containing a "poisonous or deleterious substance which may render it injurious to health"). In the interpretation of the Act by the courts, aflatoxin was considered to be an "added substance", and consequently it was necessary only to prove that it was, in fact, "poisonous and deleterious," without having to show that the quantity present in any particular food would "render it injurious to health." In applying this law to aflatoxin, the Food and Drug Administration (FDA) set an "action level" of 20 ppb for total aflatoxin in all foods and feeds, and of 0.5 ppb for aflatoxin M_1 in milk. With action levels set, the job of regulatory control of foods and feeds in general then revolved primarily around voluntary compliance activities by the food industry itself with the FDA monitoring such activities by collecting and analyzing food samples. These activities have been effective in lowering the average human exposure to aflatoxin in the United States.

II. METHODS FOR DETECTION OF MYCOTOXINS

A. General Requirements

Since 1962 and the discovery of the aflatoxins, a great deal of effort has been applied to the development of analytical methods, particularly methods for the determination of the aflatoxins and their metabolites. This effort has resulted in the publication of over 1300 papers describing a "method" for one or more mycotoxins; 38% of these methods were related to aflatoxins [49]. Several excellent reviews of the currently available methodology have been published [13, 50-53].

In selecting and using a particular method it is well to consider the following factors, any one of which could be a major determinant for selection.

Purpose

Many analytical methods are developed for a specific analyte in a particular substrate for a narrowly defined research goal. Such methods are rarely applicable to another type of substrate without modification. Many procedures are designed to screen large numbers of samples of a particular type; these methods give a qualitative or only a roughly quantitative answer, and may have some incidence of false positives. On the other hand, such screening procedures are designed to be rapid and inexpensive, and can be extremely useful in quality control. Other procedures are "research" in nature in that they tend to give precise and accurate results, are time consuming, and require the services of an experienced analyst. For regulatory purposes it may be necessary to resort to such procedures; in such cases it is desirable that the method be evaluated in an interlaboratory collaborative study and it is essential that the method include a confirmation of identity.

Sampling and sample preparation

In conducting analyses of foods and feeds it is absolutely essential to consider carefully the importance of the manner in which the sample is collected and prepared for analysis. One must be aware of the fact that if the analytical sample is not representative of the lot, the analytical result, no matter how accurate, is meaningless. Sampling/subsampling errors can be so large that the error of the analytical method becomes insignificant. For example, as Lillehoj has reported [54], in the analysis of peanuts for aflatoxin it has been estimated statistically that, using a 48 lb sample, 98% of the total error is due to sampling/subsampling errors, and only 2% is due to analysis error. As far as the analysis error is concerned, the major contribution to this error lies in the manner of preparation of the sample for quantitation (i.e., in the extraction-cleanup step) [55]. A realization of the importance of these factors has led to the development of sampling plans designed to minimize sampling/subsampling errors [53, 56-58].

Integrity of the analytical standard

In a recent study the Smalley Committee of the American Oil Chemists' Society distributed, as part of its aflatoxin check sample series, a standard solution of aflatoxins B_1, B_2, G_1, and G_2 as one of the samples to be analyzed by measurement against the analysts' own reference standard. The major source of error in the analysis, therefore, should have been that associated with calibration of the standard (C.V. ±5%), and that associated with visual estimation of the fluorescence intensity of the thin layer chromatography (TLC) spot (C.V. ±20%) (i.e., a total expected C.V. of ±21%). Instead, the between-laboratory C.V. was found to be about ±90% [59]. These results emphasize the necessity for controlling the integrity of the reference standards; the concentrations of such standards must be established accurately and their integrity checked regularly.

Confirmation of identity

A good analytical method should include a procedure for confirmation of identity of the analyte. This step is frequently ignored. A rigorous confirmation needed for a regulatory analysis, for example, might involve some type of mass spectral or infrared analysis. On the other hand, many other less rigorous confirmatory techniques have been developed which are perfectly satisfactory, for example, for screening purposes. These include various bioassay procedures (e.g., the chick embryo bioassay for aflatoxin [60] and the brine shrimp assay for trichothecenes [61]), the use of absorbance ratioing (as in the case of the high-pressure liquid chromatography (HPLC) method for zearalenone [62]), or the use of two separate detectors based on the measurement of different physical properties (as in the case of roquefortine, where both ultraviolet (UV) and electrochemical detectors were used [63]).

With these general concerns in mind, the following discussion relates to the methodology developed for the eight mycotoxins selected for in-depth review (see introduction) and briefly summarizes methodology available for detection of a group of mycotoxins which have not been studied extensively, but which, in our opinion, should be investigated.

B. Aflatoxin

Over 500 papers have been published describing methodology for the aflatoxins [49] and this information has been summarized frequently in the literature [17, 20, 50-53, 64]. The reader is referred to this extensive literature for an in-depth discussion of the subject. Only a brief review will be presented here.

The earliest methods for detection of the aflatoxins were bioassay procedures; the most common of these used the fertile chicken egg as the test organism. Many other systems have been used, including ducklings, a variety of microorganisms (e.g., *Bacillus megaterium*), and brine shrimp, to mention a few. The major drawback of all these tests was the lack of specificity and accurate quantitation.

The earliest chemical determinations involved measuring fluorescence intensity on TLC. These TLC methods have evolved to our present-day TLC methods, which are capable of detection limits for most practical purposes of about 0.1 ng/g for meat, milk, and eggs; 1.0 ng/g for basic susceptible commodities; and 10 ng/g for mixed feeds [19].

Recent years have seen the rapid growth of HPLC methods of analysis, both normal and reverse phase. Particularly interesting have been the development of specialized detectors for HPLC, including sensitive fluorescence detectors and fluorescence detectors containing flow cells packed with silica gel [49].

A tremendous amount of effort has been applied to the development of sensitive screening procedures (particularly the use of minicolumns) and extremely sensitive radioimmunoassay (RIA) procedures for detection of aflatoxins in samples of biological origin [49]. These efforts have been complemented by activity aimed at developing confirmatory techniques for the aflatoxins and their metabolites.

C. Citrinin

Citrinin is a β-hydroxy-α, β-unsaturated acid; its chemical properties reflect this unique structural feature [13]. Although it is only very sparingly soluble in water, it is readily extracted into dilute base; acidification then regenerates the free acid. Citrinin readily undergoes thermal decomposition in acidic or basic solutions, probably undergoing decarboxylation; it has been observed that heating contaminated corn results in loss of citrinin, although the toxicity of the product remains [65]. It has also been reported to be unstable photochemically, both in solution and in the solid state [13]. Several color reactions of citrinin are known [13], including the formation of a brown color in the presence of $FeCl_3$, a deep wine-red color with H_2O_2/H^+, a green color with $TiCl_4$, a deep blue color with Folin's reagent, and a yellow-green fluorescence under long-wave UV light upon exposure to formic acid on a TLC plate; these color reactions have frequently been used for analytical purposes.

The methodology for analysis of citrinin in foods and feeds has not been well developed. The earliest methods relied upon a colorimetric determinative step; these methods were relatively insensitive and nonspecific. Later methods relied upon a thin layer chromatographic determinative step; these methods were uniformly unsatisfactory, in general because the recovery of citrinin was poor, most interferences were not removed, and the citrinin spot on TLC invariably showed excessive streaking.

In recent years several attempts have been made to solve these severe analytical problems. The recently published methods [66-68] resulting from these studies are still not satisfactory in terms of detection, freedom from interferences, speed, and accuracy of analysis; however, they are the best methods currently available (Table 6).

One of the major problems involves recovery (extraction) of citrinin from the natural substrate. This problem is partially resolved by using an acidic extraction solvent [66]; given the known instability of citrinin [65], care must be taken to avoid heating the extracts.

A second problem involves the presence of co-extractants which interfere with the determinative step. This problem has been partially solved by introducing a defatting step (isooctane) followed by partition into sodium bicarbonate, reacidification and extraction into chloroform, and by introducing a reverse-phase HPLC determinative step [66]. Another problem which has been partially resolved is that of spreading (streaking) of the citrinin spot on the TLC plate. Several novel techniques have been proposed. In one case [66] the TLC plate is impregnated with oxalic acid; in another [68] the plate is impregnated with the disodium salt of ethylenediaminetetraacetic acid. Both of these modifications tend to reduce streaking or tailing of the citrinin spot.

Our own experience with these methods has led to the conclusion that none are completely satisfactory and that there is a good deal of room for improvement. We recommend a method which, although not completely satisfactory, has considerable utility. It is a combination of the methods proposed by Marti et al. [66] and the TLC procedure developed by Stubblefield [67].

Table 6 Analytical Methods for Citrinin

Determinative step	Substrate	Derivative	Determination limit (ng/g)	Recovery (%)	Reference
HPLC	Corn	-	50	60-80	66
TLC	Barley				
TLC	Corn		50	40-100	65
TLC	-		-	-	67
TLC	Feed	HCO_2H	500	75-92	68

Table 7 Analytical Methodology for the Ochratoxins

Determinative step	Substrate	Derivative	Determination limit (ng/g)	Recovery (%)	Reference
TLC	Corn, barley	NaOH spray	100	-	69
TLC	Cereals	Et_3N/MeOH	25	80-100	70
TLC	Grains, peanuts	-	20	80-100	71
TLC	Nuts, cheese	-	ca. 50	40-60	72
	Cocoa, coffee, soybeans, pepper, dairy products, meats, sugars, corn, cottonseed, beverages, rice, sorghum				
TLC	Cereals	-	10-50	85	73
TLC	-	NH_3	-	-	74
TLC	Grains	-	45-90	86-100	75
TLC	Barley	alc. $NaHCO_3$	12	81.2	76
TLC	Cocoa beans	-	<20	68-100	77
Minicolumn	Barley	-	12-64	60-100	78
RIA	Body tissues, fluids	-	20	-	79
TLC	Green coffee	-	-	69.1	80
Spectrophotometric	Barley	-	4	90	81
HPLC	Cereals	-	1-5		82
Spectrophotometric	Blood, plasma	-	2	60	83
HPLC	Kidney	NH_3	<1	78	84

D. Ochratoxin [13, 31]

Methods for detecting and quantitating the ochratoxins have improved steadily since the first TLC method was developed in 1966 [69]. Most of the methods developed are based on TLC (see Table 7); the food or feed is first extracted with an organic solvent, usually chloroform, and the extract is then purified through partition of the ochratoxin into aqueous bicarbonate followed by reacidification and partition back into an organic solvent. On the TLC plate ochratoxin A is seen as a blue-green fluorescent spot under long-wave UV light; on exposure to base (amines, NH_3, OH^-, $NaHCO_3$), a more intense, blue fluorescent spot is observed. This technique, together with formation of the ethyl ester derivatives for confirmation of identity, forms the basis of the official AOAC method for ochratoxin [76].

In recent years some specialized methods have been developed, including a rapid minicolumn screening procedure [78], a spectrophotometric procedure for analysis of barley and physiological fluids that involves enzymatic hydrolysis of ochratoxin A to ochratoxin α and measurement of the loss of fluorescence intensity at 380 nm [81-83], a radioimmunoassay technique for analysis of body tissues and fluids [79], and several HPLC procedures [83, 84]. Of particular interest is the method developed by Hunt et al. [84] for analysis of pig kidney. In this procedure the sample extract is purified through enzymic hydrolysis and dialysis. The ochratoxin α formed is separated by reverse-phase HPLC and detected by using a post-column ammoniation reaction followed by measurement of the fluorescence intensity of the resulting derivative. A detection limit of less than 1 ng/g has been claimed.

E. Patulin

Patulin is a highly reactive, low molecular weight mycotoxin containing an unusually large number of functional groups, including an unsaturated lactone function and a cyclic hemiacetal function. Excellent analytical methods have been designed based on the physical/chemical properties of these functional groups. For example, the strong UV absorption at 276 nm of the unsaturated lactone function provides the basis for several good HPLC procedures using UV detectors. The hemiacetal function is readily opened in the presence of acid, forming an aldehyde which is readily derivatized to form phenylhydrazones, dinitrophenylhydrazones, and other carbonyl derivatives that have been used extensively for paper and thin layer chromatographic visualization. Alternatively, the free hydroxyl function has been derivatized (acetates, trifluoroacetates, etc.); these derivatives are used in a variety of gas chromatographic separations and determinations using flame ionization or electron capture detectors. Some of these methods are summarized in Table 8.

Table 8 Analytical Methods for Patulin

Determinative step	Substrate	Derivative	Determination limit (ng/ml)	Recovery (%)	Reference
GLC	Apple juice	Acetate, chloroacetate, silyl ether	700	90	85
TLC	Corn, wheat, rye, oats, sorghum	None	40	-	86
HPLC	Apple juice	None	11	785	87
TLC	Apple juice	MBTH[a]	25	60	88
GLC	Grains	TMS	200	73-79	89
GC-MS	Apple juice	TMS	1	-	90
HPLC	Apple butter	-	-	98	91
GLC	Rice, grains, flour, soybeans	TMS	20	90	92
TLC	Apple products	NH_3	1000	97.5	93
TLC	Apple products	2,4-DNP	50	60	94
TLC	Tomatoes, pears, apples, cucumbers, plums	-	40	80-95	95
TLC	Apple juice	MBTH	20	-	96
HPLC	Grape juice	-	5	-	-
HPLC	Apple juice	-	1	83	97
TLC	Apple juice	Aniline	50	100	98

[a] MBTH, 0.5% 3-methyl-2-benzothiazolinone hydrazone hydrochloride.

F. Penicillic Acid

Although there are a large number of screening procedures for penicillic acid, few quantitative methods are available for this mycotoxin. One would expect, on the basis of its structural features (see Figure 1), that the molecule would be quite soluble in water and polar organic solvents, and that it would easily react with the appropriate reagent to form derivatives suitable for use in an analytical method. This has been found to be the case. Penicillic acid readily forms acetate, trifluoroacetate, and silyl ether derivatives which have been used in GLC methods. It reacts with phenylhydrazine to form an intensely yellow, fluorescent pyrazoline derivative, with p-anisaldehyde to form a distinctive green color that when heated on a TLC plate yields an intensely blue fluorescent compound, and with ammonia, to form an intensely blue fluorescent product. All of these reactions have been used in sensitive TLC methods for determination of penicillic acid. Some of the more recently developed methods are described in Table 9.

Although penicillic acid has been found in whole grains and beans freshly ground for analysis, recoverable penicillic acid decreases measurably in a matter of hours after grinding and mixing, probably as a result of interaction with sulfhydryl (bond-SH) groups to which the compound is thus exposed. Selection of commodities to be analyzed (e.g., whole grains versus flours) and preparation of samples for analysis should be carried out with this in mind.

G. Roquefortine

Roquefortine is one of several alkaloids, including isofumigaclavines A and B, which have been isolated from cultures of *Penicillium roqueforti*. Several procedures have been described for the isolation of roquefortine and other metabolites from cultures grown on liquid media. These procedures have generally favored chloroform, chloroform-methanol, or ethyl acetate-ammonia (pH 10) as the extraction solvent, but one study indicated that acetone was the most efficient solvent [107]. Only two methods have been reported for the determination of roquefortine in samples of blue cheese [63, 108]. The procedure described in this chapter, which is a combination of these methods, permits detection of roquefortine and isofumigaclavine A by TLC and determination of roquefortine by HPLC with UV and for electrochemical detectors.

H. Sterigmatocystin

A variety of analytical methods have been developed for the analysis of foods and feeds for sterigmatocystin (see Table 10). These analytical methods are modeled after those developed for aflatoxin analysis; they are based upon a strong UV absorption at 326 nm (methanol)

Table 9 Analytical Methods for Penicillic Acid

Determinative step	Substrate	Derivative	Determination limit (ng/ml)	Recovery (%)	Reference
GLC-EC	Corn, dried beans, apple juice	TFA	4	80	99
GLC-EC[a]	Grains	TMS	20	90 (50 ng/g)	100
GLC-EC[a]	-	TMS	-	-	101
TLC	Sausage	p-Anisaldehyde	-	-	102
TLC	Culture medium, corn	NH_3	-	-	103
GLC-FI[a]	Corn, rice	TMS or underivatized	(0.025 μg)	-	104
HPLC	Meat, dairy products, cereals	-	500	-	105
HPLC	Grains, dried beans, Swiss cheese	TFA	25	70-80	106

[a] Also concurrently analyzes for patulin.

Table 10 Analytical Methods for Sterigmatocystin

Determinative step	Substrate	Derivative	Determination limit (ng/g)	Recovery (%)	Reference
TLC	Grain, oilseed	Acetate	(2.5 ng)	-	109
TLC	Cereals, groundnuts	KOH spray	200	-	110
TLC	Grains	$AlCl_3$ spray	30	90	111
GLC	Rice	-	50	-	112
HPLC	Corn, oats	-	25	Corn, 59 Oats, 74	113
TLC	-	I_2 vapor	(0.0325 μg)	-	114
HPLC	Culture media	-	-	-	115
GC-MS	Wheat, rice, corn barley		1	-	116
TLC	Cereal grains, soybeans	$AlCl_3$ spray	50	92-134	117
HPLC	Culture media	-	-	-	118
TLC	Grains	$AlCl_3$ spray	50	86-96	119
2D-TLC	Vegetable foods	$AlCl_3$ spray	-	-	120
2D-TLC	Cheese	$AlCl_3$ spray	5	30-80	121

Table 11 Analytical Methods for Trichothecenes

Determinative step	Substrate	Derivative	Determination limit (ng/g)	Recovery (%)	Reference
TLC	Media	p-Anisaldehyde	-	-	126
GLC	Grain	TMS	9000 (T-2)	80-100	127
TLC-GLC	Cereal grains	H_2SO_4/TMS	-	-	128
TLC	Media	H_2SO_4	-	-	129
GC-MS	Feeds	TMS	1000	-	130
Photometric	Feeds	GSH/enzyme	1000	-	131
TLC	Feeds	H_2SO_4	1000-4000	-	132
TLC	Media	H_2SO_4/2,4-DNP	6000	-	133
GC-MS	Milk, corn	TMS	100	65	134
GC-MS	Mixed feed	TMS	-	-	135
GC-MS	Rice cultures	TMS	200	-	136
GC-MS and TLC	Foods, feeds	-	1000	-	137
GC	Corn, mixed feeds	Hexafluoro-butyrate	100 T-2 25 DAS	105 97	138
GC	-	TMS, hexafluoro-butyrate	0.9 T-2 0.3 DAS	-	139
Photometric	-	Chromotropic acid	-	-	140

Table 12 Selected Methods for "Other Mycotoxins"

Mycotoxin	Determinative step	Substrate	Determination level (ng/g)	Reference
Altenuene	HPLC	Sorghum	<100	141
Alternariol	HPLC	Sorghum	<100	141
Amanitin	TLC	Mushrooms	Screening	142
Butenolide	TLC	Culture medium	Screening	143
Citreoviridin	TLC	Culture medium	Screening	144
Cyclochlorotine	TLC	Wheat	Screening	145
Cyclopiazonic acid	TLC	Rice, corn, wheat	Screening	146
Cytochalasins	TLC	Culture medium	Screening	147
Ergot alkaloids	HPLC	Culture medium	Screening	148
	RIA	Plasma	100-250 (pg/ml)	149
Fumitremorgen A				150
Fusarenon-X	GLC	Rice, corn, wheat	100	150
Gliotoxin	TLC		Screening	151
Griseofulvin	GLC	Plasma	20	152

Kojic acid	TLC	Culture medium	Screening	153
Luteoskyrin	TLC	Rice	Screening	154
Malformin A	TLC	Onions	Screening	155
Moniliformin	TLC	Corn	Screening	156
Mycophenolic acid	TLC	Blue cheese	Screening	157
Nivalenol	GLC	Rice, corn, wheat	100	151
Penitrems	TLC	Cream cheese	Screening	158
PR toxin	TLC	Blue cheese	250	159
Rubratoxin B	RIA			160
Rugulosin	TLC	Grains	100	161
Satratoxins	HPLC	Wheat, oats, barley, corn	100	162
Secalonic acid	TLC		Screening	151
Sporidesmins	GLC	Culture medium		163
Tenuazonic acid	GLC	Sorghum		164
Verruculogen	TLC	Oats	Screening	165
Xanthomegnin	HPLC	Corn	750	166
Zearalenone	HPLC	Corn	10	167
Zearalenol	GLC	Corn, oats		168

and the formation of intensely fluorescent derivatives. Sterigmatocystin itself fluoresces a dull, brick-red color under long-wave UV light; its fluorescent intensity is only about one-thousandth that of aflatoxin B_1. However, treatment with acetic anhydride and pyridine leads to formation of a highly fluorescent (blue) derivative. Unfortunately, this derivative is not stable on a TLC plate. Various other reagents (KOH, $AlCl_3$, I_2) form more stable, fluorescent products; the most commonly used reagent has been $AlCl_3$, which forms a bright yellow, fluorescent compound. The coupling of excellent extraction-cleanup steps with a two-dimensional TLC determinative step using an $AlCl_3$ spray reagent has recently been reported in a method for the determination of sterigmatocystin in cheese, with a limit of detection of about 5 ng/g [121]; this method also includes a confirmation of identity involving the formation of a "water adduct" in the presence of trifluoroacetic acid, a reaction frequently used in confirmatory procedures for aflatoxin.

In recent years several HPLC methods for sterigmatocystin have been developed which show excellent potential, as well as a gas chromatographic-mass spectrometric procedure with an estimated detection limit of about 1 ng/g.

I. Trichothecenes

Extensive reviews of trichothecene methodology have been published [42, 122, 123]. On the one hand, the trichothecenes contain a number of functional groups around which a sensitive analytical method might be built, including free hydroxyl and carbonyl groups which may be readily derivatized, ester functions which are readily hydrolyzed, and a relatively stable epoxide function; on the other hand, the molecule does not exhibit fluorescent properties, nor does it absorb strongly in the UV. The problem of analysis for the trichothecenes is compounded by the fact that more than 45 known mold metabolites contain the trichothecene nucleus, many of which have quite similar chemical and physical properties.

Nevertheless, steady progress has been made in the development of analytical methods for low levels of the trichothecenes, including some simple (but nonspecific) bioassay procedures [61, 124, 125]; a series of TLC procedures in which the trichothecene is visualized by spraying the plate with H_2SO_4 and charring to yield a blue-fluorescent product; and some excellent GC methods based upon formation of trimethylsilyl ether or heptafluorobutyrate ester derivatives coupled with a mass spectrometric confirmation (see Table 11). None of these methods is completely satisfactory for a variety of reasons and new methods based upon formation of UV-absorbing or colored derivatives which could be quantitated by HPLC are certain to appear shortly. It is known that in the presence of acid and heat, many of the trichothecenes liberate formaldehyde, which can then be determined photometrically [140]; it is conceivable that this type of reaction could be used to develop a method for the trichothecenes as a group. Alternatively, a method might be developed around the selective hydrolysis of the trichothecene to the alcohol from which the various esters are derived.

J. Other Mycotoxins

Analytical methods are available for many other mycotoxins (see Table 12). Most of these methods are not well developed, have not been extensively tested for precision or accuracy, have not been widely used, and in many cases were developed for screening purposes only.

III. SELECTED ANALYTICAL METHODS

A. Aflatoxins

TLC and HPLC methods

Summary. Samples of peanuts and peanut products, hard nuts, corn, and soybeans are extracted with chloroform. Samples containing cottonseed are extracted with acetone-water; the extracts are purified using a preliminary cleanup step involving lead acetate precipitation, followed by silica gel-acid alumina column chromatography. The aflatoxins are isolated by silica gel column chromatography and the determination is carried out using thin layer chromatography (TLC) or normal- or reverse-phase high-pressure liquid chromatography (HPLC) with fluorescence detectors. The TLC procedure includes a step for confirmation of the presence of aflatoxins B_1 and G_1 by derivative formation on a TLC plate.

The TLC procedure has a limit of determination of about 5 ng/g. The normal-phase HPLC procedure requires a fluorescence detector which has a silica gel packed flow cell and has a limit of determination of about 2.5 ng/g. The reverse-phase HPLC procedure includes a step for derivative formation and has a limit of determination of about 1 ng/g. Overall recoveries of aflatoxins added to samples at levels of 5 ng/g should average greater than 75%.

Apparatus. (1) Mechanical shaker; (2) glass chromatographic columns 350 × 22 mm i.d. with a 300 ml reservoir and stopcock; (3) Butt column (for samples of cottonseed and cottonseed products) 125 × 32 mm i.d.; (4) thin layer chromatographic equipment: glass plates, 20 × 20 cm; applicator; mounting board; spotting template;

10 μl syringe; desiccating storage cabinet; chromatographic tank; long-wave UV lamp (use with UV-absorbing eyeglasses) or viewing cabinet equipped with long-wave UV lamps; (5) liquid chromatograph capable of delivering 1 ml/min, pulseless flow with high-pressure injection valve (25 μl loop) and equipped with fluorescence detector; for determination by normal phase, the detector flow cell must be packed with 10 to 30 μm silica having a surface area which is the same as that of the liquid chromatographic silica column (Varian Fluorichrom, Varian Associates, Walnut Creek, CA 94598, or equivalent); (6) liquid chromatographic column: for determination by normal-phase HPLC, 250 × 3 to 4 mm i.d. stainless steel column packed with 5 or 10 μm silica; for determination by reverse-phase HPLC, 250 × 3 to 4 mm i.d. stainless steel column packed with 5 or 10 μm of C-8 or C-18 packing.

Reagents. (1) Solvents: ACS grade chloroform, acetone, benzene, cyclohexane, anhydrous ethyl ether ($\leq$ 0.01% ethanol), acetonitrile, methanol, absolute ethanol; (2) acetic acid, trifluoroacetic acid; (3) diatomaceous earth: Hyflo Super-Cel or equivalent; (4) lead acetate solution (for samples containing cottonseed): dissolve 100 g of $Pb(OAc)_2 \cdot 3H_2O$ in water with warming, add 1.5 ml of acetic acid, and dilute to 500 ml; (5) acidic alumina (for samples containing cottonseed) Fisher A-948 (80-200 mesh): add 3% water by weight, shake well, and equilibrate overnight; (6) silica gel for column chromatography; silica gel 60, 0.063 to 0.200 mm (EM Laboratories, Inc., Elmsford, NY 10523) or equivalent; (7) silica gel (for TLC): the following have been found to be satisfactory: Macherey-Nagel GMR (distributed by Brinkmann Instruments, Inc.), Applied Science Adsorbosils 1 or 5, and Mallinckrodt Silic AR 4G or 7G; test each lot with aflatoxin standard solution using conditions described under "Determination by TLC"; the aflatoxins should separate into four distinct spots and resist fading; (8) aflatoxin standards: (a) Prepare individual solutions of aflatoxins B_1, B_2, G_1, and G_2 in benzene-acetonitrile (98:2) having concentrations of 8 to 10 μg/ml. Determine actual concentrations of the individual aflatoxins by scanning the solutions on a UV spectrometer from 380 to 300 nm, recording the absorption maximum (A) near 350 nm, and calculating the concentrations using the following equation:

$$\mu\text{g aflatoxin/ml} = \frac{(A \times MW \times 1000 \times CF)}{E}$$

where CF is a correction factor specific for each instrument (can be taken as 1 for most modern instruments) and MW and E are as follows:

Aflatoxin	MW	E
B_1	312	19,800
B_2	314	20,900
G_1	328	17,100
G_2	330	18,200

(b) Standard solution for TLC (0.5 μg of aflatoxins B_1 and G_1 and 0.2 μg of aflatoxins B_2 and G_2/ml). Using the solutions prepared above, pipet quantities calculated to contain 12.5 μg of aflatoxins B_1 and G_1 and 5.0 μg of aflatoxins B_2 and G_2 into a 25 ml volumetric flask and dilute to the mark with benzene-acetonitrile (98:2). (c) Standard solution for normal-phase HPLC (0.1 μg of aflatoxins B_1 and G_1 and 0.04 μg of aflatoxins B_2 and G_2/ml). Pipet 5.0 ml of the standard solution for TLC [reagent 8(b) above] into a 25 ml volumetric flask and dilute to the mark with benzene-acetonitrile (98:2). (d) Standard solution for reverse-phase HPLC (10 ng of aflatoxins B_1, B_2, G_1, and G_2/ml). Using the standard solutions prepared in reagent 8(a), pipet quantities calculated to contain 1 μg of each of the four aflatoxins B_1, B_2, G_1, and G_2 into a 100 ml volumetric flask and dilute to the mark with benzene-acetonitrile (98:2).

Sample Preparation and Extraction

Peanut butter and meal, peanuts, hard nuts, corn and soybeans. Peanut butter and meal do not require preparation unless they contain large particles. Grind samples of raw and roasted peanuts, hard nuts, corn, and soybeans to pass a 0.85 mm opening (20 mesh sieve).

Weigh 50 g of prepared sample into a 500 ml glass-stoppered Erlenmeyer flask; add 25 ml of water, 25 g of diatomaceous earth, and 250 ml of chloroform. Secure stopper and shake vigorously with mechanical shaker for 30 min. Filter through 24 cm folded filter paper and collect the first 50 ml of filtrate for column chromatography.

Cottonseed products. Grind whole seed, kernels, or meals to pass a 1 mm opening (18 mesh sieve).

For conventional samples, weigh a 25 g sample into a 500 ml glass-stoppered Erlenmeyer flask, add 250 ml of acetone-water (85:15), secure the stopper, and shake vigorously for 30 min. on a mechanical shaker. Filter through 24 cm folded filter paper and collect 100 ml of filtrate.

For ammoniated cottonseed meals, weigh a 25 g sample into a 500 ml glass-stoppered Erlenmeyer flask, add 40 ml of 0.1 N HCl solution and allow to soak 5 min. Add 210 ml of acetone, secure the stopper, and shake vigorously for 30 min. on a mechanical shaker. Filter through 24 cm folded filter paper and collect 100 ml of filtrate.

For all cottonseed samples, transfer 100 ml of filtrate from the extraction step to a 250 ml beaker, add 80 ml of water and 20 ml of 20% $Pb(OAc)_2$ solution (reagent 4), stir well, and allow to stand for 5 min. Add about 5 g of diatomaceous earth, stir well, and filter through 24 cm folded filter paper, collecting 100 ml of filtrate.

Transfer the 100 ml of filtrate to a 250 ml separatory funnel, add 50 ml of methylene chloride, shake vigorously for 30 sec., and allow the layers to separate. Prepare the Butt column by tamping a small plug of glass wool into the bottom of the column and adding successive layers of 2 cm of anhydrous Na_2SO_4, 5 g of acidic alumina, 5 g of silica gel 60, and 2 cm of anhydrous Na_2SO_4. Drain the lower methylene chloride layer through the Butt column and collect the filtrate in a 250 ml beaker. Add a second 50 ml portion of methylene chloride to the separatory funnel and shake; after the layers have separated, pass the lower layer through the Butt column into the beaker. Wash the Butt column with 50 ml of chloroform-acetone (9:1) and add this to the beaker. Evaporate the combined eluates just to dryness on a steam bath, taking care not to overheat the dry extract. Dissolve the extract in 50 ml of chloroform for the column chromatography step.

Column Chromatography. Add chloroform until the 300 × 22 mm chromatographic column is about one-half full. Tamp a small plug of glass wool in the bottom of the column and add 5 g of anhydrous sodium sulfate. Add 10 g of silica gel 60 to the column, stir with a long rod to remove any bubbles, and drain a few milliliters of solvent to aid settling. Add 15 g of anhydrous sodium sulfate and drain the solvent just to the top of the packing. Add a 50 ml sample extract to the column and drain at the maximum flow rate until the solvent just reaches the top of the packing. For ammoniated cottonseed meals only, add 100 ml of benzene-acetic acid (9:1) and drain to the top of the packing. For all samples add 200 ml of ethyl ether-hexane (3:1) and drain to the top of the packing. Discard washes. Add 200 ml of chloroform-acetone (4:1) and collect the eluate in a 250 ml beaker. Evaporate this to a few milliliters on a steam bath and transfer to a 4 dram vial, using 3 to 5 ml of chloroform to rinse the beaker. Evaporate the eluate just to dryness under a stream of nitrogen.

The determination of aflatoxins may be carried out by TLC or by normal- or reverse-phase HPLC or by combinations of these techniques. For determination by TLC alone, dissolve samples other than those containing cottonseed in 0.2 ml of benzene-acetonitrile (98:2); dissolve samples of cottonseed or cottonseed products in 0.1 ml of benzene-acetonitrile (98:2). If the determination is to be made by normal-phase HPLC, dissolve the sample in 0.5 ml (0.25 ml for samples containing cottonseed) of the HPLC mobile solvent. If the determination is to be made by reverse-phase HPLC, prepare the hemiacetal derivatives of aflatoxins B_1 and G_1 with trifluoroacetic acid as described in the reverse-phase HPLC determination step. If the determination is to be made by a combination of two of the techniques described, dissolve the sample extract in 2.0 ml of chloroform, pipet 1.0 ml of this solution into a separate 3 dram vial, and evaporate both solutions just to dryness under a stream of nitrogen. Dissolve these sample extracts in one-half the amount of solvent listed above for the determination. When dissolving a sample extract in a solvent for final determination, shake the vials vigorously to ensure that all components go into solution.

Determination by TLC. Prepare 20 × 20 cm glass plates of silica gel (0.25 mm wet thickness) using 30 g of any of the adsorbents listed under Reagents with the amount of water specified by the manufacturer. Activate the plates by heating them at 110°* for 1 hr. and store them in a desiccating cabinet until just before use. To prepare plate for chromatography, scribe a line 16 cm from the bottom edge as a solvent stop and scribe lines 0.5 cm in from each edge to prevent edge effects. If plates are to be scanned with a densitometer, score the plates to provide separate channels. Prepare developing solvent of chloroform-acetone (9:1).

Spot 2, 5, and two 10 µl spots of the sample extract and 2, 5, and 10 µl of the mixed aflatoxin standard solution on an imaginary line about 4 cm from the bottom of the plate. In addition, spot 5 µl of the standard solution on top of one of the 10 µl standard spots as an internal standard. Develop the plate in a closed, unlined, equilibrated tank with the developing solvent to the stop line. Remove the plate and air dry. View the plate under long-wave UV light in a darkened room or in a viewing cabinet. The aflatoxin standard should show four spots clearly separated from one another, which in order of decreasing R_f are B_1, B_2, G_1, and G_2. Identify aflatoxins in the sample by comparing the R_f values of sample spots with those of the standards. If sample spots have the same intensity as the standard spots, calculate the amount of aflatoxin in the sample directly. If sample spots do not have the same intensity as standard spots, estimate the amount of dilution required, taking into account the amount of sample used in the analysis.

Evaporate the sample solution to dryness under a stream of nitrogen and redissolve in the calculated volume of benzene-acetonitrile (98:2). For quantitative determination spot 3.5, 5.0, and two 6.5 µl portions of the redissolved sample extract and 3.5, 5.0, and 6.5 µl of the aflatoxin standard solution on separate spots about 1.5 cm apart on a new plate. In addition, spot 5.0 µl of standard on top of one of the

---

*All temperature data are in degrees Celsius.

6.5 μl sample spots. Develop the plate as previously described and view the plate under long-wave UV light. Compare the fluorescence intensities of the B_1 spots in the sample with those of the standards and determine which sample portion matches one of the sample spots. Compare B_2, G_1, and G_2 spots in the same manner.

Calculate the concentration of aflatoxin B_1 in the sample using the following formula:

$$\text{ng aflatoxin } B_1/\text{g} = \frac{S \times C \times V}{X \times W}$$

where

S = μl of aflatoxin B_1 standard equal to unknown,
C = concentration (μg/ml) of aflatoxin B_1 standard,
V = final volume of sample extract (μl),
X = μl of sample extract spotted giving fluorescence intensity equal to S,
W = amount (g) of sample represented by extract

Calculate the amount of aflatoxins B_2, G_1, and G_2 in the same manner.

The TLC determination may be carried out by densitometric analysis of the spots. In this case scan the plate with the densitometer according to the instructions of the manufacturer. Irradiate with a 365 nm source and measure the emission intensity at 420 to 460 nm. Calculate the amount of each aflatoxin present using the following formula:

$$\text{ng aflatoxin/g} = \frac{A \times S \times C \times V}{B \times X \times W}$$

where

A = area of aflatoxin peak in sample,
S = μl of aflatoxin standard spotted,
C = concentration (μg/ml) of aflatoxin standard,
V = final volume (μl) of sample extract,
B = area of aflatoxin peak in standard,
X = μl of sample extract spotted,
W = amount (g) of sample represented by extract

Confirmation of Aflatoxin B_1 and G_1 by Derivative Formation on a TLC Plate. Divide a prepared TLC plate in two equal sections by scoring a line down the plate. Cover one section with a clean glass plate. On the uncovered side spot two aliquots of the sample extract calculated to contain 0.5 to 5 ng of aflatoxins B_1 and G_1. On top of one of these spots add a portion of the aflatoxin standard solution which contains about the same amount of B_1 and G_1; also spot an equal amount of the standard on a separate spot. To each of these spots add 1 μl of trifluoroacetic acid (TFA) and allow the plate to set for 5 min. at room temperature. Remove excess reagent by directing a stream of warm air over the spots. Uncover the second section of the plate and spot sample extract and standard in the same manner as on the first section but do not add TFA. Develop the plate with chloroform-acetone (85:15). Remove the plate, air dry, and view the plate under long-wave UV light. Unreacted aflatoxins appear near the top of the plate. Derivatives of aflatoxins B_1 and G_1 (B_{2a} and G_{2a}) appear as blue fluorescent spots having R_f values about 0.25 of those of unreacted B_1 and G_1. The presence of the aflatoxin derivatives in the sample extract confirms the presence of aflatoxins B_1 and G_1 in the sample.

Determination by Normal-Phase HPLC. Prepare HPLC mobile solvent of water-saturated chloroform-cyclohexane-acetonitrile-absolute ethanol (75:22.5:3.0:1.5). The amount of absolute ethanol in the mobile solvent may be varied to obtain optimum resolution of the aflatoxins with different silica gel columns; however, increasing the amount of ethanol will reduce the fluorescence intensity of the aflatoxins. Set the liquid chromatographic flow rate at 1.0 ml/min. Set the fluorescence detector excitation at 350 to 360 nm and the emission at 410 to 420 nm cutoff.

Pipet 0.5, 1.0, 2.0, 3.0, 4.0, and 5.0 ml of the aflatoxin HPLC standard solution (100 ng of aflatoxins B_1 and G_1/ml and 40 ng of aflatoxins B_2 and G_2/ml) into separate 2 dram vials and evaporate just to dryness under a stream of nitrogen. Pipet 1.0 ml of the HPLC mobile solvent into each vial to give respective final concentration of 50 and 20, 100 and 40, 200 and 80, 300 and 120, 400 and 160, and 500 and 200 ng of aflatoxins B_1 and G_1/ml and B_2 and G_2/ml. Inject 25 μl of the most dilute standard solution into the liquid chromatograph and set the sensitivity controls so that the aflatoxin B_1 peak (first of the four aflatoxin peaks) gives a response of about 10% of full scale. Inject 25 μl of each of the standard solutions into the liquid chromatograph and prepare a standard curve for each of the four aflatoxins by plotting peak heights versus concentration (ng/ml).

Inject 25 μl of the sample solution into the liquid chromatograph under the same conditions used in preparing the standard curve. Identify the aflatoxin peaks in the sample by comparison of retention times with those of the standards; the aflatoxins elute in the order B_1, B_2, G_1, and G_2. If any of the aflatoxin peaks in the sample are larger than the highest corresponding standard peak, quantitatively dilute the sample with the mobile solvent and reinject. Determine the concentration of the individual aflatoxins in the sample extract directly from the standard curve. Calculate the amount of each aflatoxin in the sample using the following formula:

$$\text{ng aflatoxins } B_1,\ B_2,\ G_1,\ \text{or } G_2/\text{g sample (ppb)} = \frac{A \times B}{C}$$

where

A = concentration (ng/ml) of the aflatoxin in the sample extract,
B = volume (ml) of sample extract,
C = amount (g) of sample represented by extract

Determination by Reverse-Phase HPLC. Prepare HPLC mobile solvent of water-acetonitrile-methanol (65:20:15). Set the liquid chromatographic flow rate at 1.0 ml/min. Set the fluorescence detector excitation (bandpass filter or monochromator) at 350 to 360 nm and the emission cutoff filter at 410 to 420 nm.

Pipet 1.0, 2.0, 3.0, 4.0, and 5.0 ml of the aflatoxin reverse-phase HPLC standard solution [reagent 8(d), 10.0 ng of aflatoxins B_1, B_2, G_1, G_2/ml] into separate 3 dram vials and evaporate just to dryness under a stream of nitrogen. Add 100 μl of trifluoroacetic acid-water (1:1) to each vial, swirl to thoroughly wet the sides, and let stand at room temperature for 10 min. Evaporate the solution just to dryness under a stream of nitrogen. Pipet 1.0 ml of water-acetonitrile (80:20) into each vial to give a final concentration of 10, 20, 30, 40, and 50 ng of aflatoxins B_{2a} (B_1), B_2, G_{2a} (G_1), and G_2/ml. Inject 25 μl of the most dilute standard solution (10 ng/ml) into the liquid chromatograph and set the fluorescence detector sensitivity and range controls so that the aflatoxins, which elute in the order G_{2a}, B_{2a}, G_2, and B_2, give a response of 15 to 20% of full scale. Inject 25 μl of each of the standard solutions into the liquid chromatograph, and prepare standard curves for each of the four aflatoxins by plotting peak heights versus concentration (ng/ml).

Add 100 μl of trifluoroacetic acid-water (1:1) to the sample extract, swirl to ensure that all of the extract comes in contact with the reagent, allow to stand for 10 min., and evaporate just to dryness under a stream of nitrogen. If the total extract is to be used for reverse-phase HPLC analysis, dissolve the extract in 1.0 ml of water-acetonitrile (1:1); if the sample extract was divided in half for separate analysis by TLC or normal-phase HPLC, dissolve the extract in 0.5 ml of water-acetonitrile (1:1). Inject 25 μl of the sample solution into the liquid chromatograph under the same conditions used in preparing the standard curve. Identify the aflatoxin peaks in the sample by comparison of retention times with those of the standards. If any of the aflatoxin peaks in the sample are higher than the corresponding standard peak, quantitatively dilute the sample with water-acetonitrile (80:20) and reinject. Determine the concentration of the individual aflatoxins in the sample extract directly from the standard curve. Calculate the amount of each aflatoxin in the sample using the following formula:

$$\text{ng aflatoxin } B_1\ (B_{2a}),\ B_2,\ G_1\ (G_{2a}),\ \text{or } G_2/\text{g sample (ppb)} = \frac{A \times B}{C}$$

where

A = Concentration (ng/ml) of the aflatoxin in the sample extract,
B = volume (ml) of the sample extract,
C = amount (g) of sample represented by the extract

Minicolumn methods

Summary. Minicolumn methods are designed to be rapid, inexpensive screening procedures for the detection and semiquantitation of aflatoxins. Two minicolumn procedures are described. The first procedure requires a more extensive sample cleanup, but may be used for a wide variety of samples, including corn and corn products, peanuts and peanut products, cottonseed meal, nuts, dried fruits, and mixed feeds. The limit of detection is generally found to be about 15 ng/g for mixed feeds and about 10 ng/g for other commodities, although experienced analysts can detect aflatoxins present at the 5 ng/g level with good accuracy in samples other than mixed feeds. The second procedure was primarily designed for the rapid analysis of corn samples and has a shorter sample cleanup step. The accepted limit of detection is about 10 ng/g. The procedures include the preparation of a reference minicolumn containing aflatoxins equivalent to the 20 ng/g level in samples. Analysts may prepare other reference minicolumns containing aflatoxins at lower levels. It is recommended that analysts periodically prepare minicolumns from samples which are known to be free of aflatoxins for comparison purposes. In all cases where minicolumn tests show a sample to be within 25% of a tolerance or guideline level, the sample should be analyzed by a quantitative procedure.

Apparatus. (1) High-speed blender with 1 quart jars and lids; (2) ultraviolet light-long-wave (365 nm) UV hand lamp (use with UV-absorbing eyeglasses) or Chromato-Vue cabinet (Ultra-Violet Products, Inc.) or equivalent; (3) minicolumn: 5.5 to 6.0 mm (i.d.) × 200 mm glass tubes tapered at one end to about 2 mm; (4) minicolumn support racks: to hold columns upright (test tube rack may be used); (5) (for procedure 1) syringe: 5 ml, with 5 in., 15 gauge needle; (6) (for procedure 2) culture tubes: 20 mm (o.d.) × 150 mm (disposable) with plastic tube closures (30 and 60 ml separatory funnels may be substituted for the culture tubes).

Reagents

For procedure 1. (1) Solvents: chloroform and acetone, ACS grade; (2) sodium hydroxide solution (0.2 M): dissolve 8.0 g of NaOH in 1 liter of distilled water; (3) ferric chloride solution: dissolve 20 g of anhydrous $FeCl_3$ (Fisher Scientific Co. No. I-89, or equivalent) in 300 ml of distilled water; (4) cupric carbonate, basic (Fisher Scientific Co. No. C-453, or equivalent); (5) sulfuric acid solution (0.03%): dilute 0.3 ml of H_2SO_4 to 1 liter with distilled water; (6) potassium hydroxide-potassium chloride solution (0.02 N KOH with 1% KCl): dissolve 1.12 g of KOH and 10 g of KCl in 1 liter of distilled water; (7) diatomaceous earth: Hyflo Super-Cel or equivalent.

For procedure 2. (1) Solvents: ACS grade benzene, chloroform, acetone, methanol; (2) zinc acetate-sodium chloride solution: dissolve 150 g of $Zn(OAc)_2 \cdot 2H_2O$ (Fisher Scientific Co. No. Z-20, or equivalent), 150 g of NaCl, and 4 ml of acetic acid in 1 liter of distilled water.

For procedures 1 and 2. (1) Minicolumn packings: (a) Florisil, 100-200 mesh (Fisher Scientific Co. No. F-101, or equivalent); (b) silica gel: silica gel 60, 70-230 mesh (E. Merck No. 7734, or equivalent); (c) alumina, neutral: 80-200 mesh, Brockmann activity I (Fisher Scientific Co. No. A-950 or J.T. Baker Chemical Co. No. 0540); (d) calcium sulfate, anhydrous: Drierite, nonindicating, 20-40 mesh (W.A. Hammond Drierite Co. Xenia, OH 45385, or equivalent). Dry all packing materials at 100° for 2 hrs. Store conditioned packings in a desiccator with active desiccant; (2) filter paper: coarse porosity, prefolded, 15 and 32 cm (Schleicher and Schuell No. 588, or equivalent); (3) standards: (a) prepare separate solutions of aflatoxins B_1 and G_1 (10 μg/ml) in either chloroform or benzene-acetonitrile (98:2); (b) stock solution (100 ng aflatoxins B_1 and G_1/ml: pipet 1.0 ml each of the aflatoxins B_1 and G_1 standards (10 μg/ml) into a 100 ml volumetric flask and dilute to mark with chloroform; (c) standard solution (10 ng of aflatoxins B_1 and G_1/ml): pipet 5.0 ml of the standard stock solution (b) into a 50 ml volumetric flask and dilute to the mark with chloroform.

Procedure 1

Preparation of minicolumn. Tamp a small plug of glass wool into the tapered end of the column. Add the following packings to the column to the height listed, in order: 8 to 10 mm of anhydrous calcium sulfate, 8 to 10 mm of Florisil, 16 to 20 mm of silica gel, 8 to 10 mm of neutral alumina, and 8 to 10 mm of anhydrous calcium sulfate. Tap the column after the addition of each packing to obtain an even interface. Tamp a small plug of glass wool onto the top of the packing.

Preparation of reference minicolumn. Pipet 2.0 ml of the aflatoxin standard solution (c) (10 ng of aflatoxins B_1 and G_1/ml) into the column and allow the solution to drain until it reaches the top of the packing. Add 3 ml of $CHCl_3$-acetone (9:1) solution to the column, and allow the solution to drain until it reaches the top of the packing. If the reference column is to be used repeatedly, force all the solvent from the column with nitrogen gas, seal both ends of the columns, and store in a freezer. Under these conditions reference columns are stable for 2 to 3 months. Repeated exposure to UV light diminishes the intensity of the fluorescent band.

Sample extraction and cleanup. Weigh 50 g of ground sample into a blender jar, add 250 ml of acetone-water (85:15), and blend at high speed for 3 min. Filter through 32 cm prefolded filter paper into a 250 ml graduated cylinder.

Add 170 ml of 0.2 N NaOH solution and 30 ml of $FeCl_3$ solution to a 600 ml beaker and mix. Transfer 150 ml of the sample filtrate to the beaker, add 3 g of basic cupric carbonate, and mix thoroughly. Add 150 ml of diatomaceous earth, mix thoroughly, and filter through 32 cm prefolded filter paper into a 250 ml graduated cylinder. Transfer 150 ml of filtrate to a 500 ml separatory funnel; add 150 ml of 0.03% H_2SO_4 and 10 ml $CHCl_3$. Shake vigorously for about 1 min., allow the layers to separate, and transfer the lower layer (13 to 14 ml) to a 125 ml separatory funnel. Add 100 ml of KOH-KCl solution, swirl gently for 30 sec. and allow the layers to separate. (If an emulsion occurs, transfer the emulsion to another 125 ml separatory funnel and wash with 50 ml of 0.03% H_2SO_4 solution.) Drain 3 ml of the lower ($CHCl_3$) layer into a 3 dram (11 ml) vial and cap.

Chromatography and determination. Transfer 2 ml of the chloroform extract to the column with the syringe. Clamp the column in an upright position and allow the solution to drain until it reaches the top of the packing. Pipet 3 ml of $CHCl_3$-acetone (9:1) solution onto the column and allow the solution to drain until it reaches the top of the packing. Do not let the column run dry during the determination.

Examine sample and reference columns in a darkened room under long-wave UV light or in a viewing cabinet. The presence of aflatoxin is indicated by a blue fluorescent band at the top of the Florisil layer (about 2.5 cm from the bottom of the column). Some uncontaminated samples show a faint white, yellow, or brown fluorescent band at the top of the Florisil layer in the sample column. If the band does not have a definite bluish tint, the sample is negative.

Procedure 2

Preparation of minicolumn. Tamp a small plug of glass wool into the tapered end of the column. Add the following packings to the column to the height listed, in order: 5 to 7 mm of anhydrous calcium sulfate, 5 to 7 mm of Florisil, 20 mm of silica gel, 10 to 15 mm of neutral alumina, and 5 to 7 mm of anhydrous calcium sulfate. Tap the column lightly after the addition of each packing to obtain an even interface. Tamp a small plug of glass wool onto the top of the column.

Preparation of reference minicolumn. Pipet 2.0 ml of the aflatoxin standard solution onto the column and allow the solution to drain until it reaches the top of the packing. Pipet 3 ml of $CHCl_3$-acetone (9:1) solution onto the column and allow the solution to drain until it reaches the top of the packing. If the reference column is to be used repeatedly, force all of the solvent from the column with nitrogen gas, seal both ends of the column, and store in a freezer. Under these conditions reference columns are stable 2 to 3 months. Repeated exposure to UV light diminishes the intensity of the fluorescent band.

Sample extraction and cleanup. Weigh 50 g of ground sample into a blender jar, add 100 ml of methanol-water (80:20), and blend at high speed for 1 min. Filter through 32 cm prefolded paper into a 100 ml graduated cylinder.

Transfer 15 ml of filtrate to a culture tube (or 60 ml separatory funnel), add 15 ml of zinc acetate-salt solution, cap, and shake vigorously for 10 sec. Filter through 15 cm prefolded paper into a 50 ml graduated cylinder. Transfer 15 ml of this filtrate to a second culture tube (or 30 ml separatory funnel). Add 3 ml of benzene, cap, shake gently for 10 sec. and allow the layers to separate.

Chromatography and determination. Pipet 1.0 ml of the benzene (upper) layer onto the column. Clamp the column in an upright position and allow the solution to drain until it reaches the top of the packing. Pipet 3 ml of $CHCl_3$-acetone (9:1) solution onto the column and allow this to drain until the solution reaches the top of the packing.

Examine sample and reference columns in a darkened room under UV light or in a viewing cabinet. The presence of aflatoxin is indicated by a blue fluorescent band at the top of the Florisil layer (about 2 cm from the bottom of the column).

Aflatoxin M_1 in dairy products

Summary. Samples of fluid milk, powdered milk, cheese, or butter are extracted with acetone-water. Samples are cleaned up by lead acetate precipitation, liquid-liquid partition, and silica gel column chromatography using small-particle-size silica gel with a centrifuge to elute the wash and final solutions.

Aflatoxin M_1 may be determined by either TLC analysis or reverse-phase HPLC with a fluorescence detector. The limit of determination by either TLC or HPLC analysis is 0.1 ng/ml for fluid milk, 0.5 ng/g for powdered milk, and 0.25 ng/g for cheeses and butter.

Both the TLC and HPLC procedures include confirmation steps which are based on formation of the acetate derivatives and subsequent analysis.

Apparatus. (1) Explosion-proof blender with a 1 quart jar and cover; (2) polypropylene columns 65 × 9 (i.d.) mm with plastic filter disks and a 12 ml extension funnel [Quick-Sep No. 15-1550 (column) and 15-1570 (funnel), BioLab Products, San Jose, CA 95128, or equivalent]; (3) test tubes 125 × 14 (i.d.) mm; (4) thin layer chromatography equipment: glass plates 20 × 20 cm; applicator; mounting board; spotting template; 10 μl syringe; desiccating storage cabinet; chromatographic tank; long-wave 15 W UV lamp (use with UV-absorbing glasses) or viewing cabinet equipped with 15 W long-wave UV lamps; (5) liquid chromatograph capable of delivering 1 ml/min pulseless flow with high-pressure injection valve and 25 μl loop; (6) fluorescence detector; (7) liquid chromatographic column, 250 × 3 to 4 (i.d.) mm packed with 5 or 10 μm of octadecyl reverse-phase packing.

Reagents. (1) ACS grade acetone, hexane, ethyl ether, chloroform, methylene chloride, ethanol, isopropanol, acetonitrile, anhydrous ethyl ether; (2) lead acetate solution: (20%) dissolve 100 g of $Pb(OAc)_2 \cdot 3H_2O$ in water with warming, add 1.5 ml of acetic acid, and dilute to 500 ml; (3) sodium sulfate solution (saturated): add 75 g of anhydrous Na_2SO_4 to 250 ml of water in a 300 ml glass-stoppered Erlenmeyer flask, and stir or shake vigorously; (4) sodium chloride solution: (5%) dissolve 25 g of NaCl in 500 ml of water; (5) silica gel for column chromatography: Adsorbosil 5 (No. 16238 Applied Science Laboratories, State College, PA 16801); (6) silica gel for TLC: Macherey-Nagel GHR (Macherey, Nagel and Co., Duren, Germany, distributed by Brinkmann Instruments, Inc.), Applied Science Adsorbosils 1 or 5 (Applied Science Laboratories, State College, PA 16801) or Mallinckrodt Silic AR 4G or 7G, Mallinckrodt Chemical Co., St. Louis, MO 63134) or equivalent; (7) aflatoxin M_1 standard solutions: (a) stock solution (12.5 μg/ml): dissolve aflatoxin M_1 standard in acetonitrile to give a concentration of 12.5 μg/ml. To determine the actual concentration, scan this solution in a recording spectrometer from 370 to 320 nm against acetonitrile. Record the maximum absorbance (A) at about 350 nm and calculate the concentration using the following equation:

$$\mu g \text{ aflatoxin } M_1/ml = \frac{A \times MW \times 1000 \times CF}{E}$$

where

A = maximum absorbance measured

MW = 328

CF = correction factor for the particular spectrometer; obtained by scanning standard potassium dichromate solutions (0.25, 0.125, and 0.0625 mM in 0.018 N H_2SO_4 with molarity calculated to three significant figures) from 380 to 320 nm against 0.018 N H_2SO_4 and determining the maximum absorbance (A) near 350 nm; the molar absorptivity (E) is calculated at each concentration: E = (A × 1000)/conc. in mM and the CF should be between 0.95 and 1.05; calculate CF using the formula CF = 3160/E, where 3160 is the value for E for $K_2Cr_2O_7$ solution

E = 19,850 for aflatoxin M_1

(b) TLC standard solution (0.5 μg/ml): pipet 1.0 ml of the aflatoxin M_1 stock solution into a 25 ml volumetric flask and dilute to mark with benzene; (c) HPLC standard solution (20 ng/ml): pipet 1.0 ml of the TLC standard solution [reagent 7(b)] into a 25 ml volumetric flask and dilute to mark with benzene-acetonitrile (99:1); (8) reagent grade pyridine and acetic anhydride; (9) 4-DMAP solution: dissolve 49 mg of 4-dimethylaminopyridine (No. 10770-0, Aldrich Chemical Co., Milwaukee, WI 53233) in 10.0 ml of dry methylene chloride.

Sample Preparation and Extraction. Cut cheese samples into small cubes. Using the table below, weigh the amount of cheese, powdered milk, or butter, or measure fluid milk into a blender jar and add the amount of water listed.

Product	Sample volume or weight	Water added before extraction (ml)
Fluid milk	100 ml	10
Powdered milk	20 g	100
Blue cheese	50 g	80
Ricotta cheese	50 g	65
Cheddar cheese	50 g	80
Butter	50 g	90

Add 10 g of diatomaceous earth and 300 ml of acetone and blend at moderate speed for 3 min. Filter through 32 cm folded filter paper into a 500 ml graduated cylinder.

Transfer 275 ml of filtrate to a 600 ml beaker. Add 20 ml of lead acetate solution (reagent 2) and 200 ml of water to the beaker, stir, and allow to stand for 5 min. Add 10 ml of saturated sodium sulfate solution (reagent 3), stir, and filter through 32 cm folded filter paper into a 500 ml graduated cylinder. Transfer 350 ml of filtrate to a 500 ml separatory funnel, add 100 ml of hexane (with annatto-colored cheese or butter use ethyl ether), and shake vigorously for 1 min. Allow the layers to separate, and drain the lower aqueous layer into a 600 ml beaker. Discard the upper hexane (or ethyl ether) layer and pour the aqueous phase back into the same 500 ml separatory funnel. Rinse the beaker with 50 ml of 5% NaCl solution (reagent 4) and add this to the separatory funnel. Add 100 ml of chloroform to the separatory funnel and shake vigorously. Allow the layers to separate and drain the lower layer into the 600 ml beaker. In the same manner, extract the aqueous solution with an additional 50 ml of chloroform, combine the chloroform extracts, and discard the aqueous solution. Transfer the chloroform extract back into the separatory funnel, rinse the beaker with 100 ml of 5% NaCl solution, and add this to the funnel. Shake vigorously, allow the layers to separate, and drain the lower layer through a layer of anhydrous sodium sulfate in a funnel into a 250 ml beaker. Discard the aqueous salt solution, rinse the separatory funnel with two 10 ml portions of chloroform, and add these to the chloroform extract in the beaker. Evaporate the chloroform to 5 to 10 ml on a steam bath, transfer to a 4 dram vial using 2 ml of chloroform to rinse the beaker, and evaporate just to dryness under a stream of nitrogen.

Column Chromatography. To prepare silica gel slurry, weigh 30 g of Adsorbosil 5 silica gel into a 250 ml glass-stoppered Erlenmeyer flask, add 90 ml of chloroform, stopper, and shake vigorously. Immediately pipet 5 ml of the slurry into the polypropylene column and insert this column into a 125 × 15 mm test tube. Place a test tube holding column into a centrifuge and centrifuge at 1000 to 1200 rpm for 2 min. Examine column; silica gel should be firmly and evenly packed in the column and all the chloroform should be in the test tube. Discard chloroform and reinsert column into test tube.

Dissolve the sample extract in 5 ml of methylene chloride and transfer to column. Centrifuge at 1000 to 1200 rpm for 2 min. In the same manner, rinse the sample vial with 5 ml of methylene chloride, add to column, and centrifuge. Discard solvent collected in test tube. Successively add 5 ml of anhydrous ethyl ether and 4 ml of chloroform to the column; after the addition of each solvent, centrifuge at 1000 to 1200 rpm for 2 min. Discard eluant collected in test tube and place column in a clean test tube. Add 8 ml of methylene chloride-absolute ethanol (96:4) to the column and centrifuge for 3 min. Evaporate the eluant collected in the test tube to about 1 ml, carefully transfer to a 2 dram vial, rinse the test tube with 1 ml of chloroform, and add this to the vial. Evaporate the extract just to dryness under a stream of nitrogen. M_1 may be determined by TLC or HPLC analysis or by both of these techniques. If the determination is to be made by TLC, dissolve the sample extract in 100 μl of chloroform; if the determination is to be made by HPLC, dissolve the extract in 500 μl of water-acetonitrile (65:35); if the determination is to be made by both TLC and HPLC, dissolve the extract in 2.0 ml of chloroform, pipet 1.0 ml to a separate 2 dram vial, and evaporate both solutions just to dryness under a stream of nitrogen; dissolve the extract in one vial in 50 μl of chloroform for TLC analysis, and dissolve the extract in the second vial in 250 μl of water-acetonitrile for HPLC analysis. After adding either solvent to the extract, shake the vial vigorously to ensure that the extract is completely dissolved.

Determination by TLC. Coat 20 × 20 cm glass plates to a thickness of 0.25 mm with an aqueous slurry of one of the silica gels listed under "Reagents." Activate the plates by heating at 110° for 1 hr and store them in a desiccating cabinet with active silica gel desiccant until just before use. Prepare developing solvent of chloroform-acetone-isopropanol (85:10:5).

Spot 2, 4, 6, 8, and 10 μl of the aflatoxin standard (0.5 μg/ml) and 20 and 10 μl of the sample extract about 1.5 cm apart on an imaginary line about 4 cm from the bottom of the plate. Develop the plate in a closed, unlined, equilibrated tank with the developing solvent to a height of about 12 cm. Remove the plate and air dry. View the plate under long-wave UV light. Aflatoxin M_1 appears as a blue fluorescent spot having an R_f of about 0.5. Compare fluorescent intensities of the sample aflatoxin M_1 spots with those of the standard spots and determine which sample portion matches one of the standards. Calculate the concentration of aflatoxin M_1 in ng/g (ppb) using the formula

$$\text{ng aflatoxin } M_1/\text{g (or ml)} = \frac{S \times C \times V}{X \times W}$$

where

S = μl of aflatoxin M_1 standard equal to sample
C = concentration (μg/ml) of aflatoxin M_1 standard
V = μl of final dilution of sample extract
X = μl of sample extract spotted giving fluorescence intensity equal to S
W = amount of sample represented by final extract in g or ml = 47.6 ml for fluid milk, 9.5 g for powdered milk, and 23.8 g for cheeses and butter if the extract from the column chromatography step was used only for the determination by TLC; if the extract from the column was divided for determination by both TLC and HPLC, W = 23.8 ml, 4.8 g, and 11.9 g for fluid milk, powdered milk, and cheeses and butter, respectively

Confirmation by Derivative Formation and TLC Analysis. Evaporate the remainder of the sample extract in the vial to dryness. Transfer 50 μl of the aflatoxin M_1 TLC standard solution [reagent 7(b), 0.5 μg M_1/ml] into a separate 2 dram (7 ml) vial and evaporate just to dryness. Add 50 μl of pyridine and 100 μl of acetic anhydride to both vials, cap with Teflon-lined caps, and shake vigorously. Allow the solutions to stand at room temperature for 15 min.; then evaporate the solutions to dryness on a steam bath under a stream of nitrogen. Dissolve the contents of both vials in 30 μl of chloroform by shaking vigorously.

Spot 20 µl of the acetate derivative solutions of the sample and standard and 4 µl of the aflatoxin M_1 standard solution [reagent 7(b)] on separate spots on a TLC plate. Develop the plate in an unlined, unequilibrated tank for about 1 hr, using chloroform-acetone (9:1) as the developing solvent. Remove the plate and air dry. Examine the plate under long-wave (365 nm) UV light. Aflatoxin M_1 and M_1 acetate appear as fluorescent spots having R_f values of about 0.11 and 0.55, respectively.

Determination by HPLC. Prepare HPLC mobile solvent of water-acetonitrile (65:35). Set the flow rate at 0.8 ml/min. Set the fluorescence detector excitation at 350 nm (or use a 320 to 380 nm bandpass filter) and the emission cutoff filter at 410 nm. Pipet 1.0, 1.0, 2.0, 3.0, and 4.0 ml of the aflatoxin M_1 HPLC standard solution (20 ng/ml) into separate 2 dram vials and evaporate just to dryness under a stream of nitrogen. Pipet 2.0 ml of the HPLC mobile solvent into the first vial and 1.0 ml into each of the four remaining vials to give concentrations of 10, 20, 40, 60, and 80 ng of aflatoxin M_1/ml. Inject 25 µl of the lowest standard solution (10 ng M_1/ml) into the liquid chromatograph and adjust the sensitivity and gain controls to give a response of 5 to 10% of full scale. Inject 25 µl of each of the standard solutions into the liquid chromatograph and prepare a standard curve by plotting peak height versus concentration (µg/ml).

Inject 25 µl of the sample solution into the liquid chromatograph under the same conditions used in preparing the standard curve. Identify the aflatoxin M_1 peak in the sample by comparison of retention times with that of the standard. If the sample peak is larger than the highest standard peak, quantitatively dilute the sample with the HPLC mobile solvent and reinject. Determine the concentration of aflatoxin M_1 in the sample extract directly from the standard curve. Calculate the amount of aflatoxin M_1 in the sample using the following formula:

$$\text{Aflatoxin } M_1\text{, ng/g (or ml) sample (ppb)} = \frac{A \times B}{C}$$

where

A = concentration (ng/ml) of aflatoxin M_1 in sample extract

B = volume (ml) of sample extract

C = amount (g) of sample represented by final extract; C = 47.6 ml for fluid milk, 9.5 g for powdered milk, and 23.8 g for cheeses and butter if the extract from the column chromatography step was used only for determination by HPLC; if the extract from the column was divided for determination by both TLC and HPLC C = 23.8 ml, 4.8 g, and 11.9 g for fluid milk, powdered milk, and cheeses and butter, respectively

Confirmation by Derivative Formation and HPLC Analysis. Evaporate the remainder of the sample solution to dryness. Pipet 2.0 ml of the aflatoxin M_1 HPLC standard solution [reagent 7(c), 20 ng M_1/ml] into a separate 2 dram (7 ml) vial and evaporate just to dryness. Add 50 μl of acetic anhydride and 500 μl of 4-DMAP solution (reagent 9) to each vial, cap with a Teflon-lined cap, and shake vigorously. Allow the solutions to sit at room temperature for 20 min.; then evaporate just to dryness under a stream of nitrogen. Dissolve the sample and the M_1 standard in 250 μl and 1.0 ml, respectively, of the HPLC mobile solvent.

Inject 25 μl of the standard M_1 acetate derivative solution into the liquid chromatograph under the same conditions used in the determination step. Aflatoxin M_1 acetate should have a retention time of about twice that of M_1. Inject 25 μl of the derivatized sample solution into the liquid chromatograph and confirm the presence of aflatoxin M_1 in the sample by comparing the retention time of the sample peak with that of the standard.

B. Citrinin

Summary

Citrinin is extracted from corn or barley with aqueous, acidified acetonitrile solution. Sample is cleaned up by liquid-liquid partition, first into chloroform and then into mild base, followed by acidification and extraction back into chloroform.

Citrinin may be determined by either of two thin layer chromatography (TLC) procedures or by high-pressure liquid chromatography (HPLC) using a fluorescence detector. The limits of determination by TLC and HPLC are 50 and 40 ng/g (ppb), respectively.

Apparatus

(1) Wrist action shaker; (2) thin layer chromatographic equipment: 20 × 20 cm glass plates, applicator, mounting board, spotting template, 10 μl syringe, desiccating storage cabinet, chromatographic tank, 15 W long-wave UV lamp (use with UV-absorbing eyeglasses); (3) fluorodensitometer: excitation 350 nm, emission cutoff filter 450 nm (SD-3000, Schoeffel Instrument Corp., Westwood, New Jersey) or equivalent; (4) liquid chromatograph capable of delivering 1 ml/min pulseless flow with high-pressure injection valve and 25 μl loop; (5) fluorescence detector: excitation, 336 nm; emission cutoff filter, 450 nm; (6) liquid chromatographic column: reverse phase, 10 μm (Partisil 10 ODS, Whatman Inc., 9 Bridewell Place, Clifton, NJ 07014) or equivalent.

Reagents

(1) Solvents: ACS grade acetonitrile, isooctane, chloroform, methanol, benzene; (2) solutions: 4% w/v KCl in water; 20% v/v H_2SO_4 in water, 5% w/v $NaHCO_3$ in water, 6N HCl, 0.25 N H_3PO_4, 10% w/v oxalic acid in methanol, 0.05 M EDTA: dissolve 18.6 g of ethylenediaminetetraacetic acid, disodium salt dihydrate ($Na_2EDTA \cdot 2H_2O$) in 1 liter of distilled water; (3) Silica Gel 60 for TLC or precoated, 0.25 mm thick plates of Silica Gel 60 (EM Laboratories, Inc., 500 Executive Boulevard, Elmsford, NY 10523); Adsorbosil-1 silica gel (Applied Science Laboratories, Inc., State College, PA 16801) or equivalent; (4) acetic acid, anhydrous sodium sulfate; (5) citrinin standard solution (10 μg/ml): weigh 1.0 mg of citrinin into a 100 ml volumetric flask and dilute to volume with chloroform (prepare this solution fresh daily).

Sample extraction and liquid-liquid partition

Grind samples of corn or barley to pass a 2 mm opening. Weigh 25 g of ground sample into a 500 ml glass-stoppered Erlenmeyer flask. Add 180 ml of acetonitrile, 20 ml of 4% KCl solution, and 2 ml of 2% sulfuric acid solution. Secure the stopper in place with masking tape and shake vigorously for 10 min. with a wrist action shaker. Filter sample through fluted filter paper into a 250 ml graduated cylinder. Transfer 100 ml of filtrate to a 250 ml separatory funnel, add 50 ml of isooctane, and shake gently for 1 min. Allow the layers to separate; then drain the lower phase into a second 250 ml separatory funnel. Discard the isooctane and rinse the funnel with chloroform. Add 25 ml of water and 50 ml of chloroform to the aqueous solution and shake gently for 1 min. Allow the layers to separate and drain the lower layer into the rinsed separatory funnel. Extract the aqueous solution with a second 50 ml portion of chloroform. Combine the chloroform extracts, discard the aqueous solution, and rinse the separatory funnel with chloroform. Add 25 ml of 5% sodium bicarbonate solution to the combined chloroform extracts and shake gently for 1 min.; allow the layers to separate. Transfer the chloroform layer to the rinsed separatory funnel, and collect the alkaline solution in a 400 ml beaker. In the same manner extract the chloroform solution with two additional portions of 5% sodium bicarbonate solution. Combine the alkaline extracts in the 400 ml beaker; discard the chloroform solution and rinse the separatory funnel with chloroform. Acidify the alkaline extract to pH 2 (pH meter or test paper) by slowly adding $HCl\text{-}H_2O$ solution (1:1) while stirring. Transfer the acidic solution to a rinsed, 250 ml separatory funnel. Shake gently for 30 sec., allow the layers to separate, and drain the lower layer into a 250 ml beaker through a glass funnel containing 30 g of anhydrous sodium sulfate. Extract the acidic solution with a second 50 ml portion of chloroform in the same manner. Combine the chloroform extracts in the beaker and evaporate to about 5 ml on a steam bath (40°) under a stream of nitrogen. Transfer the extract to a 4 dram vial, using a few milliliters of chloroform to rinse the beaker, and evaporate just to dryness under a stream of nitrogen.

Citrinin may be determined by either of two TLC procedures or by HPLC analysis or by both of these techniques. For determination by TLC only, dissolve the sample extract in 500 μl of chloroform; for determination by HPLC only, dissolve the sample extract in 500 μl of 0.25 N H_3PO_4-acetonitrile (75:25). For determination by TLC and HPLC, dissolve the sample extract in 2.0 ml of chloroform, pipet 1.0 ml into a separate 3 dram vial, and evaporate both solutions just to dryness under a stream of nitrogen. Dissolve one extract in 250 μl of chloroform for TLC analysis and the second extract in 250 μl of 0.25 N H_3PO_4-acetonitrile (75:25) for HPLC analysis.

Determination by TLC (procedure 1)

Prepare 20 × 20 cm glass plates of silica gel 60 (0.25 mm thick) or use precoated plates. Dip the plates in a solution of 10% (w/v) oxalic acid in methanol for 2 min., remove, and air dry overnight. Prepare developing solvent of chloroform-hexane-methanol (64:35:1) just prior to use.

Spot 2, 5, and 10 μl of the sample extract and 1, 2, 4, 6, and 8 μl of the citrinin standard (10 μg/ml in chloroform) about 1.5 cm apart on an imaginary line about 4 cm from the bottom of the plate. In addition, spot 5 μl of the standard solution on top of a separate 5 μl spot of the extract. Develop the plate in a closed, unlined, equilibrated tank with the developing solvent to a height of about 15 cm. Remove the plate and air dry. View the plate under long-wave UV light. Citrinin appears as a yellow fluorescent spot with an R_f of about 0.6. If the weakest sample spot is more intense than the strongest standard spot, quantitatively dilute the sample extract and re-chromatograph.

Calculate the amount of citrinin in the sample by comparing the citrinin sample spot with a standard spot of equal intensity using the following formula:

$$\text{ng citrinin/g sample (ppb)} = \frac{S \times C \times V}{X \times W}$$

where

S = μl of standard equal to sample
C = concentration (μg/ml) of standard
V = final volume (μl) of sample
X = μl of sample spot which had fluorescence intensity equal to the standard spot
W = amount of (g) sample represented by final extract

Determination by TLC (procedure 2)

Prepare 20 × 20 cm glass plates by mixing 55 g of Adsorbosil-1 silica gel with 65 ml of the 0.05 M EDTA solution, spreading the slurry to a wet thickness of 0.5 mm. Air dry the plates for 30 min., activate them by heating at 110° for 1 hr, and store them in a desiccating cabinet with active silica gel desiccant until just before use. Prepare developing solvent of benzene-acetic acid (95:5).

Spot 2, 5, and 10 µl of the sample extract and 1, 2, 4, 6, and 8 µl of the citrinin standard (10 µg/ml in chloroform) about 1.5 cm apart on an imaginary line about 4 cm from the bottom of the plate. In addition, spot 5 µl of the standard solution on top of a separate 5 µl spot of the sample. Develop the plate in an unlined, unequilibrated tank with the developing solvent to a height of about 15 cm. Remove the plate and air dry. View the plate under long-wave UV light. Citrinin appears as a yellow fluorescent spot with an R_f of about 0.8. If the weakest sample spot is more intense than the strongest standard spot, quantitatively dilute the sample and re-chromatograph.

For quantitative determinations, scan the plates with a fluorodensitometer with excitation set at 365 nm and emission set at 505 nm. Prepare a standard curve of response (integrator counts or peak heights) versus amount of citrinin per spot (ng). Determine the amount of citrinin in the sample spot directly from the standard curve. Calculate the amount of citrinin in the sample using the following formula:

$$\text{Citrinin, ng/g sample (ppb)} = \frac{A \times V}{B \times W}$$

where

A = ng of citrinin in sample spot (from standard curve)
V = volume (µl) of sample extract
B = volume (µl) of extract spotted
W = amount (g) of sample represented by extract

Alternatively, the amount of citrinin in the sample may be calculated by visual comparison, under long-wave UV light, of sample spots with standard spots of equal intensity and use of the formula given in TLC procedure 1.

Determination by HPLC

Standard Curve. For analysis of corn samples, prepare mobile solvent of 0.25 N H_3PO_4-acetonitrile (50:50); for analysis of barley samples prepare mobile solvent of methanol-0.25 N H_3PO_4 (55:45). Set the liquid chromatograph flow rate at 1.0 ml/min.

Pipet 5.0 ml of the citrinin standard solution (10 µg/ml) into a 50 ml volumetric flask and dilute to mark with chloroform. Pipet 1.0, 2.0, 3.0, 4.0, and 5.0 ml of this solution into separate 3 dram vials and evaporate to dryness under a stream of nitrogen at room temperature. Pipet 1.0 ml of 0.25 N H_3PO_4-acetonitrile (75:25) into each vial to give final concentrations of 1.0, 2.0, 3.0, 4.0, and 5.0 µg of citrinin/ml.

Inject 20 μl of the most dilute standard (1 μg/ml) into the liquid chromatograph and adjust the fluorescence detector sensitivity controls so as to give a response of 15 to 20% of full scale. Inject 20 μl of each of the standard solutions into the liquid chromatograph, and prepare a standard curve by plotting response versus concentration (μg/ml).

Determination. If sample extract was divided and one-half used for TLC determination, dissolve the second portion in 250 μl of 0.25 N H_3PO_4-acetonitrile (75:25); otherwise, dissolve the sample extract in 500 μl of 0.25 N H_3PO_4-acetonitrile (75:25). Inject 20 μl of the sample solution into the liquid chromatograph under the same conditions used for preparing the standard curve. Identify the citrinin peak in the sample by comparison of retention times with those of the standard. If the sample peak is larger than the highest standard peak, quantitatively dilute the sample and reinject. Determine the concentration of citrinin in the sample extract directly from the standard curve. Calculate the amount of citrinin in the sample using the following formula:

$$\text{citrinin ng/g sample (ppb)} = \frac{A \times B}{C \times 1000}$$

where

A = concentration (μg/ml) of citrinin in sample
B = volume (ml) of sample extract
C = amount (g) of sample represented by extract

C. Ochratoxins

Introduction

Ochratoxins A and B are extracted from grain samples with chloroform-aqueous H_3PO_4 or from green coffee samples with chloroform-water. Samples are cleaned up by adding the chloroform extract to a column containing aqueous $NaHCO_3$-diatomaceous earth, washing the column with hexane and chloroform to remove extraneous compounds and eluting the ochratoxins with 2% acetic acid in benzene. The determination of ochratoxins is carried out using either thin layer chromatography (TLC) analysis, with a determination limit of 40 ng/g, or analysis by reverse-phase HPLC with a fluorescence detector which has a limit of determination of 10 ng/g. The TLC procedure includes a confirmation step in which the plates may be sprayed with reagents which will alter the color and intensity of the ochratoxin spots. Confirmation of the ochratoxins may be carried out by forming the methyl ester derivatives and determining the derivatized samples by HPLC.

Apparatus

(1) Chromatographic column: 250 × 22 mm i.d. with stopcock; (2) thin layer chromatography (TLC) equipment: 20 × 20 cm glass plates, ap-

plicator, spotting template, desiccating storage cabinet, chromatographic tank, long- and short-wave UV lamp (use with UV-absorbing eyeglasses), densitometer; (3) liquid chromatograph with high-pressure injection valve and 25 μl loop; (4) liquid chromatographic column: 25 cm × 3 mm i.d. stainless steel, packed with 5 μm Spherisorb ODS (Applied Science Labs) or equivalent; (5) fluorescence detector: variablo-wavelength excitation with 425 nm emission cutoff filter (Schoeffel Instrument Corporation, Westwood, NJ 07675, Model 970, or equivalont).

Reagents

(1) Solvents: ACS grade chloroform, benzene, methanol, toluene, hexane; (2) reagents: phosphoric acid, sodium bicarbonate, acetic acid, aluminum chloride; (3) bicarbonate-diatomaceous earth mixture: soak acid-washed Celite 545 in methanol for 2 hr, filter through Buchner funnel, wash thoroughly with water, and dry at 150° overnight. Add 25 ml of 5% aqueous sodium bicarbonate to 50 g of the dry diatomaceous earth and mix well; (4) silica gel for TLC: Adsorbosil 1 or 5 (Applied Science Laboratories, State College, PA 16801) or Silic AR 4G or 7G (Mallinckrodt Chemical Co., St. Louis, MO 63134); (5) standard solutions: (a) stock solutions: weigh 2.5 mg of ochratoxin A (or B) into separate 50 ml volumetric flasks and dilute to the mark with benzene-acetic acid (99:1). Determine the concentration of these solutions from the UV spectrum by scanning these solutions from 350 to 300 nm with a spectrophotometer, using 1 cm cells with benzene-acetic acid (99:1) in the reference cell. Calculate the concentration of ochratoxins using the following formula:

$$\mu\text{g ochratoxin A (or B)/ml} = \frac{A \times MW \times 1000 \times CF}{E}$$

where

A = absorption at the wavelength of maximum absorption
MW = molecular weight (403 for ochratoxin A and 369 for ochratoxin B)
CF = correction factor for a particular instrument as determined by using standard potassium dichromate solutions (may be taken as 1 for most modern instruments)
E = molar absorptivity (5550 for ochratoxin A and 6000 for ochratoxin B)

(b) working solution: pipet 2.0 ml of each of the stock solutions into a 100 ml volumetric flask and dilute to the mark with benzene-acetic acid to give a final concentration of 1.0 μg of ochratoxin A and B/ml; (6) boron trifluoride-methanol, 14% BF_3 (w/v) (No. 18002, Applied Science Laboratories, State College, PA 16801, or equivalent).

Sample preparation and extraction

Grind samples of grain (corn, oats, wheat, or barley) or green coffee to pass a 2 mm opening. Weigh 25 g of ground sample into a 250 ml glass-stoppered Erlenmeyer flask. Add 125 ml of chloroform and 12.5 ml of 0.05 M H_3PO_4 (for green coffee, add 12.5 ml of water); secure the stopper with masking tape. Shake 30 min. on a wrist action shaker and filter through 32 cm fluted filter paper into a 250 ml graduated cylinder.

Column chromatography

Place a small plug of glass wool in the bottom of the 250 × 22 mm i.d. glass column. Transfer 6 g of the $NaHCO_3$-diatomaceous earth mixture to the column and tamp it firmly to form an even layer at the bottom of the column. Transfer 100 ml of the sample extract to the column and elute until the solution just reaches the top of the packing. Wash the column with 70 ml of hexane followed by 70 ml of chloroform; discard the washings. Add 100 ml of benzene-acetic acid (98:2) to the column and collect the eluate in a 150 ml beaker. Evaporate this solution to about 5 ml on a steam bath ($\leq$40°) under a stream of nitrogen, and quantitatively transfer to a 4 dram vial, using a few milliliters of chloroform to rinse the vial. Evaporate to dryness under a stream of nitrogen.

If determination of ochratoxins is to be carried out by TLC, dissolve sample in 1.0 ml of benzene-acetic acid (99:1). If determination is to be carried out by HPLC, dissolve the sample in 1.0 ml of the mobile solvent. If the determination is to be carried out by both TLC and HPLC, pipet 2.0 ml of chloroform into the sample vial, swirl to dissolve the contents, pipet 1.0 ml of this solution into a separate 4 dram vial, and evaporate the solution in both vials to dryness. Dissolve the contents of one vial in 0.5 ml of benzene-acetic acid (99:1) for analysis by TLC; dissolve the contents of the second vial in 0.5 ml of the mobile solvent for analysis by HPLC.

Analysis by TLC

Coat 20 × 20 cm glass plates to a thickness of 0.25 mm with an aqueous slurry of one of the silica gels listed under "Reagents." Activate the plates by heating at 110° for 1 hr and store in a desiccating cabinet with active silica gel desiccant until just before use. Prepare developing solvent of benzene-methanol-acetic acid (90:5:5) [alternative solvent: toluene-ethyl acetate-formic acid (5:4:1); this is the preferred solvent for samples of green coffee].

Spot 2, 6, and 10 μl of the sample extract and 5, 7.5, and 10 μl of the ochratoxin A and B standard solution (1 μg/ml each) on separate spots about 1.5 cm apart on an imaginary line about 4 cm from the bottom of the plate. Develop the plate in a closed, unlined, unequilibrated tank with the developing solvent to a height of about 15 cm.

Remove the plate, air dry, and view under long- and short-wave UV light. Ochratoxin A and B appear as greenish-blue fluorescent spots with R_f values of about 0.65 and 0.5, respectively. Ochratoxin A appears most intense when viewed under long-wave UV light; ochratoxin B appears most intense under short-wave UV light. If the weakest sample spot is more intense than the strongest standard spot, quantitatively dilute the sample and rechromatograph. Calculate the amount of ochratoxins A and B in the sample by comparing the ochratoxin spot in the sample with a standard spot of equal intensity using the following formula:

$$\text{ng ochratoxin A (or B)/g sample (ppb)} = \frac{S \times C \times V}{X \times W}$$

where

S = μl of standard solution equal to the sample
C = concentration (μg/ml) of the standard
V = final volume (μl) of the sample
X = μl of the sample extract which had fluorescence intensity equal to the standard spot
W = amount (g) of sample represented by final extract

The amount of ochratoxin A and B in the sample may be determined by fluorodensitometric analysis of the TLC plates. Scan the plate with the densitometer according to the instructions of the manufacturer. Optimum spectral settings for ochratoxins A and B are: excitation, 300 to 365 nm; emission cutoff, 450 nm.

Confirmation by TLC

Spray the TLC plate with either alcoholic sodium bicarbonate solution [6 g of $NaHCO_3$ in water-ethanol (100:20)] or alcoholic aluminum chloride solution (20 g of $AlCl_3 \cdot 6H_2O$ in 100 ml of ethanol) or expose the plate to ammonia fumes. Air dry the plate and view under long-wave UV light. The fluorescence of ochratoxin changes from greenish blue to bright blue and increases in intensity.

Determination by HPLC analysis

Prepare mobile solvent as follows: Dissolve 1.36 g of monobasic potassium phosphate in 500 ml of distilled water, add 500 ml of acetonitrile, and mix. Adjust the pH of this solution to 3.0 (pH meter) with 1 M H_3PO_4 solution. Deaerate this solution. Set the fluorescence detector excitation at 323 nm (or use a 300 to 360 nm bandpass filter) and emission cutoff filter at 425 nm.

Pipet 1.0, 1.0, 2.0, 3.0, 4.0, and 5.0 ml of the ochratoxin A and B standard solution (1 μg/ml each) into separate 4 dram vials and evaporate just to dryness under a stream of nitrogen. Pipet 2.0 ml of the mobile solvent into the first vial and 1.0 ml into each of the remaining five vials to give final concentrations of 0.5, 1.0, 2.0, 3.0, 4.0, and 5.0 μg ochratoxin A and B/ml. Set the liquid chromatographic flow rate at 1.0 ml/min. and the range and sensitivity controls so that a 20 μl injection of the most dilute standard solution (0.5 μg/ml) gives a response of 5 to 10% of full scale for ochratoxin A and B. Inject 20 μl of each of the standard solutions into the liquid chromatograph and prepare standard curves by plotting response versus concentration (μg/ml).

Inject 20 μl of the sample solution into the liquid chromatograph under the same conditions as those used for preparing the standard curve. Identify the ochratoxin A and B peaks in the sample by comparison of retention times with those of the standard. If the sample peak is larger than the highest standard peak, quantitatively dilute the sample with the mobile solvent and reinject. Determine the concentration of ochratoxin A and B in the sample extract directly from the standard curve: Calculate the amount of ochratoxin A and B in the sample using the following formula:

$$\text{ng ochratoxin A (or B)/g sample (ppb)} = \frac{A \times B}{C \times 1000}$$

where

A = concentration (μg/ml) of ochratoxin A (or B) in sample extract
B = volume (ml) of sample extract
C = amount (g) of sample represented by extract

Confirmation by HPLC

Pipet 3.0 ml of the ochratoxin A and B standard solution [reagent 5(b)] into a 3 dram vial and evaporate to dryness under a stream of nitrogen. Add 1.0 ml of 14% BF_3 in methanol (reagent 6), cap the vial, and heat on a steam bath at 50 to 60° for 10 min. Transfer the solution to a 60 ml separatory funnel using two 5 ml portions of water to rinse the vial. Add 15 ml of $CHCl_3$ to the funnel and shake gently for 1 min. Transfer the lower layer to a 50 ml beaker. In the same manner extract the aqueous solution with a second 15 ml portion of $CHCl_3$ and combine the extracts in the beaker. Evaporate the $CHCl_3$ extracts to a few milliliters, transfer the solution to a 3 dram vial, and evaporate to dryness. Dissolve the derivatized standards in 1.0 ml at the HPLC mobile solvent.

Evaporate the sample extract to dryness. Prepare the methyl ester derivatives, using 14% BF_3 in methanol, and following the procedure described for the ochratoxin standards.

Inject 20 μl of the ochratoxin A and B methyl ester standard solution into the liquid chromatograph under the same conditions used in analyzing for ochratoxins. In the same manner, inject 20 μl of the derivatized sample extract into the liquid chromatograph and confirm the presence of ochratoxin in the sample by comparing the retention time of the sample peaks with those in the standard.

D. Patulin

Summary

Patulin is extracted from apple juice, apple butter, or other apple-based products with ethyl acetate. Sample is cleaned up by silica gel column chromatography; patulin is than determined by either thin layer chromatography (TLC) or high-pressure liquid chromatography (HPLC). The TLC procedure includes a confirmation step which is based on isolating patulin from the sample by preparative TLC and rechromatographing the extracted material on three additional TLC plates with different solvent systems. The limit of determination for patulin in apple juice by TLC analysis is about 20 to 25 ng/ml. The HPLC procedure includes an optional step for collecting the patulin peak for confirmation by UV absorption spectroscopy or mass spectrometric analysis. The limit of determination for patulin in apple juice by HPLC analysis is about 10 ng/g.

When apple juice containers are opened and the contents exposed to air, a compound is rapidly formed which interferes with the determination of patulin by TLC analysis, and also to some degree by HPLC analysis. For this reason apple juice and other apple-based products should be analyzed immediately after opening the container.

Apparatus

(1) Wrist action shaker; (2) glass chromatographic columns, 350 mm × 22 mm i.d. with 300 ml reservoir and stopcock; (3) thin layer chromatographic equipment: glass plates, 20 × 20 cm; applicator; mounting board; spotting template; 10 μl syringe; desiccating storage cabinet; chromatographic tank; long-wave 15 W UV lamp (use with UV-absorbing eyeglasses) or viewing cabinet equipped with 15 W, long-wave UV lamps; spray bottle; sample streaker for preparative TLC; (4) liquid chromatograph capable of delivering 1 ml/min., pulseless flow with high-pressure injection valve, 50 μl loop and 254 nm UV detector; (5) liquid chromatographic column, 250 mm × 2.1 mm i.d. stainless steel, packed with 5 μm of silica or equivalent.

Reagents

(1) Solvents: ACS grade benzene, ethyl acetate, ethyl ether (containing 2% ethanol as a preservative), toluene, chloroform, isooctane; (2) silica gel 60 (for column chromatography), 0.063 to 0.200 mm (EM Laboratories, Inc., Elmsford, NY 10523), or equivalent; (3) Adsorbosil-5 silica gel for TLC (Applied Science Laboratories, State College, PA 16801) or one of the following precoated plates: E. Merck silica gel G Uniplate (Analtech, Inc., Newark, DE 19711), Camag silica gel precoated plate No. 30079 (Mondrag Ltd., Montreal, Quebec, Canada) or

equivalent; (4) MBTH-3-methyl-3-benzothiazolinone hydrochloride (Aldrich Chemical Co., Milwaukee, WI 53233); (5) formic acid, 90% w/w, anhydrous sodium sulfate; (6) patulin standard solutions: (a) stock solution (100 μg/ml); weigh 5.0 mg of patulin into a 50 ml volumetric flask and dilute to mark with chloroform (b) standard solution for TLC (10 μg/ml); pipet 5.0 ml of the stock solution into a 50 ml volumetric flask and dilute to the mark with chloroform; (c) standard solution for HPLC (4 μg/ml); pipet 2.0 ml of the stock solution into a 50 ml volumetric flask and dilute to the mark with ethyl acetate.

Extraction

Analyze samples immediately after opening the can or bottle. (1) Apple juice: transfer 50 ml of juice to a 250 ml separatory funnel and extract with three 50 ml portions of ethyl acetate. Pass the ethyl acetate extracts through 30 g of anhydrous sodium sulfate in a glass funnel into a 250 ml beaker; wash the sodium sulfate with 20 ml of ethyl acetate, and evaporate the combined ethyl acetate solutions to 15 to 20 ml on a steam bath under a stream of nitrogen. (Caution: Do not evaporate to dryness.)

Column chromatography

Transfer the sample extract to a 100 ml graduated cylinder. Rinse the beaker with 5 ml of ethyl acetate, and add this rinse to the graduated cylinder; adjust the volume to the 25 ml mark with ethyl acetate. Add 75 ml of benzene to the graduated cylinder and stir to mix the solution.

Place a small plug of glass wool in the bottom of the column. Add 25 ml of benzene; then add a slurry of 15 g of silica gel 60 in 25 ml of benzene to the column. Stir the silica gel with a long rod to remove any bubbles and let the silica gel settle. Add 15 g of anhydrous sodium sulfate to the column, and drain the solvent to the top of the packing. Add the sample extract to the column, drain to the top of the packing, and discard the eluate. Elute patulin from the column with 200 ml of benzene-ethyl acetate (75:25); collect the eluate in a 250 ml beaker. Evaporate the eluate to about 55 ml on a steam bath under a stream of nitrogen; then transfer the residue to a 4 dram vial. Rinse the beaker with 2 ml of ethyl acetate and add this to the vial. Evaporate the extract to dryness under a stream of nitrogen.

Patulin may be deterined by TLC or HPLC or both. For determination by TLC only, immediately dissolve the sample extract in 500 μl of chloroform; for determination by HPLC only, dissolve the sample extract in 500 μl of ethyl acetate; for determination by both procedures, dissolve the sample extract in 2.0 ml of ethyl acetate, pipet 1.0 ml into a separate 2 dram vial, and evaporate both solutions just to dryness under a stream of nitrogen at room temperature. Dissolve one sample extract in 250 μl of chloroform for TLC determination and dissolve the second extract in 250 μl of ethyl acetate for HPLC determination. If the TLC or HPLC determination are not to be performed on the same day, store the extracts in a freezer to prevent evaporation of the solvent.

Determination by TLC

Prepare 20 × 20 cm plates of Adsorbsil-5 silica gel (0.25 mm wet thickness) using 50 g of the adsorbent to 55 ml of distilled water or use any of the precoated plates listed under "Apparatus." Activate the plates by heating them at 110° for 1 hr., and store them in a desiccating cabinet with active silica gel desiccant until just before use. Prepare developing solvent of toluene-ethyl acetate-90% formic acid (5:4:1). Prepare TLC spray solution by dissolving 0.5 g of MBTH in 100 ml of distilled water. Store this solution in a refrigerator and prepare fresh every 3 days.

Spot 2, 5, and 10 μl of the sample extract and 1, 3, 5, 7, and 10 μl of the patulin standard (10 μg/ml in chloroform) about 1.5 cm apart on an imaginary line about 4 cm from the bottom of the plate. In addition, spot 5 μl of the standard solution on top of a separate 5 μl spot of the extract. Develop the plate in a closed, unlined, equilibrated tank with the developing solvent to a height of about 15 cm. Remove the plate and air dry. Spray the plate with the 0.5% MBTH solution until the layer appears wet; then heat the plate at 130° for 15 min. View the plate under long-wave UV light. Patulin appears as a yellow-brown fluorescent spot with an R_f of about 0.5. If the weakest sample spot is more intense than the strongest standard spot, dilute the sample extract and re-chromatograph.

The amount of patulin in the sample may be calculated by comparing the patulin spot in the sample with a standard spot of equal intensity using the following formula:

$$\text{ng patulin/ml (or g) of sample} = \frac{S \times C \times V}{X \times W}$$

where

S = μl of the standard solution equal to the sample
C = concentration (μg/ml) of the standard
V = final volume (μl) of the sample
X = μl of the sample extract spotted which had fluorescence intensity equal to the standard spot
W = amount (g) of sample represented by the final extract

Confirmation by TLC

Spot 5 μl of the standard solution as one spot and overlay 5 μl of the standard solution on top of a 10 μl spot of the sample as the second spot, on one side of a TLC plate. Streak the remainder of the sample extract on the rest of the TLC plate. Develop the plate as described above. Dry the plate in air; cover most of the plate with a second plate and spray the standards and about 1 cm of the sample-streak portion of the plate with the 0.5% MBTH solution. Heat the plate at 130° for 15 min. Remove the unsprayed patulin band with a suction and filter device or scrape the band into a small glass funnel containing a small plug of Pyrex wool. Elute patulin from the silica gel with 10 ml of chloroform-acetone (2:1) into a 4 dram vial. Evaporate the eluate just to dryness under a stream of nitrogen and immediately dissolve in 100 μl of chloroform. Spot 10 and 20 μl of the sample solution and 5 μl of the standard solution on three separate TLC plates. Develop the plates in unlined, unequilibrated tanks with the following solvents: hexane-anhydrous ethyl ether (1:3), chloroform-methanol (95:5), and chloroform-acetone (90:10). Air dry, spray with the 0.5% MBTH solution, and heat the plates as described above. The patulin in the sample should have the same R_f as that of the standard for confirmation.

Determination by HPLC

Standard Curve. Prepare HPLC mobile solvent of isooctane-ethyl ether-acetic acid (750:250:0.5). Set the liquid chromatographic flow rate at 0.5 ml/min. and the detector range at 0.01 AUFS.

Pipet 0.5, 1.0, 2.0, 3.0, and 4.0 ml of the patulin standard solution (4.0 μg/ml) into separate 2 dram vials, and evaporate to dryness under a stream of nitrogen at room temperature. Pipet 1.0 ml of ethyl acetate into each vial to give final concentrations of 2.0, 4.0, 8.0, 12.0, and 16.0 μg of patulin/ml. Inject 20 μl of each of the standard solutions into the liquid chromatograph, and prepare a standard curve by plotting peak height versus concentration (μg/ml).

Determination. Inject 20 μl of the sample solution into the liquid chromatograph under the same conditions used for preparing the standard curve. Identify the patulin peak in the sample by comparison of retention volumes with those of the standard. If the sample peak is larger than the highest standard peak, quantitatively dilute the sample with ethyl acetate and reinject. Determine the concentration of patulin in the sample extract directly from the standard curve. Calculate the amount of patulin in the sample using the following formula:

$$\text{Patulin ng/ml sample (ppb)} = \frac{A \times B}{C \times 1000}$$

where

A = concentration (μg/ml) of patulin in sample extract
B = volume (ml) of sample extract
C = amount (g) of sample represented by extract (50 g if TLC analysis was not carried out, 25 g if sample extract was divided and one-half used for TLC)

Confirmation

After determination of the patulin content, concentrate the remaining sample solution to about 100 μl. Inject 50 μl of this solution into the liquid chromatograph under the same conditions used for determining the patulin content except set the detector range at 0.1 AUFS. Collect the peak with the same retention time as patulin. Inject a second 50 μl portion of the sample solution and collect the patulin peak. Combine the collected peaks and evaporate just to dryness. Confirm the presence of patulin in the sample by mass spectrometric analysis. Alternatively, dissolve the patulin isolated from the sample in sufficient ethyl alcohol to give a concentration of 5 to 10 μg/ml. Scan this solution with a UV spectrophotometer from 350 to 250 nm and compare the spectrum obtained to that of a standard patulin solution in the same solvent.

E. Penicillic Acid

Summary

Penicillic acid is extracted from samples of grains, dried beans, or cheese with ethyl acetate, partitioned into mild base, acidified, and partitioned back into ethyl acetate. At this point an aliquot of the extract may be screened for penicillic acid by thin layer chromatographic (TLC) analysis. The limit of determination for the TLC procedure is 50 ng/g. Some samples may contain compounds which interfere with the determination; with these, the sample extract is further cleaned up by silica gel column chromatography.

Penicillic acid may be determined by either high-pressure liquid chromatography (HPLC) or gas-liquid chromatography (GLC) after formation of the trifluoroacetate (TFA) derivative. Determination by HPLC requires a variable-wavelength UV detector set at 270 nm or a fixed-wavelength detector at 254 nm. The limit of determination by HPLC analysis is 20 ng/g. Determination by GLC analysis requires an electron capture detector and has a limit of determination of 4 ng/g. Overall recovery of added penicillic acid at levels of 20 ng/g and above exceeds 80%. Penicillic acid is known to react with other sample constituents after samples have been ground: consequently, the extraction and cleanup through the liquid-liquid partitioning steps should be carried out as quickly as possible.

Apparatus

(1) Explosion-proof blender with 1 liter jar and cover; (2) pH meter (standardized at pH 3) or pH test paper; (3) glass chromatographic columns 250 × 14 mm i.d. with a 250 ml reservoir and stopcock; (4) thin layer chromatographic equipment: 20 × 20 cm glass plates;

applicator; mounting board; spotting template; 10 μl syringe; desiccating storage cabinet; chromatographic tank; long-wave UV lamp or viewing cabinet; spray bottle; (5) liquid chromatograph capable of delivering 1 ml/min. pulseless flow with a high-pressure injection valve and a 50 μl loop; (6) variable-wavelength liquid chromatographic detector or fixed-wavelength 254 nm detector; (7) liquid chromatographic column, 10 μm, C-18 reverse phase; (8) gas chromatograph with electron capture detector and recorder. GLC conditions: 6 ft × 2 to 3 mm i.d. glass column packed with 3% OV-17 on Gas Chrom Q (100-120 mesh) or equivalent packing; nitrogen gas flow rate, 70 to 80 ml/min; temperature (°C): injector, 160; detector, 215; column, 140 to 160 to elute penicillic acid TFA derivative in 6 to 8 min.

Reagents

(1) Solvents: ethyl acetate, benzene, isooctane, toluene, hexane; (2) silica gel for TLC: Adsorbosil-5 (Applied Science Laboratories, State College, PA 16801) or equivalent; (3) TLC developing solvent: toluene-ethyl acetate-90% formic acid (6:3:1); (4) TLC spray reagent: dissolve 0.5 ml of p-anisaldehyde (Aldrich Chemical Company, Inc., Milwaukee, WI 53233) in a solution of methanol-glacial acetic acid-concentrated sulfuric acid (70:10:5); (5) silica gel for column chromatography: silica gel 60, 0.063 to 0.200 mm (EM Laboratories, Inc., Elmsford, NY 10523); (6) column chromatography eluting solvent: hexane-ethyl acetate-glacial acetic acid (750:250:1); (7) penicillic acid standard solutions: (a) stock solution (100 μg/ml): weigh 10.0 mg of penicillic acid into a 100 ml volumetric flask and dilute to the mark with ethyl acetate containing 0.1% glacial acetic acid; (b) standard solution for HPLC and GLC analysis (1 μg/ml): pipet 1.0 ml of the penicillic acid stock solution into a 100 ml volumetric flask and dilute to the mark with ethyl acetate containing 0.1% glacial acetic acid.

Sample preparation

Grind samples of grain or dried beans to pass a 2 mm opening. Cut cheese samples into cubes of about 0.5 cm and mix. Weigh a 50 g sample into a blender jar; add 25 ml of 0.01 N HCl and 250 ml of ethyl acetate. Blend for 3 min at moderate speed. Filter the sample through folded filter paper into a 250 ml graduated cylinder.

Liquid-liquid partition

Transfer 200 ml of the sample extract to a 250 ml separatory funnel, add 25 ml of 3% sodium bicarbonate solution, shake gently for 30 sec, and allow the layers to separate. Drain the lower layer into a 150 ml beaker. In the same manner extract the sample solution with two additional 25 ml portions of 3% sodium bicarbonate solution and combine the alkaline extracts in the 150 ml beaker. Carefully add 1 N HCl solution to the alkaline solution with stirring until a pH of 3 is reached (pH meter or pH test paper). Transfer the acidic solution to a 250 ml separatory funnel, add 50 ml of ethyl acetate, and shake gently for 30 sec. Transfer the lower layer into another 250 ml separatory funnel and extract with a second 50 ml portion of ethyl acetate. Discard the aqueous solution, combine the ethyl acetate extracts, and drain them through 30 g of anhydrous sodium sulfate in a glass funnel into a 150 ml beaker. Wash the sodium sulfate with an additional 10 ml of ethyl acetate and add it to the beaker. Evaporate the ethyl acetate to about 5 ml on a steam bath and transfer to a 4 dram vial using a few milliliters of ethyl acetate to rinse the beaker. Evaporate the extract just to dryness under a stream of nitrogen at room temperature.

TLC screening procedures (optional)

Prepare 20 × 20 cm plates of Adsorbosil-5 (0.25 mm thick) silica gel and activate them at 110° for 2 hr.

Dissolve the sample extract in 4.0 ml of ethyl acetate. Transfer 1.0 ml of this solution to a 2 dram vial and evaporate to dryness under a stream of nitrogen at room temperature. Dissolve the extract in 100 μl of chloroform and gently swirl the vial to dissolve the contents. Spot 2, 5, and 10 μl of the sample and 1, 3, and 5 μl of the penicillic acid standard (100 μg/ml in chloroform) about 1.5 cm apart on an imaginary line about 4 cm from the bottom of the plate. Develop the plate in a closed, unequilibrated tank with the developing solvent to a height of about 15 cm. Remove the plate and allow the solvent to evaporate. Spray the plate with the p-anisaldehyde spray solution and then heat it at 130° for 8 min. View the plate under long-wave UV light. Penicillic acid appears as a blue spot with an R_f of about 0.5.

Column chromatography

Place a small plug of glass wool at the bottom of the column; then add 20 ml of the eluting solvent. Add 3 g of anhydrous sodium sulfate; then add 5 g of silica gel 60 and stir to remove any bubbles. Drain a few milliliters of solvent from the column to settle the silica gel; then add 3 g of anhydrous sodium sulfate to the top of the column. Dissolve the sample extract in 3 ml of the eluting solvent, shake gently to dissolve the contents, and add it to the column. Drain the solvent to the top of the column packing and collect the eluate in a graduated cylinder; do not allow the column to go dry. Rinse the vial with two 2 ml portions of the eluting solvent; add these to the column and drain the solution to the top of the packing. Add 245 ml of the eluting solvent to the column and drain the solution at about 3 ml/min. Discard the first 120 ml of eluate and collect the next 130 ml in a 150 ml beaker. Evaporate the eluate to about 5 ml on a steam bath; then transfer the sample to a 4 dram vial, rinsing the beaker with 2 ml of ethyl acetate. Evaporate the extract just to dryness under a stream of nitrogen.

Analysis by HPLC

Standard Curve. Pipet 1.0, 2.0, 3.0, 4.0, and 5.0 ml of the penicillic acid standard solution (1 μg/ml) into separate 3 dram vials and evaporate just to dryness under a stream of nitrogen. Prepare the trifluoroacetate (TFA) derivatives by adding 200 μl of trifluoroacetic anhydride to each vial, capping the vials immediately with Teflon-lined caps and allowing the vials to stand at room temperature for 15 min. with periodic swirling to wet the sides of the vials. Carefully evaporate off excess reagent, using a gentle stream of nitrogen. Dissolve each standard in 1.0 ml of the liquid chromatographic mobile solvent to give final concentrations of 1.0, 2.0, 3.0, 4.0, and 5.0 μg of penicillic acid as the trifluoroacetate per milliliter.

Set the liquid chromatographic flow rate at 1.0 ml/min, the variable-wavelength UV detector at 270 nm (a 254 nm fixed-wavelength UV detector may be used), and the detector sensitivity at 0.02 AUFS. Inject 25 μl of each standard solution into the liquid chromatograph and prepare a standard curve by plotting peak height versus concentration of the standard solution in μg/ml.

Determination. Form the penicillic acid TFA derivatives in the same manner described for the standards, adding 100 μl of trifluoroacetic anhydride to the dry sample extract. After evaporating the excess derivatization reagent, dissolve the sample extract in 1.0 ml of the liquid chromatographic mobile solvent. Inject 25 μl of this solution into the liquid chromatograph under the same conditions used in preparing the standard curve. Identify the penicillic acid TFA peak in the sample by comparison of retention times with the standard. If the sample peak is larger than the highest standard peak, quantitatively dilute the sample and reinject. Determine the concentration of penicillic acid in the sample extract directly from the standard curve. Calculate the amount of penicillic acid in the sample using the following formula:

$$\text{ng penicillic acid/g sample} = \frac{A \times B}{C \times 1000}$$

where

A = concentration (μg/ml) of penicillic acid in the sample extract
B = volume (ml) of sample extract
C = amount (g) of sample represented by the extract

Analysis by GLC with EC detector

Standard Curve. Pipet 0.5, 1.0, 1.5, 2.0, and 2.5 ml of the penicillic acid standard solution (1 μg/ml) into separate 3 dram vials and evaporate just to dryness under a stream of nitrogen. Prepare penicillic acid TFA derivatives by adding 200 μl of trifluoroacetic anhydride to each vial, capping the vials with caps lined with an inert material, and allowing the vials to stand at room temperature for 15 min. with swirling at 5 min. intervals to mix the solution. Carefully evaporate off the excess reagent under a stream of nitrogen. Dissolve each standard in 1.0 ml of isooctane to give final concentrations of 0.5, 1.0, 1.5, 2.0, and 2.5 μg of penicillic acid TFA/ml.

Set the GLC carrier gas flow rate at 60 to 70 ml/min. Inject 3.0 μl of the lowest standard (0.5 μg/ml) into the gas chromatograph and set the electrometer sensitivity to give a recorder response of 10 to 20% full scale deflection. Inject 3.0 μl of each of the standard solutions into the gas chromatograph, and prepare a standard curve of micrograms of penicillic acid (as the TFA derivative) versus response (peak height or integrator counts).

Determination. Form the penicillic acid-TFA derivative of the sample extract obtained from the column cleanup step in the same manner as described above. Inject 3.0 μl of the derivatized extract into the gas chromatograph under the same conditions used in obtaining the standard curve and identify the penicillic acid-TFA derivative in the sample by comparing the retention time of the sample peak with that obtained for the standards. If the peak from the sample extract is larger than the highest standard peak, quantitatively dilute the sample with isooctane and reinject. Determine the concentration of penicillic acid in the sample extract directly from the standard curve. Calculate the amount of penicillic acid in the sample using the following formula:

$$\text{ng penicillic acid/g sample (ppb)} = \frac{A \times B}{C \times 1000}$$

where

A = concentration (μg/ml) of penicillic acid in the sample extract
B = volume (ml) of sample extract
C = amount (g) of sample represented by the extract

F. Roquefortine and Isofumigaclavine A in Blue Cheese

Summary

Roquefortine and isofumigaclavine A are extracted from blue cheese with ethyl acetate. Samples are cleaned up by liquid-liquid partition, first into dilute aqueous HCl and then, after the aqueous solution is made alkaline, back into ethyl acetate. The determination of isofumigaclavine A is carried out by a TLC procedure. The limit of determination for this procedure is 100 ng/g. Roquefortine may be determined by either TLC or HPLC with ultraviolet (UV) and/or electrochemical (EC) detectors. The limits of determination by TLC and HPLC are 200 and 16 ng/g, respectively. In determining roquefortine in samples by HPLC, coupling the UV and EC detectors in series provides a rapid check of the amount of roquefortine present.

Apparatus

(1) Explosion-proof blender with 1 quart blender jar; (2) thin layer chromatography (TLC) equipment: 20 × 20 cm glass plates, applicator, spotting template, desiccating storage cabinet, chromatographic tank, spray bottle, 10 μl syringe; (3) liquid chromatograph with high-pressure injection valve and 25 μl loop; (4) liquid chromatographic column: 25 cm × 3 to 4 mm i.d. stainless steel column packed with 10 μm of LiChrosorb RP-2 (EM Laboratories, Inc., Elmsford, NY 10523) or equivalent; (5) UV detector with monochromator or 312 mm filter; (6) electrochemical detector: thin layer detector cell with amperometric controller (Bioanalytical Systems Inc., West Lafayette, IN 47906) or equivalent.

Reagents

(1) Solvents: ethyl acetate, methanol, chloroform; (2) HCl solution: dissolve 1.0 ml of concentrated HCl (35 to 38%) in 1 liter of distilled water; (3) silica gel for TLC: Adsorbosil I (Applied Science Labs., Inc., State College, PA 16801) or equivalent or silica gel F 1500/LS 254 thin layer sheets (Schleicher and Schuell); (4) liquid chromatograph mobile phase: dissolve 5.75 g of monobasic ammonium phosphate (0.05 M) in 1 liter of distilled water-methanol (50:50); (5) roquefortine standard solutions: (a) TLC solution (100 μg/ml): dissolve 2.5 mg of roquefortine in 25 ml of chloroform; (b) HPLC solution (1 μg/ml): pipet 1.0 ml of the TLC solution into a 100 ml volumetric flask and dilute to volume with ethyl acetate; (6) isofumigaclavine A standard solution (50 μg/ml): dissolve 1.0 mg of isofumigaclavine A in 20 ml of methylene chloride.

Sample extraction and liquid-liquid partition

Cut cheese samples into small cubes, mix, and transfer about 100 g to a 250 ml beaker. Warm on steam bath until cheese melts and stir to obtain a homogeneous mixture. Weigh 25 g of this sample into a blender jar, add 10 g of diatomaceous earth, and 250 ml of ethyl acetate and blend at high speed for 5 min. Filter sample through fluted paper into a 250 ml graduate cylinder. Transfer 100 ml of filtrate to a 250 ml separatory funnel, add 50 ml of the HCl solution (reagent 2), shake gently for about 20 sec., and allow the layers to separate. Transfer lower layer to another 250 ml separatory funnel and extract ethyl acetate solution with a second 50 ml portion of HCl solution. Combine acidic solutions in a second separatory funnel; slowly add 50 ml of 3% $NaHCO_3$ in distilled water and 50 ml of ethyl acetate. Shake gently for about 20 sec., allow the layers to separate, and transfer the lower layer to another separatory funnel. In the same manner extract the aqueous solution with a second 50 ml portion of ethyl acetate. Discard the aqueous layer, combine ethyl acetate extracts in a 250 ml Erlenmeyer flask, add a few boiling chips, and evaporate to 4 to 5 ml on a steam bath. Quantitatively transfer this solution to a 4 dram vial, rinsing the flask with 2 ml of ethyl acetate, and evaporate just to dryness on a steam bath under a gentle stream of nitrogen.

TLC screening procedure

Prepare 20 × 20 cm glass plates of silica gel (0.25 mm thick) and activate them at 110° for 1 hr. or use precoated plates.

Dissolve sample extract in 200 μl of methylene chloride. Spot 2, 5, and 10 μl of the sample extract and 5 and 10 μl of standard solutions of roquefortine (100 μg/ml in methylene chloride) and isofumigaclavine A (50 μg/ml in methylene chloride) on separate spots about 1.5 cm apart on an imaginary line about 4 cm from the bottom of the plate. Develop the plate in a closed, lined, equilibrated tank with chloroform-methanol-28% ammonium hydroxide (90:10:1) developing solvent to a height of about 15 cm. Remove the plate and air dry. Spray the plate with a methanol-sulfuric acid solution (1:1) until the plate appears wet. Allow the plate to air dry; then heat it at 110° for 10 min. Roquefortine appears as a light blue-gray spot at an R_f of about 0.40; isofumigaclavine A appears as a violet spot at an R_f of about 0.60. The amount of roquefortine and isofumigaclavine A in the sample may be estimated by comparing the sample spots with standard spots of similar intensity. Other developing solvents which may be used for confirmation together with R_f values, obtained by using these solvents in unlined tanks, for roquefortine and isofumigaclavine A, respectively, are chloroform-diethylamine (8:1) (R_f values 0.35 and 0.80) and chloroform-methanol (9:1) (R_f values 0.40 and 0.45).

Procedure for analysis of sample extract for Roquefortine by HPLC with UV and/or electrochemical detector

Standard Curve. Pipet 0.25, 0.5, 1.0, 2.0, 4.0, and 8.0 ml of roquefortine standard solution (1 μg/ml) into separate 4 dram vials and evaporate just to dryness under stream of nitrogen. Pipet 1.0 ml of HPLC mobile solvent into each vial; this gives standard concentration of 0.25, 0.5, 1.0, 2.0, 4.0, and 8.0 μg of roquefortine/ml. Set the liquid chromatographic flow rate to 1.0 ml/min. If the UV detector is to be used, set the wavelength at 312 nm and the sensitivity to 0.02 AUFS. If the electrochemical detector is to be used, set the applied potential to + 1.0 V versus silver-silver chloride reference and the current sensitivity to 50 nA/V. If both detectors are to be used in series, connect the UV detector inlet to the liquid chromatograph column outlet and the UV detector outlet to the inlet of the electrochemical detector. Inject 25 μl of each standard solution into the liquid chromatograph. Prepare standard curves by plotting peak heights versus concentration (μg/ml) of the standard solutions.

Determination. Dissolve the sample extract in 0.5 ml of the liquid chromatograph mobile phase. Inject 25 μl of the sample extract into the liquid chromatograph under the same conditions used in preparing the standard curve. Identify the roquefortine peak in the sample by comparison of retention time with that of the standard. If the sample peak is higher than the highest standard peak, quantitatively dilute the sample and reinject. Determine the concentration of roquefortine in the sample extract directly from the standard curve obtained from a UV and/or electrochemical detector. Calculate the amount of roquefortine in the sample using the following formula:

$$\text{ng roquefortine/g sample (ppb)} = \frac{A \times B}{C \times 1000}$$

where

A = concentration (μg/ml) of roquefortine in sample extract
B = volume (ml) of sample extract
C = amount (g) of sample represented by extract

If both the UV and electrochemical detectors were connected in series, compare the results obtained from the two determinations; close agreement (i.e., within 5%) provides confirmation of the amount of roquefortine in the sample.

G. Sterigmatocystin

Summary

Sterigmatocystin is extracted from samples of corn, oats, wheat, or barley with acetonitrile-aqueous KCl solution. Samples are cleaned up by liquid-liquid partition and silica gel column chromatography.

Sterigmatocystin may be determined by either silica gel thin layer chromatography (TLC) or normal-phase high-pressure liquid chromatography (HPLC) with a variable-wavelength UV detector set at 320 nm. The limits of determination by TLC and HPLC analysis are 80 and 50 ng/g, respectively. Recovery of sterigmatocystin added to grains at the 100 to 200 ng/g level should exceed 80% by either of the determinative procedures. The TLC procedure includes optional confirmation steps based on forming derivatives of sterigmatocystin.

Apparatus

(1) Wrist action shaker; (2) glass chromatographic columns: 300 × 22 mm i.d. with a 300 ml reservoir and stopcock; (3) thin layer chromatographic equipment: 20 × 20 cm glass plates; applicator, mounting board; spotting template; 10 μl syringe; desiccating storage cabinet; chromatographic tank; long- and short-wave UV lamps (use with UV-absorbing eyeglasses) or viewing cabinet equipped with long- and short-wave UV lamps; spray bottle; (4) liquid chromatograph capable of delivering 1 ml/min. pulseless flow with high-pressure injection valve and 25 μl loop; (5) variable-wavelength liquid chromatograph UV de-

tector; (6) liquid chromatograph column, 250 × 3.5 mm i.d. stainless steel packed with 5 or 10 μm of silica.

Reagents

(1) Solvents: ACS grade acetonitrile, chloroform, cyclohexane, benzene, ethyl acetate, methanol, ethanol, acetone, methylene chloride; (2) pyridine, acetic anhydride, acetic acid; (3) silica gel for column chromatography: silica gel 60, 0.063 to 0.200 mm (EM Laboratories, Inc., Elmsford, NY 10523) or equivalent; (4) silica gel for TLC: Adsorbosil 1 (Applied Science Laboratories, State College, PA 16801) or equivalent; (5) aluminum chloride spray solution (20%): dissolve 20 g of $AlCl_3 \cdot 6H_2O$ in 100 ml of ethanol; (6) potassium hydroxide spray solution (20%): dissolve 20 g of KOH pellets in 100 ml of methanol; (7) sterigmatocystin standard solutions: (a) stock solution (100 μg/ml): weigh 5.0 mg of sterigmatocystin into a 50 ml volumetric flask and dilute to the mark with benzene; (b) standard solution for TLC and HPLC (5 μg/ml); pipet 5.0 ml of the sterigmatocystin stock solution into a 100 ml volumetric flask and dilute to mark with benzene.

Extraction

Weigh 50 g of ground sample into a 500 ml glass-stoppered Erlenmeyer flask, add 180 ml of acetonitrile and 20 ml of 4% KCl in water, and secure the stopper with masking tape. Shake the sample for 30 min. using a wrist action shaker. Filter through 32 cm folded paper into a 250 ml graduated cylinder. Transfer 150 ml of the filtrate to a 250 ml separatory funnel, add 50 ml of hexane, and shake vigorously for 30 sec. Transfer the lower layer to a second 250 ml separatory funnel; discard the hexane solution. Add 50 ml of water and 50 ml of chloroform to the funnel, shake gently, and allow the layers to separate. Transfer the lower layer to another 250 ml separatory funnel. In the same manner extract the aqueous solution with a second 50 ml portion of chloroform and combine the chloroform extracts in the separatory funnel. Add 25 ml of 3% $NaHCO_3$ in water to the chloroform extracts, shake gently, and allow the layers to separate. Drain the lower layer into a 150 ml beaker and evaporate to 5 to 10 ml on a steam bath. Transfer the solution to a 4 dram vial and evaporate just to dryness under a stream of nitrogen.

Column chromatography

Add cyclohexane to the chromatographic column until it is about one-half full. Tamp a small plug of glass wool into the bottom of the column; then add 5 g of anhydrous sodium sulfate. Add 10 g of silica gel to the column; stir this layer with a long rod to remove any bubbles and drain a few milliliters of solvent from the column to aid in settling the packing. Finally, add 15 g of anhydrous sodium sulfate to the column and drain the solvent just to the top of the packing.

Dissolve the sample extract in 1 ml of benzene and transfer this to the column. Rinse the vial with 1 ml of benzene and add this to the column. Drain the column until the solvent reaches the top of the packing. Add 200 ml of cyclohexane-ethyl acetate (4:1) to the column and collect the entire eluate in a 300 ml Erlenmeyer flask. Evaporate the eluate to 5 to 10 ml on a steam bath and quantitatively transfer this to a 4 dram vial. Rinse the flask with 1 to 2 ml of chloroform and add this to the vial. Evaporate the solvent just to dryness on a steam bath under a stream of nitrogen.

Sterigmatocystin may be determined by TLC or HPLC analysis or by both of these techniques. For determination by TLC only dissolve the sample extract in 1.0 ml of benzene; for determination by HPLC only, dissolve the sample extract in 1.0 ml cyclohexane-methylene chloride (3:1); for determination by both procedures, dissolve the sample extract in 2.0 ml of chloroform, pipet 1.0 ml into a separate 4 dram vial, and evaporate both solutions just to dryness under a stream of nitrogen. Dissolve one sample extract in 500 μl of benzene for analysis by TLC and dissolve the second extract in 500 μl of cyclohexane-methylene chloride (3:1) for analysis by HPLC.

Determination by TLC

Prepare 20 × 20 cm silica gel plates (0.25 mm wet thickness) using 50 g of the adsorbent to 55 ml of distilled water or use precoated plates. Activate the plates by heating them at 110° for 1 hr. and store them in a desiccating cabinet with active silica gel desiccant until just before use. Prepare developing solvent of benzene-methanol-acetic acid (90:5:5). Prepare TLC spray solution by dissolving 20 g of $AlCl_3 \cdot 6H_2O$ in 100 ml of ethanol.

Spot 3.5, 5.0, and 6.5 μl of the sample extract and 3.5, 5.0, and 6.5 μl of the sterigmatocystin standard (5 μg/ml in benzene) about 1.5 cm apart on an imaginary line about 4 cm from the bottom of the plate. In addition, spot 5 μl of the standard solution on top of a separate 5 μl spot of the extract. Develop the plate in a closed, lined, equilibrated tank with the developing solvent to a height of about 15 cm. Remove the plate and air dry. Spray the plate with the 20% $AlCl_3$ solution until the layer appears wet; then heat the plate at 80° for 10 min. View the plate under short-wave UV light. Sterigmatocystin appears as a yellow fluorescent spot with an R_f of about 0.6. If the weakest sample spot is more intense than the strongest standard spot, quantitatively dilute the sample and re-chromatograph.

The amount of sterigmatocystin in the sample may be calculated by comparing the sterigmatocystin spot in the sample with a standard spot of equal intensity using the following formula:

$$\text{ng sterigmatocystin/g sample (ppb)} = \frac{S \times C \times V}{G \times X}$$

where

- S = µl of standard solution which gives a spot equal to that of the sample
- C = concentration (µg/ml) of the standard
- V = final volume (µl) of the sample
- G = amount (g) of sample represented by the final extract
- X = µl of the sample extract spottod which had intensity equal to sample spot S

Confirmation by TLC

Prepare TLC plates as described under the determination step. Spot twelve 10 µl spots of the sample extract about 0.5 cm apart on an imaginary line about 4 cm from the bottom of the plate. Spot 10 µl of the sterigmatocystin stock solution (100 µg/ml) about 1.5 cm on either side of the sample spots. Draw a vertical line the length of the plate between the sample and standard spots to prevent contamination of the sample during development. Develop the plate as described under the determination step. View the plate under long-wave UV light. Sterigmatocystin standard spots in end channels fluoresce red. Mark a band about 1.5 cm wide in the sample area of the plate at the same R_f as the sterigmatocystin standard spots, taking care not to include any standard sterigmatocystin. Scrape the sterigmatocystin standard spots off the plate and discard. Scrape the marked sample area into 9 cm folded filter paper in a glass funnel. Wash the silica gel in the filter paper with 4 ml of methanol followed by 4 ml of chloroform, collecting the eluants in a 4 dram vial. Evaporate this solution to about 2 ml; then pipet 1 ml into a second 4 dram vial and evaporate both solutions to dryness. Transfer 5 µl of the sterigmatocystin stock solution (100 µg/ml) into two other 4 dram vials and evaporate to dryness under a stream of nitrogen. Treat one sample and one standard as a pair. Add 500 µl of 0.1 N HCl to each vial of the first pair, cap, shake, and heat on steam bath for 30 min. Evaporate the solvent to dryness on steam bath under a stream of nitrogen. Treat the other sample and standard as a second pair and add 250 µl of pyridine and 250 µl of acetic anhydride to each vial. Heat these vials on a steam bath for 30 min.; then evaporate to dryness under a stream of nitrogen.

Add 25 µl of chloroform to each vial. Spot 10 µl from each vial on a silica gel TLC plate in the following order: (1) standard from first pair, (2) sample from first pair, (3) standard from second pair, (4) sample from second pair, and (5) 10 µl of sterigmatocystin stock solution (100 µg/ml). Develop plate in lined, equilibrated tank with acetone-chloroform (5:95).

Examine the developed plate under long-wave UV light and compare the sample and standard spots. Acetate derivatives (second pair) appear as blue fluorescent spots at an R_f of about one-half of that of the red sterigmatocystin spot. Remove the plate and spray with

20% KOH in methanol and reexamine under long-wave UV light. The sterigmatocystin derivatives formed by treatment with HCl solution (first pair) appear as yellow fluorescent spots at an R_f of about one-fourth of that of the standard sterigmatocystin spot, which also fluoresces yellow after spraying with KOH solution. Some unreacted sterigmatocystin spots may appear above the derivative spots. If the spots from the derivatized samples have the same color and R_f values as the corresponding standard derivatives, the presence of sterigmatocystin in the samples is confirmed.

Determination by HPLC

Prepare HPLC mobile solvent of cyclohexane-methylene chloride (25% water saturated)-acetic acid (75:25:0.1). Set the liquid chromatographic flow rate at 0.5 ml/min., the variable-wavelength UV detector at 320 nm, and the detector range at 0.02 AUFS.

Pipet 0.5, 1.0, 1.5, and 2.0 ml of the sterigmatocystin standard solution (5 μg/ml) into separate 2 dram vials and evaporate to dryness under a stream of nitrogen at room temperature. Pipet 1.0 ml of the HPLC mobile solvent into each vial to give final concentrations of 2.5, 5.0, 7.5, and 10.0 μg sterigmatocystin/ml. Inject 20 μl of each of these solutions into the liquid chromatograph and prepare a standard curve by plotting peak height versus concentration (μg/ml).

Inject 20 μl of the sample solution into the liquid chromatograph under the same conditions used for preparing the standard curve. Identify the sterigmatocystin peak in the sample by comparison of retention volumes with those of the standard. If the sample peak is larger than the highest standard peak, quantitatively dilute the sample with the mobile solvent and reinject. Calculate the amount of sterigmatocystin in the sample using the following formula:

$$\text{Sterigmatocystin, ng/g sample (ppb)} = \frac{A \times B}{C \times 1000}$$

where

A = concentration (μg/ml) of sterigmatocystin in the sample extract
B = volume (ml) of sample extract
C = amount (g) of sample represented by the extract

H. T-2 Toxin and Diacetoxyscirpenol

Summary

Samples of ground grain (corn, oats, barley, or wheat) are extracted with ethyl acetate-water. The sample is cleaned up by ammonium sulfate precipitation, liquid-liquid partition, and silica gel column chromatography. T-2 toxin and diacetoxyscirpenol (DAS) may be determined by thin layer chromatography (TLC) or gas-liquid chromatography (GLC) using either flame ionization (FI) or electron capture (EC) detectors. The limit of determination for T-2 toxin and DAS by TLC analysis is 50 to 75 ng/g; the limit of determination for analysis by GLC-FI or GLC-EC is 25 and 10 ng/g, respectively. Overall recovery of T-2 toxin and DAS added to grains at the 50 to 100 ng/g level should exceed 75%.

Apparatus

(1) Explosion-proof blender with a 1 quart blender jar; (2) rotary evaporator; (3) chromatographic column: 250 mm × 10 mm i.d. with a 200 ml reservoir and stopcock; (4) thin layer chromatography (TLC) equipment: 20 × 20 cm glass plates, applicator, spotting template, desiccating storage cabinet, chromatographic tank, long-wave UV lamp (use with UV-absorbing eyeglasses); (5) gas chromatograph with flame ionization or electron capture detectors and recorder (preferably with temperature-programming capability).

Reagents

(1) Solvents: ACS grade ethyl acetate, methanol, methylene chloride, acetone, hexane, toluene; (2) silica gel 60, 0.063 to 0.2 mm (E. Merck, Darmstadt, Germany); (3) Adsorbosil-1 TLC silica gel (Applied Science Laboratories, State College, PA 16801) or equivalent; (4) chemicals: reagent grade ammonium sulfate, anhydrous sodium sulfate, sodium bicarbonate, acetic acid, sulfuric acid; (5) N,O-bis(trimethylsilyl) trifluoroacetamide containing 1% trimethylchlorosilane as a catalyst (BSTFA + 1% TMCS) (Pierce Chemical Company, Rockford, IL 61105).

Sample preparation and extraction

Grind samples of grain to pass a 2 mm opening. Weigh 60 g of ground sample into a 1 quart blender jar; add 25 ml of water and 300 ml of ethyl acetate. Blend at moderate speed for 3 min. Filter sample through 32 cm fluted filter paper (S&S No. 588 or equivalent) in a glass funnel into a 500 ml graduated cylinder. Transfer 250 ml of filtrate to a 500 ml round-bottom flask and evaporate to dryness on a rotary evaporator at 40°. (If a rotary evaporator is not available, evaporate filtrate to dryness in a 400 ml beaker on a steam bath at 40° under a stream of nitrogen. Add 15 ml of absolute ethanol to the flask and swirl to dissolve the contents.) Add 75 ml of 1% acetic acid in water and 10 ml of an aqueous solution saturated with ammonium sulfate to the flask and swirl to mix. Allow the solution to stand for 2 min.; then add 5 g of Hyflo SuperCel (filter aid) and filter through 24 cm fluted filter paper (S&S No. 588 or equivalent) in a glass funnel into a 100 ml graduated cylinder.

Transfer 75 ml of filtrate to a 250 ml separatory funnel, add 15 ml of methylene chloride, shake vigorously for 30 sec., and allow the layers to separate. Transfer the lower layer to a second separatory funnel. In the same manner extract the aqueous solution with a second 15 ml portion of methylene chloride. Combine the methylene chloride extracts in the second separatory funnel, add 50 ml of hexane, and stir. Pour this solution through 20 g of anhydrous sodium sulfate in a glass funnel into a 150 ml beaker. Wash the sodium sulfate with 20 ml of methylene chloride and combine the solutions in the beaker.

Column chromatography

Add methylene chloride until the column is about half full; then gently tamp a small plug of glass wool into the bottom of the column. Add 1 g of anhydrous sodium sulfate and allow it to settle; then add 2 g of silica gel 60 and stir this layer with a long-handled rod to remove any bubbles; finally, add 1 g of anhydrous sodium sulfate. Drain the methylene chloride just to the top of the packing; do *not* let the column go dry. Add the sample extract to the column and drain the solution to the top of the packing, collecting the eluate in a 150 ml beaker. Add 25 ml of 5% acetone in methylene chloride to the column and drain to the top of the packing. Discard eluate. Add 30 ml of 20% acetone in methylene chloride and collect eluate in a 50 ml beaker. Concentrate this solution to about 5 ml on a steam bath (40°) under a stream of nitrogen. Transfer the solution to a 3 dram vial, rinse the beaker with 1 ml of methylene chloride, and add this to the vial. Evaporate this solution just to dryness on a steam bath (40°) under a stream of nitrogen.

TLC screening procedure (optional)

Prepare 20 × 20 cm glass plates of Adsorbosil-1 silica gel (0.25 mm thick) and activate them at 120° for 1 hr. Store the plates in a desiccating cabinet with active silica gel until just before use.

Dissolve sample extract in 100 μl of methylene chloride. Spot 2, 5, and 10 μl of the sample extract and 1, 2, 5, and 10 μl of a standard solution of T-2 toxin and diacetoxyscirpenol (20 μg/ml each in methylene chloride) on separate spots about 1.5 cm apart on an imaginary line about 4 cm from the bottom of the plate. Develop the plate in a closed, unlined, equilibrated tank with developing solvent of ethyl acetate-toluene (3:1) to a height of about 15 cm. Remove the plate and air dry. Spray the plate with a methanol-sulfuric acid solution (1:1) until the plate appears wet. Allow the plate to air dry, then heat at 125° for 10 min. View the plate under long-wave UV light. T-2 toxin appears as a gray-green fluorescent spot at an R_f of about 0.75; diacetoxyscirpenol appears as a violet fluorescent spot at an R_f about 0.50. The amount of T-2 toxin and diacetoxyscirpenol in the sample may be estimated by comparing the sample spots with standard spots of equal intensity.

Evaporate sample solution to dryness for analysis by GLC.

Derivative formation

Prepare the T-2 toxin and diacetoxyscirpenol TMS derivatives by adding 100 μl of BSTFA + 1% TMCS to dry sample extract with a 250 μl syringe, rinsing the sides of the vial with the reagent. Let the sample stand at room temperature for 45 min., swirling the vial gently every 15 min. to wet the sides.

Column chromatography

Add methylene chloride until the column is about half full; then gently tamp a small plug of glass wool into the bottom of the column. Add 1 g of anhydrous sodium sulfate and allow it to settle; then add 2 g of silica gel 60 and stir this layer with a long-handled rod to remove any bubbles; finally, add 1 g of anhydrous sodium sulfate. Drain the methylene chloride just to the top of the packing; do not let the column go dry. Add the derivatized sample to the column, rinse the sample vial with three 5 ml portions of hexane, and add these to the column. Drain the column just to the top of the packing, collecting the eluate in a beaker. Add 15 ml of methylene chloride to the column and drain to the top of the packing. Discard the combined eluates. Add 20 ml of 5% acetone in methylene chloride to the column and collect this eluate in a 50 ml beaker. Evaporate to about 5 ml on a steam bath; then transfer the sample to a 3 dram vial. Rinse the beaker with 2 ml of methylene chloride and add this to the vial. Evaporate the sample solution just to dryness under a stream of nitrogen.

Detection/quantitation by GLC with FI or EC detectors

Standard Curve. Weigh 2.0 mg each of T-2 toxin and diacetoxyscirpenol into a 100 ml volumetric flask and add methylene chloride to the mark to give concentrations of 20 μg of T-2 toxin and diacetoxyscirpenol/ml.

For analysis using the FI detector, pipet 4.0, 3.0, 2.0, 1.0, and 1.0 ml of the T-2 toxin and DAS standard solution into separate 3 dram vials and evaporate just to dryness under a stream of nitrogen. Add 100 μl of BSTFA + 1% TMCS reagent to each vial with a 250 μl syringe, rinsing the sides of the vial with the reagent. Cap the vials with Teflon-lined caps and allow them to stand at room temperature for 45 min., with gentle swirling every 15 min. Evaporate the solutions just to dryness under a stream of nitrogen. Pipet 1.0 ml of methylene chloride into each of the first four vials and 2.0 ml into the fifth vial to give final concentrations of 80.0, 60.0, 40.0, 20.0, and 10.0 μg of T-2 toxin and diacetoxyscirpenol/ml.

For GLC analysis with the FI detector use a 4 ft × 2 mm i.d. glass column packed with 3% OV-17 on 80/100 mesh Gas Chrom Q or equivalent. Set the nitrogen flow rate at 30 ml/min., the injector and detector temperatures at 220° and 280°, respectively, and the initial column temperature at 180°, with temperature programming at 2°/min. to a final temperature of 240°. Under these conditions the TMS ether derivatives of diacetoxyscirpenol and T-2 toxin have retention times of about 16 and 24 min., respectively. (If a gas chromatograph with temperature-programming capability is not available, determine the toxins separately, using column temperatures of 200° for diacetoxyscirpenol and 240° for T-2 toxin.) Set the range and attenuation controls so that a 3 μl injection of the most dilute standard (10 μg/ml) gives a response of 5 to 10% of full scale.

Inject 3 μl of each standard solution into the gas chromatograph. Prepare standard curves by plotting peak heights (or integrator counts) versus concentration (μg/ml).

For analysis using the EC detector, pipet 1.0 ml of the T-2 toxin diacetoxyscirpenol standard solution (20 μg/ml) into a 100 ml volumetric flask and dilute to the mark with methylene chloride to give concentrations of 0.20 μg of T-2 toxin and diacetoxyscirpenol/ml. Pipet 4.0, 3.0, 2.0, 1.0, and 1.0 ml of this solution into separate 3 dram vials, and evaporate just to dryness under a stream of nitrogen. Form the TMS ether derivatives in the same manner as described above using 100 μl of BSTFA + 1% TMCS reagent per vial. After evaporation of the reagent, pipet 1.0 ml of hexane into the first four vials and 2.0 ml of hexane into the fifth vial to give final concentrations of 0.8, 0.6, 0.4, 0.2, and 0.1 μg of T-2 toxin and diacetoxyscirpenol/ml. For GLC analysis with the EC detector, use the same column and the same detector, injector, initial and final column temperatures, and temperature-programming rate as described for analysis with FI detector above. Use high-purity nitrogen or 5% methane in argon as the carrier gas with a flow rate of 30 ml/min. Set the range and attenuation controls so that a 3 μl injection of the most dilute standard (0.1 μg/ml) gives a response of 5 to 10% of full scale.

Inject 3 μl of each standard solution into the gas chromatograph. Prepare a standard curve by plotting peak heights (or integrator counts) versus concentration (μg/ml).

Determination. For GLC determination with the FI detector, dissolve the derivatized sample extract in 100 μl of methylene chloride. Inject 3 μl of this solution into the gas chromatograph under the same conditions used for preparing the standard curve. For GLC determination with the EC detector, dissolve the derivatized sample extract in 10.0 ml of hexane. Inject 3 μl of this solution into the gas chromatograph under the same conditions used for preparing the standard curve. For either determination, identify T-2 toxin and diacetoxyscirpenol peaks by comparing retention times with those of the standards. If the peaks from the sample extract are larger than the highest standard peak, quantitatively dilute the sample with the appropriate solvent and reinject. Determine the concentration of T-2 toxin and diacetoxyscirpenol in the sample extract from the appropriate standard curve. Calculate the amount of the toxins in the sample using the following formula:

$$\text{T-2 toxin or diacetoxyscirpenol ng/g sample (ppb)} = \frac{A \times B}{C \times 1000}$$

where

A = concentration (μg/ml) of toxin in sample extract
B = volume (ml) of sample extract
C = amount (g) of sample represented by extract (37.5 g if TLC screening was not carried out)

REFERENCES

1. T.D. Wyllie and L.G. Morehouse (Eds.). *Mycotoxic Fungi, Mycotoxins, and Mycotoxicoses*, Vol. 3: *Mycotoxicoses of Man and Plants: Mycotoxin Control and Regulatory Practices*. Marcel Dekker, New York, 1978.
2. C.J. Mirocha and S.V. Pathre. Identification of the toxic principle in a sample of poaefusarin. Appl. Microbiol. *26*, 719-724 (1978).
3. K. Apostolov, P. Spasic, and N. Bojanic. Evidence of a viral aetiology in endemic (Balkan) nephropathy. Lancet *2*(7948), 1271-1273 (1975).
4. P. Krogh. Mycotoxic porcine nephropathy: a possible model for Balkan endemic nephropathy In *Endemic Nephropathy* (A. Puchley, Ed.). Bulgarian Academy of Sciences, Sofia, Bulgaria, (1974), pp. 266-270.
5. P. Krogh, B. Hald, R. Plestina, and S. Ceovic. Balkan (endemic) nephropathy and foodborn ochratoxin A: preliminary results of a survey of foodstuffs. Acta Path. Microbiol. Scand. Sect. B *85*, 238-240 (1977).
6. K. A. V. R. Krishnamachari, V. Nagarajan, R.V. Bhat, and T. B. G. Tilak. Hepatitis due to aflatoxicosis. An outbreak in Western India. Lancet *1* (7915), 1061-1063 (1975).
7. K. A. V. R. Krishnamachari, R.V. Bhat, V. Nagarajan, and T. B. G. Tilak. Investigations into an outbreak of hepatitis in parts of Western India. Indian J. Med. Res. *63*(7), 1036-1048 (1975).
8. C.A. Linsell. Decision on the control of a dietary carcinogen-aflatoxin. In *IARC Sci. Publ. 25*, 111-122 (1979).
9. F.G. Peers. Aflatoxin in relation to the epidemiology of human liver cancer. In *Gsundheitsgefahrdung durch Aflatoxine*. Int. Toxikol. ETH and Univ. Zurich, Zurich, (1978), pp. 90-108.
10. T.D. Wyllie and L.G. Morehouse (Eds.). *Mycotoxic Fungi, Mycotoxins, and Mycotoxicoses*, Vol. 2; *Mycotoxicoses of Domestic and*

Laboratory Animals, Poultry and Aquatic Invertebrates and Vertebrates. Marcel Dekker, New York (1978).
11. L. Stoloff. Occurrence of mycotoxins in foods and feeds. In *Mycotoxins and Other Fungal Related Products* (J.V. Rodricks, Ed.), Adv. Chem. Ser. No. 149. American Chemical Society, Washington, D.C. (1976).
12. *Conference on Mycotoxins in Animal Feeds and Grains Related to Animal Health.* U.S. Department of Commerce, NTIS. PB-300 300, 1979.
13. T.D. Wyllie and L.G. Morehouse (Eds.). *Mycotoxic Fungi, Mycotoxins, and Mycotoxicoses*, Vol. 1: *Mycotoxic fungi and chemistry of mycotoxins.* Marcel Dekker, New York, 1978).
14. J.V. Rodricks and L. Stoloff. Aflatoxin residues from contaminated feed in edible tissues of food producing animals. In *Mycotoxins in Human and Animal Health* (J.V. Rodricks, Ed.). Pathotox Publishers, Park Forest South, Ill., 1977, pp. 67-79.
15. A.W. Hayes. Biological activities of mycotoxins. *Mycopathologia 65*, 29-41 (1979).
16. K. Uraguchi and M. Yamazaki (Eds.). *Toxicology, Biochemistry and Pathology of Mycotoxins.* Wiley, New York, 1978.
17. J.V. Rodricks, C.W. Hesseltine, and M.A. Mehlman (Eds.). *Mycotoxins in Human and Animal Health.* Pathotox Publishers, Park Forest South, Ill., 1977.
18. *IARC Monographs on the Evaluation of Carcinogenic Risk of Chemicals to Man*, Vol. 10: *Some Naturally Occurring Substances.* International Agency for Research on Cancer, Lyon, France, 1976.
19. L. Stoloff, Aflatoxins: an overview. In *Mycotoxins in Human and Animal Health* (J.V. Rodricks, Ed.). Pathotox Publishers, Park Forest South, Ill., 1977, pp. 7-28.
20. J.G. Heathcote and J.R. Hibbert. *Aflatoxin: Chemical and Biological Effects.* Elsevier, New York, 1978.
21. M.R. Pai and T.A. Venkiatsubramanian. Aflatoxins: a review. J. Sci. Ind. Res. *38*, 73-80 (1979).
22. G.R. Hogan, N.J. Ryan, and A.W. Hayes. Aflatoxin B_1 and Reye's syndrome. Lancet *1*(8063), 561 (1978).
23. N.R. Ryan, G.R. Hogan, A.W. Hayes, A.D. Unger, and M.Y. Siraj. Aflatoxin B_1: its role in the etiology of Reye's syndrome. Pediatrics *64*(1), 71-75 (1979).
24. A.C. Hetherington and H. Raistrick. Studies in the biochemistry of micro-organisms: XIV. On the production and chemical constitution of a new yellow coloring matter, citrinin, produced from glucose by *Penicillium citrinum* Thom. Phil. Trans. R. Soc. (Lond.) Ser. B *220*, 269-275 (1931).
25. H. Raistrick and G. Smith. Antibacterial substances from mold: I. Citrinin, a metabolic product of *Penicillium citrinum* Thom. Chem. Ind. *60*, 828 (1941).

26. A.M. Ambrose and F. DeEds. Acute and subacute toxicity of pure citrinin. Soc. Exp. Biol. Med. *59*, 289-291 (1945).
27. P. Krogh, B. Hald, and C.J. Pedersen. Occurrence of ochratoxin A and citrinin in cereals associated with mycotoxic porcine nephropathy. Acta Pathol. Microbiol. Scand. *B81*, 689-695 (1973).
28. P. Krogh. Epidemiology of mycotoxic porcine nephropathy. Nord. Vet. Med. *28*, 452-458 (1976).
29. G.A. Sansing, E.B. Lillehoj, R.W. Detroy, and M.A. Miller. Synergistic toxic effects of citrinin, ochratoxin A and penicillic acid in mice. Toxicon *14*, 213-220 (1976).
30. W.T. Roberts and E.C. Mora. Toxicity of *Penicillium citrinum* AVA-532 contaminated corn and citrinin and broiler chicks. Poult. Sci. *57*, 1221-1226 (1979).
31. W.W. Carlton and P. Krogh. Ochratoxins. In *Conference on Mycotoxins in Animal Feeds and Grains Related to Animal Health*. U.S. Department of Commerce NTIS. PB-300 300, 1979, pp. 165-287.
32. P. Krogh. Ochratoxins. In *Mycotoxins in Human and Animal Health* (J.V. Rodricks, Ed.). Pathotox Publishers, Park Forest South, Ill., 1977, pp. 489-498.
33. M. Kanisawa and S. Suzuki. Induction of renal and hepatic tumors in mice by ochratoxin A, a mycotoxin. Gann *69*, 599-600 (1978).
34. M. Kanisawa, S. Suzuki, Y. Kozuka, and M. Yamazaki. Histopathological studies on the toxicity of ochratoxin A in rats: I. Acute oral toxicity. Toxicol. Appl. Pharmacol. *42*, 55-64, (1977).
35. A. Ciegler. Patulin. In *Mycotoxins in Human and Animal Health* (J.V. Rodricks, Ed.). Pathotox Publishers, Park Forest South, Ill., 1977, pp. 609-624.
36. F. Dickens and H. E. H. Jones. Carcinogenic activity of a series of reactive lactones and related substances. Br. J. Cancer *15*, 85-100 (1961).
37. F. Dickens and H. E. H. Jones. Further studies on the carcinogenic and growth-inhibitory activity of lactones and related substances. Br. J. Cancer *17*, 100-108 (1963).
38. F. Dickens and H. E. H. Jones. Further studies on the carcinogenic action of certain lactones and related substances in the rat and mouse. Br. J. Cancer *A*, 392-403 (1965).
39. P.S. Steyn. Mycotoxins, excluding aflatoxin, zearalenone and the trichothecenes. In *Mycotoxins in Human and Animal Health* (J.V. Rodricks, C.W. Hesseltine, and M.A. Mehlman, Eds.). Pathotox Publishers, Park Forest South, Ill., 1977, pp. 419-467.
40. J.J. van der Watt. Sterigmatocystin. In *Mycotoxins* (I. F. H. Purchase, Ed.). Elsevier, New York, 1974, pp. 369-382.
41. T. Hamaski and Y. Hatsuda. Sterigmatocystin and related com-

pounds. In *Mycotoxins in Human and Animal Health* (J.V. Rodricks, C.W. Hesseltine, and M.A. Mehlman, Eds.). Pathotox Publishers, Park Forest South, Ill., 1977, pp. 597-607.
42. J.V. Rodricks (Ed.). *Mycotoxins in Human and Animal Health*. Pathotox Publishers, Park Forest South, Ill., 1977, pp. 185-340.
43. C.J. Mirocha. Trichothecene toxins produced by *Fusarium*. In *Conference on Mycotoxins in Animal Feeds and Grains Related to Animal Health*, U.S. Dept. of Commerce, NTIS PB-300 300, 1979, pp. 289-373.
44. R. Schoental, A.Z. Jaffe, and B. Yagen. The induction of tumours of the digestive tract and of certain other organs in rats given T-2 toxin, a secondary metabolite of *Fusarium sporotrichioides*. Br. J. Cancer *38*, 171 (1978).
45. R. Schoental. The role of *Fusarium* mycotoxins in the aetiology of tumors of the digestive tract and of certain other organs in man and animals. Front. Gastrointest. Res. *4*, 1-6 (1979).
46. R. Schoental, A.Z. Jaffe, and B. Yagen. Cardiovascular lesions and various tumors found in rats given T-2 toxin, a trichothecene metabolite of *Fusarium*. Cancer Res. *39*, 2179-2189 (1979).
47. W. F. O. Marasas, S. J. van Rensburg, and C. J. Mirocha. Incidence of *Fusarium* species and the mycotoxins, deoxynivalenol and zearalenone, in corn produced in esophageal cancer areas in Transkei. J.Agric. Food Chem. *27*, 1108-1112 (1979).
48. L. Stoloff. Aflatoxin control, past and present. J. Assoc. Off. Anal. Chem., *63*, 1067-1073 (1980).
49. A.E. Pohland, C.W. Thorpe, and S. Nesheim. Newer developments in mycotoxin methodology. Pure Appl. Chem. *52*, 213-223 (1979).
50. S. Nesheim. Methods of aflatoxin analysis. In *National Bureau of Standards Special Publication No. 519. Trace Organic Analysis: A New Frontier in Analytical Chemistry*. Gaithersburg, Md., 1979, pp. 355-372.
51. T. Romer. Methods of detecting mycotoxins in mixed feed ingredients. Feedstuffs *48*(16), 18-46 (1976).
52. W. Horwitz, (Ed.). Natural poisons. In *Official Methods of Analysis of the AOAC*, 13th ed. Association of Official Analytical Chemists, 1980 Washington, D.C., Chapter 26.
53. P.L. Schuller, W. Horwitz, and L. Stoloff. A review of sampling plans and collaboratively studied methods of analysis for aflatoxins. J. Assoc. Off. Anal. Chem. *59*(6), 1315-1343 (1976).
54. E.B. Lillehoj. Natural occurrence of mycotoxins in feeds-pitfalls in determination. In *Interactions of Mycotoxins in Animal Production*. National Academy of Sciences, Washington, D.C., 1979, pp. 139-153.
55. W.A. Pons, Jr., L.S. Lee, and L. Stoloff. Revised method for aflatoxins in cottonseed products, and comparison of thin layer and high performance liquid chromatography determinative steps: collaborative study. J. Assoc. Off. Anal. Chem. *63*, 899-906, (1980).

56. N.D. Davis, J.W. Dickens, R.L. Freie, P.B. Hamilton, O.L. Shotwell, T.D. Wyllie, and J.F. Fulkerson. Protocols for surveys, sampling, post-collection handling, and analysis of grain samples involved in mycotoxin problems. J. Assoc. Off. Anal. Chem. *63*(1), 95-101 (1980).
57. A.E. Waltking. Sampling and preparation of samples of peanut butter for aflatoxin analysis. J. Assoc. Off. Anal. Chem. *63*(1), 103-106 (1980).
58. A.D. Campbell. Sampling foodstuffs for mycotoxin analysis. Pure Appl. Chem. *52*, 205-211 (1979).
59. J.D. McKinney. Private communication.
60. M.J. Verrett, J.P. Marliac, and J.M. McLaughlin. Use of the chicken embryo in the assay of aflatoxin toxicity. J. Assoc. Off. Anal. Chem. *47*, 1003-1006 (1964).
61. R.M. Eppley. Sensitivity of brine shrimp (*Artemia saliva*) to trichothecenes. J. Assoc. Off. Anal. Chem. *57*(3), 618-620 (1974).
62. G.M. Ware and C.W. Thorpe. Determination of zearalenone in corn by high pressure liquid chromatography and fluorescence detection. J. Assoc. Off. Anal. Chem. *61*, 1058-1062 (1978).
63. G.M. Ware, C.W. Thorpe, and A.E. Pohland. Determination of roquefortine in blue cheese and blue cheese dressing by high pressure liquid chromatography with ultraviolet and electrochemical detectors. J. Assoc. Off. Anal. Chem. *63*, 637-641 (1980).
64. S. Nesheim. Factors affecting the thin-layer chromatography of aflatoxins. In *Symposium on Chemical and Environmental Application of Quantitative Thin Layer Chromatography* (J. Touchstone and D. Rogers, Eds.). Wiley-Interscience, New York, 1980.
65. L.K. Jackson and A. Ciegler. Production and analysis of citrinin in corn. Appl. Environ. Microbiol. *36*(3), 408-411 (1978).
66. L.R. Marti, D.M. Wilson, and B.D. Evans. Determination of citrinin in corn and barley. J. Assoc. Off. Anal. Chem. *61*(6), 1353-1358 (1978).
67. R.D. Stubblefield. Thin layer chromatography determination of citrinin. J. Assoc. Off. Anal. Chem. *62*(1), 201-202 (1979).
68. R.V. Chalane and H.M. Stahr. Thin layer chromatographic determination of citrinin. J. Assoc. Off. Anal. Chem. *62*(3), 570-572 (1979).
69. P.S. Steyn and K. J. v.d. Merve. Detection and estimation of ochratoxin A. Nature (Land.) *211*, 418 (1966).
70. P.M. Scott and T.B. Hand. Method for the detection and estimation of ochratoxin A in some cereal products. J. Assoc. Off. Anal. Chem. *50*(2), 366-371 (1967).
71. L.J. Vorster. A method for the analysis of cereals and groundnuts for three mycotoxins. Analyst *94*, 136-142 (1969).

72. R.M. Eppley. Screening method for zearalenone, aflatoxin and ochratoxin. J. Assoc. Off. Anal. Chem. *51*(1), 74-78 (1968).
73. F.S. Chu and M.E. Butz. Spectrophotofluorodensitometric measurement of ochratoxin A in cereal products. J. Assoc. Off. Anal. Chem. *53*(6), 1253-1257 (1970).
74. H.L. Trenk and F.S. Chu. Improved detection of ochratoxin A on thin layer plates. J. Assoc. Off. Anal. Chem. *54*(6), 1307-1309 (1971).
75. L. Stoloff, S. Nesheim, L. Yin, J.V. Rodricks, M. Stack, and A.D. Campbell. A multimycotoxin detection method for aflatoxins, ochratoxin, zearalenone, sterigmatocystin and patulin. J. Assoc. Off. Anal. Chem. *54*, 91-97 (1971).
76. S. Nesheim, N.F. Hardin, O.J. Francis, Jr., and W.S. Langham. Analysis of ochratoxins A and B and their esters in barley, using partition and thin layer chromatography: I. Development of the method. J. Assoc. Off. Anal. Chem. *56*(4), 817-821 (1973).
77. P.M. Scott. Modified method for the determination of mycotoxins in cocoa beans. J. Assoc. Off. Anal. Chem. *56*, 1028-1030 (1973).
78. B. Hald and P. Krogh. Detection of ochratoxin A in barley using silica gel minicolumns. J. Assoc. Off. Anal. Chem. *58*, 156-158 (1975).
79. O. Aalund, K. Brunfeldt, B. Hald, P. Krogh, and K. Paulsen. A radioimmunoassay for ochratoxin A: a preliminary investigation. Acta Pathol. Microbiol. Scand. Sec. C *83*, 390-392 (1975).
80. C.P. Levi. Collaborative study of a method for the determination of ochratoxin A in green coffee. J. Assoc. Off. Anal. Chem. *58*(2), 258-262 (1975).
81. K. Hult and S. Gatenbeck. A spectrophotometric procedure, using carboxypeptidase A, for the quantitative measurement of ochratoxin A. J. Assoc. Off. Anal. Chem. *59*(1), 128-129 (1976).
82. E. Josefsson and T. Moller. High pressure liquid chromatographic determination of ochratoxin A and zearalenone in cereals. J. Assoc. Off. Anal. Chem. *62*(5), 1165-1168 (1979).
83. K. Hult, Ochratoxin A in pig blood: method of analysis and use as a tool for feed studies. Appl. Environ. Microbiol. *38*, 772 (1979).
84. D.C. Hunt, L.A. Philip, and N.T. Crosby. Determination of ochratoxin A in pig's kidney using enzymic digestion, dialysis and high-performance liquid chromatography with post-column derivatization. Analyst *104*, 1171-1175 (1979).
85. A.E. Pohland, K. Sanders, and C.W. Thorpe. Determination of patulin in apple juice. J. Assoc. Off. Anal. Chem. *53*(4), 692-695 (1970).
86. A.E. Pohland and R. Allen. Analysis and chemical confirmation of patulin in grains. J. Assoc. Off. Anal. Chem. *53*, 686-687 (1970).
87. G.M. Ware, C.W. Thorpe, and A.E. Pohland. Liquid chromato-

graphic determination of patulin in apple juice. J. Assoc. Off. Anal. Chem. *57*(5), 1111-1113 (1973).

88. P.M. Scott and B. P. C. Kennedy. Improved method for the thin layer chromatographic determination of patulin in apple juice. J. Assoc. Off. Anal. Chem. *56*(4), 813-816 (1973).
89. S.T. Suzuki, Y. Fujimoto, Y. Hoshino, and A. Tanaka. Simultaneous determination of patulin and penicillic acid in grains by gas chromatographic method. Agric. Biol. Chem. *38*(6), 1259 1260 (1974).
90. J.D. Rosen and S.R. Pareles. Quantitative analysis of patulin in apple juice. J. Agric. Food Chem. *22*(6), 1024-1026 (1974).
91. G.M. Ware. High pressure liquid chromatographic method for the determination of patulin in apple butter. J. Assoc. Off. Anal. Chem. *58*(4), 754-756 (1975).
92. Y. Fujimoto, T. Suzuki, and Y. Hoshino. Determination of penicillic acid and patulin by gas-liquid chromatography with an electron capture detector. J. Chromatogr. *105*, 99-106 (1975).
93. T.E. Salem and B.G. Swanson. Fluorodensitometric assay of patulin in apple products. J. Food Sci. *41*, 1237-1238 (1976).
94. E.E. Stenson, C.N. Huhtanen, T.E. Zell, D.P. Schwartz, and S.F. Osman. Determination of patulin in apple juice products as the 2,4-dinitrophenylhydrazone derivative. J. Agric. Food Chem. *25*(5), 1220-1222 (1977).
95. K. Polzhofer. Determination of patulin in foodstuffs: II. Determination of patulin in tomatoes, pears, apples, cucumbers and plums. Z. Lebensm. Unters. Forsch. *163*, 272-273 (1977).
96. U. Leuenberger, R. Gauch, and E. Baumgartner. The quantitative analysis of the mycotoxin patulin in fruit juices by high-pressure liquid or thin layer chromatography. J. Chromatogr. *161*, 303-309 (1978).
97. H. Stray. High pressure liquid chromatographic determination of patulin in apple juice. J. Assoc. Off. Anal. Chem. *61*(6), 1359-1362 (1978).
98. J.C. Young. Fluorescence detection and determination of patulin by thin layer chromatography of its aniline imine. J. Environ. Sci. Health *B14*(1), 15-26 (1979).
99. C.W. Thorpe and R.L. Johnson. Analysis of penicillic acid by gas-liquid chromatography. J. Assoc. Off. Anal. Chem. 57(4), 861-865 (1974).
100. Y. Fujimoto, T. Suzuki, and Y. Hoshino. Determination of penicillic acid by gas-liquid chromatography with an electron-capture detector. J. Chromatogr. *105*, 99-106 (1975).
101. T. Suzuki, Y. Fujimoto, Y. Hoshino, and A. Tanaka. Trimethylsilylation of penicillic acid and patulin, and the stability of the products. J. Chromatogr. *105*, 95-98 (1975).
102. A. Ciegler, H.J. Mintzlaff, D. Weisleder and L. Leistner. Potential production and detoxification of penicillic acid in mold-fer-

mented sausage (Salami). Appl. Microbiol. *24*(1), 114-119 (1972).

103. A. Ceigler and C.P. Kurtzman. Fluorodensitometric assay of penicillic acid. J. Chromatogr. *51*, 511-516 (1970).

104. R.W. Pero, D. Harvan, R.G. Owens, and J.P. Suoro. A gas chromatographic method for the mycotoxin penicillic acid. J. Chromatogr. *65*, 501-506 (1972).

105. D.C. Hunt, A.T. Bourdou, and N.T. Crosby. Use of HPLC for the identification and estimation of zearalenone, patulin and penicillic acid in food. J. Sci. Food Agric., 239-244 (1978).

106. C.W. Thorpe. Determination of penicillic acid in grains, dried beans and swiss cheese by HPLC with a UV detector presented at the 92nd Annual Meeting of the AOAC, Washington, D.C., (1978), Abstr. No. 129.

107. P.M. Scott, B. P. C. Kennedy, J. Harwig, and B.J. Blanchfield. Study of conditions for production of roquefortine and other metabolites of *Penicillium roqueforti*. Appl. Environ. Microbiol. *33*(2), 249-253 (1977).

108. P.M. Scott and P. B. C. Kennedy. Analysis of blue cheese for roquefortine and other alkaloids from *Penicillium roqueforti*. J. Agric. Food Chem. *24*, 865-868 (1976).

109. L.J. Vorster and I. F. H. Purchase. A method for the determination of sterigmatocystin in grain and oilseed. Analyst *93*, 694-696 (1968).

110. L.J. Vorster. A method for the analysis of cereals and groundnuts for three mycotoxins. Analyst *94*, 136-142 (1969).

111. M. Stack and J.V. Rodricks. Method for analysis and chemical confirmation of sterigmatocystin. J. Assoc. Off. Anal. Chem. *54*(1), 87-90 (1971).

112. M. Manabe, M. Minamisawa, and S. Matsuura. Extraction and clean-up method for the sterigmatocystin analysis of rice (gas-liquid chromatographic assay of sterigmatocystin, Part II). J. Agric. Chem. Soc. (Jap.) *47*, 204-215 (1973).

113. M.E. Stack, S. Nesheim, N.L. Brown, and A.E. Pohland. Determination of sterigmatocystin in corn and oats by high-pressure liquid chromatography. J. Assoc. Off. Anal. Chem. *59*(5), 966-970 (1976).

114. G. Sullivan, D.D. Maness, G.J. Yakatan, and J. Scholler. Thin-layer chromatography separation of sterigmatocystin, 5-methoxysterigmatocystin and O-methylsterigmatocystin. J. Chromatogr. *116*, 490-492 (1976).

115. D. G. I. Kingston, P.N. Chen, and J. R. Vercellotti. High-performance liquid chromatography of sterigmatocystin and other metabolites by *Aspergillus versicolor*. J. Chromatogr. *118*, 414-417 (1976).

116. A.S. Salhab, G.F. Russell, J.R. Coughlin, and D. P. H. Hsieh. Gas-liquid chromatography and mass spectrometric ion selective

detection of sterigmatocystin in grains. J. Assoc. Off. Anal. Chem. *59*(5), 1037-1044 (1976).
117. G.N. Shannon and O.L. Shotwell. Thin layer chromatographic determination of sterigmatocystin in cereal grains and soybeans. J. Assoc. Off. Anal. Chem. *59*(5), 963-965 (1976).
118. K. Ito, A. Yamane, T. Hamaschi, and Y. Hatsuda. An assay of sterigmatocystin and related metabolites of *Aspergillus versicolor* by high speed liquid chromatography. Agric. Biol. Chem. *40*(10), 2099-2100 (1976).
119. A.K. Athnasios and G.O. Kuhn. Improved thin layer chromatographic method for the isolation and estimation of sterigmatocystin in grains. J. Assoc. Off. Anal. Chem. *60*(1), 104-106 (1977).
120. R. Schmidt, K. Neunhoeffer, and K. Dose. Quantitative determination of sterigmatocystin in moldy vegetable foods. Z. Anal. Chem. *299*, 382-384 (1979).
121. H.P. Van Egmond, W.E. Paulsch, E. Deijll, and P.L. Schuller. Thin layer chromatographic method for analysis and chemical confirmation of sterigmatocystin in cheese. J. Assoc. Off. Anal. Chem. *63*(1), 110-119 (1980).
122. S.V. Pathre and C.J. Mirocha. Assay methods for trichothecenes and review of their natural occurrence. In *Mycotoxins in Human and Animal Health* (J.V. Rodricks, Ed.). Pathotox Publishers, Park Forest South, Ill., 1977, pp. 229-253.
123. R.M. Eppley. Trichothecenes and their analysis. J. Am. Oil Chem. Soc. *56*(9), 824-829 (1979).
124. Y. Ueno, M. Hosoya, and Y. Ishikawa. Inhibitory effects of mycotoxins on the protein synthesis in rabbit reticulocytes. J. Biochem. *66*, 419-422 (1969).
125. C.W. Chung, M.W. Trucksess, A.L. Giles, Jr., and L. Friedman. Rabbit skin test for estimation of T-2 toxin and other skin-irritating toxins in contaminated corn. J. Assoc. Off. Anal. Chem. *57*(5), 1121-1127 (1974).
126. P.M. Scott, J.W. Lawrence, and W. van Walbeek. Detection of mycotoxins by thin-layer chromatography: application to screening of fungal extracts. Appl. Microbiol. *20*(5), 839-842 (1970).
127. C.O. Ikediobi, I.C. Hsu, J.R. Bamburg, and F.M. Strong. Gas-liquid chromatography of mycotoxins of the trichothecene group. Anal. Biochem. *43*, 327-340 (1971).
128. J.R. Bamburg. The biological activities and detection of naturally occurring 12,13-epoxy-Δ^9-trichothecenes. Clin. Toxicol. *5*(4), 495-515 (1972).
129. Y. Ueno, N. Sato, K. Ishii, K. Sakai, H. Tsunoda, and M. Enomoto. Biological and chemical detection of trichothecene mycotoxins of *Fusarium* species. Appl. Microbiol. *25*(4), 699-704 (1973).
130. T. Tatsuno, K. Ohtsubo, and M. Saito. Chemical and biological

detection of 12,13-epoxytrichothecenes isolated from *Fusarium* species. Pure Appl. Chem. *35*(3), 309-313 (1973).

131. F. M. D. Foster, T.F. Slater, and D. S. P. Patterson. A possible enzymic assay for trichothecene mycotoxins in animal feedstuffs. Biochem. Soc. Trans. *3*, 875-878 (1975).
132. B.A. Roberts and D. S. P. Patterson. Detection of twelve mycotoxins in mixed animal feedstuffs using a novel membrane cleanup procedure. J. Assoc. Off. Anal. Chem. *58*(6), 1178-1181 (1975).
133. W.G. Sorenson, M.R. Sueller, and H.W. Larsh. Qualitative and quantitative assay of trichothecin: a mycotoxin produced by *Trichothecium roseum*. Appl. Microbiol. *29*(5), 653-657 (1975).
134. S.R. Pareles, G.J. Collins, and J.D. Rosen. Analysis of T-2 toxin (and HT-2 toxin) by mass fragmentography. J. Agric. Food Chem. *24*(4), 872-875 (1976).
135. C.J. Mirocha, S.V. Pathre, B. Schauerhamer, and C.M. Christensen. Natural occurrence of *Fusarium* toxins in feedstuff. Appl. Environ. Microbiol. *32*(4), 553-556 (1976).
136. S.V. Pathre and C.J. Mirocha. Analysis of deoxynivalenol from cultures of *Fusarium* species. Appl. Environ. Microbiol. *35*(5), 992-994.
137. H.M. Stahr, A.A. Kraft, and M. Schuh. The determination of T-2 toxin, diacetoxyscirpenol and deoxynivalenol in foods and feeds. Appl. Spectrosc. *33*(3), 294-297 (1979).
138. T.R. Romer, T.M. Boling, and J.L. MacDonald. Gas-liquid chromatographic determination of T-2 toxin and diacetoxyscirpenol in corn and mixed feeds. J. Assoc. Off. Anal. Chem. *61*(4), 801-808 (1978).
139. N. Milama and H. LeLievre. Qualitative and quantitative determination of two 12,13-epoxytrichothecenes (T-2 toxin and diacetoxyscirpenol) by gas-liquid chromatography. Analyst *7*(5), 232-235 (1979).
140. T. Kato, Y. Asabe, M. Suzuki, and S. Takitani. Spectrophotometric and fluorimetric determinations of trichothecene mycotoxins with reagents for formaldehyde. Anal. Chem. Acta *106*, 59-655 (1979).
141. L.M. Seitz and H.E. Mohr. Analysis of *Alternaria* metabolites by high pressure liquid chromatography. Anal. Biochem. *70*, 224-230 (1976).
142. C. Andary, F. Enjalbert, G. Privat, and B. Mandrou. Assay for amatoxins in *Amanita phalloides* Fries (Basidiomycetes) with direct spectrometric measurements of chromatograms. J. Chromatogr. *132*, 525-532 (1977).
143. E. Romvary-Szailer and G. Sellyey. A rapid method to determine toxin production of mould strains isolated from local feedstuff. Magy. Allatorv. Lapja *31*(8), 521-524 (1976).

144. G. Engel. Investigations on the production of mycotoxins and their quantitative analysis. J. Chromatogr. *130*, 293-297 (1977).

145. A.C. Ghosh, A. Manmade, J.M. Townsend, A. Bousquet, J.F. Howes, and A.L. Demain. Production of cyclochlorotine and a new metabolite, simatoxin, by *Penicillium islandicum* Sopp. Appl. Environ. Microbiol. *35*(6), 1074-1078 (1978).

146. J. LeBars. Cyclopiazonic acid production by *Penicillium camemberti* Thom and natural occurrence of this mycotoxin in cheese. Appl. Environ. Microbiol. *38*(6), 1052-1055 (1979).

147. R.A. Zabel, C.A. Miller, and S.W. Tanenbaum. Convenient procedures for the biosynthesis, isolation, and isotope labeling of cytochalasins. Appl. Environ. Microbiol. *37*(2), 208-212 (1979).

148. M. Wurst, M. Flieger, and Z. Rehacek. Analysis of ergot alkaloids by high performance liquid chromatography: II. Cyclol alkaloids (ergo-peptines). J. Chromatogr. *174*, 401-407 (1979).

149. H.F. Schran, H.J. Schwarz, K.C. Talbot, and L.J. Loeffler. Specific radioimmunoassay of ergot peptide alkaloids in plasma. Clin. Chem. *25*(11), 1928-1933 (1979).

150. H. Kamimura, M. Nishijima, K. Saito, S. Takahashi, A. Ibe, S. Ochiai, and Y. Naoi. Studies on mycotoxins in foods: VIII. Analytical procedure of trichothecene mycotoxins in cereals. J. Food Hyg. Soc. (Jap.) *19*, 443-448 (1978).

151. Z. Durachova, V. Betinia, and P. Nemec. Systematic analysis of mycotoxins by thin-layer chromatography. J. Chromatogr. *116*, 141-154 (1976).

152. H. Kamimura, Y. Omi, Y. Shiobara, N. Tamaki, and Y. Katogi. Simultaneous determination of griseofulvin and 6-desmethylgriseofulvin in plasma by electron-capture gas chromatography. J. Chromatogr. *163*, 271-279 (1979).

153. A.H. Moubasher, M. I. A. Abdel-Kader, and I.A. El-Kady. Toxigenic fungi isolated from Roquefort cheese. Mycopathologia *66*(3), 187-190 (1978).

154. A.C. Ghosh, A. Manmade, B. Kobbe, J.M. Townsend, and A.L. Demain. Production of luteoskyrin and isolation of a new metabolite, pibasterol, from *Penicillium islandicum* Sopp. Appl. Environ. Microbiol. *35*(3), 563-566 (1978).

155. R.W. Curtis, W.R. Stevenson, and J. Tuite. Malformin in *Aspergillus niger*-infected onion bulbs (Allium cepa). Appl. Microbiol. *28*(3), 362-365 (1974).

156. H.R. Burmeister, A. Ciegler, and R.F. Vesonder. Moniliformin, a metabolite of *Fusarium moniliforme* NRRL 6322: purification and toxicity. Appl. Environ. Microbiol. *37*(1), 11-13 (1979).

157. P. Lafont, M.G. Siriwardana, I. Combernale, and J. Lafont. Mycophenolic acid in marketed cheese. Food Cosmet. Toxicol. *17*, 147-149 (1979).

158. J.L. Richard and L.H. Arp. Natural occurrence of the mycotoxin penitrem A in moldy cream cheese. Mycopathologia *67*(2), 107-109 (1979).
159. P.M. Scott and S.R. Kanhere. Instability of PR-toxin in blue cheese. J. Assoc. Off. Anal. Chem. *62*(1), 141-147 (1979).
160. R.M. Davis and S.S. Stone. Production of anti-rubratoxin antibody and its use in a radioimmunoassay for rubratoxin B. Mycopathologia *67*(1), 29-33 (1979).
161. Y. Takeda, E. Isohata, R. Amano, and M. Uchiyama. Simultaneous extraction and fractionation and thin layer chromatographic determination of fourteen mycotoxins in grains. J. Assoc. Off. Anal. Chem. *62*(3), 573-578 (1979).
162. M.E. Stack and R.M. Eppley. High pressure liquid chromatographic analysis of cereal grains for satratoxins G and H. J. Assoc. Off. Anal. Chem. *63*(6), 1278-1281 (1980).
163. C.A. Pyle, S.D. Aust, J.W. Ronaldson, P.T. Holland, and E. Payne. Analysis of sporidesmin by gas chromatography. N.Z.J. Sci. *21*, 379-382 (1978).
164. D.B. Sauer, L.M. Seitz, R. Burroughs, H.E. Mohr, J.L. West, R.J. Milleret, and H.D. Anthony. Toxicity of *Alternaria* metabolites found in weathered sorghum grain at harvest. J. Agric. Food Chem. *26*(6), 1380-1383 (1978).
165. R.T. Gallagher and G. C. M. Latch. Production of the tremorgenic mycotoxin verruculogen and fumitremorgen B by *Penicillium piscarium* Westling. Appl. Environ. Microbiol. *33*(3), 730-731 (1977).
166. M.E. Stack, N.L. Brown, and R.M. Eppley. High pressure liquid chromatographic determination of xanthomegnin in corn. J. Assoc. Off. Anal. Chem. *61*, 590-592 (1978).
167. G.M. Ware and C.W. Thorpe. Determination of zearalenone in corn by high pressure liquid chromatography and fluorescence detection. J. Assoc. Off. Anal. Chem. *61*(5), 1058-1062 (1978).
168. W.M. Hagler, C.J. Mirocha, S.V. Pathre, and J.C. Behrens. Identification of the naturally occurring isomer of zearalenol produced by *Fusarium roseum* Gibbosum in rice culture. Appl. Environ. Microbiol. *37*(5), 849-853 (1979).

6

N-Nitrosamines and N-Nitroso Compounds

IRA S. KRULL* and DAVID H. FINE New England Institute for Life Sciences, Waltham, Massachusetts

I. INTRODUCTION

It has long been known that amines can react with various nitrosating agents, under a variety of conditions, to form a wide array of N-nitroso derivatives [1,2]. The reaction of diethyiamine hydrochloride with sodium nitrite at an acidic pH to form N-nitrosodiethylamine (NDEA) has been known since 1863 [3]. It was generally assumed that only secondary amines can effectively form stable N-nitroso derivatives (i.e., N-nitrosamines). However, it has now become apparent that primary and tertiary amines, as well as tetralkylammonium salts, can all form N-nitroso derivatives under the appropriate reaction conditions [4,5]. In addition to the reaction with nitrite under acidic conditions, nitrosation of amines and/or amine derivatives (amides, ureas, carbamates, guanidines, etc.) can also occur via reaction with nitrogen oxides (NO, NO_2, N_2O_3, N_2O_4). In addition, nitrosation can occur via transnitrosation from preformed X-nitroso [6,7] or X-nitro [8] derivatives (N-, C-, O-, etc.). It has become apparent, therefore, that there are many amines and/or amine derivatives that can form N-nitroso derivatives, and that there are several possible pathways available for the formation of the same N-nitrosamine. In this chapter, we use the terms N-nitroso derivatives and N-nitrosamines interchangeably; however, to be perfectly correct, these terms may refer to different classes of organic compounds.

Not only are N-nitrosamines readily formed under laboratory conditions, as well as in the environment, but they are also readily formed

*Present affiliation: Northeastern University, Boston, Massachusetts.

under in vivo conditions [9-11]. In vivo formation of N-nitrosamines has been demonstrated to occur in humans following the ingestion of a bacon-spinach-beer meal [12].

In view of the various possible pathways for nitrosation of amines and/or amine derivatives, it is not unexpected for N-nitroso compounds to be found in many different areas of the human environment [4,5]. The list of items that have now been demonstrated to contain measurable levels of preformed N-nitroso compounds has grown considerably over the past decade. The occurrence of N-nitrosamines in foodstuffs has been extensively reviewed [13-15]. N-Nitrosamines have been found in tobacco and tobacco smoke, and in indoor atmospheres under conditions of excessive tobacco smoking [16-18]. Formulations of the drug Aminopyrine, a widely used over-the-counter drug in Germany, have been shown to possess varying levels of N-nitrosodimethylamine (NDMA) [19], and in this country a large number of drugs have been screened for possible N-nitroso compounds, with only a small percentage being positive [20]. Fan et al. have reported percentage levels of N-nitrosodiethanolamine (NDEIA) to be present in various commercial samples of cutting fluids [21]. Other investigators have also reported on the presence of various N-nitrosamines in European brands of cutting fluids [22,23]. With regard to cosmetic products, Fan et al. have discussed the presence of varying levels of NDEIA in certain formulations of cosmetics, lotions, and shampoos [24]. Many agricultural chemicals have been shown to contain a wide variety of N-nitroso derivatives [25,26].

The greatest exposure of humans to N-nitrosamines is in the workplace [27]. Recently it has been demonstrated that the air in tire factories contains high levels of N-nitrosomorpholine (NMOR) [28,29]. The tire industry has long been known to have a higher than average rate of cancer incidence among its workers, and it may be possible to relate this to the presence of a known animal carcinogen in the workers' environment. Some leather tanners have the largest daily exposure to a N-nitrosamine (NDMA) yet known [28,30]. Along similar lines, NDMA has been found as a pollutant in the air of a factory producing dimethylamine [31,32], in air samples taken in the vicinity of a plant manufacturing a rocket propellant [33,34], and in the neighborhood of a factory making amines [33,34].

The current widespread interest in the chemistry and analysis of N-nitrosamines stems from the observation of severe liver necrosis in sheep fed a diet containing fishmeal preserved with nitrite [35], and the identification of NDMA as the toxic agent in such products [36]. N-nitroso compounds have been studied extensively with regard to mutagenicity and carcinogenicity in animals [9,37-47]. Over 100 of the approximately 130 different N-nitroso compounds tested in animals have been now shown to be carcinogenic in various animal species. As an example, NDEA has been tested for carcinogenic properties in at least 14 different animal species, and has been found to be active in all species that have been tested. The site of the tumor produced depends on the chemical structure of the N-nitroso compound, the route of administration, and the particular animal being tested. In the case of NDMA, NDEA, and N-nitrosopyrrolidine (NPYR), dose-response studies with less than 100 rats at low doses has indicated that between 1 and 5 ppm of these N-nitrosamines in the diets is marginally carcinogenic. It has been demonstrated that the in vivo metabolism of NDMA is similar in both human and rat liver [48]. Samples of human liver and lung are capable of forming alkylating and mutagenic metabolites from N-nitrosamines [49,50]. Furthermore, the rate of metabolism in human liver slices is comparable to that in the rat liver, with the levels of nucleic acid methylation being similar in both species. In humans it is known that excessive exposure to NDMA causes acute toxic liver damage [51].

The question arises regarding the carcinogenic properties of N-nitroso compounds in humans. There is a substantial amount of indirect evidence, which taken together, is suggestive that, indeed, N-nitrosamines may be carcinogenic to humans. However, a cause-and-effect relationship between exposure to low levels of N-nitrosamines and the incidence of human cancer has not yet been made.

The understanding that humans may be exposing themselves to relatively large amounts of various N-nitroso compounds is a fairly recent development. If N-nitroso compounds indeed cause cancer in humans, then reducing high exposures could significantly reduce the incidence of cancer in humans. This goal can be accomplished only by the continued determination of major routes of exposure for humans to N-nitroso compounds, and by the subsequent elimination of such exposures. In essence, this is a problem of methods of analysis for N-nitrosamines, and it is the intention of this chapter to describe the most recent advances in methods, instrumentation, and techniques for the analysis of both volatile and nonvolatile N-nitrosamines.

II. CHEMISTRY

A. Formation of N-Nitrosamines

The in vitro preparation of N-nitroso compounds in the laboratory has traditionally involved the reaction between a secondary amine and sodium nitrite under acidic conditions [1,2]. This basic nitrosation reaction has been studied in considerable detail by a number of investigators, and has been extended to include reactions with various amine derivatives, such as amides, ureas, guanidines, carbamates, peptides, nucleosides, and lactams. The basic kinetics and mechanism of the reaction with nitrite under acidic conditions has been discussed [2,5,10, 11]. Not only can secondary amines undergo nitrosation by nitrite, but it has long been known that primary amines can also partake in this reaction [2]. Most recently, Tannenbaum et al. have demonstrated the formation of N-nitrosamines from primary amines and nitrite, as well as catalytic effects by inorganic thiocyanate [52]. The overall yields for these types of reactions, in the absence of a catalyst, are generally low (0.1 to 0.5%). A general review of the reactions of primary amines with nitrous acid is available [53], and possible reaction pathways have been proposed [54].

The N-nitrosation reaction is generally slow at neutral or alkaline pH, owing to the low equilibrium concentration of the active nitrosating intermediate, nitrous anhydride (N_2O_3). However, it has been demonstrated that an appreciable nitrosation rate for secondary amines can occur at pH 6 to 11 in the presence of suitable catalysts, such as chloral or formaldehyde [55]. Keefer has also shown that various metal ions can catalyze the reaction of nitrous acid under basic conditions [56]. N-Nitrosamine formation has also been shown to be accelerated by certain microorganisms at acidic pH values [57]. Still other catalysts have been recently elucidated with regard to the basic nitrous acid reaction [58]. Inhibition of the nitrous acid nitrosation reaction has been shown with a wide variety of inorganic and organic compounds, such as ascorbic acid, sulfamic acid, tocopherol, and others [59-62].

Tertiary amine-type compounds also undergo the nitrosation reaction with nitrous acid, and this subject has been extensively reviewed [2,10,63]. Although most tertiary amines possess low rates of nitrosation under the usual reaction conditions, examples have been shown to undergo a rather rapid formation of N-nitrosamines [64,65]. A detailed study of the mechanisms of nitrosation of tertiary amines by nitrous acid has recently been presented by Ohshima and Kawabata [66]. They also discuss the formation of N-nitrosamines from two tertiary amine oxides.

For many years it was assumed that the most important system for nitrosation of amines was nitrous acid (or nitrous anhydride, N_2O_3). It is now apparent that several other routes are available for the efficient conversion of amines to their N-nitroso derivatives. Thus Challis and Kyrtopoulos have demonstrated that under oxygen-rich conditions, nitric oxide itself can nitrosate both primary and secondary amines in organic solvents [67,68]. However, under these reaction conditions, nitric oxide itself is a poor nitrosating agent, and presumably it is the oxidation product, nitrogen dioxide and subsequent products, that are the effective nitrosating agents. Challis et al. have also demonstrated a catalytic effect on the reaction with nitric oxide by inorganic metal salts and molecular iodine [68]. Some of the salts effective in these reactions were those of zinc, copper, iron, and silver, but the most effective catalyst was I_2. These metal salt-catalyzed reactions in organic solvents are considerably faster in the rate of N-nitrosamine formation than comparable reactions with nitrous acid.

It has been known for many years that certain oxides of nitrogen, N_2O_3 (nitrous anhydride) and N_2O_4 (dinitrogen tetroxide) can readily nitrosate amines and amine derivatives [2,68]. However, it has only been recently demonstrated that both primary and secondary amines react in neutral and alkaline aqueous media (pH 7 to 14) to form the corresponding N-nitrosamines [67-70]. The mechanisms of nitrosation by complex nitrogen oxides have been discussed by Challis and Kyrtopoulos [69,70].

Another route for the formation of N-nitrosamines involves a reaction termed transnitrosation, whereby the nitrosyl group of a N-nitrosamine may be transferred to a secondary amine. Thus in the case of N-nitrosodiphenylamine and morpholine, under the appropriate solvent and temperature conditions, it is possible to generate N-nitrosomorpholine and diphenylamine. Transnitrosations involving N-nitrosamines have been extensively studied by Buglass et al. [6] and more recently by Singer et al. [7,71]. Transnitrosation by aromatic N-nitroso derivatives appears to be rapid under elevated thermal conditions in nonpolar, organic solvents, polar solvents, and under aqueous acidic conditions. It is possible that transnitrosation can also occur from other nitrosyl donor compounds, such as C-nitroso and S-nitroso. The nitrosation reactions by organic nitrites (—O—NO) have been known for some time, and constitute one of the basic methods for the preparation of N-nitrosamines [1,2]. This may be a transnitrosation reaction, since it presumably involves the transfer of the nitrosyl group from a donor molecule (—O—NO) to an acceptor molecule, the secondary amine. The mechanism of nitrosation by organic nitrites (—O—NO) may also involve the intermediacy of nitric oxide, this being oxidized to nitrogen dioxide. Thus the basic mechanism may involve the intermediate dinitrogen tetroxide (N_2O_4) as the active nitrosating species [67, 68].

Nitrosation of amines by aliphatic C-nitro compounds has been known for the past 50 years [2]. Tetranitromethane, for example, effectively nitrosates amines to form the corresponding N-nitrosamines. This type of reaction has recently been studied in greater depth by Fan et al., both with regard to the generality of the reaction and its application to other amines [8]. It would seem that many aliphatic C-nitro and aromatic C-nitro compounds can nitrosate secondary amines, as well as tertiary amines, to varying extents.

From a synthetic point of view, there are many other methods for the preparation of N-nitrosamines in the laboratory. These may involve the use of nitrosyl halides, nitrosonium tetrafluoroborate, and other nitrosyl donor reagents [1,2]. However, in general, these methods for the formation of N-nitrosamines are not as widely employed as those previously mentioned.

B. Reactions of N-Nitrosamines That Affect Analysis

In the analysis of N-nitrosamines, we must be concerned with those factors that may adversely affect the successful outcome of the analytical method. N-Nitrosamines are, unfortunately, extremely reactive. Thus they are sensitive to prolonged thermal treatment as well as to photochemical irradiation [2]. In addition, certain N-nitroso derivatives are not stable to excessive conditions of pH, and β-hydroxynitrosamines undergo a fragmentation reaction under alkaline conditions [72]. Most, if not all, N-nitroso derivatives undergo reactions with inorganic acids, and this has formed the basis for the denitrosation of such compounds [73]. The acids active in denitrosation of N-nitrosamines are halogen acids, such as HCl, HBr, and HI [74]. With regard to photochemical reactivity, Fiddler et al. have shown that most volatile N-nitrosamines, and presumably nonvolatile ones also, are rapidly destroyed by the action of ultraviolet light [75].

The reduction of the nitroso group to the amino group is one of the characteristic reactions of N-nitroso compounds [2], and this reaction can be used as the basis of a chemical test for the presence of N-nitrosamines. Thus NDMA can be readily converted to dimethylhydrazine by the reaction with zinc dust and acetic acid. Lithium aluminum hydride (LAH) can also be used as an effective reducing agent for the synthesis of di-n-propyl, di-n-butyl, and di-n-pentylhydrazines. Other effective reducing agents are also known for the conversion of various N-nitrosamines to hydrazines [1,2].

N-Nitroso derivatives can be readily converted to their N-nitro analogs via various oxidizing agents. One of the most effective oxidizing agents known for this reaction is trifluoroperacetic acid. The simplicity of the method, and the purity and high yields of the final N-nitramines, have made the oxidation of N-nitrosamines with this reagent a valuable preparative method in the laboratory. Several other organic reagents are known that will also effectively convert N-nitrosamines into the corresponding N-nitramines [2]. This oxidation reaction of N-nitrosamines has also formed the basis for various analytical methods for N-nitrosamines, some of which will be discussed later.

One of the most significant physical properties of N-nitroso derivatives is the relative ease of dissociation of the —N—NO. For example, in N-nitrosodiphenylamine, the energy required to break the C—N bond is 105 kcal/mol, whereas the bond dissociation energy for the N—NO bond is only 11 kcal/mol. For other simple dialkylnitrosamines, the energy required for the N—NO bond dissociation is on the order of 40 to 60 kcal/mol. This relatively low energy requirement for release of nitric oxide from N-nitrosamines means that exposure of gaseous N-nitroso compounds to high temperatures (400 to 500°)* can be a selective method for the removal of nitric oxide without causing other major rearrangements or dissociations in the remainder of the molecule. It is this physical property of N-nitrosamines that allowed for the successful development of the Thermal Energy Analyzer (TEA), an instrument relatively specific for N-nitrosamines [76].

---

*All temperature data are in degrees Celsius.

III. SENSITIVITY REQUIREMENTS

The screening of the environment for N-nitroso compounds can be a costly and time-consuming process. Improved analytical techniques are currently available for the rapid screening of various samples for N-nitroso compounds. However, the important question of sensitivity limits and their adequacy still remains. Without a sensitivity limit, negative results, with their finite lower limit of detection, do not provide rigorous answers. Furthermore, negative results that do not contribute to a systematic, general model can only be taken as negative results for the single, unique circumstance that is examined. Similarly, the significance of positive results becomes difficult to assess if there is no knowledge about background levels.

Analytical data by themselves cannot speak to the issue of hazard. Only if hazard associated with a particular sample is based on toxicological data can the analytical results provide a reasonable basis for the setting of priorities.

Ambient levels of N-nitrosamines in human blood have been estimated to be equivalent to 1 to 7 μg/day [12], which is slightly greater than the exposure from nitrite-preserved foodstuffs. Based on this knowledge, it is possible to conclude that human exposure to less than 0.1 μg/day of N-nitrosamines is probably only of marginal interest. Using 0.1 μg/day of human exposure as the goal of the analytical technique, the sensitivity limits to meet this goal can be calculated. Thus, for air sampling, a sensitivity limit of 0.05 $\mu g/m^3$ is needed, whereas 100 ppb is needed for a facial cosmetic and 1000 ppb for a pepper cure that is ingested in minute quantitites.

There are very few known methods of detection for N-nitrosamine analysis that can routinely provide a sensitivity limit of 0.05 ppb. At the present time, only the Thermal Energy Analyzer and high-resolution mass spectrometry with peak matching are accepted as being sufficiently specific and sensitive for the accurate and reliable analysis of complex samples for N-nitrosamines [77,78].

IV. METHODOLOGY

A. Gas Chromatography-Thermal Energy Analysis

Many of the lower molecular weight N-nitrosamines are sufficiently volatile to allow for their analysis by gas chromatography (GC). Because the instrumentation for GC is so readily available in most analytical laboratories, over 95% of the published studies on the environmental occurrence of N-nitroso compounds have employed GC equipment. Most of the common detectors for GC are not specific for N-nitrosamines, and in the analysis of complex samples for trace levels of these materials, interferences from other compounds has presented a major problem in the routine use of the common GC detectors.

In 1973, Fine and Rufeh proposed the use of chemiluminescence to detect N-nitrosamines via the formation of the nitrosyl radical, after thermal cleavage of the N—NO bond [79]. This system has been successfully developed by Fine et al. [76, 79, 80] and has been commercially available for the past few years from Thermo Electron Corporation. Any gas chromatograph, operated isothermally or with temperature programming, can be interfaced to the Thermal Energy Analyzer (TEA) [81-83].

The GC-TEA interface operates by having gaseous samples swept through a catalytic pyrolyzer by a carrier gas, usually argon. All N-nitroso compounds present in the sample entering the pyrolyzer are cleaved at the N—NO bond, thereby releasing the nitrosyl radial (NO). The yield of NO is approximately stoichiometric for most N-nitrosamines. Solvent vapor, pyrolysis products, and NO pass through a cold trap at -150° which, in principle, removes all materials other than the permanent gases. The NO and the carrier gas are then swept into a low-pressure reaction chamber, where the NO reacts with ozone to generate electronically excited singlet state nitrogen dioxide (NO_2^*). The key reactions occurring in the reaction chamber are:

$$RR'\text{—N—NO} \xrightarrow[350\text{-}550^\circ]{\text{pyrolysis}} R\text{—}\dot{N}\text{—}R' + \dot{N}O$$

$$\dot{N}O + O_3 \longrightarrow NO_2^* + O_2$$

$$NO_2^* \longrightarrow NO_2 + h\nu$$

The excited NO_2^* then decays back to its ground state with the concomitant emission of light in the near infrared region of the spectrum (0.6 to 2.8 μm). The intensity of the light emitted is a direct measure of the amount of N-nitroso compound present in the sample. The Thermal Energy Analyzer system is selective because it produces a response only if a compound meets several requirements. Thus pyrolysis must occur within a few seconds within the catalytic pyrolysis tube at a moderate temperature, to give a product that survives a cold trap and reacts with ozone at reduced pressure. The product of this reaction must then emit light in the near-infrared region of the spectrum. The chemiluminescent reactions must be sufficiently rapid for the emission to occur before the reactants leave the reaction chamber. Because of the relative selectivity of the TEA, it is possible to analyze N-nitroso compounds quantitatively at high sensitivity, even in the presence of many co-eluting compounds. This reduces the cleanup procedures for samples prior to the GC-TEA step. The detection limit in GC-TEA is routinely less than 100 pg (10^{-12} g) for NDMA or NPYR.

It should be mentioned that the TEA is not totally specific for N-nitrosamines alone [8,84,85]. Thus several other classes of organic compounds will also respond to the TEA, to varying molar extents, depending on the structure of such compounds. Organic nitrites

(O—NO), N-nitramines (N—NO_2), C-nitroso (C—NO), poly C-nitro (C—NO_2), nitrates (O—NO_2), and inorganic nitrite may produce responses on the TEA. It is also probable that other classes of organic compounds (e.g., S-nitroso and S-nitro) will also be found to respond to the TEA. Thus the presence of a response by GC-TEA for a new sample cannot necessarily be taken as proof of the presence of an N-nitroso compound. Confirmation of positive results is necessary, either by the use of chemical tests to be described shortly, and/or by the use of high-resolution mass spectrometry. There is strong evidence that high-resolution mass spectrometry with continuous peak matching is a reliable confirmatory technique for the identification of N-nitrosamines [77,82].

Various applications of GC-TEA for the determination of volatile N-nitrosamines have been reported in the literature. Collaborative studies conducted by the International Agency for Research on Cancer (IARC) employing widely differing analytical methods in different laboratories have been reported [82,83]. Results obtained, both qualitatively and quantitatively, agree reasonably well with those obtained by TEA and high-resolution mass spectrometry with continuous peak matching. The TEA has two major advantages over other detectors for N-nitroso compounds. It is generally up to 100 times more sensitive than alternative, routine GC detectors such as mass spectrometry and flame ionization or alkali flame ionization types. Also, the TEA is more selective for the N-nitroso moiety than other detectors. This selectivity, with the reservations already mentioned, allows the TEA to be used at maximum sensitivity, even for the most complex and crude samples. Such a feature allows for only minimal sample cleanup and preconcentration prior to analysis. This greatly reduces the possibility for artifact formation and/or loss.

Gough et al. have described a chemiluminescent detector, analogous to the TEA, for the determination of volatile N-nitrosamines in various foodstuffs [86]. Although similar in principle to the Thermal Energy Analyzer, their detector is considerably less sensitive by at least two orders of magnitude.

B. Gas Chromatography-Mass Spectrometry

Mass spectrometry (MS) combined with gas chromatography has customarily been used for the analysis of GC amenable N-nitrosamines. The spectral fragmentation patterns of many N-nitrosamines have been documented, and several papers detail the fragmentation pathways for a number of N-nitroso compounds [87-95]. Gadbois et al. [90] and Gaffield et al. [91] have presented information on chemical ionization mass spectrometry. Mass spectrometric techniques for the analysis of volatile N-nitrosamines have been reviewed recently by Gough [92,95].

It has been observed by Gough and Webb [93] and Dooley et al. [94] that even with high resolution, a potentially interfering fragment [$^{29}Si(Me)_3$] with a retention time close to that of NDMA may be encountered. A resolution of 70,000 is required for complete separation, and a mismatch between the two compounds can be observed even at a resolution of 7000. Other potentially undesirable effects have been observed by Gough et al. [77] and may arise from the method of displaying the high-resolution signal. Under certain conditions, coeluted materials on the GC may suppress the mass spectrometer response and hence affect quantitation [96]. This, and other problems, can be overcome by the use of a peak-matching technique. Here, the mass region in the vicinity of the reference fragment (usually derived from a fluorinated hydrocarbon) and the N-nitrosamine fragment of the same approximate mass are alternatively scanned every few seconds. The method allows for the observance of the reference peak as well as the rise and fall of the N-nitrosamine peak. Monitoring only the precise mass of the parent N-nitrosamine ion using high-resolution mass spectrometry can lead to erroneous results [77]. One of the most reliable procedures for identifying N-nitrosamines is by mass spectrometry, using selective ion monitoring and continuous peak matching with high resolution, after initial GC separation [77,92]. Low-resolution mass spectrometers are less costly and more widely available, and they can be used successfully on relatively clean extracts, particularly for compounds having long GC retention times and complex fragmentation patterns. It should be noted that parent ion monitoring at high resolution with peak matching requires considerable operator skill. Also, not all commercially available multi-ion monitoring units are suitable for use at high resolution, and they cannot normally be used with a wide mass range without a loss of sensitivity at the higher mass region.

Gough et al. [77] recently compared the various mass spectrometric methods which are being used for the confirmation of data for GC-amenable N-nitrosamines. A wide variety of food and biological samples was used in this study. Low-resolution mass spectrometry (LRMS) was performed by monitoring two ions. High-resolution mass spectrometry with precise ion monitoring was performed with a resolution of 7000. The instrument was focused directly on the appropriate parent ion. High-resolution mass spectrometry (HRMS) with peak matching (PM) was done as above, with the mass range in the vicinity of the appropriate parent ion being continuously scanned with respect to a suitable internal standard. Thermal Energy Analysis was carried out using a Thermo Electron Model 502 instrument. Only the high-resolution method with precise peak matching gave data which was in agreement with that obtained using the TEA. The discrepancies between the various mass spectrometric results arose partly because interfering compounds giving ions of similar mass may be present, and also because co-eluting materials of any mass altered the mass spectrometric response. This problem may be practically overcome if high-efficiency capillary columns are used on the gas chromatograph, or by using continuous peak-matching techniques. Peak matching has the additional advantage of minimizing problems associated with both instrument instability and co-eluting peaks. It is to be concluded from the study of Gough et al. that all GC-MS (low-resolution) data for the presence of volatile N-nitrosamines in complex environmental systems are suspect, and some of these may be in error. Similarly, GC-MS (high-resolution) data are acceptable only if continuous peak-matching methods have been employed.

In the case of N-nitrosodiethanolamine, a nonvolatile N-nitrosamine, Arsenault and Biemann introduced the purified sample directly into the mass spectrometer with a solid probe, and used high-resolution MS equipped with a photographic plate [21,24]. N-nitrosodiethanolamine was the first "nonvolatile" N-nitroso compound in the environment to be identified.

C. High-Pressure Liquid Chromatography-Thermal Energy Analysis

Samples can be introduced into the TEA in one of three modes. First, samples can be introduced directly into the detector. Second, samples can be introduced into a GC which is interfaced to the TEA. Third, samples can be introduced into a high-pressure liquid chromatograph (HPLC) which is interfaced to the TEA [97-99]. Most HPLC detectors currently available are not specific to a particular class of compounds, and will not allow for their estimation in the presence of co-eluting materials. The TEA is unique in that it represents the only practical HPLC detector that can be routinely used for the analysis of N-nitrosamines in complex sample matrices.

The TEA, when operated in the HPLC mode, operates on the same basic principles as discussed above with regard to GC-TEA. However, here a liquid sample is swept through the catalytic pyrolyzer by argon carrier gas, and all organic materials are quickly vaporized and/or pyrolyzed. Following the pyrolyzer, the solvents are condensed out inside large (300 ml) vacuum cold traps, prior to entering the chemiluminescent chamber. If the temperature of the traps is too low, some of the solvent mixture will solidify, thereby blocking the flow of carrier gas. Alternatively, if the temperature of the traps is too high, some of the HPLC solvents may be swept over into the reaction chamber. This may adversely affect the sensitivity and selectivity of the instrument. In practice, the temperature of the first cold trap is chosen so that it will effectively condense out all of the carrier solvent, but not solidify it. The temperature of the second trap may then be kept low enough to condense out any escaping solvent vapors from the first trap, and also to contain other materials that might cause an interference within the reaction chamber.

At the low temperatures used in the cold traps, only the carrier gas, the nitrosyl radical (NO), and a very few, low molecular weight organic species pass through both cold traps. The use of a small, stainless steel cartridge, packed with Tenax-GC, placed after the second cold trap and before the reaction chamber, has been found useful in removing traces of small organic moieties and reactive species which survive the cold traps. The remaining TEA operations are identical to those already described for the GC-TEA mode.

Flow programming can be used in HPLC-TEA analyses and is analogous to flow-programming methods in HPLC-UV. This method has been utilized in going from 0.2 ml/min to 2.0 ml/min, without producing more than a slight baseline drift during the entire chromatogram [97]. In flow programming, the flow rate of the HPLC solvent is slowly increased during the analysis, allowing for a decreased overall time between each injection of sample. The detector response in HPLC-TEA has been determined to be linear over four orders of magnitude, from as low as 500 pg, with N-nitroso compounds as diverse as N-nitrosocarbazole, N-nitroso-N-ethylaniline, and N-nitrosopiperidine.

Solvent programming has been utilized in a number of HPLC-TEA analyses. Baseline drift can become more of a problem with solvent programming than with any other method in HPLC-TEA, but this can be minimized by a careful choice of the solvent mixture and the temperatures of the cold traps employed.

There are some restrictions when using the TEA in combination with HPLC. Nitric acid cannot be used as part of the HPLC solvent, nor can solvents be used which are buffered with organic or inorganic salts. If such salts are used, or if the sample itself is an organic salt, the HPLC injection nozzle inside the furnace, as well as the furnace itself, may become clogged with unvaporized solids [100]. Eventually, the sample will not be able to enter the pyrolysis chamber, and the flow of solvent through it will be restricted. On column injection is not possible with the TEA, because the "stopped flow" technique upsets the TEA vacuum. Therefore, a valve-type injector for HPLC must be used. Taking the restrictions above into consideration, the TEA can be successfully interfaced to any HPLC system [24,97-102].

With the HPLC-TEA, screening procedures for background N-nitroso compounds can proceed relatively rapidly, and a large number of samples can be studied in a short period of time. Exhaustive extraction of environmental or industrial products, followed by HPLC-TEA determinations, allows for the rapid establishment of upper limits to background N-nitroso compound levels. With HPLC-TEA, the limits of detection for most N-nitrosamines are in the range 0.1 to 1.0 ng per injection. This allows for a sensitivity range of approximately 10 to 100 ppb for most compounds, but this depends on the particular sample preparation and chromatographic conditions employed in any given analysis.

Finally, it should be noted that the TEA is compatible with most, but not all modes of HPLC. Thus it is possible to employ liquid-solid adsorption, liquid-liquid partition, gel permeation, and reverse-phase HPLC, but not ion exchange or paired-ion chromatography. Also, polar N-nitroso compounds with hydroxyl or carboxyl groups, such as N-nitrosamino acids and N-nitrosodiethanolamine, have relative molar response factors on the TEA of less than 1.0. Esterification of the free hydroxyl groups or carboxylic acid moieties results in a derivative having a relative response factor closer to 1.0, which is similar to that obtained from the more volatile N-nitrosamines.

D. High-Pressure Liquid Chromatography-Ultraviolet Spectrometry and Colorimetry

Most N-nitroso derivatives exhibit a characteristic UV absorption spectrum, with a strong absorption band at or near 230 nm (pi-pi*), and a much weaker absorption band at higher wavelengths (330 to 350 nm) (n-pi*) [103,104]. The absorption band of N-nitrosamines is considerably stronger at the shorter wavelengths (230 nm), with an extinction coefficient for many materials between 5000 and 10,000. Thus it is this region that is of interest for the HPLC-UV analysis of N-nitrosamines, and many workers have successfully used the technique for measuring the concentrations of N-nitrosamines in model systems, as well as in extracts of environmental samples containing high levels of N-nitrosamines [105,106]. Because of interferences from other components that absorb in the same region, this technique is not generally suitable for trace analysis in complex food extracts or other environmental samples. For similar reasons, the IR and NMR techniques, although useful for characterizing pure N-nitrosamines [107,108], have found little use in trace analysis. Heyns and Roper have described the HPLC-UV analysis of various types of N-nitroso compounds, including N-nitroso-N-alkylureas and N-nitroso-N-alkylurethans [109]. In this instance, separation was achieved by HPLC using reverse-phase partitioning and detection by UV at 254 nm. The lowest detection limit in these cases was 10 ng per injection. Similarly, Montgomery et al. [110] have discussed the HPLC-UV analysis of various N-nitrosoureas and their metabolites, again using a reverse-phase system. Direct HPLC-UV analysis for N-nitrosamines has also been applied by Iwaoka and Tannenbaum, in the separation of the syn and anti conformers of N-nitrosamino acids [111]. This method has also been applied by Iwaoka et al. for either the quantitation of N-nitrosamines in relatively clean food samples or for a rapid column cleanup procedure prior to final confirmation and quantitation by GC-MS [112]. Cox has demonstrated the use of HPLC-UV for the estimation of volatile N-nitrosamines in complex food samples, with a reduction in the chromatographic analysis time as compared to GC [113]. However, as generally observed by most workers, the method is prone to interference from other extracted materials in comparison with other methods of analysis. For the routine analysis of foods that do not give rise to interfering peaks, this method can be quite useful. Cox also describes a derivatization method that employs eventual HPLC-UV detection of the final derivatized N-nitrosamines [113]. Hecht et al. have also applied variable-wavelength UV detection with HPLC separations for the analysis of various N-nitroso derivatives of tobacco alkaloids [18,114]. Rao and McLennon have reported on the HPLC-UV analysis of the N-nitroso derivatives of piperazine formed from the in vivo reaction of this drug with inorganic nitrite [115]. Green et al. have compared HPLC-UV with HPLC-TEA for the analysis of N-nitroso species produced in the nitrosation reaction of spermidine and in food extracts [116]. The HPLC-UV method revealed the presence of many interfering species, whereas the HPLC-TEA methods were relatively specific for the N-nitroso compounds present [101,116].

Preussmann et al. have recently reported on the analysis of urine for N-nitrosodiethanolamine utilizing HPLC-UV [117]. These workers made use of a variable-wavelength UV detector, with detection at 248 nm. The use of such variable UV detectors for the analysis of N-nitrosamines may offer certain advantages over fixed-wavelength apparatus [114,118].

The use of direct HPLC-UV analysis for N-nitrosamines is difficult for most environmental samples, especially with regard to co-eluting, interfering substances. For these reasons, HPLC-UV for the direct analysis of N-nitrosamines has not gained widespread acceptance.

In colorimetric methods of analysis, the N-nitrosamines are first cleaved. The resulting fragment (NO, NO_2, NO_2^-, or an amine) is then determined colorimetrically following a reaction with a suitable chromophor. The cleavage can be brought about by exposure to UV light [119,120], by treatment with hydrobromic acid in glacial acetic acid [121], or by heat [122]. Sander observed that if the irradiation is carried out with long-wavelength irradiation (360 nm) at an alkaline pH, the technique is more specific for N-nitrosamines [123]. Fan and Tannenbaum developed an automated technique based on this same principle [124]. This automated technique was further extended by Singer et al., who interfaced it with a high-pressure liquid chromatograph [122]. Their HPLC system utilizes reverse-phase chromatography, and is, in principle, capable of detecting 0.5 nmol. Several compounds are known to interfere with the method [125] and particularly with the dyes that are used. The most extensively used colorimetric method is that of Eisenbrand and Preussmann [121], in which the liberated nitrosating species, formed after treatment with hydrobromic acid in glacial acetic acid, is captured by diazotization with sulfanilic acid. This is subsequently coupled with N-(naphthyl)ethylenediamine. This technique is satisfactory for the analysis of 17 N-nitrosamines, with an average recovery of 99.5%. Since it determines only nitrite, the method is suitable for group analysis of N-nitrosamines but is incapable of distinguishing between different N-nitrosamines unless it is coupled with HPLC. Another method developed by Eisenbrand and Preussmann is based on the determination and quantitation of secondary amines produced by the cleavage of the original N-nitrosamines present in a sample. This colorimetric method has been used for measuring N-nitrosamines present in food extracts [126].

E. Polarography and Electrochemical Detection

One of the more interesting physical properties of N-nitroso compounds is their ability to be readily oxidized and reduced by other than chemical means. Thus Heath and Jarvis were the first to use polarography for the detection of NDMA in animal tissues [127], their limit of detection being 500 μg/liter. Volatile N-nitrosamines can be distinguished from each other on the basis of the differences in their half-wave potentials. Although several other workers have used this technique, it is now generally accepted that the method is not sufficiently specific for the analysis of complex mixtures [127,128]. Thus interferences were shown to occur from furfural and pyrazines, common constituents of many foodstuffs [128,129]. This technique can be used for the analysis of N-nitrosamines in less complex systems, such as in model experiments.

Chang and Harrington, as well as Hasebe and Osteryoung, have recently described the use of differential pulse polarography in model systems [130,131]. An electrochemical method has been described for the analysis of N-nitrosamines in foodstuffs and is reported to detect these compounds at levels as low as 0.2 ppb [132]. In this procedure Snider and Johnson first remove interfering substances by ion exchange chromatography. The N-nitrosamines are photochemically converted to nitrite anion, which is adsorbed on another ion exchange column for the removal of contaminating materials. Eventually, the nitrite generated photochemically from the N-nitrosamines is detected electrochemically using a platinum electrode for the conversion of nitrite to nitric oxide. From the current-time curves which are obtained, the amount of N-nitrosamine can be determined by a comparison with known standards. In general, interference by other compounds is not a problem, but the most serious interference being due to organic nitro compounds ($O{-}NO_2$, $C{-}NO_2$, $N{-}NO_2$). The method of Snider and Johnson has not been interfaced with any chromatography apparatus. It may be applicable to the screening of complex samples for total N-nitroso content rather than for the identification and quantitation of individual N-nitrosamines. Those samples that are positive for N-nitroso derivatives must still be analyzed further using either GC or HPLC with additional specific detectors (MS, TEA, etc.).

In recent years, electrochemical detection with HPLC has been developed for a large number of organic compounds. An example is the work of Kissinger's group [133,134]. Liquid chromatography electrochemical detection (LCEC) has been successfully applied for the routine analysis of materials, such as catecholamines, phenols, and aniline derivatives [135-137]. However, despite its potential for N-nitrosamine analysis, there have been no literature reports applying the method to the detection of N-nitroso compounds in complex environmental samples.

F. Thin Layer Chromatography

Thin layer chromatography (TLC) has been used by many workers for both qualitative and quantitative determination of N-nitrosamines. The major advantage of the technique are its simplicity and relatively low cost. However, with only a few exceptions, the technique is only semi-quantitative, and not sufficiently selective to distinguish N-nitrosamines of closely related structure and similar R_f.

Preussmann et al. was the first to report on the use of a TLC method for detecting N-nitrosamines in microgram amounts [138]. This method used a diphenylamine spray reagent together with UV light and formed a colored complex with palladium chloride [139]. Preussmann et al. also described a different TLC technique whereby the N-nitrosamines were detected on TLC plates by spraying with the Griess reagent after initial exposure to UV light [140]. A positive response to both of the foregoing reagents was then considered positive for the presence of a particular N-nitrosamine. In other methods, the secondary amines formed by photolysis of the N-nitrosamines with UV light were detected by the classical ninhydrin reagent [139,141]. The detection limits for these TLC methods range from 0.2 to 2 μg per compound, depending on the particular structure of the N-nitrosamines. Young has recently described a highly sensitive method whereby N-nitrosamines can be detected by TLC as fluorescent spots after exposure to UV irradiation followed by spraying with fluorescamine reagent [142,143]. The detection limit here varied between 10 and 500 ng per compound. The majority of the 24 N-nitrosamines analyzed afforded fluorophors.

Rao and Bejnarowicz have reported a direct TLC analysis for a certain N-nitroso derivative of sarcosine, together with its N-lauroyl ester [144]. This method utilizes various detection systems, such as (1) direct UV (254 nm) observations, (2) exposure to iodine vapors, and (3) spraying with a sulfuric acid-ethanol solution (1:1) and heating on a hot plate for 10 min.

In several methods, N-nitrosamines are chromatographed after formation of their derivatives. Such derivatives include the nitramines [145], fluorescent dansyl derivatives of the corresponding secondary amines [146], and fluorescent hydrazones [147]. Another method involves the formation of hydrazines from the N-nitrosamines, which are then converted to the hydrazides, and these are analyzed by two-dimensional TLC [148]. The zones containing the fluorescent hydrazones can then be removed from the TLC plates, extracted from tho adsorbent, and identified by their characteristic UV and mass spectra [147]. Sen et al. have reported that the ninhydrin reaction product of N-nitrosopyrrolidine on TLC plates (silica gel) is highly fluorescent when viewed under UV light, giving a detection limit of 10 ng per spot [149]. Wolfram et al. utilized the HBr in acetic acid denitrosation reaction on N-nitrosoproline, followed by formation of the highly fluorescent NBD (7-chloro-4-nitro-benzo-2-oxas-1,3-diazole) derivative of the amino product [150]. The fluorescent derivative (NBD-proline) is then detected and quantitated by either thin layer chromatography or HPLC. Using this method, it was possible to detect less than 10 ng of N-nitrosoproline. A comprehensive review of thin layer chromatography methods for N-nitrosamines, and the use of derivatives for the analysis of N-nitrosamines is available [151].

Despite the fact that TLC methods appear to be versatile and sensitive, they are generally of questionable reliability. The single exception is probably Sen's procedure for NPYR in bacon [149]. TLC methods have not found general acceptance as a routine procedure for the trace analysis of N-nitrosamines in complex samples. However, recent developments in TLC have accomplished greatly improved separations, especially the use of programmed multiple development (PMD) [152], high-performance radial chromatography [153], and ultramicro TLC on cylindrical supports [154]. These methods could perhaps be coupled with newer procedures for the quantitative determination of TLC plates [155,156]. Finally, TLC has now been automated, suggesting that this method might eventually be utilized, in certain select instances, for the routine analysis of some N-nitrosamines [157].

G. Gas Chromatography-Flame Ionization, Alkali Flame Ionization, Coulson, and Hall Detection

The application of common GC detectors for the analysis of N-nitrosamines has recently been reviewed [151]. Perhaps because GC instrumentation is available in most analytical laboratories, it has been the principal method of analysis for volatile N-nitrosamines. This may also be the reason that most of the literature on the analysis of N-nitroso compounds deals with volatile materials. The conventional flame ionization detectors (FID) have been found to be of limited value for N-nitrosamines. Before the advent of the TEA, most workers in the field employed one of the more selective nitrogen specific detectors [158,159].

The alkali flame ionization detector (AFID) and the Coulson electrolytic conductivity detector (CECD) are the two major detectors of this type. The AFID is made relatively specific to nitrogen compounds by placing a ring or coil coated with $RbSO_4$ or KCl on or around the hydrogen flame [160-162]. The sensitivity here is generally greater than with conventional FID, with a limit of detection for NDMA of about 4 ng. The AFID has been successfully used for routine screening of foodstuffs for the presence of volatile N-nitrosamines [162-164]. The sensitivity of the AFID can be adversely affected by organochlorine solvents [105]. Sensitivity is also affected by the condition of the salt tip [165].

In the CECD method, the GC column effluent is mixed with a stream of hydrogen gas, and then passed through a hot quartz pyrolysis tube containing a nickel wire as the catalyst. In this manner, all nitrogen-containing compounds present in the original sample are reduced to ammonia. The ammonia is then detected and quantitatively measured by the change in the conductivity of water in a special detector cell assembly [166]. The FID and AFID methods are useful for screening, but they are not specific to N-nitrosamines, and independent confirmation is therefore essential for every analysis.

There are restrictions on the routine use of these detectors for the analysis of N-nitrosamines. Many other nitrogen, as well as phosphorus compounds give a positive response on the AFID [167]. Rhoades and Johnson have used the pyrolytic mode of the CECD to enhance the selectivity to N-nitrosamines [168]. Although the pyrolytic mode is not as sensitive as the conventional mode [167,169], because of the increased selectivity, the pyrolytic mode became the CECD mode of choice [167,170-173]. Palframan et al. have compared the performance characteristics of an AFID with those of a CECD, and concluded that the sensitivity of the two detectors was virtually identical [167].

The modified Hall detector [174] is more useful than the conventional CECD. Eisenbrand et al. have used this detector for the analysis of N-nitrosamines in a variety of foodstuffs such as wheat, rice, bread, cured ham, and fermented sausages [175]. The principle of operation of the Hall detector is the same as that of the CECD, but the former is more sensitive than the latter, owing to improved geometric design of the electrolytic conductivity cell and other working parameters. In principle, about 50 pg of NDMA can be detected using this method.

H. Derivatization for Gas Chromatography and Liquid Chromatography

Several references have already been made to the use of various derivatives for the analysis of N-nitroso compounds, and this subject has recently been extensively reviewed [151]. There are many ways by which N-nitroso materials may be chemically modified to generate derivatives which can then be determined more easily, and with increased sensitivity and/or specificity than the parent compound. In the following discussion, we indicate the use of specific reagents for the conversion of N-nitrosamines into other organic compounds; however, it should be understood that additional reagents are available which will effect the identical conversions [139,176]. Thus anyone interested in utilizing the formation of derivatives should be aware not only of what has already been accomplished in this area, but that other reagents and methods can also be utilized [177-179].

Hydrazines

N-Nitroso compounds can be easily reduced to their hydrazines, which are then further derivatized. Several standard reducing agents have been used for this purpose, such as zinc in hydrochloric acid [180], and metal hydrides ($LiAlH_4$) [147,181,182]. The unsymmetrical hydrazine thus formed is further condensed with various derivatizing reagents, aldehydes [147,180,183] or acid chlorides [148,182]. The most satisfactory approach was the conversion of the hydrazine to its 3,5-dinitrobenzaldehyde hydrazone, which was then analyzed using GC-electron capture detection (ECD) [17].

Amines

Analogous to the formation of hydrazines from N-nitrosamines is their conversion to secondary amines. Several methods are available for effecting this denitrosation reaction [2], one of the more popular being the use of hydrobromic acid (HBr) in glacial acetic acid [73,146]. Alliston et al. have used electrolysis in alkali medium to effect the same conversion [184]. Also of use are the reactions of the N-nitrosamines with cuprous chloride in hydrochloric acid, as well as the reaction with titanium [111] chloride in glacial acetic acid [185]. The secondary amine produced by these various methods can then all be converted to appropriate derivatives for either GC, TLC, or HPLC analysis. For GC analysis [178], one of the most common derivatives used is the heptafluorobutyryl amide (HFB-amide), formed by the reaction of the HFB-acid chloride and the amine. This derivative can then be analyzed by GC-electron capture or GC-mass spectrometry [82,175,184,186]. Other amine derivatives have also been used. For example, Cox [113], formed the 2,4-dinitrophenyl derivative of his amines, and then used HPLC-UV in the range 340 to 360 nm for the quantitative and qualitative determinations. This particular method was applied to the analysis of N-nitrosamines in pork luncheon meat and fried pig liver. Interfering compounds could be distinguished by running a blank determination with the sample, but leaving out the reduction step on the N-nitrosamine. Eisenbrand hydrolyzed N-nitrosamines and then formed the fluorescent dansyl derivatives of the secondary amines. These were than analyzed by TLC with UV detection of the final derivatives [146]. Sen et al. formed the ninhydrin derivative of the N-nitrosopyrrolidine amine, pyrrolidine, and detected this by TLC with UV light [149]. Still other amine derivatives have been described [151,179].

Nitramines

Virtually all N-nitroso compounds can be converted to their oxidation products, the nitramines ($N—NO_2$), by several different oxidative pathways. Thus Sen prepared dimethylnitramine by the oxidation of NDMA with trifluoroacetic acid in hydrogen peroxide (50%) [187]. Althorpe et al. investigated the conversion of a series of N-nitrosamines into the nitramines by similar oxidation with peroxytrifluoroacetic acid formed from hydrogen peroxide and trifluoroacetic acid [188]. The nitramines were then detected by GC-electron capture detection, which was 100 to 1000 times more sensitive than with flame ionization. Nitramines have also been detected by TLC, as in the determination of N-nitrosamines in various alcoholic beverages [145]. Confirmation of nitramines can also be obtained by GC-mass spectrometry [189]. Hotchkiss et al. describe the use of newer reaction conditions for the conversion of N-nitrosamines to the nitramines, followed by GC-TEA analysis of both compounds simultaneously [190].

Miscellaneous derivatives

A recent method for the analysis of N-nitrosamines involves a report by Gaffield and Lundin [191]. These workers studied the formation of hexafluoroacetone derivatives of certain nitrosamino alcohols and amines. These adducts could then be determined by determination of the ^{19}F NMR spectroscopy. As little as 0.3 μg of certain N-nitrosamines could be detected by conversion to their hexafluoroacetone derivatives (NMR concentration = 6.9×10^{-6} M). This probably represents the limits of detection for ^{19}F NMR analyses, which represents a limit of about 1 ppm in actual samples. The method has not been used for environmental samples.

Eisenbrand et al. have used the trimethylsilyl (TMS) derivatives of N-nitroso amino acids for the GC-TEA analysis of N-nitrosoproline, N-nitrosohydroxyproline, and N-nitrososarcosine [192]. This method has been used with a wide variety of foodstuffs. N-nitrosodiethanolamine can also be silylated to yield a volatile derivative suitable for GC analysis.

Sen et al. have reported on a method whereby N-nitrosamino acids are converted into their methyl ethers and then analyzed by GC-MS [193]. This method has been applied to the analysis of a N-nitrosopyrrolidine derivative, as well as in the analysis of N-nitrosodiethanolamine in cutting fluids [21,173]. Both the trimethylsilyl and the methyl ether methods are particularly valuable, because they convert nonvolatile N-nitroso derivatives into volatile materials suitable for analysis by GC.

V. CONFIRMATORY TECHNIQUES

As in all analyses at the part-per-billion level, there are no methods that are entirely specific for N-nitroso compounds under all circumstances. However, the analyst concerned with trace levels of N-nitroso compounds is better equipped than in the analysis of most other organic species. There are two entirely different problems to be considered, one in the analysis of routine samples using well-established methods, and the other for identification of a compound of unknown origin. These two cases are considered separately.

A known nitrosamine

For routine analyses involving known N-nitrosamines, most currently accepted methods involve some cleanup of the sample or its extract, followed by analysis by GC-TEA for the volatile N-nitrosamines, and by HPLC-TEA in the case of nonvolatile N-nitrosamines. Depending on the nature of the problem, the following confirmatory procedures can be used.

1. GC-TEA analysis on two vastly different GC columns, including coinjection of the known N-nitrosamine(s) standard (Section IV.A).
2. Combined GC-TEA and HPLC-TEA analysis (Section V.A). Quantitation by GC and HPLC should agree within experimental error.
3. GC-MS (Section IV.B). Suitable care should be used in the choice of the MS method.

TEA peak of unknown origin

If there is a sizable peak on the GC-TEA or HPLC-TEA which does not co-elute with a known standard, it then becomes necessary to characterize the material giving rise to the TEA response. If there is sufficient material, and the unknown is amenable to GC and can be readily isolated in a relatively clean state, GC-MS is the initial, preferred method of structure identification. If this is not possible, or if the material is amenable only to HPLC analysis (is nonvolatile), the isolation and structure characterization becomes time consuming and expensive. To prevent wasted effort in characterizing compounds which are not N-nitroso compounds, a series of tests can be carried out for the presence of the N-nitroso group. Although none of the tests is definitive, when taken together it is possible to be reasonably certain that the compound contains the N-nitroso functional group.

The tests are:

1. Use of general TEA confirmatory techniques (Section V.B)
2. Use of UV irradiation (Section V.C)
3. Use of chemical tests for N-nitrosamines (Section V.D)

If, as a result of these tests, the unknown material appears to be an N-nitroso compound, appropriate artifact experiments and structure identification should be attempted. The following steps are suggested as a general guide for the analysis of unknown N-nitrosamines:

Application of appropriate artifact experiments should be conducted to ensure that the compounds determined are present in the original sample at the observed levels (Section VI). Only if these experiments indicate that the unknown is present at the observed level in the original sample, and that it has not been formed during the analysis, is it worth proceeding as follows. If the material is volatile, it should be concentrated sufficiently for initial GC-MS analysis (Section IV.B).

In the case of nonvolatile materials, it must be isolated by either open column chromatography or HPLC in sufficient quantity and purity for characterization by standard methods in natural product identification (Section V.E).

Structure identification by MS alone may not be sufficient in the case of previously unreported N-nitroso derivatives, and additional structural information may have to be obtained. This can include spectroscopic analysis by IR, NMR, UV-VIS, and other methods, as deemed appropriate or necessary (Section V.E).

Enough data should be accumulated to confirm the structure beyond a reasonable doubt.

If additional structure identification is needed, this can involve the formation of appropriate derivatives, and the subsequent characterization of the derivatives (Section IV.H).

A. Combined GC-HPLC Methods

If an environmental sample produces a TEA response on GC-TEA, it is possible to confirm the presence of a known N-nitrosamine by using a combination of GC-TEA and HPLC-TEA on the same sample.

In GC, compounds elute as a function of their relative vapor pressures and solubility in the stationary phase. In HPLC, compounds elute according to their size, polarity, solubility in the mobile phase, attraction to the stationary phase, ionic properties, and other physical parameters. Because of these basic differences between GC and HPLC, the elution order of a series of compounds is usually quite different. If a relatively selective detector is used for both GC and HPLC, the possibility of two compounds co-eluting in both systems is fairly small.

The possibility of incorrect identification is further reduced by physically isolating a single peak from HPLC-TEA, which is then concentrated and reinjected onto GC-TEA. Positive identification versus a known N-nitrosamine standard is then made. First, the peak must elute at the known GC or HPLC retention time of the standard, and co-injection must produce only a single peak. Second, the magnitude (quantitation) of the HPLC-TEA and GC-TEA peaks must be within experimental error. Internal TEA confirmation has been used successfully to identify NDMA in air [81,194], and NDMA and NDPA in herbicides [25]. In all cases, GC-high-resolution mass spectrometry also confirmed the presence of the N-nitrosamine. The parallel HPLC-TEA and GC-TEA technique was also used to confirm the presence of NDMA and NDEA in human blood following ingestion of cooked bacon and spinach [12]. In this instance, an insufficient amount of the N-nitrosamine was available to confirm by any other technique. Parallel TEA confirmation is especially valuable when the availability of the sample is limited.

B. General TEA Methods

In the use of the TEA for the detection of N-nitroso compounds, false positive artifacts are known to be caused by compounds with labile nitrosyl groups, those with labile nitro groups, and those containing certain substituted olefins which chemiluminesce with ozone [97,99, 195].

Substituted olefins are readily distinguished from N-nitroso compounds on the TEA by use of a low-temperature (-150°) cold trap, in combination with an in-line Tenax-GC filled cartridge [102]. A N-nitroso compound should produce a TEA peak height identical with that obtained in the absence of the Tenax-GC cartridge, and at all trap temperatures above -150°. However, other compounds with labile nitrosyl or nitro groups, such as organic nitrites and nitrates [5,85], aliphatic C-nitroso compounds [84], N-nitramines [85,190], and certain organic C-nitro compounds [8] cannot be distinguished from N-nitroso compounds on the TEA [195]. False-positive responses due to labile nitroso or nitro groups, other than N-nitroso, can only be demonstrated to be false by a combination of several experiments, as outlined below (Sections V.C and V.D).

C. Ultraviolet Photolysis

One of the simplest confirmatory tests to apply to the material producing a response of unknown origin on the TEA, either by GC or HPLC, involves analyzing the sample extract both before and after it has been exposed to UV light [196,197]. Ideally, the sample under analysis is first spiked with a known N-nitrosamine as an internal standard. The internal standard should elute close to the unknown peak of interest.

It is important for this method that the solvent itself does not absorb the light; otherwise, complications can arise from either quenching or sensitization of the basic photolysis reactions. The use of an internal standard should draw attention to this problem. A portion of the sample is then irradiated with a broad-spectrum UV light source or a sunlamp [75]. If the TEA response from the standard N-nitrosamine decreases in peak height, but that for the unknown material remains constant, the TEA response was probably not due to an N-nitroso compound. This test is not foolproof, however, because C-nitroso compounds, which also produce a TEA response, can be destroyed under the same irradiation conditions [198]. If a Pyrex filter is used for the irradiations, simple olefins should not be affected, and they will not exhibit a decrease in their TEA response.

It is also possible that a compound which is not an N-nitroso material can produce a TEA response, and under irradiation conditions, this can be changed to another material that does not produce a TEA signal. This was found to be the situation in the case of sodium saccharin, an organic salt that does indeed yield a TEA signal when analyzed by HPLC [100]. Irradiation experiments by UV must be reviewed critically [75,195].

It might prove possible to differentiate between C-nitroso and N-nitroso compounds by careful use of the photochemical test. Under identical solvent and irradiation conditions, typical N-nitroso derivatives, such as N-nitrosodiphenylamine, N-nitrosocarbazole, N-nitrosopiperidine, NDMA, NDEA, NPYR, and NDEIA, undergo disappearance of their HPLC-TEA response within 60 min. In the case of C-nitroso compounds, such as 2-methyl-2-nitrosopropane, nitrosobenzene, 4-nitrosodiphenylamine, and p-nitrosodimethylaniline, there is a very large difference in their photochemical reactivities. Some of these undergo disappearance of their HPLC-TEA signal upon irradiation within 60 min, but the p-aniline derivatives are stable. Thus it may be possible to differentiate C-nitroso versus N-nitroso compounds on this basis. Further work in this area is continuing in our laboratory [198].

D. Denitrosation with Hydrobromic Acid in Acetic Acid (HBr-HOAc) and Glacial Acetic Acid (HOAc) Alone

The use of hydrobromic acid (HBr) in glacial acetic acid (HOAc) as a denitrosation reagent (HBr-HOAc) for the analysis of N-nitrosamines was first applied by Eisenbrand and Preussmann [121]. It has been modified and improved by Johnson and Walters [199], Downes et al. [73], and Krull et al. [20].

The HBr-HOAc denitrosation test is applied as follows. The sample is extracted into an organic solvent such as acetone, ethyl acetate, or methylene chloride. The solvent must be of the highest purity, and free of water and alcohols. A known standard N-nitroso compound is then added to the extract to serve as an internal control. The retention time of the standard and the unknown should be similar. A small amount of the organic extract is then diluted with an excess of 10% HBr in glacial acetic acid (freshly prepared) and in glacial acetic acid alone. Typically, the ratio of organic extract to the acetic acid reagent is about 4:1 or 5:1. The reaction mixtures are then heated in sealed vials for 20 min at about 40°, after which time all three mixtures are analyzed by HPLC-TEA. Peak heights for the unknown TEA and the internal control are then compared. If the unknown material is an N-nitroso compound, it should behave as does the internal control. These methods are difficult to apply to GC, where acetic acid may adversely affect the packing materials.

The denitrosation test with HBr-HOAc and the HOAc test are not completely specific for N-nitroso compounds alone. We have studied several classes of organic compounds in these two tests, including N-nitroso, C-nitroso, O-nitroso and C-nitro derivatives. In the case of N-nitroso compounds, we have analyzed N-nitrosocarbazole, N-nitrosodiphenylamine, N-nitrosodimethylurea, N-nitroso-N-methyl-p-toluene sulfonamide, N-nitroso-N-methyl-N'-nitroguanidine, and several typical N-nitroso dialkylamines (NDMA, NDEA, etc.). With regard to the HBr-HOAc test, all of the N-nitroso standards exhibited a disappearance of their HPLC-TEA response. In the case of the HOAc alone, none of the N-nitroso compounds showed a decrease in their HPLC-TEA response.

In the case of O-nitroso compounds, we have studied iso-pentyl nitrite, t-butyl nitrite, and n-butyl nitrite. These materials undergo a loss of their HPLC-TEA response with both HBr-HOAc and HOAc. Thus O-nitroso compounds exhibit a different response than for N-nitroso and C-nitroso materials, in the HOAc procedure.

The C-nitroso derivatives studied have included 2-nitro-1-propanol, 1,5-difluoro-2,4-dinitrobenzene, and 2,3-dimethyl-2,3-dinitrobutane. All of these showed no change in their TEA responses using either HBr-HOAc or HOAc. Thus C-nitro materials behave differently as compared with N-nitroso compounds.

We have studied four C-nitroso compounds, 2-methyl-2-nitrosopropane, p-nitrosodiphenylamine, nitrosobenzene, and p-nitrosodimethylaniline. In the HBr-HOAc test, there is a disappearance of the HPLC-TEA response for all four C-nitroso compounds. With HOAc alone, there is no change in the HPLC-TEA response. Thus both N-nitroso and C-nitroso compounds produce the same responses in the denitrosation test with HBr-HOAc and with HOAc.

In summary, for the majority of those organic compounds that produce significant TEA responses, it is possible to differentiate C-nitroso and N-nitroso materials from other false positives. It is not yet possible to differentiate C-nitroso from N-nitroso compounds.

However, C-nitroso compounds have not been reported to be present in the environment, and they are usually unstable to environmental conditions. Also, we have found the C-nitroso materials can show different photochemical properties as compared with N-nitroso compounds. Using a combination of photolysis, HBr-HOAc, and HOAc alone, it is possible to be reasonably secure in the assignment of an N-nitroso structure to an unknown material.

It is to be expected that simple olefins may also undergo a loss of their TEA response after treatment with HBr-HOAc reagent by addition of HBr across the double bond. However, this class of compounds can be distinguished from N-nitrosamines by some of the methods already described (Sections V.B and V.C).

Walters et al. have now developed a method, again making use of the HBr-HOAc denitrosation step, as well as other chemical reactions, as a rapid screen for N-nitrosamines in complex food and environmental samples [200]. This new method, apparently, can differentiate N-nitroso compounds from most, if not all, other classes of organic and inorganic compounds that are capable of producing a TEA response. The approach utilizes a series of chemical reactions in conjunction with chemiluminescence detection for nitric oxide generated from the sample.

E. Isolation of the Unknown by Open Column Chromatography or HPLC

The identification of an N-nitrosamine in a new sample ultimately relies on conventional techniques of chemical and/or spectroscopic structure elucidation.

We have already mentioned the use of various forms of mass spectrometry for the structural identification of unknown N-nitroso derivatives (Section IV.B). However, the isolation of sufficient quantities from environmental samples, often available in limited amounts, can be a difficult and complex task. This is particularly true for nonvolatile compounds where GC-MS systems cannot be used. In the isolation of N-nitrosodiethanolamine from cutting fluids [21] and beauty products [24], in the isolation of glycerol dinitrate from drinking water at the sub-ppb level [201], in the isolation of N-nitrosomorpholine from air samples [29], and various N-nitrosamines from pesticides [25], we have employed initial cleanup of the crude sample extracts, followed by repetitive isolation of a narrow peak from HPLC-UV or HPLC-TEA as the final step prior to solid probe or GC-mass spectrometry. Often, several sequential HPLC isolations on different chromatographic supports and with different solvent systems are necessary to obtain a sufficiently pure sample. Final concentration of relatively nonvolatile samples is best carried out under vacuum. It is important to monitor the isolation procedure at each step, to ensure that the material of interest is still present, and to ensure that it is indeed being purified from one step to the next. Contamination problems are critical, and suitable measures must be employed to prevent this from occurring even in the final stages. All glassware, HPLC columns, solvents, and any other materials that may come into contact with the sample must be carefully cleaned and protected from contamination. Contaminants in HPLC solvents, nitrogen gas bottles, column packings, and elsewhere can result in the amount of the contaminant exceeding that of the material of interest. Unfortunately, experience borne of failures is the best instructor in this area, and there are few references that specifically deal with isolation procedures for trace levels of N-nitroso materials [202].

It is also useful to have a sample blank available. In this way it is possible to subtract the mass spectrum of the blank from that of the sample, and thus to arrive at a final spectrum for the material of interest. Proper blanks must be run in precisely the same manner as done for the sample, with the same volumes of solvent, columns, conditions, and so on.

F. Derivatization of the Unknown N-Nitrosamine

Derivatization of an isolated N-nitroso material is another method for the confirmation of its identity. Many easily prepared derivatives of N-nitrosamines are described in the literature, together with suitable methods for their preparation (Section IV.H). As an example of the derivatization method of confirmation, Fan et al. have described the derivatization of N-nitrosodiethanolamine (NDEIA) [21]. After isolation from an actual sample, this material was converted to its dehydration product, N-nitrosomorpholine. This derivative was identified by combined GC-TEA and HPLC-TEA, as well as by its high-resolution mass spectrum. In a second approach, the isolated NDEIA was converted to its O-methyl ether derivative, by methylation with sodium hydride and methyl iodide. This material was compared with an authentic sample of the O-methyl ether of NDEIA by GC-CECD.

VI. ARTIFACT PROBLEMS

A. Contamination Control

The problem of artifacts in the analysis for N-nitrosamines has been reviewed recently by Krull et al. [195]. General contamination control has been extensively discussed by Zief and Mitchell [202].

A specific detector, such as the TEA, enables the analyst concerned with trace amounts to limit concern to contamination by compounds that can release the nitrosyl moiety and their precursors. This reduces the overall problem of contamination to more manageable levels. However, when performing routine analyses in the ppm-ppb range, the problem of contamination is still present. The problem can be reduced by destroying any N-nitroso compounds present in one of three ways. First, by washing all glassware in chromic acid, followed by repeated washings with distilled water, and then a series of organic solvents. Second, by treating all glassware with a freshly prepared solution of 5 to 10% HBr in glacial HOAc at 40° for at least 1 to 2 hr in the absence of even trace amounts of water or methanol [73]. The glassware is then rinsed as above. Third, by use of continuous, ultraviolet light exposure (germicidal lamps).

Demonstration of the efficacy of any method for the prevention of trace contamination depends on the performance of suitable negative controls. When low levels of N-nitroso materials are being determined, such blank experiments should be carried out regularly and should include every step used in the analysis, including the same batches of chromatographic materials and chemicals. Unless the blanks themselves are free of N-nitrosamines, it is not possible to perform a meaningful analysis. Contamination control is a daily requirement, and checks for it must be run routinely.

B. False Positives

We divide the problem of artifacts into two main sections, false positives and false negatives. False positives are generally caused by the formation during the sample workup and/or analysis of precisely those materials that one is analyzing for. If a N-nitroso compound is found to be present in an entirely new sample, serious consideration must be given to the possibility of a false positive. This section deals with ways to prevent the artifactual formation of N-nitroso derivatives, and with methods designed to show, as definitely as possible, that a positive artifact has not been formed during the analysis.

Angeles et al. have recently described the artifactual formation of various N-nitrosamines during extraction of environmental samples [203]. They have shown that inorganic nitrite in the solid phase can serve as a nitrosating agent for solutions of organic amines in nonaqueous solvents (CH_2Cl_2, CHClBr, Ch_2Br_2, etc.). Logsdon et al. have also recently reported on the artifactual formation of N-nitrosamines during the analysis of water samples for organic matter [204].

Minimum number of analytical procedures

A simple precaution to minimize the possibility of artifact formation is to use the bare minimum number of analytical steps. This approach is feasible with the GC-TEA and HPLC-TEA methods of N-nitroso analysis, provided that the sample is in a form suitable for direct introduction into the apparatus. For example, Ross et al. have directly introduced aqueous pesticide formulations into both GC-TEA and HPLC-TEA in order to show that NDMA was present in the formulation itself [25].

In the case of cutting fluids, Fan et al. introduced crude formulations of up to 40% triethanolamine and 18% sodium nitrite directly into HPLC-TEA, in order to confirm the presence of NDEIA [21].

If a particular sample cannot be introduced directly into the TEA, it should be extracted and worked up with as few analytical operations as possible. In the case of air samples, Fine et al. were able to directly analyze by GC-TEA materials isolated using cryogenic trapping, without any extraction or concentration [205]. Thus the possibility of artifactual formation was limited to the method of sampling and/or the chromatrographic or detector conditions employed.

Addition of precursors

The source of the nitrosating agent that could be responsible for a positive artifact has included nitrite contamination of the sample itself [21,206], open column chromatography on nitrite contaminated packing materials for GC and LC columns [207], use of too high an injection port temperature in GC analysis of a complex sample [208], absorption of nitrogen oxides from ambient air [65]. N-nitrosamine contaminated deionized water [209] and organic solvents [19]. The most frequent source of the amine precursors is the sample itself. In order to determine if all or part of the N-nitroso compounds present are a result of the analytical methods, a number of experiments are routinely employed. The type and sequence of these control experiments is arranged so that they yield maximum information with a minimum of time and effort.

The first such experiment is the addition of a readily nitrosatable amine, together with a nitrosating agent (inorganic nitrite and/or oxides of nitrogen) to the original sample. At this point it becomes necessary to choose the correct amine precursor. Usually, there are several possible candidates, although with more complex N-nitroso derivatives the choice is often easier. Another problem arises with regard to the chemical form and physical state that amine (or the nitrosating agent) should take. This is then followed by the same sequence of analytical steps as for the analysis itself. If there is an increase found in the amount of N-nitroso compound(s) present, artifact formation may have occurred. Two additional precursor control experiments then become necessary. Excess amine(s) is then added to the sample, without any added nitrosating agent, and the amount of N-nitroso derivative determined. If additional N-nitroso compounds are observed, it is likely that artifact formation has occurred. If no increased formation of the N-nitroso material is observed, a third experiment is carried out with added nitrosating agent alone, in the absence of added amine(s). If additional N-nitroso compounds are not formed, it can be reasonably assumed that there was no artifact formation in the original analysis. If, on the other hand, enhancement is observed, artifact formation may have occurred. If artifact formation has indeed occurred, the analytical method must be modified to avoid this.

To reduce the number of precursor experiments required, initial work should be done with rather high concentrations of amine(s) and nitrosating agent or amine (nitrosating agent) alone. The amounts of precursors added to the sample in these initial experiments should be from 10 to 100 times the amount of N-nitroso compound determined originally. If, with these large concentrations, enhancement is not observed, there is no need to use lower precursor concentrations. However, if high concentrations lead to enhancement, further experiments are needed at progressively lower concentration.

In the case of air monitoring, where nitrogen oxides are always present, collection of samples in unsuitable traps creates additional routes for artifact formation of N-nitroso compounds [68]. Validation procedures for air sampling have been described [205], in which the most useful positive artifact control experiment involved the use of gaseous amines added to the air prior to the trap. If the addition of the precursor amine does not lead to enhancement, positive artifact formation of the N-nitroso compound is probably absent. The use of deuterated amine precursors has been used to resolve the question of artifact formation in air sampling [205].

Use of added inhibitors

Several workers routinely add nitrosation inhibitors such as ascorbate [210], or sulfamic acid [24] to all samples prior to analysis. Nitrosation inhibitors are effective, because at the proper pH they compete with amines for available nitrite [10,59]. Care is required to ensure that the inhibitor is added in excess so as to account for all the available nitrite. If addition of an inhibitor decreases the amount of N-nitroso compound observed, it is probable that some or all of the N-nitroso material originally determined was due to artifact formation.

Artifact formation via transnitrosation

Artifact formation due to transnitrosation within the sample can be detected by the use of control experiments already discussed. Also, the use of combined GC-TEA and HPLC-TEA can usually eliminate the possibility of artifact formation due to transnitrosation, if this occurs during the chromatographic process itself [208]. Often, a temperature above ambient is required to produce significant transnitrosation. Thus, by working at room temperature, as is done with most HPLC, this problem might be entirely prevented.

Artifact experiments involving the chromatographic-detector system

False positives are known in gas chromatography [208,211] and to a lesser extent in HPLC [207,212]. The formation of an N-nitroso material on-column during HPLC on nitrite-free packings is unlikely. If an N-nitroso material is shown to be present using a variety of HPLC columns and conditions, it is indicative that no positive artifact formation has occurred during HPLC. For volatile N-nitrosamines, a combination of GC and HPLC techniques has been used to eliminate positive artifact formation during chromatography [25,205,208]. Although false positives due to the TEA itself are possible, they can generally be eliminated by a combination of photochemical, chemical, and TEA modifications.

C. False Negatives

Effect of heat, light, and excessive pH conditions

Accidental destruction of N-nitroso compounds can occur in sunlight, and even under fluorescent lighting [101]. The problem can be avoided by the use of yellow or incandescent lights, or by working in the dark with photographic red lights. Excessive heat should generally be avoided during the extraction and/or workup. Solvent reduction steps, liquid-liquid extractions, and the chromatographic analysis should all be carried out at or below room temperature. In the case of thermally labile N-nitroso compounds, the isolation and workup must be carried out in the cold. The use of very basic or acidic pH conditions can result in the destruction of part or all of certain N-nitroso compounds [72]. However, even water at neutral pH can lead to the destruction of compounds such as N-nitroso carbamates, amides, and so on, and low recoveries of such materials might be due to hydrolysis reactions. Perhaps the best method for minimizing negative artifacts is to minimize the number of analytical steps.

Accidental loss and inappropriate analytical methodology

Although most routes for loss of sample are obvious, N-nitroso material can be destroyed during gas chromatography or high-pressure liquid chromatography.

In GC, the use of a high temperature in the inlet or oven can lead to the partial or complete destruction of many N-nitroso materials. In HPLC, a portion of the N-nitroso compound may be irreversibly adsorbed onto the column packing material. It is also possible that the material of interest will not be stable to certain HPLC stationary phases and/or solvent conditions. This problem might be avoided by the use of several different HPLC columns, together with widely differing solvent conditions for the same sample. However, false negatives are always a possibility, and whether or not an N-nitroso material has been detected, it is necessary to perform suitable recovery experiments.

Recovery studies can be carried out with the original N-nitroso material added to the sample directly, or by using a close analog of the compound of interest. In most instances, the actual material is the preferred substance, but this requires analyzing the sample and the spiked sample separately. This not only requires time but can also lead to repetitive artifacts. Alternatively, ^{14}C-labeled internal standards, together with scintillation counting, can be used [210].

False negatives due to the detector

In the TEA itself, a false-negative response to an N-nitroso compound has not yet been observed. However, it should be noted that N-nitroso compounds with free bond-OH groups, such as NDEIA and N-nitrosamino acids, give a submolar response, presumably due to intramolecular OH bonding to the NO group. If the bond-OH group is first methylated, a molecular response is then observed [21].

VII. METHODS OF ANALYSIS

A. Foodstuffs

The analysis of foodstuffs for N-nitrosamines has been reviewed recently [5,13,14,53,101]. Several methods are available, both for volatile and nonvolatile N-nitroso compounds. For volatile N-nitrosamines, the most rapid and most sensitive is distillation from mineral oil, followed by analysis on GC-TEA. This technique was selected as one method of choice in the FDA's meat screening program [213]. Confirmation is by GC-MS or HPLC-TEA. Alternative extraction techniques for volatile N-nitrosamines include steam distillation and alkali distillation. Comprehensive solvent extraction procedures for both volatile and nonvolatile N-nitroso compounds are available; however, these are still relatively complex and tedious.

Distillation from mineral oil

The mineral oil technique for volatile N-nitrosamine analysis is attributable to Fine et al. [214]. This method involves the use of readily available USP mineral oil and can be used with samples as diverse as fish, meat, oil, bread, cheese, whole blood, laboratory animals, biological samples, and soil. A necessary condition for the successful application of the procedure is that the volatile N-nitroso compounds can be transferred, under vacuum, from the original sample to a receiving flask maintained at liquid nitrogen temperatures. The mineral oil procedure cannot be used for the analysis of nonvolatile N-nitroso compounds. Figure 1 illustrates the mineral oil distillation apparatus as

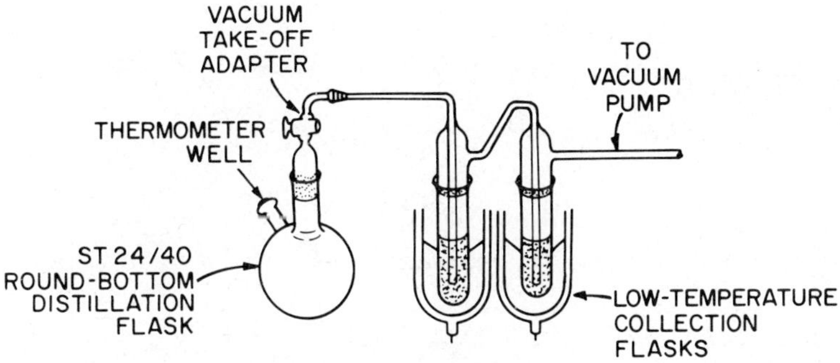

Figure 1 Mineral oil distillation apparatus. (From Ref. 247.)

originally employed in our laboratory. Figure 2 shows an improved version of the apparatus attributable to the International Agency for Research on Cancer in Lyon, France [215]. The first step is to homogenize the sample with a nitrosation inhibitor, such as ascorbic acid, sulfamic acid, or tocopherol. Ideally, a combination of ascorbic acid (or sulfamic acid) should be used together with tocopherol, to ensure a lack of artifactual N-nitrosamine formation during the actual distillation step. If 10 to 30 g of a sample is to be distilled, approximately 0.5 g of each of the nitrosation inhibitors should be added to the sample before homogenization. The homogenized sample plus inhibitors are added to a two-necked round-bottom flask (500 ml), and about 60 to 70 ml of USP mineral oil is added to the sample so as to cover it completely. If the sample is dry, 5 to 10 ml of water is added to the flask. Water is essential if high recoveries are to be obtained. The flask is attached to a vacuum distillation apparatus through the liquid nitrogen cold trap. A single cold trap, maintained at liquid nitrogen temperatures, is sufficient to trap all volatile N-nitrosamines. The pressure is reduced to about 1.5 to 2.0 mmHg throughout the system. The temperature of the distilling flask is then raised slowly over a period of about 40 to 50 min to a maximum of 110°. This can be maintained for another 10 to 15 min if less volatile N-nitrosamines are being determined. If frothing occurs, the heat source to the distilling flask is removed until the frothing decreases. A slightly modified procedure, using a dry ice-acetone cold trap instead of liquid nitrogen, has been described by Spiegelhalder [216]. Here the connection to the vacuum pump is disconnected as soon as the pressure reaches 2.0 mmHg. Because the system is not being continuously evacuated, the higher-temperature cold trap is adequate.

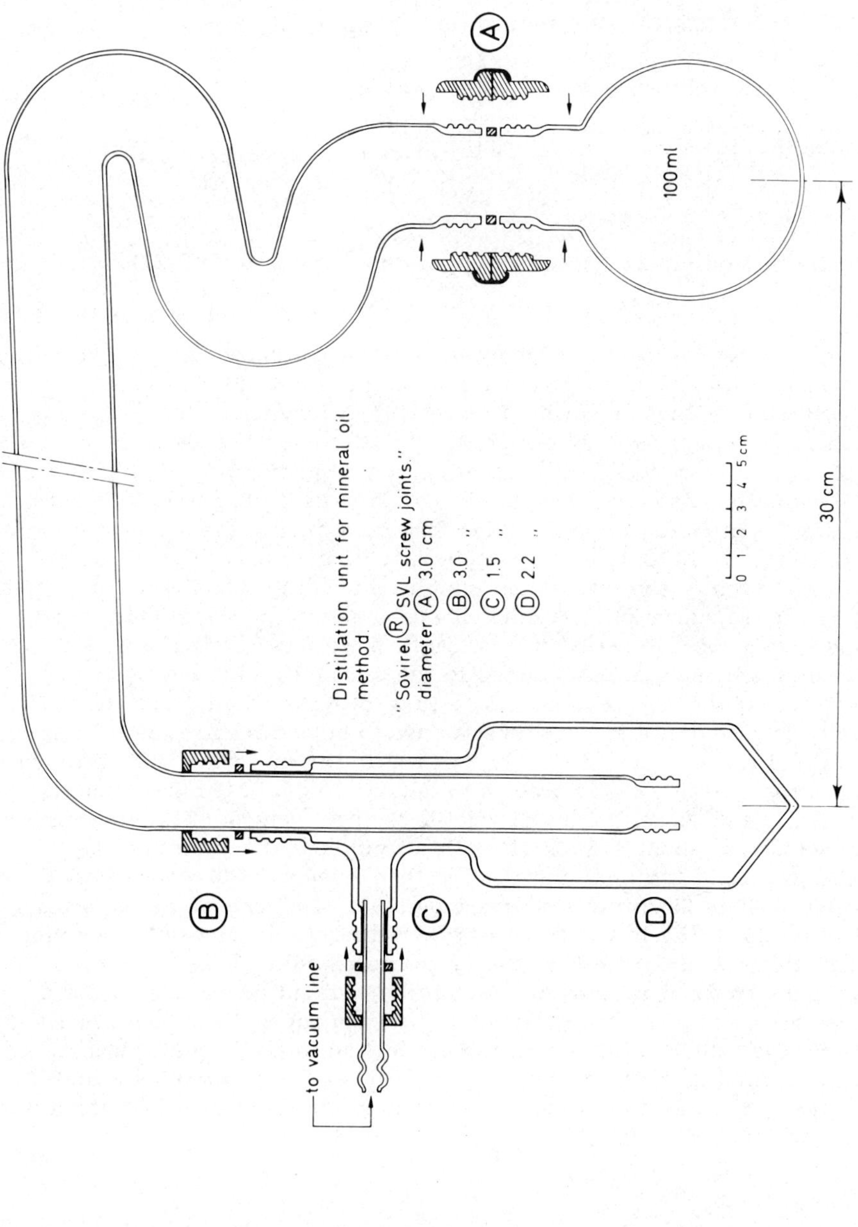

Figure 2 Improved mineral oil distillation apparatus. (From Ref. 215.)

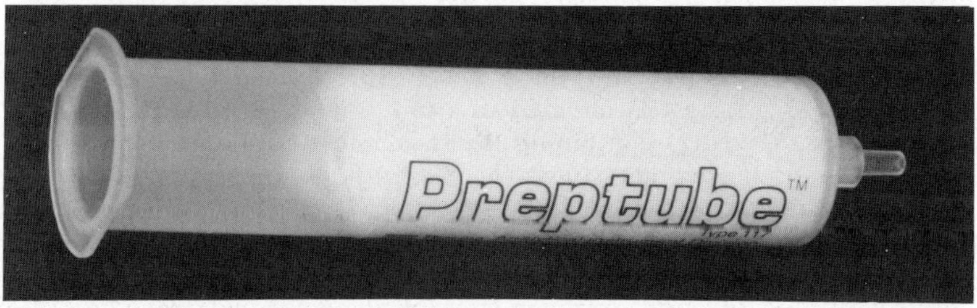

Figure 3 Photograph of the Preptube. (Courtesy of Thermo Electron Corp.)

At the end of the distillation, the distillate in the traps is thawed and made up to a constant volume (usually 15 ml) with water. It is then extracted with 3 × 25 ml of DCM, dried over 25 g of sodium sulfate, and the filter cake washed with DCM. A much more rapid extraction and drying procedure is to pour the 15 ml of water onto a Preptube (Thermo Electron), and then to flush the tube with 4 to 6 × 10 ml of DCM. The Preptube technique not only solvent-solvent extracts the N-nitrosamines, but also dries the DCM. A photograph of a Preptube is shown in Figure 3. Whichever extraction technique is employed, the DCM is concentrated on a Kuderna-Danish evaporator fitted with a Snyder column, with 0.2 to 0.3 ml of isooctane being added as a keeper. The water bath temperature is set at 52 to 53°. The concentration is stopped when the final volume is about 0.5 to 1.0 ml. Aliquots of the final concentrate are injected directly onto either GC-TEA or HPLC-TEA. The concentrate can also be used for capillary column GC-MS (high resolution with peak matching) [95].

Steam distillation and/or alkaline digestion

Prior to the use of the mineral oil procedure, volatile N-nitrosamines were generally extracted from foodstuffs by steam distillation [78,93, 164,167,213]. The technique works well for NDMA, but recovery of NPYR and relatively large molecular weight N-nitrosamines is poor. Fazio et al. [217] used steam distillation following digestion in alkali, and this was for a time the standard FDA procedure. However, it has been shown by Loeppky and Christiansen [72] that lower molecular weight N-nitrosamines can be formed by base-catalyzed decomposition of higher molecular weight precursors. Techniques involving steam distillation have been replaced in most laboratories by the more rapid and more efficient mineral oil procedure [83].

Following distillation, the aqueous fraction is further cleaned up for subsequent analysis by GC.

Solvent extraction with acetonitrile and/or methylene chloride

In this method, developed by Fine et al. [101] for nonvolatile N-nitrosamines, a 25 g sample is blended to a uniform slurry in a stainless steel blender (Waring) containing liquid nitrogen. Acetonitrile (100 ml) is added in small portions (10 ml each) with additional liquid nitrogen. Powdered anhydrous sodium sulfate (5 g) is then added, with additional homogenization, and the residual mixture allowed to warm to ambient temperature without stirring. The resultant acetonitrile slurry is gravity filtered through granular anhydrous sodium sulfate. The filter cake is washed sequentially with 2 × 40 ml of acetonitrile. Combined acetonitrile extracts are washed sequentially with 2 to 15 ml portions of isooctane. If phase separation does not occur, it is facilitated by cooling to -20°. The isooctane washings are discarded, and the acetonitrile extract is taken to dryness under vacuum at 35°. The residue is taken up in a few milliliters of a suitable solvent, such as DCM, transferred to a small concentration tube, and reduced to a final volume of about 0.5 ml with a stream of dry nitrogen in the cold. The solution is then used for both GC-TEA and HPLC-TEA analyses. Because N-nitrosamines vary in their solubility in different organic solvents, if an inappropriate solvent is chosen for the final solution, some or all of the material of interest may be left behind. It is best to use a range of solvents, particularly if both nonpolar and polar N-nitroso compounds may be present. The overall sensitivity of the procedure is about 10 μg/kg for a 25 g sample.

A modification of the acetonitrile procedure has been described by Young [218], wherein uncooked bacon was analyzed for N-nitrosamino acids. Uncooked bacon was extracted for 10 min with acetonitrile in a blender. The extract was then filtered through glass wool to remove all solids, washed with heptane, evaporated, and cleaned up on an acidic alumina column. The final extract was analyzed by TLC, followed by UV irradiation of the developed plate, and spraying with fluorescamine reagent followed by triethanolamine [142,143,218]. Accurate quantitative analyses were possible by employing spectrodensitometric determinations and appropriate instrumentation. For confirmation, the N-nitrosamino acids were resolved by two-dimensional TLC, and the eluted spots analyzed by GC-MS. The minimum detectable level was 20 to 30 ng of the N-nitrosamino acid.

Depending on the N-nitrosamines of interest, DCM may be added to the frozen-homogenized food slurry. The mixture is then filtered through fluted filter paper containing 15 g of anhydrous sodium sulfate. The filter cake is washed with 2 × 25 ml portions of DCM, and the combined filtrates are concentrated under vacuum at ambient temperature. Volatile N-nitrosamines are lost during this step. The final concentrate, about 0.5 ml, can be analyzed directly by HPLC-TEA, or it can be taken to dryness, and the residue taken up in the HPLC carrier solvent of choice. If oils are a problem in the final concentration step, it is necessary to take up the residue in a solvent such as acetonitrile. This is back-extracted with several small portions of isooctane, and then the remaining acetonitrile solution can be concentrated to a small volume for HPLC. The overall sensitivity of this method is about 10 μg/kg for a 25 to 30 g sample.

Comprehensive analytical procedures

Fan et al. have recently presented a comprehensive analytical method for the analysis of N-nitroso compounds in biological or environmental samples [102]. It is summarized in Figure 4. Complex matrices such as foodstuffs often require extensive treatment to remove all possible N-nitroso compounds present. A portion of the sample is first analyzed for volatile N-nitrosamines (class I) using the mineral oil distillation method. A second portion of the sample is extracted with methylene chloride (DCM) for nonvolatile, low-polarity compounds (class II). A third portion is extracted with acetone-water (2:1). The acetone is removed by rotary evaporation, and the remaining aqueous extract is saturated with sodium chloride. This is then washed with pentane, adjusted to pH 8 to 9 with potassium hydroxide, and then extracted with ethyl acetate. The ethyl acetate extract contains the nonvolatile, nonionic, polar N-nitroso compounds (class III). The same aqueous residue is adjusted to pH 1 to 2 with dilute sulfuric acid, and extracted with ethyl acetate. The ethyl acetate extract contains the nonvolatile ionic N-nitroso compounds (class IV). Class I compounds can be analyzed by either GC-TEA or HPLC-TEA, but classes II to IV can be analyzed only by HPLC-TEA using the appropriate chromatographic conditions. These have been detailed by Fan et al. [102] and are presented in the Appendix.

B. Drugs

Pharmaceutical products have recently been screened for N-nitroso compounds. Eisenbrand et al. [19,65], using the mineral oil technique, studied the widely used European analgesic Aminopyrine. Krull et al. [20] using solvent extraction, surveyed 73 U.S. pharmaceutical products.

Eisenbrand et al. [19,65] homogenized tablets or liquid (1 g) together with ascorbic acid (1 g), mineral oil (20 ml), water (10 ml) 5 N sulfuric acid (0.5 ml), cellulose (6 g), and an internal standard (200 ng of NDPA). The homogenate was then analyzed using a modification of the mineral oil technique described in Section VII.A.

Krull et al. [20] analyzed pharmaceutical preparations by first pulverizing (1 to 3 g) in the presence of sulfamic acid (500 mg), and then extracting with acetone or methylene chloride (1 to 3 ml). Insoluable materials were centrifuged down and the supernatant liquid removed for direct chromatographic analysis. Initial analysis was by GC-TEA. If a sample gave a peak on GC-TEA, or if there was a large "solvent" front, it was taken to indicate the presence of a possible N-nitroso material. The absence of a large "solvent" front by GC-TEA does not necessarily mean the absence of a N-nitroso compound, since it is possible that at the relatively low temperature of the GC injection port, the N-nitroso materials will not be sufficiently volatile or not decompose to produce a response. Samples of interest were further analyzed by HPLC-TEA, applying general HPLC procedures [99]. The HPLC conditions used are presented in the Appendix.

C. Blood

Fine et al. have described the recovery of volatile N-nitrosamines from blood samples, making use of the mineral oil distillation method [12]. Blood samples (20 ml) were taken and immediately poured into liquid nitrogen. Mineral oil was then added to the whole blood, and this was subjected to the standard mineral oil procedure (Section VII.A). Control experiments were performed by recovering NDMA, NDEA, and N-nitrosopyrrolidine at the 1 ppb level from whole human blood. The overall sensitivity of the method is about 0.1 ng/ml on a 30 g sample (0.1 ppb). The presence of the N-nitrosamines was confirmed by parallel GC-TEA, HPLC-TEA procedures.

Bruce has greatly simplified the procedure by pouring the whole blood (15 ml), to which ethylenediamine tetraacetic acid (EDTA) had been added, directly onto a Preptube [219] and eluting with DCM in the conventional manner [220] and analyzing by GC-TEA. Sensitivity was at the 0.1 ppb level.

D. Feces

Bruce's group recently reported on the isolation of various volatile N-nitrosamines from human feces [221]. These were recovered from feces by vacuum distillation using a freeze-drying apparatus. The freeze-drier condensate was extracted with DCM and the extract then injected onto GC-TEA and HPLC-TEA.

Bruce et al. have discussed the presence of a particular mutagen in the feces of normal humans [222,223]. At the time of writing all evidence available suggests that the active mutagen present in normal human feces is an N-nitroso derivative. However, a firm structural assignment has not, as yet, been made.

Feces samples were freeze-dried and stored at -70°. Extracts were prepared by taking the freeze-dried materials and stirring 20 to 100 g samples with 10 times their weight of peroxide-free diethyl ether. The mixture was filtered and evaporated under vacuum at about 30°. The extract was reconstituted in ether (0.5 ml/g of starting material),

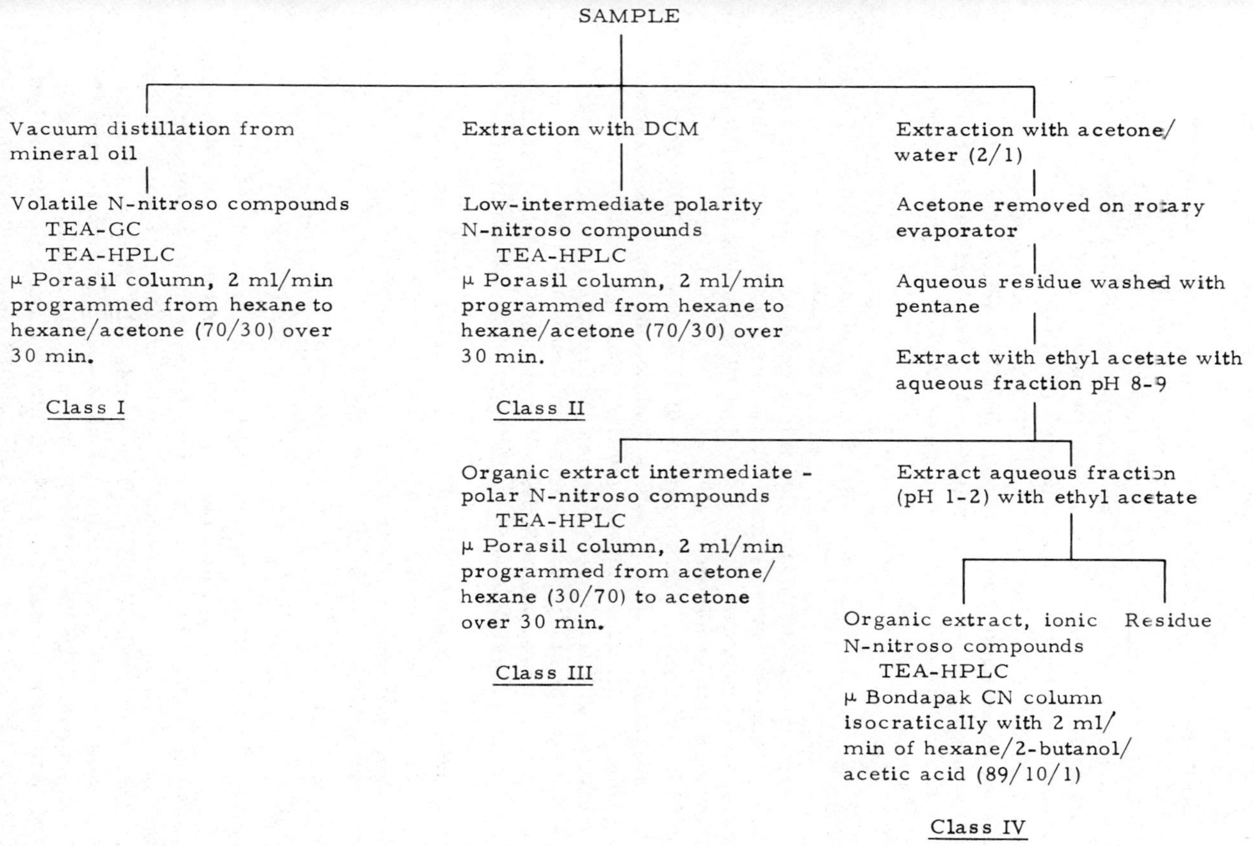

Figure 4 Exhaustive, comprehensive analytical technique for the analysis of N-nitroso compounds in biological or environmental samples. (From Ref. 102.)

and left at -20° for 30 min. This was then centrifuged at 500 gauss for 10 min to remove the precipitated material which contained no mutagenic activity. The solution was filtered further (0.5 μm, type FH, Millipore Corp.), and the filtrate was analyzed by HPLC-TEA methods [222].

A further cleanup of the crude extract was accomplished on the ether extract by concentrating the solution to 50 ml. This was applied on a silica gel column (50 × 4 cm) for preliminary purification. The column was eluted with 2000 ml of benzene, followed by 1000 ml of ether to recover the mutagenically active material. The ether eluate was concentrated to 10 ml and subjected to HPLC separation using a Porasil-type column (Waters) with ethyl acetate as the solvent. Fractions were collected at 1 min intervals from the HPLC apparatus, and each fraction was assayed for mutagenicity. For further purification, the active fraction was pooled, and again chromatographed using the same column and solvent.

E. Urine

Urine, to which suitable nitrosation inhibitors have been added, can be rapidly analyzed for volatile N-nitrosamines by pouring 15 ml onto a Preptube, eluting with 4 to 6 × 10 ml of DCM, and concentrating on a Kuderna-Danish evaporator [219]. The final concentrate is then analyzed by GC-TEA. The sensitivity of the method is 80 ng/ml (0.08 ppm). The mineral oil distillation method has also been used successfully [220], as have ion exchange resins [215].

Hicks et al. [224] have described the use of direct solvent extraction with methylene chloride. For the simple dialkyl and volatile heterocyclic N-nitrosamines, quantitative extraction can be achieved. Urine (0.6 to 1 liter) to which is added 10% (w/v) of sodium chloride, is extracted three times with 3 × 50 ml of methylene chloride. The organic extracts are concentrated using a Kuderna-Danish apparatus and analyzed either by GC-MS or GC-TEA. If it is desired to analyze for nonvolatile N-nitroso compounds from urine, then another, more polar solvent (acetonitrile) can be used for the extraction step.

F. Water

Several studies have been reported with regard to the nitrosamine content of various water systems [205,225-228]. Fan et al. have described the isolation of ethylene glycol dinitrate from drinking water supplies at trace levels [201]. The sensitivity obtained for most water analyses is less than 0.01 μg/liter for a 1 liter sample. In the case of water samples it is necessary to routinely analyze sample extracts by both GC-TEA and HPLC-TEA in order to determine both volatile and nonvolatile N-nitroso compounds [102]. There are basically two methods that can be used for the analysis of N-nitroso compounds in water samples. These are (1) liquid-liquid extraction with an organic solvent, using either a separating funnel or a Preptube, and (2) adsorption on a sorbent material such as an XAD resin.

Liquid-liquid extraction

In this method a large volume of fresh or salt water (500 to 1000 ml) is repeatedly extracted with 3 × 50 ml of dichloromethane [205]. The combined extracts are dried over anhydrous sodium sulfate (75 g), filtered, and the sodium sulfate cake extracted further with 2 × 35 ml of additional, fresh DCM. Alternatively, the DCM extracts can be dried by passage through a Preptube. The combined, dried extracts plus washings are concentrated on a Kuderna-Danish apparatus, as described previously, using isooctane as a keeper, to a final volume of approximately 0.5 to 1.0 ml. Aliquots of the final concentrate are analyzed by both GC-TEA and HPLC-TEA. Chromatrographic conditions for the most commonly occurring N-nitroso derivatives have been reported, and these are described in the Appendix.

A simpler and more rapid procedure would be to pour 15 ml of water on a Preptube, and wash the Preptube with 3 × 15 ml of DCM. The DCM can be concentrated for analysis. A single Preptube would provide enough sample to obtain a sensitivity of 0.08 μg/liter. The sensitivity can be improved by combining the extracts from multiple Preptubes.

Adsorption on solid supports

Several types of solid sorbent materials have been utilized for the removal of N-nitrosamines from water samples. These have included active carbon (charcoal) [229], and XAD-4 (XAD-8) resins (Rohm and Haas Co.). In the case of carbon adsorption, water is drawn at a known flow rate through several cylindrical columns packed with activated, purified carbon. The carbon is then partly dried by flushing the columns with purified nitrogen to remove most residual water. The charcoal columns are extracted with chloroform [229], until the chloroform extracts prove blank for N-nitrosamines. Concentration of the organic extracts can be accomplished on a rotary evaporator under reduced pressure, at ambient or slightly above ambient temperatures. It is advisable to dry the organic extracts with an inorganic drying agent prior to any final concentration steps. This approach can be utilized only for the less volatile N-nitrosamines unless care is taken during the concentration step to avoid loss of NDMA or NDEA.

In the case of XAD-type resins [201], the crude XAD-4 material requires extensive washing and sizing before it can be used for water analysis. This can be done by first treating the resin with 5% aqueous sodium bicarbonate for several hours. The slurry is filtered, and the resin rinsed successively with 0.1 N hydrochloric acid and then water.

The resin is washed in a Soxhlet apparatus for 8 hr with each of the following solvents: water, methanol, acetone, and DCM in sequence. Finally, it is sleved as an aqueous slurry to retain particles of 20 to 40 mesh size.

The resin cartridge is prepared by packing a mixture of XAD-4 and XAD-8 resins (2:1, v/v) in glass columns. A stainless steel screen of mesh small enough to retain the resin, gravel, and glass wool are placed at each end of the resin bed. During actual water sampling, it may be necessary to periodically change the glass wool when large particles clog the flow of water through the cartridge.

For the collection of large samples, upward of 20,000 gal of water can be extracted on 40 × 12 cm columns. At the end of the water sampling, the cartridge is allowed to drain at ambient pressure. The resin is washed out of the column with one resin volume of acetone, and the slurry is allowed to stand for about 1 hr. The slurry is filtered, and the resin washed with one-half a resin volume of acetone, followed by one resin volume of methylene chloride. When the acetone and DCM washings are combined, a phase separation occurs because of the water present. The organic phase is separated, and the aqueous phase is extracted twice with an equal volume of DCM. All the organic extracts are combined and reduced in volume, after first drying over anhydrous sodium sulfate. Alternatively, the Preptube can be used for the final DCM extraction and drying step.

After appropriate concentration on a rotary evaporator at low temperatures (40° or below), the final solution can be analyzed directly by HPLC-TEA and/or GC-TEA. Alternatively, it may be necessary to perform a further cleanup of this extract prior to actual TEA analysis. This will depend largely on the nature of the water samples extracted, and the complexity of the organic materials present. A detailed method for the further cleanup of water extracts has been described [201].

Lake water and sewage effluent have been analyzed for the possible presence of volatile N-nitrosamines by Nikaido et al. [230]. In this study the crude samples were first filtered through glass wool to remove suspended particles, and then passed through a column of Amberlite XAD-2 resin (24 cm × 1 cm) at a flow rate of 11 to 15 ml/min. A mixture of methylene chloride:diethyl ether (75:25), 100 ml, was used to desorb the organic compounds retained by the XAD-2 resin. The solvent was dried over anhydrous $MgSO_4$ and concentrated to 2.0 ml with a Kuderna-Danish evaporator. The concentrated extract from the Amberlite resin was placed on a basic alumina column (3 cm × 1 cm, 2.4 g) and eluted at a flow rate of 1 drop/sec. Hexane (20 ml) was first passed through the column at 3 ml/min, and then 200 µl of ethyl acetate was added to the top of the column followed by 60 ml of hexane at 3 ml/min. Finally, 50 ml of a solution of 1% ethyl acetate in methylene chloride was passed through the column at 1.5 ml/min. The final fraction was concentrated on a Kuderna-Danish evaporator at 65° and analyzed by GC [230].

The claimed recoveries of volatile N-nitrosamines using a salting-out procedure and a basic alumina column were as follows: dimethylnitrosamine (96%), diethylnitrosamine (82%), and di-n-propylnitrosamine (61%). These percent recoveries were determined with the N-nitrosamines spiked at the 180 to 260 ppb levels in water samples. The use of a basic salt (K_2CO_3) for the salting-out step also provides the water with a high pH, possibly preventing acid-catalyzed formation of the N-nitrosamines of interest from precursor amines and nitrite [230].

G. Alcoholic Beverages

A simple and rapid method for the analysis of wines, brandies, whiskeys, and so on, has been developed by Goff [231] and involves the use of the Preptube. Alcoholic beverages with less than 20% (v/v) alcohol content are extracted directly by this method, but those containing greater than this percentage alcohol are first diluted with water. An aliquot (15 ml) of the beverage to be analyzed is poured onto the Preptube and then analyzed in the conventional manner. The recoveries for the commonly occurring volatile N-nitrosamines ranged from 60 to 100%, with a detection limit of 0.4 to 1.2 ppb.

Spiegelhalder et al. have recently utilized the mineral oil distillation procedure for the analysis of NDMA from beer and ale samples in Germany [232]. Recovery efficiencies in most instances ranged from 80 to 95%, with a limit of detection of about 0.5 ppb.

Walker et al. have discussed another method of analysis for alcoholic beverages with a low or high alcohol content [233]. The method utilizes either steam or vacuum distillation of the N-nitrosamines from the beverage sample, followed by extraction of the distillate with methylene chloride. This extract is then concentrated, and taken up in n-hexane, after which it is further purified by column chromatography. The N-nitrosamines recovered are oxidized to N-nitramines, and these are extracted and purified by column chromatography. Final analysis is performed by gas chromatography with electron capture detection combined with confirmation by GC-CECD. Detailed steps for the entire procedure are presented elsewhere [233].

Bassir and Maduagwu have recently reported on the analysis for NDMA in some fermented Nigerian beverages [234]. Their method involved the use of steam distillation of the palm wines, followed by methylene chloride extraction of the distillate. The organic extract was cleaned up and concentrated to about 0.5 ml by the method of Sen and Dalpe [145]. NDMA was detected by TLC, using the procedure of Preussmann et al. [138]. Additional confirmation for the presence of NDMA was obtained by GC-FID, with a detection limit of 2 ng together with mass spectrometric identification of the TLC isolated material.

H. Cosmetics, Hand Lotions, and Shampoos

Fan et al. [24] described the analysis of cosmetic products for N-nitrosodiethanolamine (NDEIA), a relatively nonvolatile N-nitrosamine. The product (5 g) is weighed into a flask to which 250 mg of ammonium sulfamate is added. The mixture is stirred with a magnetic stirrer for 1 min until all the ammonium sulfamate crystals are dissolved. Ethyl acetate (100 ml) is added, and the mixture is stirred at room temperature for 15 min. The stirred mixture is filtered through 40 g of anhydrous sodium sulfate, and this is further washed with 50 ml of ethyl acetate. Alternatively, the ethyl acetate solution can be filtered and dried simultaneously by pouring it through a Preptube. This crude ethyl acetate extract after concentration on a roto-evaporator can be directly analyzed by HPLC-TEA; however, for most samples, it is too crude for analysis at this stage. The filtrate and washings are combined, and passed through a 25 × 1 cm chromatography column packed with 20 g of silica gel. The ethyl acetate fraction is discarded, and the column is then washed with 100 ml of acetone. The acetone fraction is collected and the column is allowed to go to dryness. The acetone is evaporated to 5 to 10 ml using a vacuum rotary evaporator operated at room temperature. The concentrate is filtered (Whatman No. 1) into a 25 ml concentration tube, and the filter is washed twice with 5 ml of acetone. The combined filtrate and washings are concentrated under a stream of nitrogen to 0.5 to 0.8 ml. A portion of the final concentrate is then analyzed by HPLC-TEA (Appendix).

Recoveries of NDEIA have been found to vary from 7 to 110%, depending on the nature of the particular sample; however, for one given sample, the recovery is consistent from analysis to analysis.

A recent development is to analyze the final extract by GC-TEA [207,235]. For this to work, it is essential that the TEA furnace be attached to the outlet of the glass GC column without the effluent coming into contact with stainless steel. It is also essential that there be no cold spots between the column and the TEA furnace. This is critical to the GC analysis of NDEIA, since even a 10° cold spot will tend to concentrate all the NDEIA at that point, leading to very broad peaks. A glass-lined injection port is also required. Chromatographic conditions are indicated in the Appendix [235].

I. Cutting Fluids

Fan et al. [21] reported that cutting fluids contained NDEIA at levels as high as 3%. These fluids are usually water based and can contain upto 18% sodium nitrite, at a pH between 8 and 11. Other reports have also appeared recently [22,23]. Because of the extraordinarily high NDEIA levels which are sometimes reported, a dilution step rather than a concentration step is often necessary.

The cutting fluid (1 g) is homogenized with sulfamic acid, (500 mg) tocopherol (500 mg), and magnesium sulfate, and extracted with a large excess (100 ml) of ethyl acetate. The extract is filtered through sodium sulfate and then analyzed by HPLC-TEA or GC-TEA [235]. Depending on the NDEIA levels that may be present, the extract may require either dilution or concentration prior to analysis. Concentration is best carried out using a rotary evaporator operating at less than 45°.

J. Soil

The analysis of soil for N-nitroso compounds was initially reported by Fine et al. [228]. There have been numerous studies recently [236-239]. Depending on the soil type, it may be possible to extract the N-nitrosamines using various solvents. The mineral oil distillation procedure can be used to extract volatile N-nitrosamines from soils that are not amenable to solvent extraction.

The soil, together with suitable nitrosation inhibitors, such as ascorbic acid and tocopherol, is homogenized with a suitable extraction solvent. The solvent is then filtered and purified prior to analysis. Ross et al. [240] extracted 50 g of soil with 60 ml of DCM. The DCM is then poured through a Preptube and concentrated and analyzed according to standard procedures. Recovery of NDPA was 80% at the 4 ppb level and 45% at the 1 ppb level. West and Day [236] extracted with a methanol-water mixture (3:1), and then purified by liquid-liquid extraction, followed by cleanup over alumina. Analysis was by GC-TEA with a sensitivity for NDPA at the 0.5 ppb level. A similar approach was used by Oliver et al. [237].

Kearney et al. analyzed for N-nitrosoatrazine in soil, using a combination of organic solvents in the extraction steps [238]. Soil (100 g) was shaken with benzene-ethyl acetate (1:3) overnight, and again with methanol (2 hr). The extracts were combined, filtered, and concentrated under nitrogen to a final volume of 0.1 ml. The N-nitrosoatrazine was analyzed by TLC on silica gel plates developed with benzene-ethyl acetate (3:1). Autoradiography was used on the TLC plates in order to determine the absolute amounts of N-nitrosoatrazine present, and as formed from ring-^{14}C atrazine originally present. The minimum limits of detection using this method were in the 10 ppb range. Recoveries were determined on the ^{14}C-atrazine using liquid scintillation counting on the final concentrate.

Khan and Young studied the formation of N-nitrosoglyphosphate in soil, and they describe another application of solvent extraction [239]. Soil (10 g) was extracted with distilled water (2 × 50 ml), centrifuged, and the combined supernatants concentrated under reduced pressure to about 10 ml. This was again centrifuged, and the supernatant washed with methylene chloride (5 × 10 ml), concentrated to 1.0 ml under reduced pressure, and diluted with 4 ml of acetonitrile. This solution was transferred to a column of Florisil and eluted with 20% water in acetonitrile (50 ml) and 60% water in acetonitrile (15 ml). The last eluate was concentrated to 10 ml, and aliquots were analyzed by TLC using the method of derivatization described by Young [142,143]. The method gave a limit of detection of 5 ng. Recovery of the N-nitroso derivative of glyphosphate from soils at the 1 and 5 ppm levels was nearly quantitative.

K. Air

Measurement of airborne N-nitrosamines often requires a sensitivity of better than 10 ng/m^3. Instrumentation is not currently available which can directly detect N-nitrosamines at this level. Recourse must be made, therefore, to removing the N-nitrosamines in a suitable trap and concentrating the sample to a more managable level. Because the N-nitrosamine precursors, amines and oxides of nitrogen, are generally present at levels 100 to 1000 times greater than the N-nitrosamines, great care must be taken to ensure that the concentration step does not also concentrate the precursors—possibly leading to catastrophic artifact formation. Several trapping techniques have been employed: Thermosorb cartridges (Thermo Electron), Tenax (Applied Science), activated charcoal, dilute alkali, and cryogenic.

Thermosorb cartridges were developed specifically for use in analyzing for N-nitrosamines in air. Air at a flow rate of up to 8 liters/min is drawn through a bed of solid adsorbent (Figure 5). After collection the cartridges are capped and sent to the laboratory for analysis. N-nitrosamines are removed from the cartridge by reverse elution with 0.5 ml of a special eluting solvent. An aliquot (typically 10 μl) of the eluate is introduced into the GC-TEA or HPLC-TEA for analysis. Concentration of the eluting solvent is not required, thereby eliminating the possibility of artifact formation during this step. Less than 2.5 ng of NDMA on the cartridge are required for analysis. Thus in an environment where the NDMA level was 100 ng/m^3, 0.025 m^3 (25 liters) of air would be needed for analysis. Thermosorb cartridges have been used in various factory environments for NDMA, NDEA, NDPA and N-nitrosomorpholine; recovery is greater than 95% for all N-nitrosamines. Because of their small size, Thermosorb cartridges are being used as personal monitors, being worn on the shirt lapel, attached by a flexible plastic hose to a small battery-driven air pump attached to the belt.

Sampling techniques for N-nitrosamines using Tenax were developed by Pellizzari et al. [241-243] and Issenberg and Sornson [244]. Air is drawn through a 1 cm o.d. glass tube, 6 cm long, packed with precleaned Tenax GC (35-60 mesh). Careful attention must be paid to the temperature of the air and the amount passed through the tube to ensure that breakthrough has not occurred. The tubes are sealed and sent to a laboratory for analysis. They are desorbed by heating in a

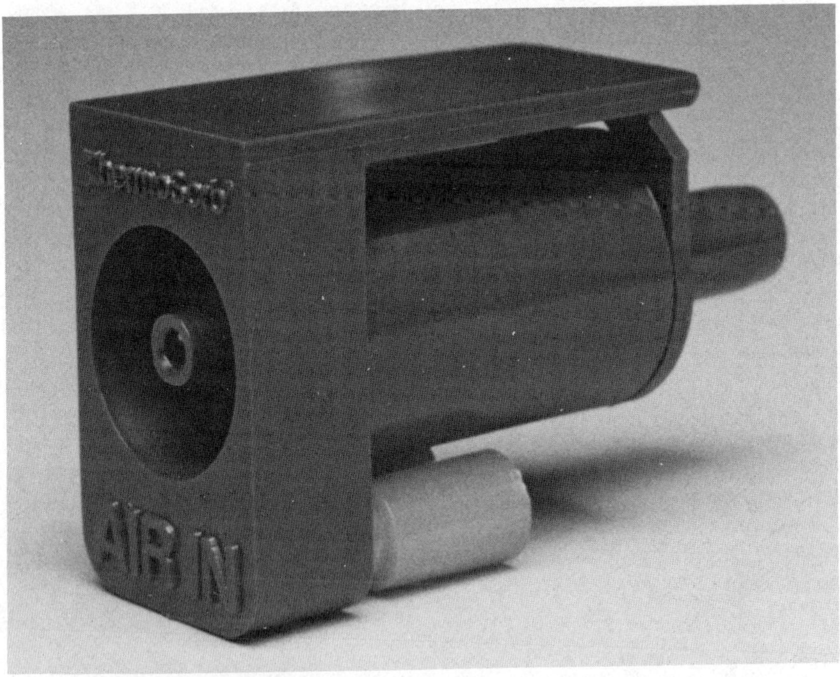

Figure 5 Photograph of the Thermosorb air sampler. (Courtesy of Thermo Electron Corp.)

stream of helium and trapping the contents in a gold-lined trap held at -192°. The gold trap is then flash heated, driving the contents directly into a capillary column (GC)-MS system. There are several drawbacks to the method. First, the Tenax may trap precursor amines and x-nitro compounds, which could form N-nitrosamines during the desorption and/or flash-heating steps. Second, Tenax has a relatively small breakthrough volume for NDMA, often the N-nitrosamine of maximum interest. These problems can be overcome by bleeding deuterated dimethylamine into the tube during analysis and ensuring that deuterated NDMA is not produced. Rounbehler [30,245] has desorbed the tubes by eluting with diethyl ether, concentrating at ambient temperature under a stream of nitrogen, and analyzing by GC-TEA and HPLC-TEA.

Activated charcoal traps were successfully used to trap NDMA by Bretschneider and Matz [31], the activated charcoal being carefully prepared and purified from pure carbon. Between 10 and 20 m^3 of air was passed through 450 mg of the active carbon, which was then eluted with 3 × 10 ml of diethyl ether. The diethyl ether was concentrated and analyzed by GC-FID. The method appears to work well for NDMA, provided that a suitable form of activated charcoal is available.

The use of dilute alkali (IN KOH) as a liquid scrubber for NDMA was introduced by Fisher et al. [246] after theoretical problems had been raised to the cryogenic trapping technique [205,229]. Air is bubbled through about 30 ml of dilute KOH at a flow rate of 2 liters/min, care being taken to avoid direct sunlight. The trap contents are extracted with DCM and dried over sodium sulfate (or poured through a Preptube and eluted with DCM), concentrated and analyzed by GC-TEA, HPLC-TEA, or GC-MS. The traps work well for NDMA, with an efficiency of 90%. However, NDEA is not trapped as well, and for NDPA the efficiency is less than 5%. Despite the potential for artifactual formation via nitrogen oxides, artifacts have not been observed for NDMA when sampling ambient air inside a rocket fuel factory, chemical factories, a leather tannery, or a tire factory. Because of its poor efficiency for N-nitrosamines other than NDMA, and because of its relative clumsiness, we have recently abandoned this trap in favor of the more convenient Thermosorb cartridge.

Cryogenic traps were used by Fine et al. in their initial work [229], but were abandoned because their liquid nitrogen requirement was difficult to meet in the field.

APPENDIX

Gas Chromatography Conditions for Volatile N-Nitrosamine Analysis

There have been many reports in the N-nitrosamine literature describing different GC columns for the successful resolution of most volatile N-nitrosamines. With an appropriate column and temperature-programming capabilities on a research grade gas chromatograph, it is indeed possible to resolve at least 14 major volatile N-nitrosamines in 15 min. We have not presented any chromatograms here, but they are largely available in the original literature. Actual conditions for GC are indicated below, with no suggestion intended regarding which methods are superior to others. Many of these methods utilized Carbowas 20M with KOH on a solid support, and thus this may signify a preference for this type of packing over others.

1. A 3.5 m × 3 mm stainless steel tube packed with 10% Carbowax 20M on Chromosorb W (80-100 mesh) operated with an argon flow of 10 ml/min at 100 psi. The column temperature is programmed from 140 to 210° at 5°/min [247].
2. A series of two columns, the first being at 2.4 m × 1.8 mm stainless steel tube packed with 15% Carbowax 20M on Chromosorb W/AW (80-100 BS mesh), DMCS treated. The second column is a 5.4 m × 1.8 mm stainless steel tube packed with

5% Carbowax 20M on Chromosorb W/AW (80-100 BS mesh), DMCS treated. The carrier gas is helium, with an injection port temperature of 160° and a column temperature of 145° (isothermal) [248].

3. Either of two columns can be used here. The first is a 34 m × 0.45 mm all-glass capillary coated column with OV-101, and the second is a 30 m × 0.45 mm all-glass capillary coated with UCON 50 HB-5100 [249].
4. A glass column, 3 m × 4 mm, packed with 10% Carbowax 20M on Chromosorb W (80-100 mesh). The carrier gas is high-purity nitrogen at 50 ml/min, and the detector temperature is 210°, with a column temperature of 140°, isothermal [235].
5. A stainless steel column, 2 m × 3.2 mm, packed with 10% Carbowax 20M on Chromosorb W (60-80 mesh), HMDS treated. This is operated with a helium gas flow of 30 ml/min, an injector temperature of 200°, and an isothermal column temperature of 190° [250].
6. A 3.5 m × 3.2 mm stainless steel tube packed with 13% Carbowax 20M-TPA on Gas Chrom P (60-80 mesh). The carrier gas is helium at a flow rate of 50 ml/min, with an injection port temperature of 185°, a detector temperature of 220°, and a column temperature programmed from 105 to 200° at 4°/min [251].
7. A 3 m × 4 mm glass column packed with 10% Carbowax 1540 and 5% potassium hydroxide on Chromosorb W/HP (100-120 mesh). This is operated with an argon flow of 70 ml/min, an injection port temperature of 200°, a detector temperature of 205°, and a column-programmed temperature of 80 to 180° at 5°/min [217].
8. A 3 m × 3.2 mm stainless steel column packed with 3% Carbowax 20M terephthalate on Gas Chrom Q (100-120 mesh). This is operated with a helium flow rate of 36 ml/min, an injection port temperature of 200°, and a column temperature held isothermal for the first 4 min at 130°, then programmed up to 200° at 8°/min [252].
9. A column 6.5 m × 2 mm stainless steel packed with 10% FFAP on Chromosorb W (80-100 mesh), acid washed, DMCS-treated. This is operated isothermally at 220° with an argon carrier gas flow of 10 to 30 ml/min [81].
10. GC analysis for NDEIA is performed with an all-glass column and inlet system, using a 180 cm × 4 mm column packed with 3% OV-225 on Chromosorb W/HP (80-100 mesh). The injection port temperature is 240 to 250°, and the column is operated either isothermally at 235° or using temperature programming from 180° to 240° at 8°/min. Argon carrier gas flow is 10 ml/min [235].

High-Pressure Liquid Chromatography Conditions for Volatile and Nonvolatile Nitrosamine Analysis

Most of the literature discussing analyses for N-nitrosamines has dealt with volatile materials, and it is only within the past several years or so that substantial information has appeared with regard to the HPLC analysis for N-nitroso derivatives. Some of these references, especially with regard to HPLC-UV methods, have been presented previously, and these can be consulted for the actual chromatographic conditions. We discuss here some of the more general HPLC-TEA conditions for the analysis of both volatile and nonvolatile N-nitrosamines [98,99,102, 253].

Several different HPLC conditions are discussed in recent publications by Krull et al. [99,253]. The actual chromatograms resulting from the sets of conditions indicated below can be found in these two references.

1. NDMA, NDEA, NDPA, and other volatile N-nitrosamines can be well resolved on a 10 μm Porasil or a 5 μm Lichrosorb Si60 (EM Labs) 30 cm × 4.2 mm column using 8% isopropanol-hexane (v/v) as the eluting solvent at a flow rate of 1 ml/min [253]. Total analysis time is about 20 min, with a sensitivity of below 1 ng per N-nitrosamine injected. Analysis time can be decreased by operating at a flow rate of 1.5 to 2.0 ml/min with the same column and conditions.
2. NDMA, NDEA, NDPA, and other volatile N-nitrosamines can be well resolved on a 10 μm Porasil or a 5 μm Lichrosorb Si60 column using a solvent mixture of hexane-methylene chloride-acetonitrile (76:23:1) at a flow rate of 1 ml/min [253]. The total time here is about 20 min, and this can also be reduced by operating at a higher flow rate of 1.5 to 2.0 ml/min with excellent resolution.
3. N^6-(methylnitroso)adenosine, an N-nitroso nucleoside, can be chromatographed in less than 6 min using a 5 μm Lichrosorb Si60 column. The solvent here is chloroform-methanol-acetic acid (300:20:5) at 1 ml/min flow rate. Detection limits are about 1-3 ng per N-nitrosamine injected [253].
4. N-nitroso derivatives of agricultural chemicals, such as N-nitrosocarbaryl and N-nitrosoatrazine, can be well resolved on a 5 μm Lichrosorb Si60 column (30 cm × 4.2 mm) with 2% acetone/isooctane at a flow rate of 1.5 ml/min. The total analysis time is less than 10 min, and by increasing the percent acetone content to 3 or 4%, the overall analysis time can be reduced further. The limits of detection here are less than 1 ng per N-nitrosamine injected [253].

5. N-nitroso derivatives of alkanolamines, such as N-nitrosodiethanolamine and N-nitrosodi-isopropanolamine, can be well resolved using again a 5 μm Lichrosorb Si60 column (30 cm × 4.2 mm) with a solvent of 47% acetone/isooctane at a flow rate of 1.5 ml/min. The overall time for analysis is less than 10 min, with a detection limit of below 1 ng per N-nitrosamine injected [21,24,253].
6. N-nitrosodiethanolamine and N-nitrosodi-isopropanolamine can also be excellently resolved on a μNH_2 column (Waters or EM Labs), 30 cm × 4.2 mm, using 3% methanol/methylene chloride as the solvent mixture. The flow rate is 1.5 ml/min, with an overall analysis time of less than 10 min [253]. The detection limits here are substantially below 1 ng per N-nitrosamine injected.
7. N-nitrosodiethanolamine can also be analyzed readily on a μNH_2 column, as above, but this time using a solvent of isopropanol-isooctane-methanol (27:63:10) at a flow rate of 3 ml/min [21,24,253].
8. N-nitrosocarbazole, N-nitroso-N-ethylaniline, N-nitrosodipropylamine, N-nitrosodiethylamine, N-nitrosopiperidine, and N-nitrosodimethylamine can all be well resolved using a μBondapak NH_2 column with solvent consisting of 85% isooctane-15% chloroform. The flow rate is 1 ml/min [97,98]. Total analysis time is less than 20 min.
9. N-nitrosamino acids, such as N-nitrosoarcosine, N-nitrosoproline, and N-nitrosohydroxyproline, can all be analyzed using a μBondapak CN (Waters) with a solvent of hexane-2-butanol-acetic acid (89:10:1) at a flow rate of 2 ml/min. The detection limit here is about 1 to 3 ng per N-nitrosamine injected [99]. The total analysis time is less than 15 min.
10. A mixture of N-nitrosocarbazole, N-nitroso-N-ethylaniline, and N-nitrosopiperidine can all be resolved on a μPorasil column (Waters), with a solvent mixture of 4% acetone-isooctane at a flow rate of 1.5 ml/min. The total analysis time here is about 12 min [98,99].

ACKNOWLEDGMENTS

The authors wish to acknowledge the assistance of Gordon Edwards of the New England Institute for Life Sciences, and Ulku Goff and Martin Wolf of Thermo Electron. Gratitude is expressed to Nancie Bornstein for secretarial assistance in the preparation of the manuscript.

Gratitude is also expressed to the U.S. National Science Foundation (NSF Grant ENV75-20802), the U.S. Environmental Protection Agency (EPA Contract 68-02-2766 and 68-02-2312, Grant R805431-01), and the

U.S. National Institute for Occupational Safety and Health (NIOSH Contract 210-77-0100) for financial support. Any opinions, findings, conclusions, or recommendations expressed are those of the authors and do not necessarily reflect the views of the NSF, NCI, EPA, and/or NIOSH.

REFERENCES

1. J. H. Boyer. Methods of formation of the nitroso group and its reactions. In *The Chemistry of the Nitro and Nitroso Groups*, Part 1, (H. Feuer, Ed.). Wiley, New York, 1969, Chapter 5.
2. A. L. Fridman, F. M. Mukametshin, and S. S. Novikov. Advances in the chemistry of aliphatic nitrosamines. Russ. Chem. Rev. *40*, 34-50 (1971).
3. A. Geuther. Ueber die Einwirklung von Saltpetrigs auren Kali auf salzsaures Diathylamin. Lieb. Ann. *128*, 515-156 (1863).
4. IARC Sci. Publ. Nos. 3, 9, 14, and 19. International Agency for Research on Cancer, Lyon, France, 1972, 1974, 1976, 1978.
5. D. H. Fine. N-Nitroso compounds in the environment. In *Advances in Environmental Science and Technology*, Vol. 9, (J. N. Pitts, R. L. Metcalf, and D. Grosjean, Eds.). Wiley-Interscience, New York, 1980.
6. A. J. Buglass, B. C. Challis, and M. R. Osborne. Transnitrosation and decomposition of nitrosamines. In *N-Nitroso Compounds in the Environment* (P. Bogovski and E. A. Walker, Eds.), IARC Sci. Publ. No. 9. International Agency for Research on Cancer, Lyon, France, 1974, pp. 94-100.
7. S. S. Singer, W. Lijinsky, and G. M. Singer. Transnitrosations: an important aspect of the chemistry of aliphatic nitrosamines. In *Environmental Aspects of N-Nitroso Compounds* (E. A. Walker, M. Castegnaro, L. Griciute, and R. E. Lyle, Eds.), IARC Sci. Publ. No. 19. International Agency for Research on Cancer, Lyon, France, 1978, pp. 175-181.
8. T. Y. Fan, R. Vita, and D. H. Fine. C-Nitro compounds: a new class of nitrosating agents. Toxicol. Lett. *2*, 5-10 (1978).
9. P. N. Magee, R. Montesano, and R. Preussmann. N-Nitroso compounds and related carcinogens. In *Chemical Carcinogens* (C. E. Searle, Ed.), ACS Monogr. 173. American Chemical Society, Washington, D.C., 1976, Chapter II.
10. S. S. Mirvish, Formation of N-nitroso compounds: chemistry, kinetics, in vivo occurrence. Toxicol. Appl. Pharmacol. *31*, 325-351 (1975).

11. S. S. Mirvish. N-Nitroso compounds: their chemical and in vivo formation and possible importance as environmental carcinogens. J. Toxicol. Environ. Health *2*, 1267-1277 (1977).
12. D. H. Fine, R. Ross, D. P. Rounbehler, A. Silvergleid, and L. Song. Formation in vivo of volatile N-nitrosamines in man after ingestion of cooked bacon and spinach. Nature (Lond.) *265*, 753-755 (1977).
13. N. T. Crosby. Nitrosamines in foodstuffs. Residue Rev. *64*, 77-135 (1976).
14. N. T. Crosby and R. Sawyer. N-Nitrosamines: a review of chemical and biological properties and their estimation in foodstuffs. Adv. Food Res. *22*, 1-71 (1976).
15. *IARC Monographs on the Evaluation of the Carcinogenic Risk of Chemicals to Humans*, Vol. 17: *Some N-Nitroso Compounds*. International Agency for Research on Cancer, Lyon, France, 1978.
16. K. D. Brunnemann and D. Hoffmann. Chemical studies on tobacco smoke: LIX. Analysis of volatile nitrosamines in tobacco smoke and polluted indoor environments. In *Environmental Aspects of N-Nitroso Compounds* (E. A. Walker, M. Castegnaro, L. Griciute, and R. E. Lyle, Eds.), IARC Sci. Publ. No. 19. International Agency for Research on Cancer, Lyon, France, 1978, pp. 343-356.
17. D. Hoffman, G. Rathkamp, and Y. Y. Liu. Chemical studies on tobacco smoke: XXVI. On the isolation and identification of volatile and nonvolatile N-nitrosamines and hydrazines in cigarette smoke. In *N-Nitroso Compounds in the Environment* (P. Bogovski and E. A. Walker, Eds.), IARC Sci. Publ. No. 9. International Agency for Research on Cancer, Lyon, France, 1974, pp. 159-165.
18. D. Hoffmann, S. S. Hecht, R. M. Ornaf, E. L. Wynder, and T. C. Tso. Chemical studies on tobacco smoke: XLII. Nitrosonornicotine: presence in tobacco, formation and carcinogenicity. In *Environmental N-Nitroso Compounds Analysis and Formation* (E. A. Walker, P. Bogovski, and L. Griciute, Eds.), IARC Sci. Publ. No. 14. International Agency for Research on Cancer, Lyon, France, 1976, pp. 307-320.
19. G. Eisenbrand, B. Spiegelhalder, C. Janzowski, J. Kann, and R. Preussmann. Volatile and nonvolatile N-nitroso compounds in foods and other environmental media. In *Environmental Aspects of N-Nitroso Compounds* (E. A. Walker, M. Castegnaro, L. Griciute, and R. E. Lyle, Eds.), IARC Sci. Publ. No. 19. International Agency for Research on Cancer, Lyon, France, 1978, pp. 311-324.
20. I. S. Krull, U. Goff, A. Silvergleid, and D. H. Fine. N-Nitroso contaminants in prescription and nonprescription drugs. Arzneim. Forsch. (Drug Res.) *28*, 870-874 (1978).

21. T. Y. Fan, J. Morrison, D. P. Rounbehler, R. Ross, D. H. Fine, W. Miles, and N. P. Sen. N-Nitrosodiethanolamine in synthetic cutting fluids: a part-per-thousand impurity. Science *196*, 70-71 (1977).
22. C. Rappe and P. A. Zingmark. Formation of nitrosamines in cutting fluids. In *Environmental Aspects of N-Nitroso Compounds* (E. A. Walker, M. Castegnaro, L. Griciute, and R. E. Lyle, Eds.), IARC Sci. Publ. No. 19. International Agency for Research on Cancer, Lyon, France, 1978, pp. 213-218.
23. R. W. Stephany, J. Freudenthal, and P. L. Schuller. N-Nitroso-5-methyl-1,3-oxazolidine identified as an impurity in a commercial cutting fluid. Recil. J. R. Neth. Chem. Soc. *97*, 177-178 (1978).
24. T. Y. Fan, U. Goff, L. Song, D. H. Fine, G. P. Arsenault, and K. Biemann. N-Nitrosodiethanolamine in cosmetics, lotions, and shampoos. Food Cosmet. Toxicol. *15*, 423-430 (1977).
25. R. D. Ross, J. Morrison, D. P. Rounbehler, S. Fan, and D. H. Fine. N-Nitroso compound impurities in herbicide formulations. J. Agric. Food Chem. *25*, 1416-1418 (1977).
26. S. Z. Cohen, G. Zweig, M. Law, D. Wright, and W. R. Bontoyan. Analytical determinations of N-nitroso compounds in pesticides by the United States Environmental Protection Agency—a preliminary study. In *Environmental Aspects of N-Nitroso Compounds* (E. A. Walker, M. Castegnaro, L. Griciute, and R. E. Lyle, Eds.), IARC Sci. Publ. No. 19. International Agency for Research on Cancer, Lyon, France, 1978, pp. 333-342.
27. P. N. Magee. Possibilities of hazard from nitrosamines in industry. Ann. Occup. Hyg. *15*, 19-22 (1972).
28. J. M. Fajen, G. A. Carson, S. Fan, D. P. Rounbehler, J. Morrison, I. S. Krull, G. Edwards, A. LaFleur, W. Herbst, U. Goff, R. Vita, K. Mills, D. H. Fine, and V. Reinhold. N-Nitroso compounds as air pollutants. Presented at the Annual Meeting of the Air Pollution Control Association, Houston, Tex., June 26, 1978.
29. J. M. Fajen, G. A. Carson, D. P. Rounbehler, T. Y. Fan, R. Vita, M. Wolf, G. S. Edwards, D. H. Fine, U. Goff, V. Reinhold, and K. Biemann. N-Nitrosamines in the rubber and tire industry. Science *205*, 1262-1264 (1979).
30. D. P. Rounbehler, I. S. Krull, U. E. Goff, K. M. Mills, J. Morrison, G. S. Edwards, D. H. Fine, J. M. Fajen, G. A. Carson, and V. Reinhold. Occupational exposure to diemethylnitrosamine in a leather tannery. Food Cosmet. Toxicol. *17*, 487-491 (1979).
31. K. Bretschneider and J. Matz. Occurrence and analysis of nitrosamines in air. In *Environmental N-Nitroso Compounds*

Analysis and Formation (E. A. Walker, P. Bogovski, and L. Griciute, Eds.), IARC Sci. Publ. No. 14. International Agency for Research on Cancer, Lyon, France, 1976, pp. 395-399.

32. D. H. Fine, J. Morrison, D. P. Rounbehler, A. Silvergleid, and L. Song. N-Nitrosamines in the air environment. In *Toxic Substances in the Air Environment* (J. G. Spengler, Ed.). Air Pollution Control Association, Pittsburgh, Pa., 1977, pp. 168-181.
33. D. H. Fine, D. P. Rounbehler, E. Sawicki, K. Krost, and G. A. DeMarrais. N-Nitroso compounds in the ambient community air of Baltimore, Maryland. Anal. Lett. *9*, 595-604 (1976).
34. D. H. Fine, D. P. Rounbehler, E. D. Pellizzari, J. E. Bunch, R. W. Berkley, J. McCrae, J. T. Bursey, E. Saweicki, K. Krost, and G. A. DeMarrais. N-Nitrosodimethylamine in air. Bull. Environ. Contam. Toxicol. *15*, 739-747 (1976).
35. N. Koppang, P. Slagsvold, M. A. Hansen, E. Sognen, and R. Svenkerud. Feeding experiments with meal produced from herring preserved with sodium nitrite and formalin. Nord. Veterinaermed. *16*, 343-362 (1964).
36. F. Ender, G. Havre, A. Helgebostad, N. Koppang, R. Madsen, L. Ceh, and O. Bjornson. Isolation and identification of a heptatoxic factor in herring meal produced from sodium nitrite preserved herring. Naturwissenschaften *51*, 637-638 (1964).
37. R. Montesano and H. Bartsch. Mutagenic and carcinogenic N-nitroso compound possible environmental hazards. Mutat. Res. *32*, 179-228 (1976).
38. S. Neale. Mutagenicity of nitrosamides and nitrosoamidines in microorganisms and plants. Mutat. Res. *32*, 229-266 (1976).
39. H. Druckrey. Chemical carcinogenesis on N-nitroso derivatives. Gann Monogr. Cancer Res. *17*, 107-132 (1975).
40. E. J. Olajos. Biological interactions of N-nitroso compounds: a review. Ecotoxicol. Environ. Safety *1*, 175-196 (1977).
41. R. C. Shank. Toxicology of N-nitroso compounds. Toxicol. Appl. Pharmacol. *31*, 361-368 (1975).
42. W. Lijinsky. Carcinogenic and mutagenic N-nitroso compounds. In *Chemical Mutagens*, Vol. 4, (A. Hollaender, Ed.). Plenum Press, New York, 1976, Chapter 41.
43. W. Lijinsky. Interaction with nucleic acids of carcinogenic and mutagenic N-nitroso compounds. Prog. Nucleic Acid Res. *17*, 247-269 (1976).
44. P. N. Magee. In vivo reactions of nitroso compounds. Ann. N.Y. Acad. Sci. *163*, 717-729 (1969).
45. P. F. Swann and P. N. Magee. Nitrosamine induced carcinogenesis. Biochem. J. *110*, 39-47 (1968).

46. P. N. Magee and J. M. Barnes. Carcinogenic nitroso compounds. Adv. Cancer Res. *10*, 163-246 (1967).
47. P. N. Magee and P. F. Swann. Nitroso compounds. Br. Med. Bull. *25*, 240-244 (1969).
48. R. Montesano and P. N. Magee. Metabolism of dimethylnitrosamine by human liver slices in vitro. Nature (Lond.) *228*, 173-174 (1970).
49. C. C. Harris, H. Autrup, G. D. Stoner, E. M. McDowell, B. F. Trump, and P. Schafer. Metabolism of dimethylnitrosamine and 1,2-dimethylhydrazine in cultured human bronchi. Cancer Res. *37*, 2309-2311 (1977).
50. H. Bartsch, A. Camus, and C. Malaveille. Comparative mutagenicity of N-nitrosamines in a semi-solid and in a liquid incubation system in the presence of rat or human tissue fractions. Mutat. Res. *37*, 149-162 (1976).
51. H. A. Freund. Clinical manifestations and studies in parenchymatous hepatitis. Ann. Intern. Med. *10*, 1144-1145 (1937).
52. S. R. Tannenbaum, J. S. Wishnok, J. S. Hovis, and W. W. Bishop. N-Nitroso compounds from the reaction of primary amines with nitrite and thiocyanate. In *Environmental Aspects of N-Nitroso Compounds* (E. A. Walker, M. Castegnano, L. Griciute, and R. E. Lyle, Eds.), IARC Sci. Publ. No. 19. International Agency for Research on Cancer, Lyon, France, 1978, pp. 155-159.
53. R. A. Scanlan. N-Nitrosamines in foods. C.R.C. Crit. Rev. Food Technol. *5*, 357-402 (1975).
54. J. J. Wartheson, R. A. Scanlan, D. P. Bills, and L. M. Libbey. Formation of heterocyclic N-nitrosamines from the reaction of nitrite and selected primary diamines and amino acids. J. Agric. Food Chem. *23*, 898-902 (1975).
55. P. P. Roller and L. K. Keefer. Catalysis of nitrosation reactions by electrophilic species. In *N-Nitroso Compounds in the Environment* (P. Bogovski and E. A. Walker, Eds.), IARC Sci. Publ. No. 9. International Agency for Research on Cancer, Lyon, France, 1974, pp. 86-89.
56. L. K. Keefer. Promotion of N-nitrosation reactions by metal complexes. In *Environmental N-Nitroso Compounds Analysis and Formation* (E. A. Walker, P. Bogovski, and L. Griciute, Eds.), IARC Sci. Publ. No. 14. International Agency for Research on Cancer, Lyon, France, 1976, pp. 153-159.
57. M. C. Archer, H. S. Yang, and J. D. Okun. Acceleration of nitrosamine formation at pH 3.5 by micro-organisms. In *Environmental Aspects of N-Nitroso Compounds* (E. A. Walker, M. Castegnaro, L. Griciute, and R. E. Lyle, Eds.), IARC Sci. Publ. No. 19. International Agency for Research on Cancer, Lyon, France, 1978, pp. 239-246.

58. R. Davies, M. J. Dennis, R. C. Massey, and D. J. McWeeny. Some effects of phenol and thiol-nitrosation reactions on N-nitrosamine formation. In *Environmental Aspects of N-Nitroso Compounds* (E. A. Walker, M. Castegnaro, L. Griciute, and R. E. Lyle, Eds.), IARC Sci. Publ. No. 19. International Agency for Research on Cancer, Lyon, France, 1978, pp. 183-198.
59. S. S. Mirvish. Blocking the formation of N-nitroso compounds with ascrobic acid in vitro and in vivo. In *Second Conference on Vitamin C* (C. G. King and J. J. Burns, Eds.). Ann. N.Y. Acad. Sci. *258*, 175-180 (1975).
60. P. J. Groenen. A new type of N-nitrosation inhibitor. In *Proceedings of the Second International Symposium on Nitrite in Meat Products* (B. J. Tinbergen and B. Krol, Eds.). PUDOC, Wageningen, 1977, pp. 171-172.
61. W. J. Mergens, J. J. Kamm, H. L. Newmark, W. Fiddler, and J. Pensabene. Alpha-tocopherol: uses in preventing nitrosamine formation. In *Environmental Aspects of N-Nitroso Compounds* (E. A. Walker, M. Castegnaro, L. Griciute, and R. E. Lyle, Eds.), IARC Sci. Publ. No. 19. International Agency for Research on Cancer, Lyon, France, 1978, pp. 199-212.
62. M. C. Archer, S. R. Tannenbaum, T. Y. Fan, and M. Weisman. Reaction of nitrite with ascorbate and its relation to nitrosamine formation. J. Natl. Cancer Inst. *54*, 1203-1205 (1975).
63. G. E. Hein. The reaction of tertiary amines with nitrous acid. J. Chem. Educ. *40*, 181-184 (1963).
64. W. Lijinsky, E. Conrad, and R. Van de Bogart. Formation of carcinogenic nitrosamines by interaction of drugs with nitrite. In *N-Nitroso Compounds Analysis and Formation* (P. Bogovski, R. Preussmann, and E. A. Walker, Eds.), IARC Sci. Publ. No. 3. International Agency for Research on Cancer, Lyon, France, 1973, pp. 130-133.
65. G. Eisenbrand, B. Spiegelhalder, J. Kann, R. Klein, and R. Preussmann. Carcinogenic N-nitrosodimethylamine as a contamination in drugs containing 4-dimethylamino-2,3-dimethyl-1-phenyl-3-pyrazolin-5-one (Amidopyrine, Aminophenazone). Arzneim. Forsch. (Drug Res.) *29*, 867-869 (1979).
66. H. Ohshima and T. Kawabata. Mechanisms of N-nitrosodimethylamine formation from trimethylamine and trimethylamineoxide. In *Environmental Aspects of N-Nitroso Compounds* (E. A. Walker, M. Castegnaro, L. Griciute, and R. E. Lyle, Eds.), IARC Sci. Publ. No. 19. International Agency for Research on Cancer, Lyon, France, 1978, pp. 143-154.
67. B. C. Challis and S. A. Kyrtopoulos. Nitrosation under alkaline conditions. J. Chem. Soc. Chem. Commun. 877-878 (1976).

68. B. C. Challis, A. Edwards, R. R. Hunma, S. A. Kyrtopoulos, and J. R. Outram. Rapid formation of N-nitrosoamines from nitrogen oxides under neutral and alkaline conditions. In *Environmental Aspects of N-Nitroso Compounds* (E. A. Walker, M. Castegnaro, L. Griciute, and R. E. Lyle, Eds.), IARC Sci. Publ. No. 19. International Agency for Research on Cancer, Lyon, France, 1978, pp. 127-142.
69. B. C. Challis and S. A. Kyrtopoulos. The chemistry of nitroso compounds: XI. Nitrosation of amines in solution by gaseous nitrogen oxides. J. Chem. Soc. Perkin Trans. II, 299-304 (1978).
70. B. C. Challis and S. A. Kyrtopoulos. The chemistry of nitroso compounds: XII. The mechanism of nitrosation and nitration of piperidine by gaseous N_2O_4 and N_2O_3 in aqueous alkaline solutions-evidence for the existence of molecular isomers of N_2O_4 and N_2O_3. J. Chem. Soc. Perkin Trans. II, 1296-1302 (1978).
71. S. S. Singer. Kinetics and mechanism of aliphatic transnitrosation. J. Org. Chem. *43*, 4612-4622 (1978).
72. R. N. Loeppky and R. Christiansen. The fragmentation reaction of beta-hydroxnitrosamines: possible environmental and biochemical significance for nitrosamine carcinogenicity. In *Environmental Aspects of N-Nitroso Compounds* (E. A. Walker, M. Castegnaro, L. Griciute, and R. E. Lyle, Eds.), IARC Sci. Publ. No. 19. International Agency for Research on Cancer, Lyon, France, 1978, pp. 117-126.
73. M. J. Downes, M. W. Edwards, T. S. Eisey, and C. L. Walters. Determination of nonvolatile nitrosamine by using denitrosation and a chemiluminescence analyzer. Analyst *101*, 742-748 (1976).
74. R. F. Eizember, K. R. Vogler, R. W. Souter, W. N. Cannon, and P. N. Wege. Reduction of nitrosamine levels in dinitroaniline pesticides. Presented at the 175th National American Chemical Society Meeting, Anaheim, Calif., March 1978, Abstr. PEST 085.
75. W. Fiddler, R. C. Doerr, and E. G. Piotrowski. Observations on the use of the Thermal Energy Analyzer as a specific detector for nitrosamines. In *Environmental Aspects of N-Nitroso Compounds* (E. A. Walker, M. Castegnaro, L. Griciute, and R. E. Lyle, Eds.), IARC Sci. Publ. No. 19. International Agency for Research on Cancer, Lyon, France, 1978, pp. 33-40.
76. D. H. Fine, F. Rufeh, D. Lieb, and D. P. Rounbehler. Description of the Thermal Energy Analyzer (TEA) for trace determinations of volatile and nonvolatile N-nitroso compounds. Anal. Chem. *47*, 1188-1191 (1975).

77. T. A. Gough, K. S. Webb, M. A. Pringuer, and B. J. Wood. A comparison of various mass spectrometric and a chemiluminescent method for the estimation of volatile nitrosamines. Agric. Food Chem. *25*, 663-667 (1977).
78. T. A. Gough. An examination of some foodstuffs for trace amounts of volatile nitrosamines using the Thermal Energy Analyzer. In *Environmental Aspects of N-Nitroso Compounds* (E. A. Walker, M. Castegnaro, L. Griciute, and R. E. Lyle, Eds.), IARC Sci. Publ. No. 19. International Agency for Research on Cancer, Lyon, France, 1978, pp. 297-304.
79. D. H. Fine and F. Rufeh. Description of the thermal energy analyzer for N-nitroso compounds. In *N-Nitroso Compounds in the Environment* (P. Bogovski and E. A. Walker, Eds.), IARC Sci. Publ. No. 9. International Agency for Research on Cancer, Lyon, France, 1974, pp. 40-44.
80. D. H. Fine, D. Lieb, and F. Rufeh. Principles of operation of the thermal energy analyzer for the trace analysis of volatile and nonvolatile N-nitroso compounds. J. Chromatogr. *107*, 351-357 (1975).
81. D. H. Fine and D. P. Rounbehler. Analysis of volatile N-nitroso compounds by combined gas chromatography and thermal energy analysis. In *Environmental N-Nitroso Compounds Analysis and Formation* (E A. Walker, P. Bogovski, and L. Griciute, Eds.), IARC Sci. Publ. No. 14. International Agency for Research on Cancer, Lyon, France, 1976, pp. 117-127.
82. M. Castegnaro and E. A. Walker. New data from collaborative studies on analyses of nitrosamines. In *Environmental Aspects of N-Nitroso Compounds* (E. A. Walker, M. Castegnaro, L. Griciute, and R. E. Lyle, Eds.), IARC Sci. Publ. No. 19. International Agency for Research on Cancer, Lyon, France, 1978, pp. 53-62.
83. D. C. Havery, T. Fazio, and J. W. Howard. Survey of cured meat products for volatile N-nitrosamines: comparison of two analytical methods. In *Environmental Aspects of N-Nitroso Compounds* (E. A. Walker, M. Castegnaro, L. Griciute, and R. E. Lyle, Eds.), IARC Sci. Publ. No. 19. International Agency for Research on Cancer, Lyon, France, 1978, pp. 41-52.
84. R. Stephany and P. L. Schuller. How specific and sensitive is the Thermal Energy Analyzer? In *Proceedings of the Second International Symposium on Nitrite in Meat Products* (B. J. Tinbergen and B. Krol, Eds.), PUDOC, Wageningen, 1977, pp. 249-255.
85. A. Lafleur, B. D. Morriseau, and D. H. Fine. Explosives identification in post-blast residues and other matrices using gas chromatography (GC) and high performance liquid chroma-

tography (HPLC) combined with a NO-specific detector. In *Proceedings of the New Concepts Symposium and Workshop on Detection and Identification of Explosives*, Reston, Va., Oct. 30-Nov. 1, 1978. U.S. Departments of Treasury, Energy, Justice, and Transportation, Washington, D.C.

86. T. A. Gough, K. S. Webb, and R. F. Eaton. A simple chemiluminescent detector for the screening of foodstuffs for the presence of volatile nitrosamines. J. Chromatogr. *137*, 293-303 (1977).
87. M. J. Saxby. Mass spectrometry of N-dialkylnitrosamines. J. Assoc. Off. Anal. Chem. *55*, 9-12 (1972).
88. W. T. Rainey, W. H. Christie, and W. Lijinsky. Mass spectrometry of N-nitrosamines. Biomed. Mass Spectrom. *5*, 395-408 (1978).
89. J. W. Pensabene, W. Fiddler, C. J. Dooley, R. C. Doerr, and A. E. Wasserman. Spectral and gas chromatographic characteristics of some N-nitrosamines. J. Agric. Food Chem. *21*, 274-277 (1972).
90. D. F. Gadbois, E. M. Ravese, R. C. Lundstrom, and R. S. Maney. N-nitrosodimethylamine in cold-smoked sablefish. J. Agric. Food Chem. *23*, 665-668 (1975).
91. W. Gaffield, R. H. Fish, R. L. Holmstead, J. Poppiti, and A. L. Yergey. Chemical ionization mass spectrometry of nitrosamines. In *Environmental N-Nitroso Compounds Analysis and Formation* (E. A. Walker, P. Bogovski, and L. Griciute, Eds.), IARC Sci. Publ. No. 14. International Agency for Research on Cancer, Lyon, France, 1976, pp. 11-20.
92. T. A. Gough. Mass spectrometric techniques. In *Environmental Carcinogens Selected Methods of Analysis*, Vol. 1: *Analysis of Volatile Nitrosamines in Food* (R. Preussmann, M. Castegnaro, E. A. Walker, and A. E. Wasserman, Eds.), IARC Sci. Publ. No. 18. International Agency for Research on Cancer, Lyon, France, 1978, pp. 29-34.
93. T. A. Gough and K. S. Webb. A method for the detection of traces of nitrosamine using combined gas chromatography and mass spectrometry. J. Chromatogr. *79*, 57-63 (1973).
94. C. J. Dooley, A. E. Wasserman, and S. Osman. A contaminant in N-nitroso-dimethylamine confirmation by high resolution mass spectrometry. J. Food Sci. *38*, 1096 (1973).
95. T. A. Gough. Determination of N-nitroso compounds by mass spectrometry. Analyst *103*, 785-806 (1978).
96. R. W. Stephany. Some critical remarks on the optimum resolution to use in trace analysis of nitrosamines with combined gas chromatography and mass spectrometry. In *Proceedings of the Second International Symposium on Nitrite in Meat Products*

(B. J. Tinbergen and B. Krol, Eds.). PUDOC, Wageningen, 1977, pp. 239-248.

97. D. H. Fine, D. P. Rounbehler, A. Silvergleid, and R. Ross. Trace analysis of polar and apolar N-nitroso compounds by combined high-performance liquid chromatography and thermal energy analysis. In *Proceedings of the Second International Symposium on Nitrite in Meat Products* (B. J. Tinbergen and B. Krol, Eds.). PUDOC, Wageningen, 1977, pp. 191-198.

98. D. H. Fine, F. Huffman, D. P. Rounbehler, and N. M. Belcher. Analysis of N-nitroso compounds by combined high-performance liquid chromatography and thermal energy analysis. In *Environmental N-Nitroso Compounds Analysis and Formation* (E. A. Walker, P. Bogovski, and L. Griciute, Eds.), IARC Sci. Publ. No. 14. International Agency for Research on Cancer, Lyon, France, 1976, pp. 43-50.

99. I. S. Krull, T. Y. Fan, M. Wolf, R. Ross, and D. H. Fine. The HPLC-TEA analysis of various biological samples for N-nitroso contaminants. In *LC Symposium I. Biological and Biomedical Applications of Liquid Chromatography* (G. Hawk, Ed.). Marcel Dekker, New York, 1979, pp. 443-474.

100. I. S. Krull, U. Goff, M. Wolf, A. M. Heos, D. H. Fine, and G. P. Arsenault. The thermal energy analysis of sodium saccharin. Food Cosmet. Toxicol. *16*, 105-110 (1978).

101. D. H. Fine, R. Ross, D. P. Rounbehler, A. Silvergleid, and L. Song. Analysis of nonionic, nonvolatile N-nitroso compounds in foodstuffs. Agric. Food Chem. *24*, 1069-1071 (1976).

102. T. Y. Fan, I. S. Krull, R. D. Ross, M. H. Wolf, and D. H. Fine. Comprehensive analytical procedures for the determination of volatile and nonvolatile, polar and non-polar N-nitroso compounds. In *Environmental Aspects of N-nitroso Compounds* (E. A. Walker, M. Castegnaro, L. Griciute, and R. E. Lyle, Eds.), IARC Sci. Publ. No. 19. International Agency for Research on Cancer, Lyon, France, 1978, pp. 3-18.

103. H. Druckrey, R. Preussmann, S. Ivankovic, and D. Schmahl. Organotrope carcinogene Wirkungen bei 65 verschiedenen N-Nitrosos-Verbindungen an BD-Ratten. Z. Krebsforsch. *69*, 103-201 (1967).

104. W. Lijinsky, L. Keefer, and J. Loo. The preparation and properties of some nitrosamino acids. Tetrahedron *26*, 5137-5153 (1970).

105. G. Eisenbrand. Recent developments in trace analysis of volatile nitrosamines. A brief review. In *N-Nitroso Compounds in the Environment* (P. Bogovski and E. A. Walker, Eds.), IARC Sci. Publ. No. 9. International Agency for Research on Cancer, Lyon, France, 1974, pp. 6-11.

106. F. Ender, G. N. Havre, R. Madsen, L. Ceh, and A. Helgebostad. Studies on conditions under which N-nitrosodimethylamine is formed in herring meal produced from nitrite preserved herring. Z. Tierphysiol. Tierernaehr. Futtermittelkd. *22*, 181-189 (1967).
107. J. W. Levin, G. W. Milne, and T. Axenrod. Raman and infrared spectra of dimethylnitrosamine. J. Chem. Phys. *53*, 2505-2512 (1970).
108. C. N. R. Rao. *Chemical Applications of Infrared Spectroscopy*. Academic Press, New York, 1964, p. 275.
109. K. Keyns and H. Roper. Analytik von N-Nitroso-Verbindungen: II. Mitt. Trennung und quantitative Bestimmung von homologen N-Nitroso-N-alkylharnstoffen und N-Nitroso-n-alkylurethanen durch schnelle Hoshdrunkflussigkeits-Chromatographie. J. Chromatogr. *93*, 429-439 (1974).
110. J. A. Montgomery, T. P. Johnston, H. J. Thomas, J. R. Piper, and C. Temple, Jr. The use of microparticulate reversed-phase packings in high-pressure liquid chromatography of compounds of biological interest. In *Advances in Chromatography* (J. C. Giddings, E. Grushka, J. Cazes, and P. R. Brown, Eds.), Vol 15, Marcel Dekker, New York, 1977, pp. 169-195.
111. W. Iwaoka and S. R. Tannenbaum. Liquid chromatography of N-nitrosamino acids and their syn- and anti-conformers. J. Chromatogr. *124*, 105-110 (1976).
112. W. T. Iwaoka, M. S. Weisman, and S. R. Tannenbaum. A solvent-partitioning high-speed, liquid chromatographic procedure for clean-up in the analysis of nitrosamines. In *N-Nitroso Compounds in the Environment* (P. Bogovski and E. A. Walker, Eds.), IARC Sci. Publ. No. 9. International Agency for Research on Cancer, Lyon, France, 1974, pp. 32-35.
113. G. B. Cox. Estimation of volatile N-nitrosamines by high-performance liquid chromatography. J. Chromatogr. *83*, 471-481 (1973).
114. S. S. Hecht, R. M. Ornaf, and D. Hoffmann. Determination of N-nitrosonornicotine in tobacco by high speed liquid chromatography. Anal. Chem. *47*, 2046-2048 (1975).
115. G. S. Rao and D. A. McLennon. High-pressure liquid chromatographic analysis of carcinogenic N-nitroso derivatives of piperazine resulting from drug-nitrite interactions. J. Anal. Toxicol. *1*, 43-45 (1977).
116. C. Green, T. J. Hansen, W. T. Iwaoka, and S. R. Tannenbaum. Specific detection systems for the chromatographic analysis of nitrosamines. In *Proceedings of the Second International Symposium on Nitrite in Meat Products*, (B. J. Tinbergen and B. Krol, Eds.). PUDOC, Wageningen, 1976, pp. 145-153.

117. R. Preussmann, G. Wurtele, G. Eisenbrand, and B. Spiegelhalder. Urinary excretion of N-nitrosodiethanolamine administered orally to rats. Cancer Lett. *5*, 207-209 (1978).
118. R. Yost, W. MacLean, and J. Stoveken. Confirmatory identification of HPLC peaks using absorbance ratios at several wavelengths. Perkin-Elmer Chromatogr. Newslett. *4*, 1-4 (1976).
119. W. Iwaoka and S. R. Tannenbaum. Photohydrolytic detection of N-nitroso compounds in high-performance liquid chromatography. In *Environmental N-Nitroso Compounds Analysis and Formation* (E. A. Walker, P. Bogovski, and L. Griciute, Eds.), IARC Sci. Publ. No. 14. International Agency for Research on Cancer, Lyon, France, 1976, pp. 51-56.
120. D. Daiber and R. Preussmann. Quantitative colorimetrische Bestimmung organischer N-Nitroso-Verbindungen durch photochemische Spaltung der Nitrosaminbindung. Z. Anal. Chem. *206*, 344-352 (1964).
121. G. Eisenbrand and R. Preussman. Eine neue Methods zur kolorometrischen Bestimmung von Nitrosaminen nach Spaltung det N-nitrosogruppe mit Bromwasserstoff in Eisessig. Arzneim. Forsch. *20*, 1513-1517 (1970).
122. G. M. Singer, S. S. Singer, and D. G. Schmidt. A nitrosamide specific detector for use with high-presssure liquid chromatography. J. Chromatogr. *133*, 59-66 (1977).
123. J. Sander. Eine methode zum Nachweiss von Nitrosaminen. Z. Physiol. Chem. *348*, 852-854 (1967).
124. T. Y. Fan and S. R. Tannenbaum. Automatic colorimetric determination of N-nitroso compounds. J. Agric. Food Chem. *19*, 1267-1269 (1971).
125. C. L. Walters, E. M. Johnson, and N. Ray. Separation and detection of volatile and nonvolatile N-nitrosamines. Analyst *95*, 485-489 (1970).
126. C. L. Walters, B. E. Newton, D. V. Parke, and R. Walker. The precursors of N-nitroso compounds in foods. In *N-Nitroso Compounds in the Environment* (P. Bogovski and E. A. Walker, Eds.), IARC Sci. Publ. No. 9. International Agency for Research on Cancer, Lyon, France, 1974, pp. 223-228.
127. D. F. Heath and J. A. E. Jarvis. The polarographic determination of dimethylnitrosamine in animal tissue. Analyst *80*, 613-616 (1955).
128. N. D. McGlashan, C. L. Walters, and A. E. M. McLean. Nitrosamines in African alcoholic spirits and oesophageal cancer. Lancet *2*, 1017-1019 (1968).
129. R. Kadar and O. Devik. The possible occurrence of nitrosamines in tobacco smoke. Beitr. Tabakforsch. *6*, 117-119 (1972).
130. S. K. Chang and G. W. Harrington. Determination of dimethyl-

nitrosamine and nitrosoproline by differential pulse polarography. Anal. Chem. *47*, 1857-1860 (1975).

131. K. Hasebe and J. Osteryoung. Differential pulse polarographic determination of some carcinogenic nitrosamines. Anal. Chem. *47*, 2412-2418 (1975).

132. B. G. Snider and D. C. Johnson. A photo-electroanalyzer for determination of volatile nitrosamines. Presented at the 176th National American Chemical Society Meeting, Miami, Fla., Sept. 1978, Abstr. ANAL.

133. P. T. Kissinger. Amperometric and coulometric detectors for high-performance liquid chromatography. Anal. Chem. *49*, 447A-456A (1977).

134. W. R. Heineman and P. T. Kissinger. Analytical electrochemistry: methodology and applications of dynamic techniques. Anal. Chem. *50*, 166R-175R (1978).

135. F. Vandemark and T. H. Ryan. Evaluation of an electrochemical LC detector. Perkin-Elmer Chromatogr. Newslett. *6*, 20-22 (1978).

136. R. J. Fenn, S. Siggia, and D. J. Curran. Liquid chromatography detector based on single and twin electrode thin-layer electrochemistry-application to the determination of catecholamines in blood plasma. Anal. Chem. *50*, 1067-1073 (1978).

137. E. M. Lores, D. W. Bristol, and R. F. Moseman. Determination of halogenated anilines and related compounds by HPLC with electrochemical and UV detection. J. Chromatogr. Sci. *16*, 358-362 (1978).

138. R. Preussmann, D. Daiber, and H. Hengy. A sensitive colour reaction for nitrosamines on thin-layer chromatograms. Nature (Lond.) *201*, 502-503 (1964).

139. *Handbook of Derivatives for Chromatography* (K. Blau and G. King, Eds.). Heyden & Son, Philadelphia, 1977.

140. R. Preussmann, G. Neurath, G. Wulf-Lorentzen, D. Daiber, and H. Hengy. Anfaerbemethoden und Dunnschift-Chromatographie von organischen N-Nitrosoverbindungen. Z. Anal. Chem. *202*, 187-192 (1964).

141. E. Kroeller. Untersuchungen zum Nachweis von Nitrosaminen in Tabakrauch und Lebensmitteln. Dent. Lebensm. Rundsch. *63*, 303-305 (1967).

142. J. C. Young. Detection and determination of N-nitrosamines by thin-layer chromatography using fluorescamine. J. Chromatogr. *124*, 17-28 (1976).

143. J. C. Young. Detection and determination of volatile and non-volatile N-nitrosamines by thin-layer chromatography using fluorescamine. In *Environmental Aspects of N-Nitroso Compounds* (E. A. Walker, M. Castegnaro, L. Griciute, and R. E. Lyle, Eds.), IARC Sci. Publ. No. 19. International Agency for Research on Cancer, Lyon, France, 1978, pp. 63-74.

144. G. S. Rao and E. A. Bejnarowicz. Thin-layer chromatography of sarcosine and its lauroyl and N-nitroso derivatives. J. Chromatogr. *123*, 486-489 (1976).
145. N. P. Sen and C. Dalpe. A simple thin-layer chromatographic technique for the semi-quantitative determination of volatile nitrosamines in alcoholic beverages. Analyst *97*, 216-220 (1972).
146. G. Eisenbrand. Determination of volatile nitrosamines at low levels in food by acid catalyzed denitrosation and formation of derivatives from the resulting amines. In *N-Nitroso Compounds Analysis and Formation* (P. Bogovski, R. Preussmann, and E. A. Walker, Eds.), IARC Sci. Publ. No. 3. International Agency for Research on Cancer, Lyon, France, 1972, pp. 64-70.
147. K. W. Yang and E. W. Brown. A sensitive analysis for nitrosamines. Anal. Lett. *5*, 293-304 (1972).
148. W. J. Serfontein and P. Hurter. Nitrosamines as environmental carcinogens: II. Evidence for the presence of nitrosamines in tobacco smoke condensate. Cancer Res. *26*, 575-579 (1966).
149. N. P. Sen, B. Donaldson, J. R. Iyengar, and T. Panalaks. Nitrosopyrrolidine and dimethylnitrosamine in bacon. Nature (Lond.) *241*, 473-474 (1973).
150. J. H. Wolfram, J. I. Feinberg, R. C. Doerr, and W. Fiddler. Determination of N-nitrosoproline at the nanogram level. J. Chromatogr. *132*, 37-43 (1977).
151. *Environmental Carcinogens: Selected Methods of Analysis. Analysis of Volatile Nitrosamines in Food*, Vol. 1 (R. Preussmann, M. Castegnaro, E. A. Walker, and A. E. Wassermann, Eds.), IARC Sci. Publ. No. 18. International Agency for Research on Cancer, Lyon, France, 1978,
152. T. H. Jupille and J. A. Perry. Programmed multiple development in thin-layer chromatography. Science *194*, 288-293 (1976).
153. R. K. Vitek and D. M. Kent. High performance radial chromatography. Am. Lab., 71-76 (Jan. 1978).
154. W. Kietz, A. A. Boulton, and V. Pollak. Ultra-micro thin-layer chromatography on a cylindrical support. J. Chromatogr. *107*, 81-89 (1975).
155. M. Gurkin and S. Gravitt. Quantitative and qualitative in situ analysis of thin-layer chromatograms. Am. Lab., (Jan. 1972).
156. U. Hezel. Quantitative photometry of thin-layer chromatograms for research and routine analysis. Am. Lab., 91-108 (May 1978).
157. M. K. Brandt. Automated thin-layer chromatography. Am. Lab., 87-94 (Sept. 1973).
158. N. P. Sen, D. C. Smith, L. Schwinghamer, and J. J. Marleau.

Diethylnitrosamine and other N-nitrosamines in foods. J. Assoc. Off. Anal. Chem. *52*, 47-52 (1969).

159. J. K. Foreman, J. F. Palframan, and E. A. Walker. Gas chromatographic determination of N-alkyl nitrosamines. Nature (Lond.) *225*, 544 (1970).

160. W. A. Aue, C. W. Gehrke, R. C. Trindle, D. L. Stalling, and C. D. Ruyle. Application of the flame-ionization detector to nitrogen-containing compounds. J. Gas Chromatogr. *5*, 381-382 (1967).

161. J. W. Howard, T. Fazio, and J. O. Watts. Extraction and gas chromatographic determination of N-nitrosodimethylamine in smoked fish: application to smoked nitrite-treated chub. J. Assoc. Off. Anal. Chem. *53*, 269-274 (1970).

162. T. Kawabata, M. Matsui, T. Ishibashi, and M. Nakamura. Analysis of N-nitrosamines by gas chromatography. Jap. Anal. *21*, 1326-1332 (1972).

163. T. Fazio, J. N. Damico, J. W. Howard, R. H. White, and J. O. Watts. Gas chromatographic determination and mass spectrometric confirmation of N-nitrosodimethylamine in smoke-processed marine fish. J. Agric. Food Chem. *19*, 250-253 (1971).

164. W. Fiddler, R. C. Doerr, J. R. Ertel, and A. E. Wasserman. Determination of N-nitrosodimethylamine in ham by gas-liquid chromatography with an alkali flame ionization detector. J. Assoc. Off. Anal. Chem. *54*, 1160-1163 (1971).

165. T. A. Gough and K. Sugden. A study of the stability of a nitrogen-selective thermionic detector. J. Chromatogr. *86*, 65-71 (1973).

166. D. M. Coulson. Electrolytic conductivity detector for gas chromatography. J. Gas Chromatogr. *3*, 134-137 (1965).

167. J. F. Palframan, J. Macnab, and N. T. Crosby. An evaluation of the alkali flame ionization detector and the Coulson electrolytic conductivity detector in the analysis of N-nitrosamines in foods. J. Chromatogr. *76*, 307-319 (1973).

168. J. W. Rhoades and D. E. Johnson. Gas chromatography and selective detection N-nitrosamines. J. Chromatogr. Sci. *8*, 616-617 (1970).

169. N. P. Sen, J. R. Iyengar, B. A. Donaldson, and T. Panalaks. Effect of sodium nitrite concentration on the formation of nitrosopyrrolidine and dimethylnitrosamine in fried bacon. J. Agric. Food Chem. *22*, 540-541 (1974).

170. K. Goodhead and T. A. Gough. The reliability of a procedure for the determination of nitrosamines in food. Food Cosmet. Toxicol. *13*, 307-312 (1975).

171. J. R. Iyengar, T. Panalaks, W. F. Miles, and N. P. Sen. A survey of fish products for volatile N-nitrosamines. J. Sci. Food Agric. *27*, 527-530 (1976).

172. N. P. Sen, J. R. Iyengar, W. F. Miles, and T. Panalaks. Nitrosamines in cured meat products. In *Environmental N-Nitroso Compounds Analysis and Formation* (E. A. Walker, P. Bogovski, and L. Griciute, Eds.), IARC Sci. Publ. No. 14. International Agency for Research on Cancer, Lyon, France, 1976, pp. 333-342.
173. N. P. Sen, B. A. Donaldson, S. Seaman, J. R. Iyengar, and W. F. Miles. Recent studies in Canada on the analysis and occurrence of volatile and non-volatile N-nitroso compounds in foods. In *Environmental Aspects of N-Nitroso Compounds* (E. A. Walker, M. Castegnaro, L. Griciute, and R. E. Lyle, Eds.), IARC Sci. Publ. No. 19. International Agency for Research on Cancer, Lyon, France, 1978, pp. 373-393.
174. R. C. Hall. A highly sensitive and selective micro-electrolytic conductivity detector for gas chromatography. J. Chromatogr. Sci. *12*, 152-160 (1974).
175. G. Eisenbrand, E. Von Rappardt, R. Zappe, and R. Preussmann. Trace analysis of volatile nitrosamines by a modified nitrogen-specific detector in the pyrolytic mode and by ion-specific determination of heptafluorobutyramides in a gas chromatography-mass spectrometry system. In *Environmental N-Nitroso Compounds Analysis and Formation* (E. A. Walker, P. Bogovski, and L. Griciute, Eds.), IARC Sci. Publ. No. 14. International Agency for Research on Cancer, Lyon, France, 1976, pp. 65-75.
176. L. F. Fieser and M. Fieser. *Reagents for Organic Synthesis*, Vols. 1-6. Wiley, New York, 1967-1977.
177. T. H. Jupille. Derivatization for detectability in HPLC. Am. Lab. 85-92 (May 1976).
178. S. Ahuja. Derivatization for gas chromatography. J. Pharm. Sci. *65*, 163-182 (1976).
179. C. R. Clark and M. M. Wells. Precolumn derivatization of amines for enhanced detectability in liquid chromatography. J. Chromatogr. Sci. *16*, 332-339 (1978).
180. F. Ender and L. Ceh. Conditions and chemical reaction mechanisms by which nitrosamines may be formed in biological products with reference to their possible occurrence in food products. Z. Lebensm. Unters. Forsch. *145*, 133-142 (1971).
181. F. W. Schueler and C. Hanna. A synthesis of unsymmetrical dimethylhydrazine using lithium aluminum hydride. J. Am. Chem. Soc. *73*, 4996 (1951).
182. W. J. Serfontein and P. Hurter. A method for identifying small amounts of nitrosamines in biological material. Nature (Lond.) *209*, 1238-1239 (1966).
183. G. Neurath, B. Piermann, and H. Wichern. Zur Frage der N-Nitrosoverbindungen in Tabakrauch. Beitr. Tabakforsch. *2*, 311-319 (1964).

184. T. G. Alliston, B. G. Cox, and R. S. Kirk. The determination of steam-volatile N-nitrosamines in foodstuffs by formation of electron-capturing derivatives from electrochemically derived amines. Analyst *97*, 915-920 (1972).

185. H. Klus and H. Kuhn. Reaktionschromatographischer Nachweis einiger N-Nitrosamine der Tabakalkaloide. J. Chromatogr. *109*, 425-426 (1975).

186. E. A. Walker and M. Castegnaro. New data on collaborative studies on the analysis of volatile nitrosamines. In *Environmental N-Nitroso Compounds Analysis and Formation* (E. A. Walker, P. Bogovski, and L. Griciute, Eds.), IARC Sci. Publ. No. 14. International Agency for Research on Cancer, Lyon, France, 1976, pp. 77-83.

187. N. P. Sen. Gas-liquid chromatographic determination of dimethylnitrosamine as dimethylnitramine at picogram levels. J. Chromatogr. *51*, 301-304 (1970).

188. J. Althorpe, D. A. Goddard, D. J. Sissons, and G. M. Telling. The gas chromatographic determination of nitrosamines at the picogram level by conversion to their corresponding nitramines. J. Chromatogr. *53*, 371-373 (1970).

189. M. Castegnaro and E. A. Walker. Developments in nitrosamine analysis. In *Proceedings of the Second International Symposium on Nitrite in Meat Products* (B. J. Tinbergen and B. Krol, Eds.). PUDOC, Wageningen, 1977, pp. 187-190.

190. J. H. Hotchkiss, J. F. Barbour, L. M. Libbey, and R. A. Scanlan. Nitramines as Thermal Energy Analyzer positive non-nitroso compounds found in certain herbicides. J. Agric. Food Chem. *26*, 884-887 (1978).

191. W. Gaffield and R. E. Lundin. Determination of nitrosamino-alcohols and amines by fluorine-19 nuclear magnetic resonance of hexafluoroacetone derivatives. In *Environmental Aspects of N-Nitroso Compounds* (E. A. Walker, M. Castegnaro, L. Griciute, and R. E. Lyle, Eds.), IARC Sci. Publ. No. 19. International Agency for Research on Cancer, Lyon, France, 1978, pp. 87-95.

192. G. Eisenbrand, C. Janzowski, and R. Preussmann. Analysis, formation, and occurrence of volatile and non-volatile N-nitroso compounds: recent results. In *Proceedings of the Second International Symposium on Nitrite in Meat Products* (B. J. Tinbergen and B. Krol, Eds.). PUDOC, Wageningen, 1977, pp. 155-169.

193. N. P. Sen, D. E. Coffin, S. Seaman, B. Donaldson, and W. F. Miles. Extraction, clean-up, and estimation as methyl ether of 3-hydroxyl-1-nitrosopyrrolidine, a non-volatile nitrosamine in cooked bacon at mass fractions of μg/kg. In *Proceedings of the Second International Symposium on Nitrite in Meat Products*

(B. J. Tinbergen and B. Krol, Eds.). PUDOC, Wageningen, 1977, pp. 179-185.

194. D. H. Fine, D. P. Rounbehler, N. M. Belcher, and S. S. Epstein. N-Nitroso Compounds: detection in ambient air. Science *192*, 1328-1330 (1976).

195. I. S. Krull, T. Y. Fan, and D. H. Fine. Problem of artifacts in the analysis of N-nitroso compounds. Anal. Chem. *50*, 698-701 (1978).

196. J. Polo and Y. L. Chow. Efficient degradation of nitrosamines by photolysis. In *Environmental N-Nitroso Compounds Analysis and Formation* (E. A. Walker, P. Bogovski, and L. Griciute, Eds.), IARC Sci. Publ. No. 14. International Agency for Research on Cancer, Lyon, France, 1976, pp. 473-486.

197. R. C. Doerr and W. Fiddler. Photolysis of volatile nitrosamines at the picogram level as an aid to confirmation. J. Chromatogr. *140*, 284-287 (1977).

198. I. S. Krull and U. Goff. Unpublished results, 1978.

199. E. M. Johnson and C. L. Walters. The specificity of the release of nitrite from N-nitrosamines by hydrobromic acid. Anal. Lett. *4*, 383-386 (1971).

200. C. L. Walters, R. J. Hart, and S. Perse. The breakdown into nitric oxide of compounds potentially derived from nitrite in a biological matrix. Z. Lebensm. Unters. Forsch. *167*, 315-319 (1978).

201. T. Y. Fan, R. Ross, D. H. Fine, L. H. Keith, and A. W. Garrison. Isolation and identification of some Thermal Energy Analyzer (TEA) responsive substances in drinking water. Environ. Sci. Technol. *12*, 692-695 (1978).

202. M. Zief and J. W. Mitchell. *Contamination Control in Trace Element Analysis*, Chemical Analysis Series, Vol. 47. Wiley-Interscience, New York, 1976.

203. R. M. Angeles, L. K. Keefer, P. P. Roller, and S. J. Uhm. Chemical models for possible nitrosamine artifact formation in environmental analysis. In *Environmental Aspects of N-Nitroso Compounds* (E. A. Walker, M. Castegnaro, L. Griciute, and R. E. Lyle, Eds.), IARC Sci. Publ. No. 19. International Agency for Research on Cancer, Lyon, France, 1978, pp. 109-116.

204. O. J. Logsdon II, K. E. Nottingham, and T. O. Meiggs. Formation of nitrosamines and cycloalkanes during analyses procedures. Presented at the 91st meeting of the Association of Official Analytical Chemists, Washington, D.C., Oct. 1977, Bastr. 215.

205. D. H. Fine, D. P. Rounbehler, E. Sawicki, and K. Krost. Determination of dimethylnitrosamine in air and water by Thermal Energy Analysis: validation of analytical procedures. Environ. Sci. Technol. *11*, 577-580 (1977).

206. D. H. Fine. An assessment of human exposure to N-nitroso compounds. In *Environmental Aspects of N-Nitroso Compounds* (E. A. Walker, M. Castegnaro, L. Griciute, and R. E. Lyle, Eds.), IARC Sci. Publ. No. 19. International Agency for Research on Cancer, Lyon, France, 1978, pp. 267-278.
207. G. Eisenbrand and B. Spiegelhalder. Personal communication, (1977).
208. T. Y. Fan and D. H. Fine. Formation of N-nitrosodimethylamine in the injection port of a gas chromatograph: an artifact in nitrosamine analysis. J. Agric. Food Chem. *26*, 1471-1472 (1978).
209. W. Fiddler, J. W. Pensabene, R. C. Doerr, and C. J. Dooley. The presence of dimethyl and diethyl nitrosamines in de-ionized water. Food Cosmet. Toxicol. *15*, 441-443 (1977).
210. S. S. Hecht, R. M. Ornaf, and D. Hoffmann. Chemical studies on tobacco smoke: XXXIII. N'-Nitrosonornicotine in tobacco: analysis of possible contributing factors and biologic implications. J. Natl. Cancer Inst. *54*, 1237-1244 (1974).
211. G. R. Umbreit. Chromatographic anomalies. Chem. Technol. *7*, 101-106 (1977).
212. D. J. Freed and A. M. Mujsce. Generation of nitrosamines by gas chromatographic analysis via direct injection. Anal. Chem. *49*, 1544-1545 (1977).
213. Food and Drug Administration (U.S.). Pre-publication bulletin on the Mineral Oil Distillation-TEA Method. FDA, Washington, D.C., (1978).
214. D. H. Fine, D. P. Rounbehler, and P. E. Oettinger. A rapid method for the determination of sub-part per billion amounts of N-nitroso compounds in foodstuffs. Anal. Chim. Acta *78*, 383-389 (1975).
215. R. W. Stephany and P. L. Schuller. The intake of nitrate, nitrite, and volatile N-nitrosamines, and the occurrence of volatile N-nitrosamines in human urine and veal calves. In *Environmental Aspects of N-Nitroso Compounds* (E. A. Walker, M. Castegnaro, L. Griciute, and R. E. Lyle, Eds.), IARC Sci. Publ. No. 19. International Agency for Research on Cancer, Lyon, France, 1978, pp. 443-460.
216. B. Spiegelhalder. Personal communication, 1978.
217. T. Fazio, J. W. Howard, and D. Havery. Analysis of volatile N-nitrosamines in food using flame thermionic detection and mass spectrometry confirmation. In *Environmental Carcinogens: Selected Methods of Analysis*, Vol. 1: *Analysis of Volatile Nitrosamines in Food* (R. Preussmann, M. Castegnaro, E. A. Walker, and A. E. Wassermann, Eds.), IARC Sci. Publ. No. 18. International Agency for Research on Cancer, Lyon, France, 1978, pp. 83-96.

218. J. C. Young. Detection and determination of N-nitrosamino acids by TLC using fluorescamine. J. Chromatogr. *151*, 215-221 (1978).
219. Thermo Electron Preptube Literature. Thermo Electron Corporation, Waltham, Mass., 1979.
220. W. R. Bruce, Personal communication, 1978.
221. T. Wang, T. Kakizoe, P. Dion, R. Furrer, A. J. Varghese, and W. R. Bruce. Volatile nitrosamines in human feces. Nature (Lond.) *276*, 280-282 (1978).
222. A. J. Varghese, P. C. Land, R. Furrer, and W. R. Bruce. Non-volatile N-nitroso compounds in human feces. In *Environmental Aspects of N-Nitroso Compounds* (E. A. Walker, M. Castegnaro, L. Griciute, and R. E. Lyle, Eds.), IARC Sci. Publ. No. 19. International Agency for Research on Cancer, Lyon, France, 1978, pp. 257-264.
223. W. R. Bruce, A. J. Varghese, R. Furrer, and P. C. Land. A mutagen in the feces of normal humans. In *Origins of Human Cancer, Cold Spring Harbor Conferences on Cell Proliferation* (H. H. Hiatt, J. D. Watson, and J. A. Winsten, Eds.). Cold Spring Harbor Laboratory, New York. 1977, pp. 1641-1646.
224. R. M. Hicks, T. A. Gough, and C. L. Walters. Demonstration of the presence of nitrosamines in human urine: preliminary observations on a possible etiology for bladder cancer in association with chronic urinary tract infection. In *Environmental Aspects of N-Nitroso Compounds* (E. A. Walker, M. Castegnaro, L. Griciute, and R. E. Lyle, Eds.), IARC Sci. Publ. No. 19. International Agency for Research on Cancer, Lyon, France, 1978, pp. 465-476.
225. D. H. Fine and D. P. Rounbehler. N-Nitroso compounds in water. Presented at the First Chemical Congress of the North American Continent, Mexico City, 1975.
226. D. H. Fine and D. P. Rounbehler. N-Nitroso compounds in water. In *Identification and Analysis of Organic Pollutants in Water* (L. H. Keith, Ed.). Ann Arbor Science Publishers, Ann Arbor, Mich., 1976, Chapter 17.
227. D. H. Fine, D. P. Rounbehler, F. Huffman, A. W. Garrison, N. L. Wolfe, and S. S. Epstein. Analysis of volatile N-nitroso compounds in drinking water at the part per trillion level. Environ. Contam. Toxicol. *14*, 404-408 (1975).
228. D. H. Fine, D. P. Rounbehler, A. Rounbehler, A. Silvergleid, E. Sawicki, K. Krost, and G. A. DeMarrais. Determination of dimethylnitrosamine in air, water, and soil by Thermal Energy Analysis: measurements in Baltimore, Md. Environ. Sci. Technol. *11*, 581-584 (1977).
229. D. H. Fine, D. P. Rounbehler, N. M. Belcher, and S. S. Epstein. N-Nitroso compounds in air and water. In *Environ-*

mental N-Nitroso Compounds Analysis and Formation (E. A. Walker, P. Bogovski, and L. Griciute, Eds.), IARC Sci. Publ. No. 14. International Agency for Research on Cancer, Lyon, France, 1976, pp. 401-408.

230. M. M. Nikaido, D. Dean-Raymond, A. J. Francis, and M. Alexander. Recovery of nitrosamines from water. Water Res. *11*, 1085-1087 (1977).

231. U. Goff. Unpublished results, 1978.

232. B. Spiegelhalder, G. Eisenbrand, and R. Preussmann. Contamination of beer with trace quantities of N-nitroso-dimethylamine. Food Cosmet. Toxicol. *17*, 29-33 (1979).

233. E. A. Walker, M. Castegnaro, and B. Pignatelli. Analysis of volatile N-nitrosmaines in food by electron capture and Coulson detection of their N-nitramine derivatives. In *Environmental Carcinogens: Selected Methods of Analysis*, Vol. 1: *Analysis of Volatile Nitrosamines in Food* (R. Preussmann, M. Castegnaro, E. A. Walker, and A. E. Wassermann, Eds.), IARC Sci. Publ. No. 18. International Agency for Research on Cancer, Lyon, France, 1978, pp. 175-187.

234. O. Bassir and E. N. Maduagwu. Occurrence of nitrate, nitrite, dimethylamine, and dimethylnitrosamine in some fermented Nigerian beverages. J. Agric. Food Chem. *26*, 200-203 (1978).

235. Thermo Electron Appl. Notes No. 1. Thermo Electron Corp., Waltham, Mass., 1979.

236. S. D. West and E. W. Day, Jr. The determination of volatile nitrosamines in crops and soil treated with dinitroaniline herbicides. Presented at the 175th National Meeting of the American Chemical Society, Anaheim, Calif., Mar. 13-17, 1978, Abstr. PEST 084.

237. J. E. Oliver, P. C. Kearney, and A. Kontson. Nitrosamines in herbicides: I. Soil degradation. Presented at the 175th National Meeting of the American Chemical Society, Anaheim, Calif., Mar. 13-17, 1978, Abstr. PEST 080, 081.

238. P. C. Kearney, J. E. Oliver, C. S. Helling, A. R. Isensee, and A. Kontson. Distribution, movement, persistence, and metabolism of N-nitrosoatrazine in soils and a model aquatic ecosystem. J. Agric. Food Chem. *25*, 1177-1181 (1977).

239. S. U. Kahn and J. C. Young. N-Nitrosamine formation in soil from the herbicide glyphosphate. J. Agric. Food Chem. *25*, 1430-1432 (1977).

240. R. Ross, J. Morrison, and D. H. Fine. Assessment of dipropylnitrosamine levels in a tomato field following application of Treflan EC. J. Agric. Food Chem. *26*, 455-457 (1978).

241. E. D. Pellizzari, J. E. Bunch, R. E. Berkley, and J. McRae. Collections and analysis of trace organic vapor pollutants in ambient atmosphere. The performance of a Tenax GC cart-

ridge sampler for hazardous vapors. Anal. Lett. *9*, 45-63 (1976).

242. E. D. Pellizzari, J. E. Bunch, J. T. Bursey, and R. E. Berkley. Estimation of N-nitrosodimethylamine levels in ambient air by capillary gas-liquid chromatograph/mass spectrometry. Anal. Lett. *9*, 579-594 (1976).

243. E. D. Pellizzari, J. E. Bunch, R. E. Berkely, and J. T. Bursey. Identification of N-nitrosodimethylamine in ambient air by capillary gas liquid chromatography/mass spectrometry/computer. Biomed. Mass Spectrom. *3*, 196-200 (1976).

244. P. Issenberg and H. Sornson. A monitoring method for volatile nitrosamine levels in laboratory atmospheres. In *Environmental N-Nitroso Compounds Analysis and Formation* (E. A. Walker, P. Bogovski, and L. Griciute, Eds.), IARC Sci. Publ. No. 14. International Agency for Research on Cancer, Lyon, France, 1976, pp. 97-108.

245. D. P. Rounbehler. Personal communication, 1978.

246. R. L. Fisher, R. W. Reiser, and B. A. Lasoski. Determination of sub-microgram per cubic meter levels of N-nitrosodimethylamine in air. Anal. Chem. *49*, 1821-1823 (1977).

247. D. H. Fine. Determination of volatile N-nitrosamines in food by chemiluminescence using the Thermal Energy Analyzer. In *Environmental Carcinogens: Selected Methods of Analysis*, Vol. 1: *Analysis of Volatile Nitrosamines in Food* (R. Preussmann, M. Castegnaro, E. A. Walker, and A. E. Wassermann, Eds.), IARC Sci. Publ. No. 18. International Agency for Research on Cancer, Lyon, France, 1978, pp. 133-140.

248. T. Gough and K. Webb. Mass spectrometric determination of volatile N-nitrosamines after screening with the Coulson electrolytic detector. In *Environmental Carcinogens: Selected Methods of Analysis*, Vol. 1: *Analysis of Volatile Nitrosamines in Food* (R. Preussmann, M. Castegnaro, E. A. Walker, and A. E. Wassermann, Eds.), IARC Sci. Publ. No. 18. International Agency for Research on Cancer, Lyon, France, 1978, pp. 141-150.

249. R. W. Stephany, J. Freudenthal, and P. L. Schuller. Meat and meat products—mass spectrometric determination of volatile N-nitrosamines. In *Environmental Carcinogens: Selected Methods of Analysis*, Vol. 1: *Analysis of Volatile Nitrosamines in Food* (R. Preussmann, M. Castegnaro, E. A. Walker, and A. E. Wassermann, Eds.), IARC Sci. Publ. No. 18. International Agency for Research on Cancer, Lyon, France, 1978, pp. 151-160.

250. N. P. Sen. Analysis of volatile N-nitrosamines using gas chromatography with Coulson detector: estimation of N-nitrosopyrrolidine by thin-layer chromatography with fluorimetric

detection. In *Environmental Carcinogens: Selected Methods of Analysis*, Vol. 1: *Analysis of Volatile Nitrosamines in Food* (R. Preussmann, M. Castegnaro, E. A. Walker, and A. E. Wassermann, Eds.), IARC Sci. Publ. No. 18. International Agency for Research on Cancer, Lyon, France, 1978, pp. 119-131.

251. W. Fiddler, J. W. Pensabene, J. C. Dooley, and A. E. Wassermann. Analysis of volatile N-nitrosamines in food using flame thermionic detection and mass spectrometry confirmation. In *Environmental Carcinogens: Selected Methods of Analysis*, Vol. 1: *Analysis of Volatile Nitrosamines in Food* (R. Preussmann, M. Castegnaro, E. A. Walker, and A. E. Wassermann, Eds.), IARC Sci. Publ. No. 18. International Agency for Research on Cancer, Lyon, France, 1978, pp. 109-118.

252. G. Eisenbrand and R. Preussmann. Analysis of volatile N-nitrosamines in food using nitrogen-specific detection and ion-specific determination of heptafluorobutyramides by gas chromatography/low resolution mass spectrometry. In *Environmental Carcinogens: Selected Methods of Analysis*, Vol. 1: *Analysis of Volatile Nitrosamines in Food* (R. Preussmann, M. Castegnaro, E. A. Walker, and A. E. Wassermann, Eds.), IARC Sci. Publ. No. 18. International Agency for Research on Cancer, Lyon, France, 1978, pp. 199-212.

253. I. S. Krull and M. H. Wolf. Thermal energy analysis for N-nitroso compounds. American Laboratory, 84-91 (May 1979).

7
Pesticides and Related Substances*

MILTON A. LUKE and HERBERT T. MASUMOTO U.S. Food and Drug Administration, Los Angeles, California

I. INTRODUCTION

Industrial chemicals employed as pesticides are normally preselected or synthesized to destroy specific biological species. Insecticides are used to kill insects, herbicides to destroy weeds, and fungicides to erradicate mold, mildew, and so on. Unfortunately, these compounds may also lead to adverse human health effects. Animal studies have indicated that many of these compounds may be carcinogenic, mutagenic, or teratogenic. It has been estimated that one-third of all the pesticides allowed for use in the United States are potential carcinogens to humans [1]. The availability of a wide variety of pesticides has been credited with increasing crop production while minimizing cost and labor. The pesticide industry uses approximately 1400 active ingredients that are formulated to produce an estimated 35,000 to 50,000 separate products for an annual volume of 1.6 billion pounds [2]. Although pesticides used in agriculture constitute less than 3% of the commonly used commercial chemicals in the United States [3], they are often highlighted as being of special concern because of their relative high intrinsic toxicity and direct application to food crops.

The permission to use such hazardous chemicals in the United States is granted by the U.S. Environmental Protection Agency (EPA). The EPA evaluates the results of animal studies and residue data sub-

*The opinions expressed in this chapter are those of the authors and do not necessarily represent the views of the U.S. Food and Drug Administration.

mitted by the manufacturers. Hazards presented by the use of the product are balanced against expected benefits. If approved, the pesticide is registered for use under specified conditions and the residue levels that are allowed (tolerances) are published. These "benefit versus hazard" decisions have become more complex as the "hazard" has shifted from acute toxicity to low-level exposure with potential health effects. As these effects have been recognized, additional chronic animal testing has become a standard requirement for all new registration.

Answers are not available on how to address low-level exposure for the pesticides and their metabolites as well as for industrial chemicals such as polychlorinated biphenyls (PCBs) and polybrominated biphenyls (PBBs). The prospect of pesticide synergistic effects adds to an otherwise complex maze of sketchy facts and figures. The authors believe that decades of time will be required before all these compounds and combinations are tested at the chronic level for the various possible adverse health effects and before conclusions can be drawn as to which residues might create unreasonable hazards to humans.

The U.S. Food and Drug Administration (FDA) is responsible for the enforcement of pesticide tolerances set by EPA for residues on food crops. A multiresidue analytical procedure has provided most of the data collected by FDA. The Mills procedure [4] has provided residue levels for the majority of the pesticides that were in use when it was developed in the early 1960s. The characteristics of the pesticides have changed from long-lived nonpolar chlorinated compounds to highly polar organophosphorus compounds and carbamates that decay rapidly. As a consequence the Mills procedure no longer is able to provide an adequate picture of the residue levels in foods and crops.

In the face of seemingly unlimited combinations of pesticides and sample types, residue analysts are faced with the restrictions of limited resources. Selection of residue methodology then becomes extremely important. Analysts must evaluate available methods and by necessity adapt them to their situation or develop new analytical techniques. Many of the earlier methods were developed around determinative procedures such as color development, thin layer chromatography, and gas chromatography with electron capture detection, which all require the absence of sample extractives which may interfere. The authors believe that modern methodology should be adapted to or developed with the highly sensitive elemental specific gas chromatographic detectors, such as the flame photometric (FPD) and the recently improved electrolytic conductivity detectors [5, 6]. The use of selective detectors can minimize the need for cleanups, which in addition to requiring additional time, also remove pesticides. As a result, the methodology of many pesticide product combinations can be revised to eliminate the cleanup procedure so that faster and more comprehensive analyses are obtained. General discussions of extractions, cleanup, and determinative techniques are presented in the following sections to provide the analyst with some insight in selecting or designing an analytical method.

II. SAMPLE EXTRACTION

The basic extraction techniques used to obtain a solution of the sample's residues are:

Solvent stripping. Sample and extracting solvent are tumbled in a jar for more than 30 min.

Blending. Sample and solvent are blended at high speeds for 2 to 5 min.

Soxhlet extraction. Sample is extracted by the use of a Soxhlet apparatus for periods greater than 8 hr.

Studies on the relative extraction efficiency of the first two techniques on sprayed field crops have shown that the solvent stripping technique cannot always provide the same sample extraction efficiency as one that is obtained by blending [7-9]. Assay values obtained by Soxhlet extractions have been used as standards against which other extraction techniques can be measured. However, the times required by this technique make Soxhlet extractions impractical for normal routine analyses. As a result, the discussion on sample extractions will be focused primarily on extractions by blending.

Formulas of many of the pesticides discussed in this chapter are presented in Figure 1. These cover a wide range in polarity and solubility. DDT, a nonpolar pesticide, is soluble in nonpolar solvents such as methylene chloride and petroleum ether but is insoluble in water. Methamidophos (Monitor), a polar pesticide, is insoluble in nonpolar solvents but is very soluble in water. Both are soluble in water-miscible solvents such as methanol, acetone, and acetonitrile. An ideal choice for a universal solvent is a water-miscible solvent. However, nonpolar solvents such as benzene and hexane were first used in sample extractions because nonpolar pesticides such as DDT and BHC were introduced first. Mixtures of nonpolar and water-miscible solvents such as isopropanol and benzene or isopropanol and hexane were used initially to reduce the problem of emulsions that occurred when only the nonpolar solvent was used [10]. Many methods used a single extraction. These extractions were assumed to be complete and the sample to be represented in the extract solution by the ratio of the weight of the sample to the volume of the extracting solvent. In the extraction of a high-moisture product such as lettuce, use of mixed solvents yielded a system with two liquid phases; a predominantly aqueous phase and a predominantly organic liquid phase. In this situation, the water-miscible solvent present in the organic liquid phase was removed by water washes. The amount of sample represented in the extract solution was assumed to be proportional to the ratio of sample to nonpolar solvent as originally measured [8].

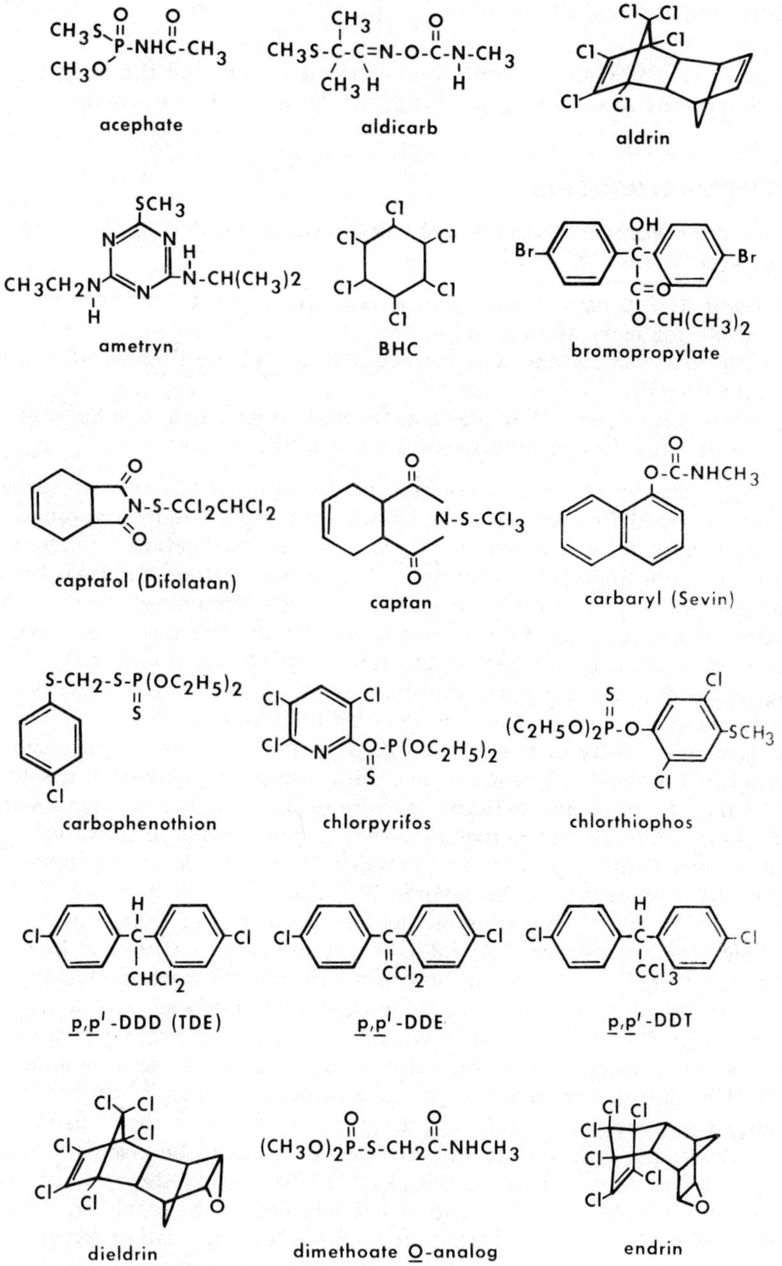

Figure 1 Formulas of various pesticides.

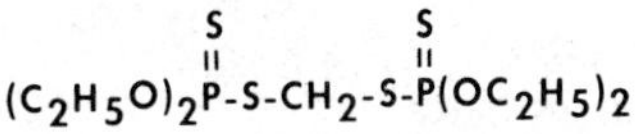

ethion

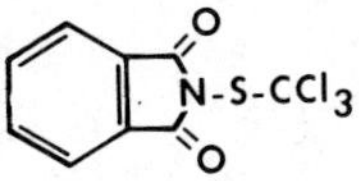

folpet

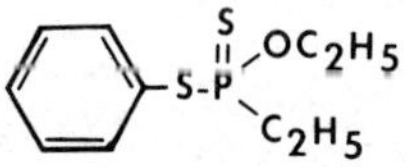

fonofos

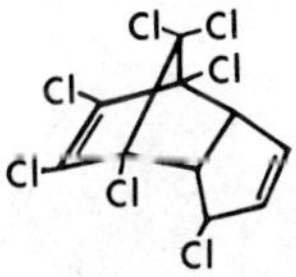

heptachlor

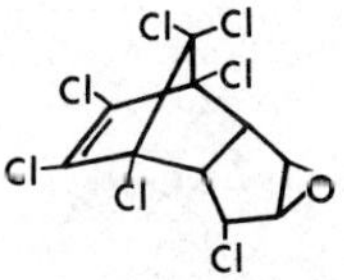

heptachlor epoxide

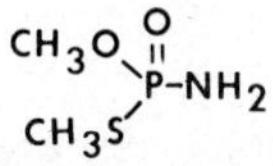

methamidophos (Monitor)

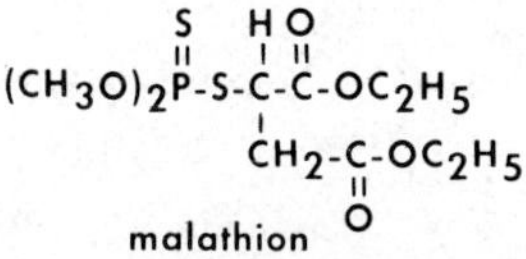

malathion

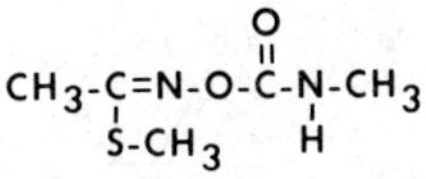

methomyl

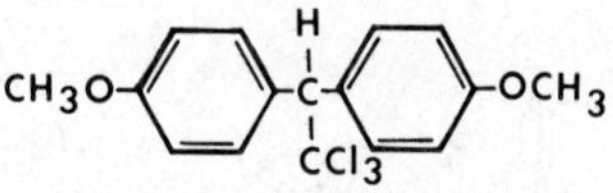

<u>p</u>,<u>p</u>′-methoxychlor

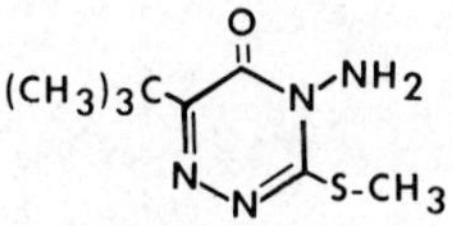

metribuzin (Sencor)

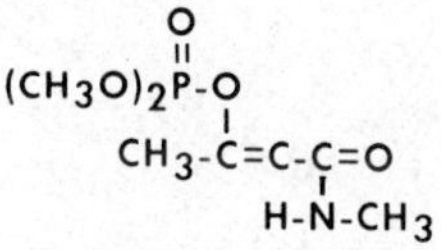

monocrotofos (Azodrin)

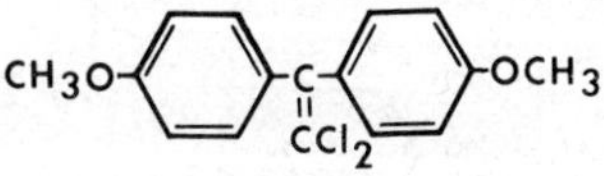

methoxychlor olefin

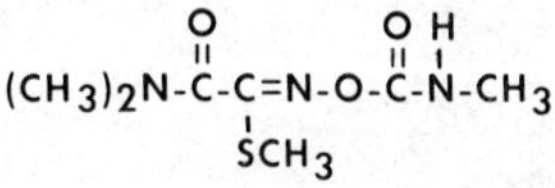

oxamyl

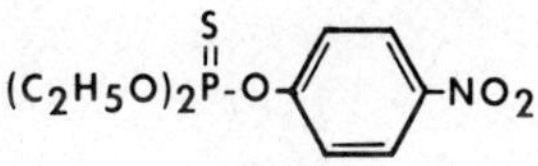

parathion

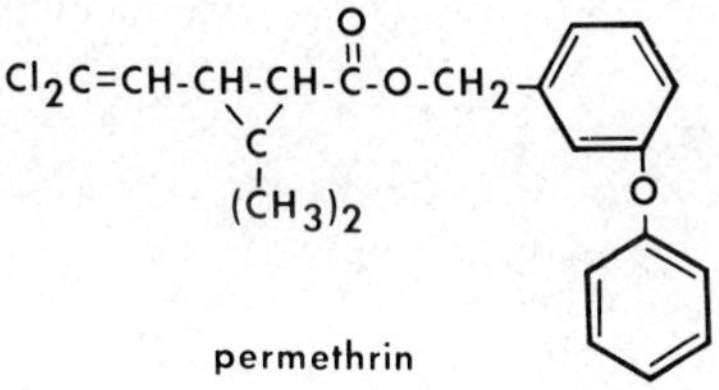

permethrin

Figure 1 (Continued)

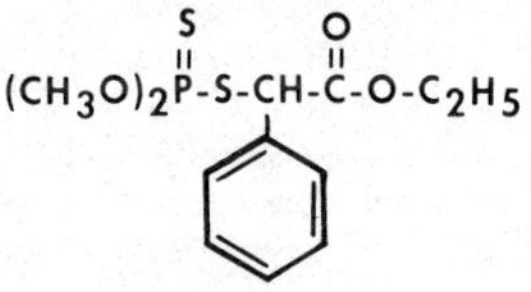

phenthoate

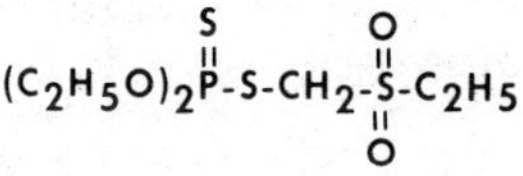

phorate sulfone

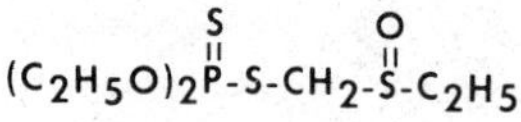

phorate sulfoxide

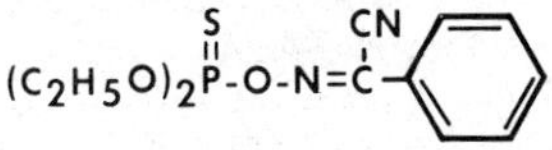

phoxim

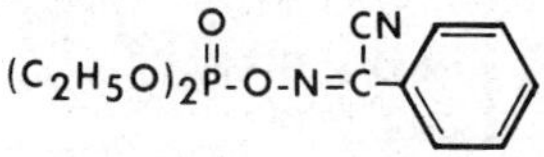

phoxim O-analog

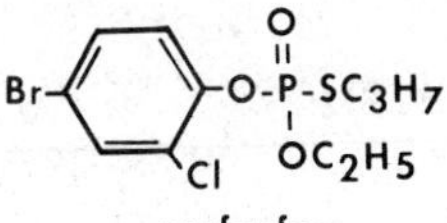

profenfos

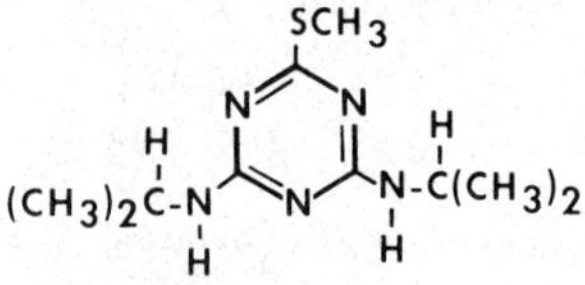

prometryn

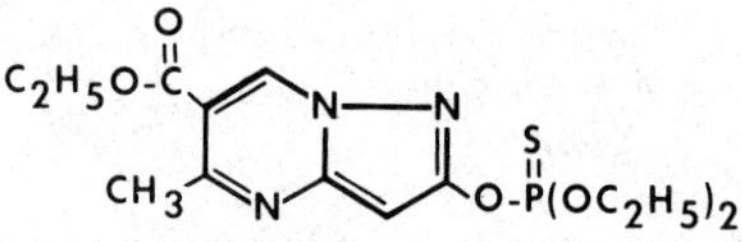

pyrazophos

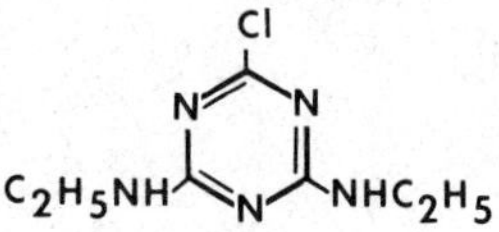

simazine

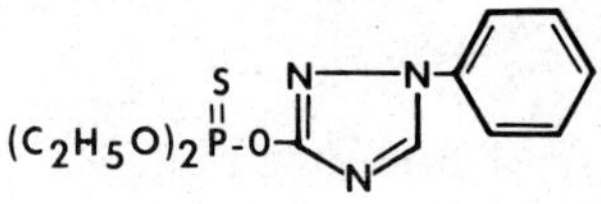

triazophos

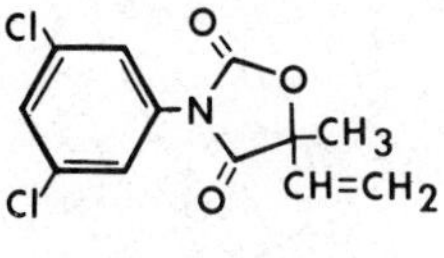

vinclozolin

Figure 1 (Continued)

Acetonitrile, a water-miscible solvent, was first used as the sole extracting solvent in an attempt to develop methodology for the organophosphorus pesticides, some members of which are water soluble [11]. This is the extracting solvent in the multiresidue procedure for organochlorine and organophosphorus residues commonly referred to as the Mills procedure [4]. The procedure has been expanded and developed by the FDA [12] and by the Association of Official Analytical Chemists (AOAC) [13]. It is based on a single extraction by acetonitrile; the amount of sample in the extract solution is proportional to the sample weight divided by the volume of acetonitrile that is used plus the volume of water present in the sample. A correction factor due to the volume contraction that occurs when acetonitrile and water are mixed is applied. A partitioning step with petroleum ether and water is used to transfer the extracted pesticides in a nonpolar solvent and to remove the water-miscible solvent. An extension of the use of the Mills acetonitrile extract has been developed to recover polar organophosphorus pesticides that are lost in the partitioning step and in a subsequent Florisil cleanup procedure [14]. A similar multiresidue procedure has been devised that uses acetone as the extracting solvent but eliminates the use of water in the partitioning step to minimize the loss of water-soluble pesticides [15].

Recoveries of samples spiked with pesticides are often undertaken to illustrate the precision and accuracy of an analytical method. The recoveries essentially consist of a combination of a blank sample with the extracting solvent that contains the pesticide in question. The recoveries show that:

1. The pesticide is not lost during the partitioning or cleanup steps.
2. Sample extractives do not interfere during the determinative step.
3. Any factors based for the analysis are correct.

The recoveries *do not* provide a measure of the total extracting efficiency of the analytical method or of the extracting solvent. Such recoveries cannot provide information on the interaction occurring between the sample and the extracting solvent. For example, in an extraction where whole carrots are tumbled with benzene in a large jar, 100% recovery would be expected when the sample is spiked by application of the spiking solution to the exterior of the carrots. Zero recovery would be expected when a syringe is used to inject the pesticide into the carrots.

Comparisons between methods or variations of methods have been used to illustrate the superiority or equivalency of a method in the analysis of sprayed field lettuce, pesticide treated soil, fish from contaminated water, and so on. However, the comparisons do not necessarily represent a measure of the efficiency of the extraction because the pesticide content of these samples is unknown. In a study with ^{14}C-labeled dieldrin, Mumma et al. [16] found that the pesticide is not completely extracted by an isopropanol-hexane blending procedure. All of the ^{14}C-labeled pesticide could be extracted by an initial extraction with isopropanol-hexane followed by a Soxhlet extraction with a methanol-chloroform mixture. A similar study of the extraction of ^{14}C-labeled dieldrin from air-dried soil indicated that extractions with mixtures of isopropanol-hexane, acetone-hexane, or acetonitrile only yield 74 to 85% recoveries of labeled pesticide [17]. Quantitative recovery was obtained by a Soxhlet extraction with a methanol-chloroform mixture. The study also illustrated that the addition of water increased the recovery of dieldrin by a 1:1 mixture of isopropanol-hexane from 74% to 97% for 20% added water (based on weight of soil). The investigator was perplexed by decreasing recoveries obtained for 30% and 100% added water. An explanation for this decrease may be related to the design of the experiment and the fact that the extracting procedure also removed the added water. When the solvents were taken to dryness by the use of a rotatory evaporator, the increasing amounts of water increased the time (after the evaporation of the more volatile solvents) that the extracted pesticide was unprotected from volatilization.

Residue values obtained by the Mumma extraction procedure have been used to compare the efficiency of the acetonitrile extraction of forage crops [18]. This study showed that acetonitrile extracted only about 15% of the dieldrin present in dry sugar beet pulp. Residue values for dieldrin, DDT, DDE, and methoxychlor comparable to those obtained by the Mumma procedure were obtained by the use of 35% water-acetonitrile extracting solvent. A lower extraction value for dieldrin was observed when a 40% water-acetonitrile solvent was used. This decrease is probably due to the decreased solubility of dieldrin in the more polar 40% water-acetonitrile solution.

A variation [19] of the Mumma extraction procedure has been used to study the effectiveness of several solvents in the extraction of a high-moisture product. The isopropanol-hexane mixture in the initial blending of the Mumma procedure was replaced by actonitrile. Table 1 lists the assay values that were obtained in the study to DDD (TDE) that had been field sprayed on kale. The 99% assay value obtained by the Mills procedure relative to the assay value obtained by the modified Mumma procedure indicates that the Mills procedure will adequately extract incurred residues from a leafy crop that contains about 83% moisture. The study also obtained lower recoveries for a triple-blending extraction procedure with acetonitrile. This lower value was probably due to an error in the design of the experimental procedure. The amount of acetonitrile present in the water-petroleum ether partitioning must be minimized to avoid the loss of pesticides [18]. (The amount of acetonitrile in the triple-extraction partitioning step was beyond the recommended upper limit.)

Table 1 Assay Values of Various Solvent Blendings for TDE from Field-Sprayed Kale

Modified Mumma[a]	Acetonitrile	Hexane and isopropanol	Ethyl acetate acetate	Methylene chloride
19.4	20	17.6	14.8	12
19.1	19.0	18.0		13
19.2	18.7	17.8		
19.2				
()				
av. 19.3	av. 19.2	av. 17.8	14.8	av. 12.5
Percent of modified Mumma	99	92	77	65

[a]Extraction by acetonitrile blending followed by Soxhlet extraction with a methanol-chloroform mixture.
Source: Ref. 19.

Although proof of the effectiveness of an extraction procedure by the use of isotope-labeled pesticides is desirable, the cost of these studies make them impractical for the residue laboratory. A reasonable approach would be to look at the extraction in terms of the following components:

1. Water
2. Nonpolar phase: fat, plant waxes, etc.
3. Adsorbents: silica in soil, cellulose, etc.

Residue analysts generally design their analyses with respect to the first two components. However, the sample's adsorbent properties are not generally considered. The increased recoveries obtained by the use of water in the extraction of soil and in the extraction of forage both indicate that adsorptive sample sites have been deactivated. The greater extraction efficiency of a methanol-chloroform mixture over an isopropanol-hexane mixture can be explained by the smaller size of the methanol molecule, which allows it to deactivate an adsorptive site by moving between the adsorptive site and the adsorbed dieldrin. Despite the fact that cellulose is a component of paper chromatography, it is not usually considered to be an adsorbent. The adsorptive properties of silica are due to folds in its surface which allow surface hydroxyl groups to approach each other more closely. The interaction between these hydroxyls results in an adsorptive site [20]. Hydroxyl groups on adjacent strands of cellulose in plant fiber could interact to form similar adsorptive sites. These adsorptive sites are deactivated by water in high-moisture products such as lettuce but must be considered in low-moisture products such as hay. Soxhlet extraction procedures need to be reevaluated as samples are often dried before extraction. Low assay values may be obtained if adsorptive sites are formed by the drying process and if methanol is not used in the extraction.

The lower residue values that are listed in Table 1 for the extraction of kale by methylene chloride and ethyl acetate illustrate the need for the use of a water-miscible solvent for better sample extraction of high-moisture products. The water-miscible solvent dissolves the sample's water and in doing so breaks up the sample's structure to provide better sample to solvent interaction. Similarly, alcohol as well as acetonitrile are used in the extraction of milk products to break the membrane of the milk fat globule [21]. Because polar and nonpolar pesticides are soluble in water-miscible solvents, there is no advantage in the use of an additional solvent (a nonpolar solvent) in the extraction of samples with a low fat content. In the analysis of fatty samples, the assay is normally made on the fat that is extracted from the sample. As a result, the use of a nonpolar solvent is required to extract the nonpolar fat, which has a limited solubility in water-miscible solvents. When a water-miscible solvent is used to extract a high-moisture product, the actual extracting reagent is the water solution of the solvent. The increased polar nature of the solution could limit the solubility of large nonpolar compounds such as waxes and fats. The presence of any insoluble nonpolar compounds presents a phase that can dissolve nonpolar pesticides. Because this situation deals with the partitioning of pesticides between two phases and not in the extraction of pesticides from a sample matrix, recovery data on spiked samples can be used to gauge the effect of this nonpolar phase. The Mills acetonitrile extraction procedure and the similar acetone extraction procedure [15] both yield good recoveries with the traditional nonpolar organochlorine pesticides for several high-moisture products.

A study on the efficiencies of acetone, methanol, and acetonitrile in the extraction of ^{14}C-labeled carbaryl (Sevin) that had been field sprayed on mustard greens and radishes has concluded that the best extracting solvent is methanol [22]. However, this conclusion is based on the total radioactivity of the compounds extracted and not on carbaryl itself. The workers found that only 50 to 75% of the extractable residue was carbaryl. Examples of percent ^{14}C extraction values are 87.3, 83.3, and 83.7% for methanol, acetone, and acetonitrile, respectively. Sample adsorption should not have been a factor as the moisture content for radishes and mustard greens are 95 and 90%, respectively.

Despite the fact that not all of the radioactivity was due to carbaryl, equivalent values would be expected for all the carbaryl-related compounds if the solvents are of equal extracting ability. An explanation for the statistical superiority that was obtained for methanol could be that methanol is able to participate in solvolytic reactions with carbaryl-related species that are chemically bound to the plant tissue and release them into solution. The use of alcohols should be avoided to avoid solvolysis of labile pesticides such as carbaryl and Monitor.

A disadvantage in the use of acetonitrile as an extracting solvent is that it cannot be used in the analysis of polar organonitrogen residues. To isolate these compounds from the sample's water in the extract requires a partitioning step similar to that used by the procedure to assay for water-soluble organophosphorus compounds [14]. In this procedure the acetonitrile is co-partitioned from the water phase. To reduce the acetonitrile level in the final assay solution so that the performance of nitrogen specific detectors are not affected is difficult. The authors feel that acetone is the best solvent for the extraction of pesticides. It is less reactive than the alcohols and does not affect the performance of the elemental specific detectors. Its boiling point of 56° versus 81° for acetonitrile and 80° for benzene results in faster solvent concentration times.* With respect to solvent concentration, the authors have not found it necessary to perform this operation with a rotatory evaporator under vacuum and at reduced temperatures to minimize the decomposition of labile residues. The use of a Kuderna-Danish concentrator fitted with a Snyder column is simpler and less expensive. A rotatory evaporator must be carefully watched to avoid the loss of pesticides that could occur when the solvent is completely removed. The Kuderna-Danish concentrator fitted with the Snyder column often is very "forgiving," even when the sample tube has been "dry" for several minutes.

A. Extraction of High Moisture-Low Fat Samples

The Mills extraction procedure is limited to pesticides that are relatively nonpolar. Low recoveries of polar pesticides are obtained due to losses that occur during the water-petroleum ether partitioning or during the Florisil cleanup of the sample extract. The acetonitrile extract can be assayed for polar organophosphorus compounds by a supplemental procedure [14]. However, this procedure is lengthy because of difficulties in the evaporation of the solvents that are used, benzene and acetonitrile. In addition, the scope of the procedure may not be applicable to the more labile pesticides because an alcohol, isopropanol, is used during solvent concentration. Low recoveries have been obtained for Monitor by this procedure.

---

*All temperature data are in degrees Celsius.

The Luke extraction procedure [15] can be used for all organochlorine, organophorphorus, organonitrogen, and hydrocarbon residues that are less polar than Monitor. Examples of the wide variety of polar and nonpolar pesticides that may be determined by this procedure are given in Appendix A. The procedure uses acetone as an extracting solvent and stresses the use of elemental specific detectors to minimize the need for sample cleanup.

Luke Extraction Procedure

Weigh 100 g of chopped or blended sample into a high-speed blender jar, add 200 ml of acetone, and blend for 2 min at high speed. Do not add Celite. Filter with suction through a Buchner funnel fitted with sharkskin filter paper. Place 80 ml of the filtrate in a 1 liter separatory funnel together with 100 ml of petroleum ether and 100 ml of methylene chloride. Shake *vigorously* for 1 min and transfer the lower aqueous layer to a second 1 liter separatory funnel. Dry the upper organic layer of the first separatory funnel by passing it through a 2 in. layer of anhydrous sodium sulfate and into a 500 ml Kuderna-Danish concentrator. To the second separatory funnel, add about 7 g of sodium chloride and extract twice with 100 ml portions of methylene chloride. Dry the lower methylene chloride layer through the layer of anhydrous sodium sulfate. Attach a Snyder column to the Kuderna-Danish concentrator and start evaporation slowly on the steam bath by placing only the tip of the receiver tube into the steam. After 100 to 150 ml of solvent has evaporated, the concentrator may be exposed to more steam. When the liquid level in the concentrator has an apparent volume (immediate volume when the concentrator is lifted from the steam bath) of about 2 ml, add 10 ml of acetone and reconcentrate to an apparent volume of 2 ml. Repeat reconcentration two more times. Cool and adjust the solvent to an appropriate volume (usually 7 ml) for gas chromatographic analysis.

The solvent reconcentration procedure is necessary only if an immediate injection is to be made into a gas chromatographic system that uses an alkali flame detector that is affected by residual methylene chloride. If a Hall electroconductivity detector is to be used, the acetone reconcentration must be replaced by a reconcentration procedure that uses 100 and 50 ml portions of petroleum ether followed by 25 ml of acetone.

The amount of sample represented in the final sample solution is calculated as follows:

$$S = W \times \frac{80}{T}$$

where

S = amount of sample in final extract
W = amount of sample weighed
T = total volume of water-acetone extract

The value of T is equal to 200 ml of acetone plus the volume due to the sample's moisture less a 10 ml contraction that occurs when 200 ml of acetone and about 85 ml of water are mixed. Obtain the sample's moisture content from Appendix B. Use 85% if the moisture content of a sample is not listed.

Mills extraction procedure

Weigh 100 g of chopped or blended sample into a high-speed blender jar, add 200 ml of acetonitrile, and blend at high speeds for 2 min. Filter with vacuum through a Buchner funnel fitted with sharkskin filter paper. Transfer a measured volume of the acetonitrile-water extract that does not exceed 170 ml of acetonitrile into a 1 liter separatory funnel together with 100 ml of petroleum ether. Shake vigorously for 1 to 2 min, add 10 ml of saturated sodium chloride solution and 600 ml of water, and shake again for 30 to 45 sec. Drain and discard the lower aqueous layer and then wash the petroleum ether layer with two 100 ml portions of water to remove residual acetonitrile. Transfer the petroleum ether to a glass-stoppered graduated cylinder and record its volume. Add anhydrous sodium sulfate to the graduate to remove any residual water. The sample solution is ready for Florisil cleanup. The amount of sample represented in the final sample solution is calculated as follows:

$$S = W \times \frac{P}{100} \times \frac{A}{T}$$

where

S = amount of sample in the final extract
W = amount of sample weighed
P = volume of petroleum ether recovered
A = volume of water-acetonitrile extract measured
T = total volume of water-acetonitrile extract

The value of T is equal to 200 ml plus the volume of water due to the sample's moisture less a 5 ml volume contraction that occurs when 200 ml of acetonitrile and about 85 ml of water are mixed. Obtain the sample's moisture content from Appendix B. Use 85% if the sample's moisture is not listed.

B. Extraction of Low Moisture-Low Fat Samples

Examples of samples in this category are forage crops and soils. The Bertuzzi extraction procedure [18] is limited to the same nonpolar compounds that are determined in the Mills procedure. The authors have obtained by the use of 35% water-acetone assay values for field-incurred residues that are comparable to those obtained by the Bertuzzi procedure. The water-acetone extracting solvent can be assayed for polar and nonpolar residues by the partitioning technique used in the Luke procedure.

Bertuzzi extraction procedure

Weigh 20 to 25 g of sample into a high-speed blender jar. Add 350 ml of 35% water-acetonitrile solution and blend at high speeds for 5 min. Continue as in the Mills procedure with "Filter with vacuum . . . ." Use 350 ml for the value of T, the total extract volume.

Extraction by water-acetone solvent

Weigh 20 to 25 g of sample into a high-speed blender jar. Add 350 ml of 35% water-acetone solution and blend at high speeds for 5 min. Continue as in the Luke procedure with "Filter with suction . . . ." Use 350 ml for the total extract volume, T.

C. Extraction of Fatty Samples

At present, the methodology for fatty samples is limited to nonpolar residues which are considered to be in the sample's fat. Many of the methods dealing with pesticides in fatty products are based on recoveries that have been made on isolated fat and not on the original product. Pesticide tolerances, besides being specified for the intact product, are sometimes expressed in terms of the isolated fat. The extraction of pesticides from fatty products has not been fully studied. The results obtained from a study [23] on the extraction of several pesticides of differing polarity illustrate the difficulty of designing a recovery procedure that truly reflects the efficiency of an extraction. When a milk sample spiked with 12 organochlorine and organophosphorus compounds was extracted by a hexane-ethyl ether solution, recoveries ranging from 10 to 92% were obtained despite the fact that less than 10% of the sample's fat had been extracted. The greater than 10% recoveries indicated that the pesticides from the spiking solution had not penetrated the matrix of the milk fat globule. The investigators surmised that the pesticides were adsorbed by hydrophobic and hydrophilic components on the milk fat globule's surface. When ethanol was used in the extraction to break the membrane of the milk fat globule, the overall recoveries ranged from 77 to 92%. The investigators ascribed the less than 100% recoveries to binding forces in the aqueous phase of the milk.

Until the extraction of pesticides from fatty samples is understood completely, a reasonable approach would be to treat the analysis of these samples in a manner that is similar to that used on milk samples. Use alcohol, acetonitrile, or perhaps acetone to break up the fat structure. In the analysis of dry fatty products such as sesame seed and nuts, the possibility of adsorption should be considered. Egg samples are presently assayed by the Mills procedure for high moisture-low fat samples by limiting the assay sample to 25 g, which is equivalent to about 3 g of fat. Fish and animal tissue could be similarly analyzed.

Fat values obtained from Appendix 2 can be used as guides in determining the sample weight that is equivalent to 3 g of fat.

Extraction of fat

A procedure for the extraction of fat from milk products is presented as a model after which extraction methods for other fatty products may be patterned. The method that is presented is not the method developed by Mills for the extraction of milk products [24], which has been adopted by the FDA and the AOAC. A disadvantage of that procedure is that it requires an explosion-proof centrifuge which is not found in most residue laboratories. The presented method is a variation of a modification [21] of the Mills fat procedure. It uses a single extraction instead of the triple extraction used by the Mills procedure. Recoveries ranging from 92 to 95% are obtainable which are comparable to those obtained by the Mills fat extraction procedure [23].

Weigh sample equivalent to about 3 g of fat into a 250 ml beaker and transfer to a 1 liter separatory funnel with the aid of water. The volume of water used in the transfer and the sample water should total to about 100 ml. Add 10 ml of 5% potassium oxalate solution and mix. Rinse the beaker with 100 ml of ethanol, transfer the rinse to the separatory funnel, and shake the mixture vigorously for 1 min. Add 200 ml of ethyl ether and shake for 2 min. Add 100 ml of petroleum ether and shake for 1 min. Let the mixture stand for 10 min and then discard the lower aqueous layer. After 1 min, discard any additional aqueous liquid that separates and elute the solvent extract through a column of anhydrous sodium sulfate (about 25 g in a 4 in. funnel with a glass wool plug) into a tared 600 ml beaker. Rinse separatory funnel with three 15 ml portions of petroleum ether. Pour each rinse through the anhydrous sodium sulfate column. Evaporate the solvent to constant fat weight on a steam bath. Take 3 g of fat through the acetonitrile-petroleum ether partitioning cleanup.

Extraction of pesticides from fatty samples

Assay values for incurred residues in milk, sesame seeds, and popcorn comparable to assays by the Mills fat extraction procedure are obtained by the following extraction procedure [25].

Weigh sample equivalent to 2 g of fat into a high-speed blender cup. Add 20 g of alumina and 350 ml of 20% water-acetonitrile (adjust volumes of acetonitrile and water to take into account the water present in the sample), and blend at high speeds for 2 min. Continue analysis as in the Mills extraction procedure for high moisture-low fat sample with "Filter with vacuum . . . . " Use 350 for the total volume of extract, T.

III. DETECTORS

The only technique that presently provides a rapid determination of pesticides with specificity and sensitivity is gas chromatography. High-pressure liquid chromatography holds some promise in the analysis of compounds such as methomyl, oxamyl, and captan that degrade during gas chromatographic analysis. This presentation is limited to the gas chromatographic detectors most useful in routine pesticide analysis. All of the detectors with the exception of the microcoulometric detector are capable of determining subnanogram amounts of compound.

A. Electron Capture Detector

The advantages of the electron capture detector are its low maintenance requirements and its high sensitivity for halogenated compounds. However, it is also responsive to compounds that have electronegative groups such as carbonyls or double bonds. Its use requires prior sample cleanup. If the detector is used in a dc mode and not in a pulsed mode, its performance can also be affected by nonelectronegative compounds that go through the cleanup procedure [26].

B. Flame Photometric Detector

The flame photometric detector is relatively specific to either organophosphorus or organosulfur compounds, depending on the light filter that is used. The detector has a linear response range of about four decades of concentration for organophosphorus compounds but has a response that is proportional to the square of the concentration of the organosulfur compounds. It is the most useful detector for the determination of organophosphorus compounds. Care should be exercised in the interpretation of the chromatograms of samples with a high sulfur background when organophosphorus compounds are being determined. The presence of large amounts of sulfur cannot be effectively filtered out and could therefore produce peaks that may be misinterpreted as being phosphorus in nature.

C. Alkali Flame Detectors

There are several commercial versions of the alkali flame detectors. Some use different alkali salts in the detector, and one does not use a flame at all but heats the alkali bead to the desired operating temperature. The detectors are more responsive to compounds that contain phosphorus or nitrogen with a greater sensitivity for organophosphorus compounds. Their performance can be affected to varying degrees, depending on the commercial detector used, by residual amounts of halogenated solvents in the sample extract.

D. Microcoulometric Detector

The microcoulometric detector is used in the residue laboratory because of its specificity to halogenated compounds. However, it has several shortcomings. It does not have the sensitivity that the electron capture and electroconductivity detectors have. Its electrolyte level must be maintained several times a day. It is a very difficult instrument to operate properly.

E. Electroconductivity Detectors

Recent design improvements by Hall and Anderson [5, 6] have resulted in electroconductivity detectors capable of determining nanograms of organoitrogen compounds and subnanogram amounts of organosulfur and organohalogen compounds. The effluent from the gas chromatographic column is either oxidized or reduced to produce a species that becomes ionic when dissolved in a suitable solvent. Organonitrogen compounds are reduced to ammonia. Organosulfur compounds are oxidized to the sulfur oxides. Organohalogen compounds can be oxidized or reduced to form the hydrogen halides. The specificity of the detectors is attained by the use of scrubbers that remove other reaction by-products and by the selection of an appropriate conducting solvent. The conducting species formed in the oxidative mods are carbon dioxide, the sulfur oxides, and the hydrogen halides. The response due to carbon dioxide is minimized by the use of a nonaqueous solvent such as n-propanol. Calcium oxide can be used to remove the sulfur oxides and silver nitrate can be used to remove the hydrogen halides. The conducting species in the reductive mode are hydrogen sulfide, ammonia, and the hydrogen halides. Hydrogen sulfide has an ionization constant that is too low to cause interference. The hydrogen halides can be removed by a basic scrubber and the effect of ammonia can be minimized by the use of a nonaqueous solvent.

The authors have found the Hall electroconductivity detector to be fairly reliable once put into operation. Its most frequent maintenance requirement is the replenishment of solvent every 2 weeks or so. Care should be exercised to avoid condensation of column bleed in the reaction tube. A cold reaction tube should never be exposed to column bleed. The use of halogenated stationary phases should also be avoided.

IV. SAMPLE CLEANUP

The primary reason for cleaning up the sample extract is to remove natural sample extractives that produce a gas chromatographic response or affect the chromatography of sample residues. The development of elemental specific detectors minimizes the need for cleanups that the

Table 2 Products with Significant Background Peaks[a]

Product	Hall-X[b]	Hall-N[c]	FPD-P[d]
Broccoli		X	X
Brussels sprouts		X	X
Cauliflower		X	X
Onions		X	X
Peas (one peak)	X	X	X
Peppers (except bell)		X	
Radish			X

[a]Luke extract.
[b]Hall electroconductivity detector in halogen mode.
[c]Hall electroconductivity detector in nitrogen mode.
[d]Flame photometric detector in phosphorus mode.
Source: Ref. 27.

nonspecific electron capture detector requires. Table 2 lists the products that have been encountered that produce significant sample peaks with the elemental specific detectors at a sensitivity range of 0.1 to 5 ng of residue. Products not listed generally have chromatograms that are relatively free of product peaks. The authors' experiences cover samples extracted by the Luke procedure for most vegetables, but for fruits is limited to melons, strawberries, grapes, and citrus products. The sample background observed for the flame photometric detector in the phosphorus mode is due to the large amounts of sulfur that these products contain.

Injections of fats and waxes accumulate in the injection port of the gas chromatographic column and cause tailing peaks as well as erratic response. This detrimental effect can be reduced by preparing the column so that injections are made into the column packing and not into the glass wool plug as is usually done. This technique allows the injection of several samples not completely free of fat before the column performance deteriorates noticeably. The original condition of the gas chromatographic column can be restored by replacing the initial column packing material.

On the other hand, injections of uncleaned sample extracts of low-fat products have a beneficial effect on the gas chromatography of many polar residues. Peak shapes as well as pesticide response often improve with injections of sample extract. Sometimes, the peak height responses of a polar residue will be reproducible for multiple sample injections but erratic for injections of the corresponding standard. The sample solution seems to have a protective effect for the residue. As a result, recoveries greater than 100 can be obtained; 130% as an example. To remedy the problem, the gas chromatographic standard is made up in the solution of a similar sample in which residues have not been found. Thus the cleanup of sample extracts for the analysis of polar residues is not necessary and may be undesirable. Examples of compounds for which this effect has been observed are: Monocrotofos (Azodrin), captan, dimethoate oxygen analog, ametryn, phenthoate, phoxim, phoxim oxygen analog, prometryn, and metribuzin (Sencor). As a rule, the enhanced response produced by the sample extract is not observed when a polar gas chromatographic column liquid phase such as diethylene glycol succinate (DEGS) is used.

The authors have found that the injections of the uncleaned extracts of the low-fat products such as fruit and vegetables will not seriously affect the performance of the gas chromatographic column. Several hundred sample injections can be made before it is necessary to replace the initial column packing material. However, after several sample injections, the deposited sample extracts can interact with pesticides present in subsequent injections. Peaks corresponding to TDE and methoxychlor olefin have been observed for DDT and methoxychlor, respectively. Decreasing response has been observed for methomyl, captan, folpet, and captafol (Difolatan). The net effect of pesticide decomposition on the gas chromatographic column is minimal and can be reduced by more frequent replacement of the initial column packing material. The presence of the decomposition peaks can sometimes be used as a confirmation of the parent compounds.

As a rule, fat and extracts of fatty samples require cleanup. Fat samples need to undergo the acetonitrile-petroleum ether partitioning cleanup. The resulting sample solution as well as the fatty sample extracts require Florisil cleanup. The more polar eluates of the Florisil cleanup, which could contain the pesticides dieldrin and endrin, may also require additional cleanup. Fatty samples extracted by the water-acetonitrile procedure are an exception. The eluate obtained does not require further cleanup. The water-acetonitrile extraction procedure for fatty samples can also be used as a cleanup procedure for fats as well. The procedure is especially useful in cleaning up fat samples that present emulsion problems during the acetonitrile-petroleum ether partitioning cleanup due to their high fatty acid content.

It is imperative that procedural background peaks be kept to a minimum. The use of a cleanup procedure does not ensure an absence of procedural contamination. The contaminant could pass through the cleanup procedure or may enter the system after and even during the cleanup procedure. A large organophosphorus background peak that seriously affected the authors' laboratory was traced to the glass wool filters of the laboratory's air-conditioning system. Organophosphorus compounds have also been found in the laboratory glass wool that is often used as a plug in the preparation of various columns. It is necessary to prewash the reagent grade anhydrous sodium sulfate and filter paper to remove traces of organonitrogen compounds when the Luke extraction procedure is used. Polychlorinated biphenyls have also been found in filter paper.

A. Acetonitrile-Petroleum Ether Partitioning

This cleanup procedure for fats [12, 13] is based on the reduced solubility that fats have in acetonitrile [28]. Most of the pesticides determined by the Mills extraction procedure for high moisture-low fat samples can be recovered by this cleanup. The determination of a compound's distribution coefficient between acetonitrile and petroleum ether can indicate if the compound will pass through the cleanup.

Weigh 3 g of fat into a 125 ml separatory funnel. Add 11 ml of petroleum ether and 30 ml of acetonitrile saturated with petroleum ether, and shake for 1 min. Drain the lower acetonitrile layer into a 1 liter separatory funnel containing 100 ml of petroleum ether, 600 ml of water, and 40 ml of saturated sodium chloride solution. Repeat partitioning with three 30 ml portions of acetonitrile saturated with petroleum ether. Shake the 1 liter separatory funnel for 1 min and drain the lower aqueous layer into a second 1 liter separatory funnel containing 100 ml of petroleum ether. Shake the second 1 liter separatory funnel for 1 min and discard the lower aqueous layer. Transfer the petroleum ether in the second 1 liter separatory funnel to the first and wash the combined pertroleum ether solution with two 100 ml portions of water. Pass the petroleum ether through a 4 in. glass funnel containing about 25 g of anhydrous sodium sulfate on a glass wool plug into a Kuderna-Danish concentrator. Fit the concentrator with a Snyder column and concentrate the solution on a steam bath. The final solution containing about 0.2 g of fat is ready for Florisil cleanup.

B. Florisil Cleanup

Florisil is an adsorbent with a fairly high load capacity. It can handle the equivalent of about 70 g of the Mills extract as well as the Luke extract (in petroleum ether) but is limited to about 0.2 g of fat. There are two basic elution systems; the standard ethyl ether-petroleum ether system [12, 13], [24, 29] and the alternative system [12, 13], [30], which uses methylene chloride, hexane, and acetonitrile. Cleaner sample eluates of fatty samples are obtained by the alternative elution system. Both systems use a 4 in. layer of Florisil in a 22 mm i.d.

chromatographic column topped by a 1/2 in. layer of anhydrous sodium sulfate. A petroleum ether solution of the sample extract is placed on the column, which is then eluted with 200 ml volumes of the following solvents in order:

Standard elution system. 6% ethyl ether-petroleum ether and 15% ethyl ether-petroleum ether (50% ethyl-petroleum ether and 100% ethyl ether have also been used)

Alternate elution system. 20% methylene chloride-hexane, 50% methylene chloride + 0.35% acetonitrile-hexane, and 50% methylene chloride + 1.5% acetonitrile-hexane

The Florisil that is used has been calcined at 677° and activated for a minimum of 5 hr at 130°. Its properties are tested by eluting 1 ml of petroleum ether containing 1 μg of heptachlor, 2 μg of heptachlor epoxide, 10 μg of ethion, 15 μg of carbophenothion, 10 μg of parathion, 3 μg of dieldrin, 3 μg of endrin, and 15 μg of malathion through a prepared column. Elution of the column by the standard elution system should result in quantitative recoveries of the first four compounds in the 6% eluate, the next three compounds in the 15% eluate, and the last compound in the 50% eluate. Florisil that behaves properly will isolate pesticides for both elution systems, as listed in Appendix C. The elution of a compound in the later eluates of either elution system requires the prior elution of the earlier elution mixtures through the Florisil column. For example, if only the 15% ethyl ether-petroleum ether mixture is used in an analysis for dieldrin, low assays may result, owing to the incomplete elution of the pesticide.

C. Carbon Cleanup

Carbon cleanup procedures are used to remove high molecular weight interferences such as plant pigments and fats [20]. The following procedure has been used on samples containing polar organophosphorus residues. Luke extracts equivalent to about 60 g of sample have been cleaned by the procedure.

Place a 1/2 in. layer of Celite in a chromatographic column (300 × 22 mm i.d. with a sintered glass frit) followed by 6 g of carbon mix (2 parts activated carbon + 8 parts Celite + 4 parts magnesium oxide). Set the carbon layer with a large glass wool plug. Add about 50 ml of methylene chloride and apply air pressure until the methylene chloride layer is at the top of the glass wool (this prewash is used to remove air pockets, which could result in channeling). Quantitatively transfer the sample into the column with methylene chloride and air pressure. Place a Kuderna-Danish concentrator below the column and elute 200 ml of 33% methylene chloride-acetone solution through the column using air pressure. Stopper and invert the Kuderna-Danish concentrator to mix the column eluate (violent bumping may occur if this is not done). Concentrate the solvent as explained in the Luke extraction procedure.

D. Saponification

Saponification [12, 13] is normally used on the 15% ethyl ether-petroleum ether eluate of the standard Florisil elution system. It removes the fat that is obtained in fatty samples or the extractives from samples such as carrots and onions, which present interferences in the electron capture chromatograms. The only compounds that elute in the 15% eluate and survive the saponification are dieldrin and endrin. The procedure cannot be applied to the 6% eluate, as most of the compounds that eluate in that fraction will be destroyed.

Evaporate the sample solution to dryness in a 125 ml Erlenmeyer flask. Add 20 ml of 2% sodium hydroxide or potassium hydroxide in ethanol, fit the flask with an air condenser, and heat on a steam bath for 30 min. Cool and transfer the solution into a 125 ml separatory funnel with three 10 ml portions of petroleum ether. Add 20 ml of water, shake vigorously for 1 min, and transfer the lower layer to a second separatory funnel containing 20 ml of petroleum ether. Shake vigorously, discard the lower layer, and transfer the petroleum ether to the first separatory funnel. Wash the combined petroleum ether layer with three 20 ml portions of 50% ethanol-water solution. Dry the petroleum ether through a column of anhydrous sodium sulfate and into a Kuderna-Danish concentrator. Rinse the sodium sulfate column with petroleum and concentrate on a steam bath to an appropriate volume for gas chromatographic determination.

E. Acid Celite Cleanup

This technique is used to remove interferences affecting the electron capture chromatography of samples such as garlic and onions. It is limited to organochlorine residues that elute in the 6% ethyl ether-petroleum ether eluate of the standard eluting system. It cannot be applied to the 15% ethyl ether-petroleum ether eluate as it destroys dieldrin and endrin.

Mix 1 ml of water with 2 g of Celite and transfer the mixture to a chromatographic column (300 × 22 mm i.d.). Use a tamping rod to form a uniform layer. Mix 6 g of Celite with 3 ml of an acid mixture containing equal volumes of sulfuric and 15 to 18% fuming sulfuric acid. Transfer the mixture to the chromatographic column in two or more portions with tamping. Place a Kuderna-Danish concentrator below the column and transfer the sample extract (in petroleum ether) quantitatively with petroleum ether. Elute 200 ml of petroleum ether through the column and concentrate the eluate to an appropriate volume for gas chromatographic analysis.

The sample solution will have about 1 to 2 ml of a petroleum-type oil which will not interfere with the electron capture analysis. The oil is a result of a sulfuric acid-catalyzed polymerization of the unsaturated hydrocarbons in petroleum ether. Its presence in the sample solution can be avoided by using petroleum ether that has previously been eluted through an acid Celite column and redistilled.

F. Alumina-Silver Nitrate Column Cleanup

This technique [31] is used to remove the carotenes from carrot extracts and the organosulfur compounds from products such as onions, cabbage, and cauliflower which interefere in their analysis by the electron capture detector. All of the common organochlorine pesticides pass through the cleanup unchanged with the exception of heptachlor, which is converted to a derivative which has relative retention times similar to aldrin on silicon and Apiezon columns.

Dissolve 0.75 g of silver nitrate in 0.7 ml of warm water and slowly add 4 ml of acetone. Add the solution to 10 g of alumina (containing 7% moisture) in an open flask and shake until the odor of acetone cannot be detected. One gram of the silver nitrate-treated alumina can be used by itself in a 8 mm i.d. chromatographic column or at the bottom of other conventional adsorption columns.

G. Miscellaneous Cleanup Procedures

The following techniques either require specialized equipment or are of limited cleanup value:

Gel permeation

The technique is used to clean the fat obtained from fatty samples. It should also be applicable to the extracts obtained from the Mills and Luke procedures.

Low-temperature precipitation

The technique [32, 33] separates fats, oils, and water from an acetone-benzene solution by cooling the temperature of the solution to -78°. It has been used on plant and animal products for several organochlorine and organophosphorus compounds. It requires a low-temperature bath, a variable vacuum pump, compressed nitrogen, and miscellaneous glassware.

Silicic acid

Silicic acid does not have the load capacity that Florisil has. Sample extracts may need a prior Florisil cleanup before applying special silicic acid separations.

Magnesium oxide

A magnesium oxide column [12, 13] is sometimes used to clean the 15% ethyl ether-petroleum ether eluate of fatty samples or to clean further the solution obtained from saponification. The authors have had erratic results with the technique and feel that it does not offer any special advantages.

Sweep co-distillation

Sweep co-distillation has official final action status by the AOAC [13] in the analysis of several organophosphorus compounds on high-moisture products such as carrots, lettuce, apples, and potatoes. However, the technique does not offer any advantage in its use, as it is also limited to the use of the alkali flame detector, which is not affected by the sample extracts. In addition, severe adsorption effects can be experienced since the technique calls for the injection of the sample extract onto uncoated gas chromatographic support.

V. GAS CHROMATOGRAPHIC DETERMINATION

Tables 3 and 4 list, respectively, the gas chromatographic columns and the gas chromatographic column-detector combinations that are used in the authors' laboratory. The authors do not regard the column or column-detector combinations as being absolute but present them to illustrate our views in residue analyses as well as our approach in maximizing the number of pesticides that may be determined. The parameters of each gas chromatographic column have been adjusted so that a chromatographic run is completed within 10 to 15 min. Note that 1 ft and 2.5 ft columns are used. Although these columns may not have the efficiency and separating power that longer columns may have, their use allows for several more injections to be made during a working day. Fortunately, complex mixtures that require greater column efficiency and separating power are seldom encountered. The simplicity of the chromatograms that are normally encountered by the use of the elemental specific detectors has allowed a single analyst to inject the extracts of up to 30 samples per working day, with each extract being injected into six to nine gas chromatographic systems.

The Luke extract can potentially contain any of the many pesticides in use, with the exception of the more polar and ionic pesticides. The injection of the extract without cleanup into gas chromatographic systems that utilize the elemental specific detectors permits the determination of compounds that might otherwise be lost in cleanup procedures. It may seem that this simplistic approach to residue analysis is made at a cost of increased instrumentation. In addition to providing increased pesticide coverage, the gas chromatographic systems of Appendix 5 also allow for the verification of pesticides determined by one system by the chromatograms obtained in the other systems. For example, simazine determined by the use of an OV-101 column combined with a Hall halogen detector is verified when a corresponding peak is observed in the chromatograms obtained by an OV-101 column with a

Table 3 Gas Chromatographic Columns Used in the Authors' Laboratory

Column	A	B	C	D	E
Liquid phase	DEGS	DEGS/H_3PO_4	DEGS/H_3PO_4	OV-101	SE-30/OV-210
Load (%)	2	2/0.5	2/0.5	2	4/6.5
Dimensions (ft × mm i.d.)	4 × 2	4 × 2	1 × 2	4 × 2	2.5/2
Column temperature (°C)	180	180	120	200	200
Flow rate (ml He/min)	60	25-30	25-30	30-60	60

Source: Ref. 27.

Table 4 Gas Chromatographic Systems Used in the Authors' Laboratory

Column[a]	Detector
B, D	Hall electroconductivity detector in halogen mode
B, D	Hall electroconductivity detector in nitrogen mode
C	Hall electroconductivity detector in sulfur mode
A, D, E	Flame photometric detector in phosphorus mode

[a]See Appendix D for columns corresponding to alphabets.
Source: Ref. 27.

Hall nitrogen detector system as well as by the DEGS column systems that use the Hall halogen and nitrogen detectors. The eight sample injections required by Table 4 are equal to the number of injections that would be required if a comprehensive analysis were to be attempted by the Mills procedure (injections of three Florisil eluates into electron capture detector and alkali flame detector gas chromatographic systems, for a total of six), by the Storherr procedure for water-soluble organophosphorus pesticides [14] (one injection), by the Holden procedure [34] for methyl carbamates (one injection), and by the Remsteiner procedure [35] for triazines (one injection). The nine injections required by the multimethod analyses do not include any additional injections that would be needed to verify the identity of any residues that are found.

The interpretation of gas chromatograms is at times difficult because of the incompleteness of the gas chromatographic tables containing residue retention data. Pesticides listed in one table are not always listed in another, and in some cases they are not listed at all. Appendices D and E list, respectively, retention and molecular formula data for gas chromatographic columns utilizing DC-200 and DC-200 with QF-1 liquid phases. Appendix F is an alphabetical listing by pesticide of the retention data for the two columns. The amounts of compound required for half-scale responses are not listed since the response is a function of the detector and the gas chromatographic conditions used. Experienced residue analysts will not experience any difficulty in identifying the older nonpolar pesticides by the use of Appendix D with the OV-101 systems and Appendix E with the SE-30/OV-210 systems. Identification of peaks occurring in a DEGS chromatogram could be more difficult because of reported differences in the DEGS liquid phases that are commercially available [36]. The relative retention times have also been observed to vary greatly with column temperature and with the age of the column, but the same general order of elution is usually maintained. Appendix G lists retention data for a DEGS column at 180° that laboratories could use as a guide in building a retention table for their DEGS column. It is recommended that laboratories start with the compounds Monitor and acephate.

The gas chromatography of polar residues such as dimethoate oxygen analog, Monitor, and acephate can be particularly difficult. For example, a laboratory that analyzes a sample that contains illegal levels of acephate may not find any of the pesticide when the sample extract is injected into a nonpolar liquid-phase gas chromatographic column. Polar residues chromatograph poorly if at all on nonpolar gas chromatographic columns such as DC-200 and OV-101. It should be noted that not all of the compounds in Appendices D and E have been properly identified as producing an erratic peak response. For example, dimethoate oxygen analog in the DC-200 system requires 20 times the amount of parathion needed to produce an equivalent peak height response despite the fact that it elutes earlier. The authors have found DEGS to be the best liquid phase for the gas chromatographic analysis of polar residues. Despite the problem of nonuniform DEGS, and the variation of relative retention times with temperatures and with column age, the authors consider it a primary GC liquid phase in the analysis of pesticide residues.

The scope of the gas chromatographic analysis of a sample can be expanded by applying the knowledge and observations of the analyst performing the gas chromatography. The 1 ft DEGS column in Table 3 was developed for the analysis of methomyl. Initial attempts to chromatograph the pesticide on a 6 ft DEGS column at 180° resulted in a peak for microgram amounts of standard, but a detector sensitivity at which nanogram amounts of compound are normally determined was required. Methomyl was apparently decomposing on the gas chromatographic column and the observed peak was due to the surviving methomyl. By decreasing the column length as well as the operating temperature, the desired sensitivity was obtained for methomyl. Ongoing work indicates that this gas chromatographic column can also be used for the related compounds, oxamyl and aldicarb. A 1 ft gas chromatographic column at elevated temperature has also been used to determine compounds that elute so slowly under normal operating conditions that they are observed in chromatograms obtained several injections later as small bumps in the baseline. The shorter column increases the sensitivity for these compounds by producing sharper and more measurable peaks. A broader than normal solvent front could also indicate the presence of early eluting compounds. In this situation the temperature of the gas chromatographic system should be lowered to analyze for these possible compounds.

VI. SUMMARY

The extraction of samples should be considered in terms of their water content, their nonpolar content (fat, waxes, etc.), and the presence of any adsorptive effects. In the extraction of low-fat products, the extraction process is simplified by the use of a water-miscible solvent or by a mixture of the solvent with water.

The use of elemental specific detector simplifies residue analyses by minimizing the need for cleanup of the sample extract. As a result, the authors' laboratory has been able to start and complete the comprehensive analyses of 30 samples a day by a team of four to six analysts. The recoveries in Appendix A for bromophropylate, profenofos, chlorpyrifos, Difolatan, chlorthiophos, fonofos, permethrin, phenthoate, phorate sulfoxide, phorate sulfone, pyrazophos, triazophos, and vinclozolin were all made after the compounds were found during routine sample analyses.

The detection of polar compounds such as Monitor, acephate, and dimethoate oxygen analog requires the use of a polar gas chromatographic column such as DEGS. The gas chromatographic behavior of some compounds is better in the presence of uncleaned sample extract. In this situation the standard solution should be made in the extract of a similar sample which does not contain the compound in question.

ACKNOWLEDGMENTS

The authors thank Donald Sawyer, Science Adviser, Food and Drug Administration, Los Angeles, Professor of Chemistry, University of California, Riverside, for his review of this chapter, and Thomas Cairns for his review and helpful comments in the preparation of this chapter.

Appendix A Recoveries Obtained by the Luke Multiresidue Procedure

Compound	Spike level[a]	Recovery	Product
Acephate (Orthene)	1.19	111	Tomato
Aldrin	0.10	101	Tomato
Ametryne	0.103	103	Cucumber
Atrazine	0.75	82	Cucumber
Azinphos-ethyl (Ethyl Guthion)	1.53	100	Bell pepper
Azinphos-ethyl	1.00	102	Tomato
Azinphos-methyl (Guthion)	0.26	100	Tomato
Bensulide (Betasan)	0.39	94	Lettuce
BHC, δ	1.00	92	Apricot puree
BHC, β	1.00	110	Apricot puree
Biphenyl	20	95	Oranges
Bromacil	6.42	88	Cucumber
Bromophos	1.00	92	Parsley
Bromopropylate (Acarol)	1.00	108	Cucumber
Captafol (Difolatan)	0.78	90	Tomato
Captan	1.04	105	Tomato
Carbaryl	5.00	104	Grapes
Carbophenothion (Trithion)	0.93	98	Lettuce
Carbophenothion sulfone	1.94	116	Cucumber
Chlorbenside	0.18	98	Tomato
Chlordane	0.55	89	Cucumber
Chlorfenvinphos	0.324	97	Bell pepper
Chlorothalonil (Daconil 2787)	1.02	81	Cucumber

Appendix A Recoveries Obtained by the Luke Multiresidue Procedure (Continued)

Compound	Spike level[a]	Recovery (%)	Product
Chlorpyrifos (Dursban)	0.10	99	Green beans
Chlorthal dimethyl (Dacthal)	1.06	89	Cucumber
Chlorthiophos	0.0918	95	Tomato
2,4-D-Isopropyl ester	1.08	94	Cucumber
DDE	1.00	90	Apricot puree
DDT	0.20	100	Tomato
DDVP	0.105	90	Tomato
DEF	0.69	105	Lettuce
Demeton-S-sulfone	5.7	115	Peppers
Dialifor	1.32	115	Potato
Diazinon	0.89	96	Lettuce
Dichloran (Botran)	1.00	80	Lettuce
Dicofol (Kelthane)	1.04	101	Oranges
Dicrotophos (Bidrin)	0.094	105	Green beans
Dieldrin	0.10	85	Lettuce
Dimethoate	0.54	108	Lettuce
Dimethoate oxygen analog	1.51	90	Grapes
Diphenamid	6.72	99	Cucumber
Endofulfan I (Thiodan I)	1.00	93	Cucumber
Endosulfan II	0.07	100	Green beans
Endosulfan sulfate	0.10	100	Green beans
Endrin	0.059	108	Tomato
EPN	1.05	105	Green beans
Ethion	0.58	97	Lettuce

Appendix A Recoveries Obtained by the Luke Multiresidue Procedure (Continued)

Compound	Spike level[a]	Recovery (%)	Product
ETU (ethylene thiourea)	0.612	48	Cucumbor
Fenamiphos (Nemacur)	0.436	97	Bell pepper
Fenitrothion (Sumithion)	1.00	88	Blueberry
Fensulfothion (Dasanit)	1.0	107	Rutabagas
Fenthion	0.14	97	Green beans
Folpet	1.08	96	Lettuce
Folpet	0.151	95	Bell pepper
Fonofos (Dyfonate)	1.00	92	Parsley
Heptachlor	0.10	90	Carrot
Heptachlor	0.10	101	Tomato
Heptachlor epoxide	1.0	92	Tomato
Lindane	0.10	77	Apricot puree
Linuron	0.50	91	Lettuce
Leptophos (Phosvel)	0.102	113	Potato
Malathion	1.00	112	Lettuce
Malathion oxygen analog	1.52	112	Potato
Mephosfolan (Cytrolane)	0.17	106	Tomato
Methamidophos (Monitor)	0.50	100	Grapes
Methidathion (Supracide)	0.862	93	Oranges
Methomyl	0.988	95	Lettuce
Methyl carbophenothion (Methyl Trithion)	0.56	118	Tomato
Methyl parathion	0.42	105	Celery
Metribuzin (Sencor)	0.19	96	Tomato

Appendix A Reoveries Obtained by the Luke Multiresidue Procedure (Continued)

Compound	Spike level[a]	Recovery (%)	Product
Mevinphos (Phosdrin)	0.70	103	Lettuce
Mirex	0.152	106	Tomato
Naled	0.406	86	Bell pepper
Naled	3.79	97	Strawberry
Nitrofen (TOK)	1.02	95	Cucumber
Oxydemeton-methyl (Metasystox R)	0.12	88	Grapes
Oxydemeton-methyl sulfone	0.113	103	Grapes
Oxythioquinox (Morestan)	0.054	107	Oranges
Parathion	0.43	107	Celery
Parathion oxygen analog	1.50	105	Tomato
PCNB	0.015	112	Tomato
Phenthoate	0.118	94	Cucumber
Phenthoate	0.0117	110	Tomato
o-Phenylphenol	10.8	104	Grapes
Phorate	0.89	106	Lettuce
Phorate sulfone	0.105	93	Lettuce
Phorate sulfoxide	0.114	116	Lettuce
Phosalone	1.80	92	Grapes
Phosmet (Imidan)	0.25	108	Tomato
Phosphamidon	1.00	91	Apple puree
Phoxim	0.10	110	Tomato
Phoxim oxygen analog	0.10	105	Tomato
Profenofos (Curacron)	0.10	102	Tomato
Prometryne	0.108	104	Cucumber

Appendix A Recoveries Obtained by the Luke Multiresidue Procedure (Continued)

Compound	Spike level[a]	Recovery (%)	Product
Pronamide (Kerb)	1.04	89	Cantaloupe
Propargite (Omite)	1.85	107	Oranges
Propham (IPC)	0.208	79	Lettuce
Propoxur (Baygon)	1125	98	Cantaloupe
Ronnel	0.10	104	Pears
Simazine	0.25	104	Tomato
Sulprofos (Bolstar)	0.105	105	Green beans
Sulprofos sulfone	0.10	105	Green beans
Sulprofos sulfoxide	0.105	106	Green beans
TDE	1.00	94	Apricot puree
Tedion	0.10	82	Apple puree
Tedion	0.054	106	Peas
Tetrachlorvinphos (Gardona)	1.08	113	Green beans
Thiabendazole	1.07	103	Oranges
Thionazin (Zinophos)	0.608	100	Tomato
Toxaphene	4.34	113	Cucumber
Triazophos (Hostathion)	0.134	106	Tomato
Trichlorfon (Dylox)	0.110	110	Oranges
Vinclozolin (Ronilan)	0.0914	98	Strawberry

[a]Parts per million.

Source: Refs. 15 and 27.

Appendix B Proximate Water, Fat, and Sugar Content in Foods and Feeds

Product	Water (%)	Fat (%)	Sugar (%)
Dairy products			
Butter	15.5	81	
Buttermilk	90.5	0.1	
Cheese			
Blue	40	30.5	
Brick	41.0	30.5	
Cheddar (American)	37	32.2	
Cheddar, pasturized, processed	40.0	30.0	
Cottage, creamed	78.3	4.2	
Cottage, uncreamed	79.0	0.3	
Cream cheese	51	37.0	
Parmesan	30	26.0	
Pasteurized process cheese food (American)	43.2	24.0	
Pasteurized process cheese spread (American)	48.6	21.4	
Swiss (domestic)	39	28.0	
Swiss, processed	40	26.9	
Cream			
Half-and-half	79.7	11.7	
Light, table or coffee	71.5	20.6	
Whipping	56.6-62.1	33.3-37.6	
Ice milk	66.7	5.1	
Sherbet (orange)	67.0	1.2	

Appendix B Proximate Water, Fat, and Sugar Content in Foods and Feeds (Continued)

Product	Water (%)	Fat (%)	Sugar (%)
Dairy products (Contd)			
Milk, cow			
Fluid, pasteurized and raw	87.2	3.7	
Chocolate drink, whole milk	81.5	3.4	
Chocolate drink, skim milk	82.8	2.3	
Condensed	27.1	8.7	
Dry, whole	2.0	27.5	
Dry, nonfat solids, instant	4.0	0.7	
Dry, nonfat solids, regular	3.0	0.8	
Evaporated	73.8	7.9	
Skim	90.5	0.1	
Milk, goat	87.5	4.0	
Fruits			
Berries			
Blackberries, dewberries, etc.	84.5	0.9	6.1
Blackberries canned in syrup	79.2	0.7	15.6
Blueberries	83.2	0.5	9.7
Cranberries	87.9	0.7	4.2
Cranberry sauce, canned, sweetened	62.1	0.2	43.0
Currants, red, white	85.7	0.2	5.7
Gooseberries	88.9	0.2	4.2

Appendix B Proximate Water, Fat, and Sugar Content in Foods and Feeds (Continued)

Product	Water (%)	Fat (%)	Sugar (%)
Fruits (Contd)			
Berries			
Huckleberries	81.9	0.6	9.7
Loganberries	83.0	0.6	6.0
Raspberries, black	80.8	1.4	7.9
Raspberries, red	84.2	0.5	7.2
Strawberries	89.9	0.5	5.3
Citrus			
Grapefruit, all varieties	88.4	0.1	6.5
Lemons, with peel	87.4	0.3	2.2
Limes	89.3	0.2	0.5
Oranges with peel	82.3	0.3	8.8
Tangerines	87.0	0.2	8.7
Melons			
Cantaloupe	91.2	0.1	4.2
Casaba	91.5	Trace	7.0
Honeydew	90.6	0.3	7.0
Muskmelons	92.7	0.2	5.4
Watermelon	92.6	0.2	6.0
Tree, vine			
Apples, not pared	83.9-84.8	0.7-0.6	11.1
Apples, summer	86.5	0.4	9.4
Apples, winter	83.6	0.3	11.2
Apples, dehydrated pieces	2.5	2.0	
Apples, dried	24.0	1.6	
Apricots, raw	85.4	0.2	10.4

Appendix B Proximate Water, Fat, and Sugar Content in Foods and Feeds (Continued)

Product	Water (%)	Fat (%)	Sugar (%)
Fruits (Contd)			
Tree, vine			
Apricots, dried	25.0	0.5	46.0
Avocado, all varieties	74.0	16.4	0.6
Bananas	75.7	0.2	19.2
Cherries, sour	83.7	0.3	9.5
Cherries, sweet	80.4	0.3	11.6
Dates, natural and dried	22.5	0.5	61.2
Figs, raw	77.5	0.3	16.2
Figs, dried	23.0	1.3	55.0
Figs, canned in syrup	68.5	0.3	28
Grapes, slip skin (American)	81.6	1.0	11.5
Grapes, adherent skin (European)	81.4	0.3	14.9
Guavas, common	83.0	0.6	
Mango	81.7	0.4	
Nectarines	81.8	Trace	11.8
Olives, Greek, cured, oil	43.8	35.8	
Olives, pickled, green	78.2	12.7	
Olives, pickled, ripe	73.0-84.4	9.5-20.1	
Papayas	88.7	0.1	
Peaches, raw	89.1	0.1	8.8
Peaches, dried	25.0	0.7	51.0
Pears, raw	83.2	0.4	8.9
Persimmons	78.2	0.4	15.9

Appendix B Proximate Water, Fat, and Sugar Content in Foods and Feeds (Continued)

Product	Water (%)	Fat (%)	Sugar (%)
Fruits (Contd)			
Tree, vine			
Pineapple	85.3	0.2	11.9
Pineapple, canned in syrup	78.0	0.1	18.6
Plums	81.1-86.6	Trace-0.2	8.3
Plums, prune type	78.7	0.2	
Plums, Damsons	78.8		8.7
Pomegranate	81.0	0.2	13.3
Prunes, dried	28.0	0.6	
Raisin, dried	18.0	0.2	
Eggs, chicken			
Raw, whole	73.7	11.5	
Raw, white	87.6	Trace	
Raw, yolk, fresh	51.1	30.6	
Dried, whole	4.1	41.2	
Dried, white	8.8-14.6	0.2	
Fish and shellfish			
Abalone, raw	75.8	0.5	
Bass, black sea, raw	79.3	1.2	
Bass, small and large mouth, raw	77.3	2.6	
Bass, striped, raw	77.7	2.7	
Bass, white, raw	78.8	2.3	
Bluefish, raw	75.4	3.3	
Buffalofish, raw	77.4	4.2	

Appendix B Proximate Water, Fat, and Sugar Content in Foods and Feeds (Continued)

Product	Water (%)	Fat (%)	Sugar (%)
Fish and shellfish (Contd)			
Bullhead, black, raw	81.3	1.6	
Butterfish, northern waters, raw	71.4	10.2	
Butterfish, gulf, raw	78.2	2.9	
Carp, raw	77.8	4.2	
Catfish, freshwater, raw	78.0	3.1	
Chub, raw	74.9	8.8	
Clams, raw, soft, meat	80.8	1.9	
Clams, raw, soft, meat and liquid	85.8	1.0	
Clams, raw, hard, round, meat	79.8	0.9	
Clams, raw, hard, round, meat and liquid	86.2	0.4	
Clams, canned, solids and liquid	86.3	0.7	
Cod, raw	81.2	0.3	
Cod, canned	78.6	0.3	
Cod, dried salt	52.4	0.7	
Crab, raw, hard-shelled	80.0	1.6	
Crab, canned	77.2	2.5	
Crayfish, spiny lobster	82.5	0.5	
Croaker, Atlantic, raw	79.2	2.2	
Croaker, white, raw	79.7	0.8	
Croaker, yellowfin, raw	79.0	0.8	
Dogfish, spiny, raw	72.3	9.0	
Drum, freshwater, raw	77.0	5.2	

Appendix B Proximate Water, Fat, and Sugar Content in Foods and Feeds (Continued)

Product	Water (%)	Fat (%)	Sugar (%)
Fish and shellfish (Contd)			
Drum, red (redfish) raw	80.2	0.4	
Flatfishes (flounder, foles, sanddabs) raw	81.3	0.8	
Froglegs, raw	81.9	0.3	
Grouper, raw	79.2	0.5	
Haddock, raw	80.5	0.1	
Hake (including whiting) raw	81.8	0.4	
Halibut, raw	76.5	1.2	
Herring, Atlantic, raw	69.0	11.3	
Herring, lake (cisco), raw	79.7	2.3	
Herring Pacific, raw	79.4	2.6	
Kingfish, raw	77.3	3.0	
Lobster, whole, raw	78.5	1.9	
Lobster, canned	76.8	1.5	
Mackerel, raw	67.2-69.8	7.3-12.2	
Mackerel, canned, solids and liquid	66.0-66.4	10.0-11.1	
Menhaden, canned, solids and liquid	67.9	10.2	
Mullet, striped, raw	72.6	6.9	
Mussels, raw, meat	78.6	2.2	
Mussels, raw, meat and liquid	83.8	1.4	
Oysters, meat, raw	79.1-84.6	1.8-2.2	
Oysters, canned, solids and liquid	82.2	2.2	

Appendix B Proximate Water, Fat, and Sugar Content in Foods and Feeds (Continued)

Product	Water (%)	Fat (%)	Sugar (%)
Fish and shellfish (Contd)			
Perch, ocean, raw	79.0-79.7	1.2-1.5	
Perch, white, raw	75.7	4.0	
Perch, yellow, raw	79.2	0.9	
Pike, various	78.3-80.0	0.9-1.2	
Pollock	77.4	0.9	
Pompano	70.9	9.5	
Rockfish, various	78.9	1.8	
Salmon, raw	63.6-76.0	3.7-15.6	
Salmon, canned, solids, bone, liquid	64.2-70.8	5.2-14.0	
Sardines, canned in oil			
Solids and liquid	50.6	24.4	
Drained solids	61.8	11.1	
Sardines, canned, natural pack, solids and liquid	65.2	13.5	
Scallops, raw	79.8	0.2	
Seabass, raw	76.3	0.5	
Shad, raw	70.4	10.0	
Sheepshead, Atlantic	75.9	2.8	
Sheepshead, freshwater, raw	77.0	5.2	
Shrimp, raw	78.2	0.8	
Shrimp, breaded, raw	65.0	0.7	
Shrimp, canned, dry pack or drained wet pack	70.4	1.1	
Skate, raw	77.8	0.7	

Appendix B Proximate Water, Fat, and Sugar Content in Foods and Feeds (Continued)

Product	Water (%)	Fat (%)	Sugar (%)
Fish and shellfish (Contd)			
Smelt, raw	79.0	2.1	
Swordfish, raw	75.9	4.0	
Trout, brook, raw	77.7	2.1	
Trout, lake, raw	70.6	10.0	
Trout, lake (siscowet), raw	36.8-64.9	54.4-19.9	
Trout, rainbow, steel-head	66.3	11.4	
Tuna, raw	70.5-71.5	4.1-3.0	
Tuna, canned in oil, solid and liquid	52.6	20.5	
Tuna, canned in water, solid and liquid	70.0	0.8	
Weakfish, raw	76.7	5.6	
Whitefish, lake, raw	71.7	8.2	
Whitefish, lake, smoked	68.2	7.3	
Nuts			
Almond, dried	4.7	54.2	4.4
Brazil	4.6	66.9	1.5
Butternut	3.8	61.2	
Cashew	5.2	45.7	6.8
Chestnuts, fresh	52.5	1.5	6.4
Chestnuts, dried	8.4	4.1	
Coconut, fresh meat with brown skin	46.9	34.7	5.1
Coconut, moist, shredded	17.3	28.6	32.0
Coconut, dried	3.5	64.9	

Appendix B Proximate Water, Fat, and Sugar Contents in Foods and Feeds (Continued)

Product	Water (%)	Fat (%)	Sugar (%)
Nuts (Contd)			
Filberts (hazelnut)	5.8	62.4	3.2
Hickory	3.3	68.7	
Macadamia nuts	3.1	71.4	2.7
Peanuts, raw with skin	5.6	47.5	
Peanuts, raw without skin	5.4	48.4	
Peanut butter	1.8-1.7	49.4-50.6	
Pecans	3.4	71.2	3.9
Pistachios	5.3	53.7	6.1
Walnuts, black	3.1	59.3	
Walnuts, English	3.5	64.0	
Oils, fats, salad dressings			
Oleomargarine	15.5	81	
Mayonnaise	15.1	79.9	
Salad dressing, mayonnaise type	40.6	42.3	
Salad dressing, other	27.5-38.8	60.0-38.9	
Salad dressing, low calorie	68.2-95.2	16-0.2	
Vegetables			
Artichoke, globe	85.5	0.2	
Asparagus	91.7	0.2	
Beans, lima, immature	67.5	0.5	
Beans, lima, dry	10.3	1.6	
Beans, pinto, dry	8.3	1.2	
Beans, red, dry	10.4	1.5	
Beans, snap, green	90.1	0.2	

Appendix B Proximate Water, Fat, and Sugar Contents in Foods and Feeds (Continued)

Product	Water (%)	Fat (%)	Sugar (%)
Vegetables (Contd)			
Beans, snap, wax or yellow	91.4	0.2	
Beans, white, dry	10.9	1.6	
Beets, common red	87.3	0.1	
Beet green	90.9	0.3	
Broadbeans, immature seeds	72.3	0.4	
Broccoli, raw spears	89.1	0.3	
Brussels sprouts	85.2	0.4	
Cabbage, common	92.4	0.2	
Cabbage, red	90.2	0.2	
Cabbage, Chinese	95.0	0.1	
Carrots	88.2	0.2	
Cauliflower	91.0	0.2	
Celery	94.1	0.1	
Chard, Swiss	91.1	0.3	
Chickpeas, garbanzos, dry	10.7	4.8	
Chicory, French endive	95.1	0.1	
Chicory, greens	92.8	0.3	
Collards, leaves and stems	86.9	0.7	
Corn, sweet, white or yellow	72.7	1.0	
Cowpeas, blackeye, dry	10.5	1.5	
Cowpeas, immature seeds	66.8	0.8	
Cress, garden	89.4	0.7	
Cucumbers, not pared	95.1	0.1	
Dandelion greens	85.6	0.7	

Appendix B Proximate Water, Fat, and Sugar Contents in Foods and Feeds (Continued)

Product	Water (%)	Fat (%)	Sugar (%)
Vegetables (Contd)			
Eggplant	92.4	0.2	
Endive, escarole	93.1	0.1	
Garlic cloves	61.3	0.2	
Horseradish, raw	74.6	0.3	
Kale, leaves and stems	87.5	0.8	
Kohlrabi	90.3	0.1	
Lettuce, headed	94.0-95.1	0.1-0.3	
Lettuce, all other	94.8	0.2	
Mushrooms	90.4	0.3	
Mustard greens	89.5	0.5	
Okra	88.9	0.3	
Onions, mature	89.1	0.1	
Onions, young, green, bulb and entire top	89.4	0.2	
Parsley	85.1	0.6	
Parsnips	79.1	0.5	
Peas, edible podded	83.3	0.2	
Peas, dry	11.7	1.3	
Peas, green, immature	78.0	0.4	
Peppers, sweet, green	93.4	0.2	
Popcorn, unpopped	9.8	4.7	
Potatoes, sweet	70.6	0.4	
Potatoes, white	79.8	0.1	
Pumpkin	91.6	0.1	
Radishes	94.5	0.1	
Rhubarb	94.8	0.1	

Appendix B Proximate Water, Fat, and Sugar Contents in Foods and Feeds (Continued)

Product	Water (%)	Fat (%)	Sugar (%)
Vegetables (Contd)			
Rutabagas	87.0	0.1	
Spinach	90.7	0.3	
Squash, summer	94.0	0.1	
Squash, winter	85.1	0.3	
Tomatoes	93.5	0.2	
Turnips	91.5	0.2	
Turnips, greens, with stems	90.3	0.3	
Watercress, with stems	93.3	0.3	
Animal feeds and grains			
Dry roughages			
Alfalfa hay	9.6	2.0	
Barley hay	8.1	2.0	
Bermuda grass hay	9.3	1.8	
Clover hay	6.7-11.8	2.0-3.6	
Corn fodder	8.9-39.3	1.4-2.2	
Corn stover	9.4-41.0	1.0-1.6	
Cottonseed hulls	9.4	0.9	
Cowpea hay	9.6-10.1	2.5-3.2	
Grass hay	11.0	3.3-2.5	
Lespedeza hay	10.9-11.0	1.4-2.6	
Native hay, western mountain states	10.0	1.4-2.1	
Oat hay	12.0-12.3	2.7-3.5	
Pasture grasses and clovers, dried	10.0	3.5	

Appendix B Proximate Water, Fat, and Sugar Contents in Foods and Feeds (Continued)

Product	Water (%)	Fat (%)	Sugar (%)
Animal feeds and grains (Contd)			
Dry roughages			
Pea hay	10.8	3.2	
Pea hulls	7.6	1.0	
Peanut hay	8.6	3.3	
Peanut ahy with nuts	8.0	12.6	
Prairie hay, western	9.6	2.4-3.4	
Red-top hay	9.0	2.3	
Rice hulls	8.0	0.8	
Sorghum fodder	10.8-34.8	2.4-2.5	
Soybean hay	8.5-12.0	1.1-6.9	
Sudan grass hay	10.8	1.6	
Sugarcane pulp, dried	5.8	0.6	
Timothy hay	11.3-12.3	2.1-4.6	
Vetch hay	8.2-12.1	1.1-2.6	
Green roughages, roots			
Alfalfa	74.6	1.0	
Beets, sugar	83.6	0.1	
Bermuda grass	65.8	1.0	
Clover	65.6-83.8	0.5-1.7	
Corn fodder	58.8-90.0	0.3-1.3	
Corn stover	77.3-78.5	0.4	
Lespedeza	63.4	1.0	
Pasture grasses	69.7-75.6	0.8-1.1	
Rape	83.6	0.6	
Rye fodder	77.7	0.8	

Appendix B Proximate Water, Fat, and Sugar Contents in Foods and Feeds (Continued)

Product	Water (%)	Fat (%)	Sugar (%)
Animal feeds and grains (Contd)			
Green roughages, roots			
Sorghum fodder, sweet	75.1	1.0	
Soybeans	75.6	1.1	
Sugarcane	78.3	1.0	
Timothy	68.7	1.0	
Silages			
Alfalfa	46.0-76.1	1.4-2.5	
Apple pomace	79.1	1.3	
Clover	60.0-75.6	0.9-1.3	
Corn	70.8-80.6	0.5-0.9	
Corn canning waste	77.6	1.0	
Ear corn	54.3	1.7	
Pea, field	72.1	1.2	
Sorghum	68.7-74.9	0.8-0.9	
Grains, concentrates, by-products			
Alfalfa seed screenings	9.7	9.9	
Apple pomace, dried	10.6	5.0	
Apple pomace, wet	78.9	1.3	
Barley, pearled	10.8-11.1	1.1-1.0	
Beet pulp, dried	8.0	0.8	
Brewers grains	7.2	6.7	
Buckwheat	9.4	2.4	
Corn, dent	11.5-30.5	3.6-4.0	
Corn, pop	9.4	5.2	

Appendix B Proximate Water, Fat, and Sugar Contents in Foods and Feeds (Continued)

Product	Water (%)	Fat (%)	Sugar (%)
Animal feeds and grains (Contd)			
Grains, concentrates, by-products			
Cornmeal, whole ground	12.0	3.9	
Cornmeal, degermed	10.2	2.5	
Cottonseed, whole	7.3	23.0	
Cottonseed, bran	8.4	1.2	
Cottonseed meal, pressed	6.5	7.2	
Crab meal	8.0	2.9	
Fish meal	7.7	7.9	
Fish meal (solvent)	8.4	2.9	
Flaxseed	6.4	36.4	
Linseed meal	8.7	6.3	
Linseed meal (solvent)	9.6	2.9	
Millet, whole-grain	9.3	3.3	
Milo grain	10.6	2.9	
Oats, various	8.5-8.9	4.7-7.2	
Peanuts	5.3-5.9	36.2-47.7	
Peanut oil meal	6.6	8.5	
Peanut oil meal (solvent)	8.4	1.4	
Rice grain, or rough rice	11.4	1.8	
Rice, polished	12.2	0.4	
Rice, bran	9.9	13.4	
Rye grain	10.0	1.7	

Appendix B Proximate Water, Fat, and Sugar Contents in Foods and Feeds (Continued)

Product	Water (%)	Fat (%)	Sugar (%)
Animal feeds and grains (Contd)			
Grains, concentrates, by-products			
Rye middlings and screenings	9.8	3.8	
Sorghum grain, all types	11.0	3.3	
Soybeans, immature seeds	69.2	5.1	
Soybeans, mature dry seeds	10.0	17.7	
Soybean oil meal	8.3	5.7	
Soybean oil meal (solvent)	8.4	1.6	
Tomato pomace, dried	5.7	14.8	
Wheat, whole grain, various	9.6-10.9	1.7-2.6	
Wheat bran, crude	9.4	5.0	
Wheat germ, crude	11.5	10.9	
Wheat bran and screenings	9.2	4.9	

Source: Ref. 12.

Appendix C Elution of Pesticides from Florisil

Compound	Standard procedure[a,c]	Alternative procedure[b,c]
Acarol	C,15%,50%	NR, 1,2,3
Alachlor (Lasso)	NR, 6%,15%	P, 3
Aldrin	6%	C, 1
Allidochlor (Randox)	NR, 6%,15%	NR, 1,2,3
Anilazine (Dyrene)	15%	C, 2
Aramite	P, 15%	
Aroclor (see Polychlorinated biphenyls)		
Aspon	6%	
Atrazine	C, 50%	NR, 1,2,3
Azinphos-ethyl (Ethyl Guthion)	P, 50%	P, 3
Azinphos-methyl (Guthion)	NR, 6%,15%	NR, 1,2,3
Azodrin (see Monocrotophos)		
Benefin (see Benfluralin)		
Benfluralin (benefin)	C, 6%	C, 2
Bensulide (Betasan, Prefar)	C, 50%	P, 3
Benzoylprop-ethyl (Suffix)	C, 100%	NR, 1,2,3
Betasan (see Bensulide)		
BHC, α	6%	C, 1
BHC, β	6%	C, 1
BHC, ∂ (lindane)	6%	C, 1
BHC, δ	6%,15%, V	C, 1
Binapacryl	P, 15%	
Bis(trichloromethyl)disulfide	6%	
Botran (see Dicloran)		
Bromacil	NR, 6%,15%,50%	NR, 1,2,3
Bromophos	6%	
Bromophos-ethyl	6%	

Appendix C Elution of Pesticides from Florisil (Continued)

Compound	Standard procedure[a,b]	Alternative procedure[b,c]
Bulan	15%	C, 2
Butoxy ethyl ester, 2,4-D	15%	
Butoxy ethyl ester, 2,4,5-T	15%	
Butyl benzyl phthalate	C, 15%,50%	
n-Butyl ester, 2,4-D	15%	
n-Butyl ester, 2,4,5-T	15%,30%	
Camphechlor (see Toxaphene)		
Captafol (Difolatan)	P, 50%	C, 3
Captan	50% V	C, 3
Captan epoxide	NR, 6%,15%	
Carbophenothion (Trithion)	6% V	P, 2
Carbophenothion oxygen analog		NR, 1,2,3
Casoron (see Dichlobenil)		
CDEC (Vegadex)	6%	C, 2
Chlorbenside	6%	C, 1
Chlordane (technical)	6%	C, 1
Chlordane, cis	6%	
Chlordane, trans	6%	
Chlordecone (Kepone)	P, 15%,50% V	NR, 1,2,3
Chlorinated napthalenes (see Polychlorinated napthalenes)		
Chlornidine (Torpedo)	C, 15%	C, 2
Chlorobenzilate	C, 15%,50%	P, 3
Chloroneb	6%	C, 2
Chloropropylate	C, 15%,50%	P, 3
Chlorothalonil (Daconil 2787)	NR, 6%,15%,50%	C, 2,3
Chlorpropham (CIPC)	15%	C, 2

Appendix C Elution of Pesticides from Florisil (Continued)

Compound	Standard procedure[a,b]	Alternative procedure[b,c]
Chlorpyrifos (Dursban)	6%	P, 2
Chlorthion	15%	
CIPC (see Chlorpropham)		
Co-Ral (see Coumaphos)		
Coumaphos (Co-Ral)	NR, 6%,15%,30%	C, 3
Counter (see Terbufos)		
Cypromid	NR, 6%,15%	P, 2
2,4-D (see the individual esters)		
Daconil 2787 (see chlorothalonil)		
Dacthal	15%	C, 2
Dasanit (see Fensulfothion)		
o,p-DDE	6%	C, 1
p,p-DDE	6%	C, 1
o,p-DDT	6%	C, 1
p,p-DDT	6%	C, 1
DDVP (see Dichlorvos)		
DEF	C, 15%,50%	P, 3
Delnav (see Dioxathion)		
Dialifor	C, 15%	C, 2
Diazinon	15%	C, 3
Di-n-butyl phthalate	C, 15%,50%	
Dicapthon	15%	C, 2
Dichlobenil (Casoron)	C, 15%	C, 2
Dichlofenthion (VC-13 Nemacide)	C, 6%	
Dichlone	NR, 6%,15%,50%	C, 2
p-Dichlorobenzene	6%	
o,p-Dichlorobenzophenone	15%	2

Appendix C Elution of Pesticides from Florisil (Continued)

Compound	Standard procedure[a,b]	Alternative procedure[b,c]
p,p-Dichlorobenzophenone	15%	2
Dichlorvos (DDVP)	NR, 6%,15%,50%	NR, 1,2,3
Dicloran (Botran)	C, 15%,20%	C, 2
Dicofol (Kelthane)	6%,15% V	C, 1,2
Dieldrin	15%	C, 2
Di-2-ethylhexyl phthalate	C, 15%,50%	
Difolatan (see Captafol)		
Diisobutyl phthalate	C, 15%,50%	
Diisohexyl phthalate	C, 15%,50%	
Diisooctyl phthalate	C, 15%,50%	
Dilan	15%	
Dimethoate		NR, 1,2,3
Dimethoate oxygen analog		NR, 1,2,3
Dimethyl phthalate	P, 6%,15%,50%	
Dinitramine	C, 6%,15%	
Dinocap (Karathane)	P, 15%	C, 2
Di-octyl phthalate	C, 15%,50%	
Dioxathion (Delnav)		P, 2
Disulfoton (Disyston)	P, 6%	NR, 1,2,3
Disyston (see Disulfoton)		
Diuron	C, 65%	NR, 1,2,3
Dursban (see Chlorpyrifos)		
Dyfonate (see Fonofos)		
Dyrene (see Anilazine)		
Endosulfan I (Thiodan I)	15%	C, 2
Endosulfan II (Thiodan II)	15%,30%	C, 2

Appendix C Elution of Pesticides from Florisil (Continued)

Compound	Standard procedure[a,b]	Alternative procedure[b,c]
Endosulfan sulfate (Thiodan sulfate)	50%	C, 2
Endrin	15%	P, 2
Endrin alcohol	C, 15%, 20%	P, 2,3
Endrin aldehyde	C, 15%, 20%	
Endrin ketone	25% (after 6% only)	C, 2
EPN	15%	P, 2
EPTC (Eptam)	P, 15%	
Ethion	6%	P, 2
Ethoprop (Mocap)	50%	NR, 1,2,3
Ethyl Guthion (see Azinphos-ethyl)		
Ethyl hexyl ester, 2,4-D	15%	
Fenchlorphos (see Ronnel)		
Fenitrothion (Sumithion)	15%	C, 1,2
Fensulfothion (Dasanit)		NR, 1,2,3
Fenthion	6%, 15%	NR, 1,2,3
Folpet (Phaltan)	C, 15%, 50% V	C, 2,3
Fonofos (Dyfonate)	6%	P, 2
Gardona (see Tetrachlorvinphos)		
Genite	C, 15%	
Guthion (see Azinphos-methyl)		
Halowax (see Polychlorinated napthalenes)		
Heptachlor	6%	C, 1
Heptachlor epoxide	6%	C, 2
Hexachlorobenzene	6%	C, 1

Appendix C Elution of Pesticides from Florisil (Continued)

Compound	Standard procedure[a,b]	Alternative procedure[b,c]
Hexachlorophene	NR, 6%,15%,50%	
Imidan (see Phosmet)		
Isobenzan (Telodrin)	6%	C, 1
Isobutyl ester, 2,4-D	15%	
Isodrin	6%	C, 1
Isooctyl ester, 2,4,5-T	15%	
Isooctyl ester, 2,4-D	15%	
Isopropalin	6%	
Isopropyl ester, 2,4,5-T	15%	
Isopropyl ester, 2,4-D	15%	
Karathane (see Dinocap)		
Kelthane (see Dicofol)		
Kepone (see Chlordecone)		
Kerb (see Pronamide)		
Korax (Lanstan)	NR, 6%,15%	
Lanstan (see Korax)		
Lasso (see Alachlor)		
Leptophos (Phosvel)	C, 6%	2
Lindane (see BHC, ∂		
Malathion	15%,50% V	C, 3
Malathion oxygen analog		NR, 1,2,3
Merphos	6%,15%,50% V	
Methidathion (Supracide)	50%	C, 3
o,p-Methoxychlor	6%	
p,p'-Methoxychlor	6%	C, 2
Methyl parathion (see Parathion-methyl)		

Appendix C Elution of Pesticides from Florisil (Continued)

Compound	Standard procedure[a,b]	Alternative procedure[b,c]
Methyl Trithion	6% V	
Mirex	6%	C, 1
MO	6%,15% V	C, 2
Mocap (see Ethoprop)		
Monocrotophos (Azodrin)		NR, 1,2,3
Monuron	C, 65%	NR, 1,2,3
Naled		NR, 1,2,3
Neburon	NR, 6%,15%,30%	NR, 1,2,3
Nemacide (see Dichlofenthion)		
Nitrofen (TOK)	C, 15%	C, 2
Oxtachlor epoxide (oxychlordane)	6%	C, 1
Octachloro-dibenzo-p-dioxin	NR, 6%,15%	C, 2,3
OMPA (see Schradan		
Ovex (Chlorfenson)	15%	C, 2
Oxadiazon	C, 15%	
Oxychlordane (see Octachlor epoxide)		
Parathion	15%	C, 2
Parathion-methyl (methyl parathion)	15%	C, 2
Parathion-methyl oxygen analog		NR, 1,2,3
Parathion oxygen analog		NR, 1,2,3
PCNB (see Quintozene)		
Pentachloroaniline	6%	C, 1
Pentachlorobenzene	C, 6%	
Pentachlorobenzonitrile	15%	
Perthane	6%	C, 1
Perthane olefin	6%	C, 1

Appendix C Elution of Pesticides from Florisil (Continued)

Compound	Standard procedure[a,b]	Alternative procedure[b,c]
Phaltan (see Folpet)		
Phenkapton	6%	
Phorate (Thimet)	6%	
Phorate oxygen analog sulfone		NR, 1,2,3
Phosalone	C, 50%	C, 2,3
Phosmet (Imidan)		P, 3
Phosphamidon		NR, 1,2,3
Phostex	6%	
Phosvel (see Leptophos)		
Photodieldrin A	15%	C, 2
Planavin	P, 50%	P, 3
Polychlorinated biphenyls	6%	C, 1
Polychlorinated napthalenes (Halowax 1099)	C, 6%	
Polychlorinated napthalenes (Halowax 1014)	C, 6%	
Polychlorinated napthalenes (Halowax 1051)	C, 6%,15%	
Prefar (see Bensulide)		
Prolan	15%	C, 2
Prometryn	P, 50%	NR, 1,2,3
Pronamide (Kerb)	C, 15%,50%	
Propachlor (Ramrod)	NR, 6%,15%	trace, 3
Propanil (Stam F-34)	NR, 6%,15%	P, 3
Propazine	C, 15%,50%	trace, 3
Quintozene (PCNB)	6%	C, 1
Ramrod (see Propachlor)		
Randox (see Allidochlor)		

Appendix C Elution of Pesticides from Florisil (Continued)

Compound	Standard procedure[a,b]	Alternative procedure[b,c]
Ronnel (Fenchlorphos)	6%	C, 2
SD 7438	C, 15%	
Simazine	C, 50%	NR, 1,2,3
Stam F-34 (see Propanil)		
Strobane	6%	C, 1
Suffix (see Benzoylprop-ethyl)		
Sulfotep	6%,15% V	P, 2
Sulphenone	25%	C, 3
Supracide (see Methidathion)		
TCNB (see Tecnazene)		
o,p-TDE	6%	C, 1
p,p'-TDE	6%	C, 1
p,p'-TDE olefin	6%	C, 1
Tecnazene (TCNB)	6%	C, 1
Tedion (see Tetradifon)		
Telodrin (see Isobenzan)		
Terbacil	NR, 6%,15%	P, 2,3
Terbufos (Counter)	6%	
Terbuthylazine	15%,50%	
2,3,4,5-Tetrachloroanisidine	6%	2
2,3,4,6-Tetrachloroanisidine	6%	2
2,3,5,6-Tetrachloroanisidine	6%	2
2,3,4,5-Tetrachloroanisole	6%	1
2,3,4,6-Tetrachloroanisole	6%	1
2,3,5,6-Tetrachloroanisole	6%	1
2,3,7,8-Tetrachlorodibenzo-p-dioxin	P, 6%,15% V	C, 1

Appendix C Elution of Pesticides from Florisil (Continued)

Compound	Standard procedure[a,b]	Alternative procedure[b,c]
2,3,4,5-Tetrachloro-nitroanisole	6%	1,2
2,3,4,6-Tetrachloro-nitoranisole	6%	1,2
2,3,5,6-Tetrachloro-nitroanisole	6%	1,2
Tetrachlorvinphos (Gardona)		NR, 1,2,3
Tetradifon (Tedion)	15%	C, 2
Tetraiodoethylene	6%	
Tetrasul	C, 6%	C, 1
Thimet (see Phorate)		
Thiodan (see Endosulfan)		
Thionazin (Zinophos)	C, 15%,50% V	
TOK (see Nitrofen)		
Toxaphene (Camphechlor)	6%	C, 1
Trichlorobenzenes	C, 6%	C, 1
Trifluralin	6%	C, 2
Trithion (see Carbophenothion)		
Vegadex (see CDEC)		
Vernolate (Vernam)	P, 15%	
Zinophos (see Thionazin)		
Zytron	6%	2

[a]Percent values are the percent ethyl ether in petroleum ether eluates.

[b]Numbers are the first, second, or third eluates of the alternative elution procedure.

[c]Quantitative data, if available, are listed by: C, recoveries greater than 80%; P, recoveries less than 80%; NR, not recovered; V, varied elution or recovery.

Source: Ref. 12.

Appendix D Retention Values for a 10% DC-200 Gas Chromatographic Column

RRT[a]	Compound	M.F.[b]
0.03	Dichlorobenzene, p-	$C_6H_4Cl_2$
0.04	DBCP	$C_3H_5Br_2Cl$
0.04[c,d]	TEPP (tetraethyl pyrophosphate)	$C_8H_{20}O_7P_2$
0.06	Trichlorobenzene, 1,3,5-	$C_6H_3Cl_3$
0.07	Trichlorobenzene, 1,2,4-	$C_6H_3Cl_3$
0.07	Dichlorvos	$C_4H_7Cl_2O_4P$
0.08	Trichlorbenzene, 1,2,3-	$C_6H_3Cl_3$
0.09	Allidochlor (Randox)	$C_8H_{12}ClNO$
0.10	Monuron	$C_9H_{11}ClN_2O$
0.10	Trichlorfon	$C_4H_8Cl_3O_4P$
0.10[c,d]	TEPP (tetraethyl pyrophosphate)	$C_8H_{20}O_7P_2$
0.11	Diuron	$C_9H_{10}Cl_2N_2O$
0.11	Neburon	$C_{12}H_{16}Cl_{12}N_2O$
0.11	Dichlobenil (Casoron)	$C_7H_3Cl_2N$
0.12	EPTC (Eptam)	$C_9H_{19}NOS$
0.13	Mevinphos (Phosdrin)	$C_7H_{13}O_6P$
0.14	Phthalate, dimethyl	$C_{10}H_{10}O_4$
0.15	Vernolate (Vernam)	$C_{10}H_{21}NOS$
0.15	Hydroxy chloroneb	$C_7H_6Cl_2O_2$
0.16[c]	BEP ester, 2,4,5-T	$C_{17}H_{23}Cl_3O_3$
0.18[c]	Propazine	$C_9H_{16}ClN_5$
0.18[c]	Simazine	$C_7H_{12}ClN_5$
0.19	Bis(trichloromethyl disulfide)	$C_2Cl_6S_2$
0.19	Chloroneb	$C_8H_8Cl_2O_2$
0.20[c,d]	TEPP (tetraethyl pyrophosphate)	$C_8H_{20}O_7P_2$
0.22	Demeton-O oxygen analog	$C_8H_{19}O_4PS$
0.23	Methyl trichlorobenzoate, 2,3,6-	$C_8H_5Cl_3O_2$

Appendix D Retention Values for a 10% DC-200 Gas Chromatographic Column (Continued)

RRT[a]	Compound	M.F.[b]
0.24	Pentachlorobenzene	C_6HCl_5
0.24	Acephate (Orthene)	$C_4H_{10}NO_3PS$
0.25	Thionazin (Zinophos)	$C_8H_{13}N_2O_3PS$
0.27	Demeton-O (Systox thiono isomer)	$C_8H_{19}O_3PS_2$
0.28	Tecnazene (TCNB)	$C_6HCl_4NO_2$
0.28	Phorate oxygen analog	$C_7H_{17}O_3PS_2$
0.28	Propachlor (Ramrod)	$C_{11}H_{14}ClNO$
0.29	Chloranil	$C_6Cl_4O_2$
0.29	Methyl ester, 2,4-D	$C_9H_8Cl_2O_3$
0.30	Dimethoate oxygen analog	$C_5H_{12}NO_4PS$
0.31	Chlorpropham (CIPC)	$C_{10}H_{12}ClNO_2$
0.32	Ethoprop (Mocap)	$C_8H_{19}O_2PS_2$
0.33	Naled	$C_4H_7Br_2Cl_2O_4P$
0.33	Sulfotep	$C_8H_{20}O_5P_2S_2$
0.33	Trifluralin	$C_{13}H_{16}F_3N_3O_4$
0.33	Dicrotophos (Bidrin)	$C_8H_{16}NO_5P$
0.34	Benfluralin (benefin)	$C_{13}H_{16}F_3N_3O_4$
0.35	Phorate (Thimet)	$C_7H_{17}O_2PS_3$
0.36	Bomyl	$C_9H_{15}PO_8$
0.37	CDEC (Vegedex)	$C_8H_{14}ClNS_2$
0.38[c]	BHC, α	$C_6H_6Cl_6$
0.38	Fonofos oxygen analog	$C_{10}H_{15}O_2PS$
0.39[c]	Simazine	$C_7H_{12}ClN_5$
0.39	Demeton-S (Systox thiol isomer)	$C_8H_{19}O_3PS_2$
0.39	Monocrotophos (Azodrin)	$C_7H_{14}NO_5P$
0.40[c]	Thiometon	$C_6H_{15}O_2PS_3$
0.40	Dicloran (Botran)	$C_6H_5Cl_2N_2O_2$

Appendix D Retention Values for a 10% DC-200 Gas Chromatographic Column (Continued)

RRT[a]	Compound	M.F.[b]
0.40	Dimethoate	$C_5H_{12}NO_3PS_2$
0.41	Atrazine	$C_8H_{14}ClN_5$
0.41	Isopropyl ester, 2,4-D	$C_{11}H_{12}Cl_2O_3$
0.42[c]	BHC, β	$C_6H_6Cl_6$
0.43	Hexachlorobenzene	C_6Cl_6
0.43[c]	Propazine	$C_9H_{16}ClN_5$
0.43	Amiben methyl ester	$C_8H_7Cl_2NO_2$
0.43	Diazinon oxygen analog	$C_{12}H_{21}N_2O_4P$
0.44	Pentachloroanisole	$C_7H_3Cl_5O$
0.44[c]	Chlordane (technical)	$C_{10}H_6Cl_8$
0.44	Methyl ester, silvex	$C_{10}H_9Cl_3O_3$
0.46	Terbuthylazine	$C_9H_{16}N_5Cl$
0.46	Dioxathion (Delnav)	$C_{12}H_{26}O_6P_2S_4$
0.47[c]	BHC, ∂ (lindane)	$C_6H_6Cl_6$
0.48	Methyl ester, 2,4,5-T	$C_9H_7Cl_3O_3$
0.49	Terbufos	$C_9H_{21}O_2PS_3$
0.49	BHC, δ	$C_6H_6Cl_6$
0.49	Schradan	$C_8H_{24}N_4O_3P_2$
0.50	Pentachlorobenzonitrile	C_7Cl_5N
0.50	Diazinon	$C_{12}H_{21}N_2O_3PS$
0.50	Quintozene (PCNB)	$C_6Cl_5NO_2$
0.50	Fonofos (Dyfonate)	$C_{10}H_{15}OPS_2$
0.50	Pronamide (Kerb)	$C_{12}H_{11}Cl_2NO$
0.51	Dinitramine	$C_{11}H_{13}F_3N_4O_4$
0.52	Chlorothalonil (Daconil 2787)	$C_8Cl_4N_2$
0.52[c]	Phosphamidon	$C_{10}H_{19}ClNO_5P$
0.53	Disulfoton (Disyston)	$C_8H_{19}O_2PS_3$

Appendix D Retention Values for a 10% DC-200 Gas Chromatographic Column (Continued)

RRT[a]	Compound	M.F.[b]
0.53[d]	Terbacil	$C_9H_{13}ClN_2O_2$
0.54	Tetraiodoethylene	C_2I_4
0.54	Dichlone	$C_{10}H_4Cl_2O_2$
0.54	Parathion-methyl oxygen analog	$C_8H_{10}NO_6P$
0.55	Chlordene	$C_{10}H_6Cl_6$
0.56	Sencor (metribuzin)	$C_8H_{14}N_4OS$
0.56	Sirmate, 2,3 isomer	$C_9H_9Cl_2NO_2$
0.56	Dichlormate (Sirmate, 3,4 isomer)	$C_9H_9Cl_2NO_2$
0.61	Isobutyl ester, 2,4-D	$C_{12}H_{14}Cl_2O_3$
0.61	Methyl ester, 4- (2,4-DB)	$C_{11}H_{12}Cl_2O_3$
0.62[c]	Chlordane (technical)	$C_{10}H_6Cl_8$
0.62	Phthalate, diisobutyl	$C_{16}H_{22}O_4$
0.63	Ronnel oxygen analog	$C_8H_8Cl_3O_4P$
0.65	Propanil (Stam F-34)	$C_9H_9Cl_2NO$
0.65	Phorate oxygen analog sulfone	$C_7H_{17}O_5PS_2$
0.66[c]	Phosphamidon	$C_{10}H_{19}ClNO_5P$
0.66	Pentachloroaniline	$C_6H_2Cl_5N$
0.66	Dichlofenthion (VC-13 Nemacide)	$C_{10}H_{13}Cl_2O_3PS$
0.66	Isopropyl ester, 2,4,5-T	$C_{11}H_{11}Cl_3O_3$
0.67[c]	BEP ester, 2,4,5-T	$C_{17}H_{23}Cl_3O_3$
0.67	Malathion oxygen analog	$C_{10}H_{19}O_7PS$
0.68[c]	BEP ester, 2,4-D	$C_{17}H_{24}Cl_2O_4$
0.68	Parathion-methyl	$C_8H_{10}NO_5PS$
0.68	Carbaryl	$C_{12}H_{11}NO_2$
0.68	Vinclozolin (Ronilan)	$C_{12}H_9Cl_2NO_2$
0.70[d]	Diamidafos (Nellite)	$C_8H_{13}N_2O_2P$
0.70	Demethon-O sulfone	$C_8H_{19}O_5PS_2$

Appendix D Retention Values for a 10% DC-200 Gas Chromatographic Column (Continued)

RRT[a]	Compound	M.F.[b]
0.71	Butyl ester, (N-), 2,4-D	$C_{12}H_{14}Cl_2O_3$
0.72[c]	Chlordane (technical)	$C_{10}H_6Cl_8$
0.74	Alachlor (Lasso)	$C_{14}H_{20}ClNO_2$
0.74	Picloram methyl ester	$C_7H_5Cl_3N_2O_2$
0.75	Prometryn	$C_{10}H_{19}N_5S$
0.76	Parathion oxygen analog	$C_{10}H_{14}NO_6P$
0.78[c]	Chlorfenethol (Dimite)	$C_{14}H_{12}Cl_2O$
0.78	Ronnel (fenchlorphos)	$C_8H_8Cl_3O_3PS$
0.79	Heptachlor	$C_{10}H_5Cl_7$
0.79[c,d]	Chlordane (technical)	$C_{10}H_6Cl_8$
0.80[c]	Dicofol, o,p- (Kelthane, o,p-)	$C_{14}H_9Cl_5O$
0.80[c]	Phostex	$C_9H_{22}O_4P_2S_4$
0.80	Chlordene, α	$C_{10}H_6Cl_6$
0.80	Dichlorobenzophenone, o,p'-	$C_{13}H_8Cl_2O$
0.81[c]	Chlordane (Compound K)	$C_{10}H_6Cl_8$
0.81	Fenitrothion (Sumithion)	$C_9H_{12}NO_5PS$
0.83[d]	Linuron	$C_9H_{10}Cl_2N_2O_2$
0.83	Phoxim oxygen analog	$C_{12}H_{15}O_4N_2P$
0.85	Phthalate, di-N-butyl	$C_{16}H_{22}O_4$
0.87	Malathion	$C_{10}H_{19}O_6PS_2$
0.87	Cyanazine (Bladex)	$C_9H_{13}ClN_6$
0.87	Phorate sulfoxide	$C_7H_{17}O_3PS_3$
0.88	Zytron	$C_{10}H_{14}Cl_2NO_2PS$
0.88	Phorate sulfone	$C_7H_{17}O_4PS_3$
0.89[c]	Phostex	$C_9H_{22}O_4P_2S_4$
0.89[c]	Phthalate, diisooctyl	$C_{24}H_{38}O_4$
0.90	Bromacil	$C_9H_{13}BrN_2O_2$

Appendix D Retention Values for a 10% DC-200 Gas Chromatographic Column (Continued)

RRT[a]	Compound	M.F.[b]
0.90	Pentachlorophenyl methyl sulfide	$C_7H_3Cl_5S$
0.92	Isobutyl ester, 2,4,5-T	$C_{12}H_{13}Cl_3O_3$
0.92	Chlorpyrifos oxygen analog	$C_9H_{11}Cl_3NO_4P$
0.94	Chlordene, ∂	$C_{10}H_6Cl_6$
0.94	Fenthion	$C_{10}H_{15}O_3PS_2$
0.95	Aspon	$C_{12}H_{28}O_5P_2S_2$
0.95[c]	Chlorfenethol (Dimite)	$C_{14}H_{12}Cl_2O$
0.95[c]	Chlordane (technical)	$C_{10}H_6Cl_8$
0.96[c]	Phostex	$C_9H_{22}O_4P_2S_4$
0.96	Chlordene, β	$C_{10}H_6Cl_6$
0.96	Desmethyl diphenamid	$C_{15}H_{15}NO$
0.96	Parathion	$C_{10}H_{14}NO_5PS$
0.97	Hydroxychlordene, 1-	$C_{10}H_6Cl_6O$
0.97[c]	Dicofol, p,p'- (Kelthane)	$C_{14}H_8Cl_5O$
0.97	Dichlorobenzophenone, p,p-	$C_{13}H_8Cl_2O$
0.98	Chlorpyrifos (Dursban)	$C_9H_{11}Cl_3NO_3PS$
0.98	Dicapthon	$C_8H_9ClNO_5PS$
0.99	Dacthal	$C_{10}H_6Cl_4O_4$
1.00	Aldrin	$C_{12}H_8Cl_6$
1.03	Parathion, amino	$C_{10}H_{16}NO_3PS$
1.03	Dacthal monoacid	$C_9H_4Cl_4O_4$
1.04	Demeton-S sulfone	$C_2H_{19}O_5PS_2$
1.05[c]	Chlorthion	$C_8H_9ClNO_5PS$
1.05	Methyl ester, 4-(2,4,5-TB)	$C_{11}H_{11}Cl_3O_3$
1.06[c]	BEP ester, 2,4,5-T	$C_{17}H_{23}Cl_3O_3$
1.06	Crufomate (Ruelene)	$C_{12}H_{19}ClNO_3P$
1.08	Diphenamid	$C_{16}H_{17}NO$

Appendix D Retention Values for a 10% DC-200 Gas Chromatographic Column (Continued)

RRT[a]	Compound	M.F.[b]
1.08	Butyl ester, N-, 2,4,5-T	$C_{12}H_{13}Cl_3O_3$
1.09	Bromophos	$C_8H_8BuCl_2O_3PS$
1.10	Isobenzan (Telodrin)	$C_9H_4Cl_8O$
1.10	Cypromid	$C_{10}H_9Cl_2NO$
1.12	Pirimiphos-ethyl	$C_{13}H_{24}N_3O_3PS$
1.12	Isopropalin	$C_{15}H_{23}N_3O_4$
1.14[c]	Chlordane (technical)	$C_{10}H_6Cl_8$
1.15	Isodrin	$C_{12}H_8Cl_6$
1.15	Chlorfenvinphos, α	$C_{12}H_{14}Cl_3O_4P$
1.17	TDE, o,p-, olefin	$C_{14}H_9Cl_3$
1.17	Captan	$C_9H_8Cl_3NO_2S$
1.19	Thiabendazole	$C_{10}H_7N_3S$
1.21[d]	Anilazine (Dyrene)	$C_9H_5Cl_3N_4$
1.21	Folpet (Phaltan)	$C_9H_4Cl_3O_2NS$
1.23	Phenthoate	$C_{12}H_{17}O_4PS_2$
1.24	Heptachlor epoxide	$C_{10}H_5Cl_7O$
1.24	Chlorfenvinphos, β	$C_{12}H_{14}Cl_3O_4P$
1.24	Sulphenone	$C_{12}H_9ClO_2S$
1.26	Octachlor epoxide	$C_{10}H_4Cl_8O$
1.26	Mephofolan (Cytrolane)	$C_8H_{16}O_3NPS_2$
1.34	Crotoxyphos (Ciodrin)	$C_{14}H_{19}O_6P$
1.36	Chlorbenside	$C_{13}H_{10}Cl_2S$
1.37	Disulfoton sulfone	$C_8H_{19}O_4PS_3$
1.38	Methidathion (Supracide)	$C_6H_{11}N_2O_4PS_3$
1.40	Photodieldrin B	$C_{13}H_9Cl_5O$
1.41	Nitrofen, amino	$C_{12}H_9Cl_2NO$
1.42	TDE, p,p'-, olefin	$C_{14}H_9Cl_3$

Appendix D Retention Values for a 10% DC-200 Gas Chromatographic Column (Continued)

RRT[a]	Compound	M.F.[b]
1.42[c]	Chlordane (technical)	$C_{10}H_6Cl_8$
1.43	Chlordane, trans	$C_{10}H_6Cl_8$
1.47	Perthane olefin	$C_{18}H_{19}Cl$
1.47	Genite	$C_{12}H_8Cl_2O_3S$
1.48	Bromophos-ethyl	$C_{10}H_{12}BrCl_2O_3PS$
1.48	DDE, o,p-	$C_{14}H_8Cl_4$
1.51[c]	Propylene glycol butyl ether ester, 2,4-D	$C_{15}H_{20}Cl_2O_4$
1.51	Tetrachlorvinphos (Gardona)	$C_{10}H_9Cl_4O_4P$
1.52	Methyl Trithion oxygen analog	$C_9H_{12}ClO_3PS_2$
1.54[c,d]	TEPP (tetraethyl pyrophosphate)	$C_8H_{20}O_7P_2$
1.55	Promecarb	$C_{12}H_{17}NO_2$
1.57	DDA, p,p'-, methyl ester	$C_{15}H_{12}Cl_2O_2$
1.58[c]	Endosulfan I (Thiodan I)	$C_9H_6Cl_6O_3S$
1.58	Ovex (Chlorfenson)	$C_{12}H_8Cl_2O_3S$
1.59[c]	Chlordane (technical)	$C_{10}H_6Cl_8$
1.60	Chlordane, cis	$C_{10}H_6Cl_8$
1.63[c]	BEP ester, 2,4-D	$C_{17}H_{24}Cl_2O_4$
1.63	Nemacur	$C_{13}H_{22}NO_3PS$
1.67	Nonachlor, trans	$C_{10}H_5Cl_9$
1.71[c]	Isooctyl ester, 2,4-D	$C_{16}H_{22}Cl_2O_3$
1.78	Butoxy ethanol ester, 2,4-D	$C_{14}H_{18}Cl_2O_4$
1.78	Profenofos (Curacron)	$C_{11}H_{15}ClBrO_3PS$
1.81	DDE, p,p'-	$C_{14}H_8Cl_4$
1.82	Merphos	$C_{12}H_{27}PS_3$
1.83	Dieldrin	$C_{12}H_8Cl_6O$
1.84[c]	Isooctyl ester, 2,4-D	$C_{16}H_{22}Cl_2O_3$

Appendix D Retention Values for a 10% DC-200 Gas Chromatographic Column (Continued)

RRT[a]	Compound	M.F.[b]
1.85	DEF	$C_{12}H_{27}OPS_3$
1.86	TDE, o,p-	$C_{14}H_{10}Cl_4$
1.86	Fensulfothion sulfone	$C_{11}H_{17}O_6PS_2$
1.93	Oxadiazon	$C_{15}H_{18}Cl_2N_2O_3$
1.95	Fensulfothion oxygen analog sulfone	$C_{11}H_{17}O_7PS_2$
1.96[c]	BEP ester, 2,4-D	$C_{17}H_{24}Cl_2O_4$
1.96[c]	Aramite	$C_{15}H_{23}ClO_4S$
1.99	Nitrofen (TOK)	$C_{12}H_7Cl_2NO_3$
2.05	Endrin	$C_{12}H_8Cl_6O$
2.07[c]	Ethyl hexyl ester, 2,4-D	$C_{16}H_{22}Cl_2O_3$
2.08[c]	Endosulfan II (Thiodan II)	$C_9H_6Cl_6O_3S$
2.09[c]	Isooctyl ester, 2,4-D	$C_{16}H_{22}Cl_2O_3$
2.09	Carbopheonthion oxygen analog	$C_{11}H_{16}ClO_3PS_2$
2.10[c,d]	TEPP (tetraethyl pyrophosphate)	$C_8H_{20}O_7P_2$
2.10	Dihydromirex, 5,10-	$C_{10}H_2Cl_{10}$
2.10[c]	Aramite	$C_{15}H_{23}ClO_4S$
2.12	Methyl Trithion	$C_9H_{12}ClO_2PS_3$
2.13	Perthane	$C_{18}H_{20}Cl_2$
2.15	Binapacryl	$C_{15}H_{18}N_2O_6$
2.26	Chlorobenzilate	$C_{16}H_{14}Cl_2O_3$
2.28[d]	Chlorpropylate	$C_{17}H_{16}Cl_2O_3$
2.28[c]	Dilan	$C_{15}H_{14}Cl_2NO_2$
2.30	Endrin aldehyde	$C_{12}H_8Cl_6O$
2.33	TDE, p,p'-	$C_{14}H_{10}Cl_4$
2.33	Leptophos photo product	$C_{13}H_{11}Cl_2O_2PS$
2.34	Chlornidine (Torpedo)	$C_{11}H_{13}Cl_2N_3O_4$
2.35	Fensulfothion (Dasanit)	$C_{11}H_{17}O_4PS_2$

Appendix D Retention Values for a 10% DC-200 Gas Chromatographic Column (Continued)

RRT[a]	Compound	M.F.[b]
2.36	Dihydromirex, 2,8-	$C_{10}H_2Cl_{10}$
2.37	Nonachlor, cis	$C_{10}H_5Cl_9$
2.40[c]	Phthalate, diisohexyl	$C_{20}H_{30}O_4$
2.42	Dihydromirex, 5,10-	$C_{10}H_2Cl_{10}$
2.44[c]	DDT, o,p-	$C_{14}H_9Cl_5$
2.44	Fensulfothion oxygen analog	$C_{11}H_{17}O_5PS$
2.46	Ethion	$C_9H_{22}O_4P_2S_4$
2.48[c]	Chlordane	$C_{10}H_6Cl_8$
2.50	Endrin alcohol	$C_{12}H_8Cl_6O$
2.50	Chlorthiophos	$C_{11}H_{15}Cl_2O_3PS$
2.51[c]	Isooctyl ester, 2,4,5-T	$C_{16}H_{21}Cl_3O_3$
2.51	Triazophos (Hostathion)	$C_{12}H_{16}N_3O_3PS$
2.56[c]	Chlordane (technical)	$C_{10}H_6Cl_8$
2.59	Tetrasul	$C_{12}H_6Cl_4S$
2.60	Famphur	$C_{10}H_{16}NO_5PS_2$
2.61[c]	Phthalate, diisohexyl	$C_{20}H_{30}O_4$
2.62	Dihydromirex, 10,10	$C_{10}H_2Cl_{10}$
2.67[c]	Endosulfan sulfate	$C_9H_6Cl_6O_4S$
2.70	Chlordecone (Kepone)	$C_{10}H_8Cl_{10}O_5$
2.75[c]	Dilan	$C_{15}H_{14}Cl_{12}NO_2$
2.79[c]	BEP ester, 2,4,5-T	$C_{17}H_{23}Cl_3O_3$
2.79	MO	$C_{12}H_6Cl_3NO_3$
2.81	Phosmet oxygen analog	$C_{11}H_{12}NO_5PS$
2.83	Carbophenothion (Trithion)	$C_{11}H_{16}ClO_2PS_3$
2.84[c]	Phthalate, diisohexyl	$C_{20}H_{30}O_4$
2.85[c]	Butoxy ethanol ester, 2,4,5-T	$C_{14}H_{17}Cl_3O_4$
2.90[c]	Isooctyl ester, 2,4,5-T	$C_{16}H_{21}Cl_3O_3$

Appendix D Retention Values for a 10% DC-200 Gas Chromatographic Column (Continued)

RRT[a]	Compound	M.F.[b]
2.91	Methoxychlor olefin	$C_{16}H_{14}Cl_2O_2$
3.0[c]	Propargite	$C_{19}H_{26}O_4S$
3.00	Phthalate, butylbenzyl	$C_{19}H_{20}O_4$
3.03[c]	DDT, p,p'-	$C_{14}H_9Cl_5$
3.05	Captafol (Difolatan)	$C_{10}H_9Cl_4NO_2S$
3.09	Cythioate	$C_8H_{12}NO_5PS_2$
3.10	Dioxin, 2,3,7,8-tetrachloro dibenzo-p-	$C_{12}H_4Cl_4O_2$
3.15	Dihydromirex, 5,10-	$C_{10}H_2Cl_{10}$
3.16[c]	BEP ester, 2,4-D	$C_{17}H_{24}Cl_2O_4$
3.19[c]	Isooctyl ester, 2,4,5-T	$C_{16}H_{21}Cl_3O_3$
3.20	Methoxychlor, o,p-	$C_{16}H_{15}Cl_3O_2$
3.21[c]	Phthalate, diisohexyl	$C_{20}H_{30}O_4$
3.24[c]	BEP, 2,4,5-T	$C_{17}H_{23}Cl_3O_3$
3.32[c]	Dilan	$C_{15}H_{15}Cl_2NO_2$
3.50	Endrin ketone	$C_{12}H_8Cl_6O$
3.60[c]	Propargite	$C_{19}H_{26}O_4S$
3.67	Monohydromirex, 8-	$C_{10}HCL_{11}$
3.70	Carbophenothion oxygen analog sulfone	$C_{11}H_{16}ClO_5PS_2$
3.70	Dieldrin chlorohydrin	$C_{12}H_9Cl_7O$
3.70	Planavin	$C_{13}H_{19}N_3O_6S$
3.90[c]	Dinocap (Karathane)	$C_{18}H_{24}N_2O_6$
3.90	Phosmet (Imidan)	$C_{11}H_{12}O_4NPS_2$
4.00[c]	Dicofol, o,p- (Kelthane, o,p-)	$C_{14}H_9Cl_5O$
4.0[a]	BEP ester, 2,4-D	$C_{17}H_{24}Cl_2O_4$
4.1	Carbophenothion oxygen analog sulfoxide	$C_{11}H_{16}ClO_4PS_2$

Appendix D Retention Values for a 10% DC-200 Gas Chromatographic Column (Continued)

RRT[a]	Compound	M.F.[b]
4.1	Leptophos oxygen analog	$C_{13}H_{10}BuCl_2O_3P$
4.18	Monohydromirex, 10-	$C_{10}HCl_{11}$
4.2[c]	Phostex	$C_9H_{22}O_4P_2S_4$
4.2	Suffix (benzoylprop-ethyl)	$C_{18}H_{17}Cl_2NO_3$
4.2[c]	Dinocap (Karathane)	$C_{18}H_{24}N_2O_6$
4.2	EPN	$C_{14}H_{14}NO_4PS$
4.22	Dihydromirex, 5,10-	$C_{10}H_2Cl_{10}$
4.3[c]	Phostex	$C_9H_{22}O_4P_2S_4$
4.3[c]	Dicofol, p,p'- (Kelthane)	$C_{14}H_9Cl_5O$
4.3	Acarol	$C_{17}H_{16}Br_2O_3$
4.3	Photodieldrin A	$C_{12}H_8Cl_6O$
4.5	Methoxychlor, p,p'-	$C_{16}H_{15}Cl_3O_2$
4.6	Phenkapton	$C_{11}H_{15}Cl_2O_2PS_3$
4.6	Tetrasul sulfoxide	$C_{12}H_6Cl_4OS$
4.7[c]	Dinocap (Karathane)	$C_{18}H_{24}N_2O_6$
4.9	Tetradifon (Tedion)	$C_{12}H_6Cl_4O_2S$
5.0[c]	Dinocap (Karathane)	$C_{18}H_{24}N_2O_6$
5.0	Azinphos-methyl (Guthion)	$C_{10}H_{12}N_3O_3PS_2$
5.0	Carbophenothion sulfone	$C_{11}H_{16}ClO_4PS_3$
5.2[c]	BEP ester, 2,4,5-T	$C_{17}H_{23}Cl_3O_3$
5.3	Carbophenothion sulfoxide	$C_{11}H_{16}ClO_3PS_3$
5.3	Phosalone	$C_{12}H_{15}ClNO_4PS_2$
5.4[c]	Phthalate, diisooctyl	$C_{23}H_{28}O_4$
5.6	Leptophos (Phosvel)	$C_{13}H_{10}BrCl_2O_2PS$
5.7	Mirex	$C_{10}Cl_{12}$
5.8[c]	Propargite	$C_{19}H_{26}O_4S$
5.8	SD 7438	$C_{11}H_{18}O_4P_2S_4$

Appendix D Retention Values for a 10% DC-200 Gas Chromatographic Column (Continued)

RRT[a]	Compound	M.F.[b]
6.1[c]	Phthalate, diisooctyl	$C_{24}H_{38}O_4$
6.2	Azinphos-ethyl (Ethyl Guthion)	$C_{12}H_{16}N_3O_3PS_2$
6.4	Phthalate, di-2-ethylhexyl	$C_{24}H_{28}O_4$
6.4	Dialifor	$C_{14}O_{17}ClNO_4PS_2$
6.5	Nitrofen, n-acetyl	$C_{14}H_{11}Cl_2NO_2$
6.6[c]	Phthalate, diisooctyl	$C_{24}H_{38}O_3$
6.9[c]	BEP ester, 2,4,5-T	$C_{17}H_{23}Cl_3O_3$
7.3	Coumaphos oxygen analog	$C_{14}H_{16}ClO_6P$
7.4[c]	Phthalate, diisooctyl	$C_{24}H_{38}O_4$
7.5	Pyrazophos	$C_{13}H_{20}O_5N_2PS$
8.8[c]	Phthalate, diisooctyl	$C_{24}H_{38}O_4$
9.3	Bensulide (Prefar)	$C_{14}H_{24}NO_4PS_3$
9.5	Hexachlorophene dimethyl ether	$C_{15}H_{10}Cl_6O_2$
9.5	Coumaphos	$C_{14}H_{16}ClO_5PS$
10.0[c]	BEP ester, 2,4-D	$C_{17}H_{24}Cl_2O_4$
10.3[c]	Phthalate, diisooctyl	$C_{24}H_{38}O_4$
11.8	Phthalate, di-n-octyl	$C_{24}H_{38}O_4$
13	Hexachlorophene	$C_{13}H_6Cl_6O_2$
30	Dioxin, octachloro-dibenzo-p-	$C_{12}Cl_8O_2$

[a]Retention time relative to aldrin at 200°.

[b]Molecular formula.

[c]One of two or more related peaks.

[d]Peak height response varies.

Source: Ref. 12.

Appendix E Retention Values for a Gas Chromatographic Column Containing a 1:1 Mixture of 10% DC-200 and 15% QF-1

RRT[a]	Compound	M.F.[b]
0.06	Dichlorobenzene, p-	$C_6H_4Cl_2$
0.06	DBCP (dibromochloropropane)	$C_3H_5Br_2Cl$
0.06	Trichlorobenzene, 1,3,5-	$C_6H_3Cl_3$
0.07	Trichlorobenzene, 1,2,4-	$C_6H_3Cl_3$
0.08	Trichlorobenzene, 1,2,3-	$C_6H_3Cl_3$
0.10	Monuron	$C_9H_{11}ClN_2O$
0.11	EPTC (Eptam)	$C_9H_{19}NOS$
0.13	Dichlorvos	$C_4H_7Cl_2O_4P$
0.14	Diuron	$C_9H_{10}Cl_2N_2O$
0.14	Neburon	$C_{12}H_{16}Cl_2N_2O$
0.15	Vernolate (Vernam)	$C_{10}H_{21}NOS$
0.17	Allidochlor (Randox)	$C_8H_{12}ClNO$
0.18	Hydroxychloroneb	$C_7H_6Cl_2O_2$
0.19	Trichorfon	$C_4H_8Cl_3O_4P$
0.19	Naled	$C_4H_7Br_2Cl_2O_4P$
0.20	Dichlobenil (Casoron)	$C_7H_3Cl_2N$
0.23	Chloroneb	$C_8H_8Cl_2O_2$
0.24	Anisole, 2,3,4,6-tetrachloro-	$C_7H_4Cl_4O$
0.24	Anisole, 2,3,5,6-tetrachloro-	$C_7H_4Cl_4O$
0.24	Pentachlorobenzene	C_6HCl_5
0.25[c]	BEP ester, 2,4,5-T	$C_{17}H_{23}Cl_3O_3$
0.26	Phthalate, dimethyl	$C_{10}H_{10}O_4$
0.26[c]	Propazine	$C_9H_{16}ClN_5$
0.26[c]	Simazine	$C_7H_{12}ClN_5$
0.31	Mevinphos (Phosdrin)	$C_7H_{13}O_6P$
0.31	Methyl trichlorobenzoate, 2,3,6-	$C_8H_5Cl_3O_2$
0.36	Demeton-O (Systox thiono isomer)	$C_8H_{19}O_3PS_2$

Appendix E Retention Values for a Gas Chromatographic Column Containing a 1:1 Mixture of 10% DC-200 and 15% QF-1 (Continued)

RRT[a]	Compound	M.F.[b]
0.38	Anisole, 2,3,4,5-tetrachloro-	$C_7H_4Cl_4O$
0.38	Thionazin (Zinophos)	$C_8H_{13}N_2O_3PS$
0.38	Tecnazene (TCNB)	$C_6HCl_4NO_2$
0.39[c,d]	TEPP (tetraethyl pyrophosphate)	$C_8H_{20}O_7P_2$
0.40	Chloranil	$C_6Cl_4O_2$
0.41	Demeton-O oxygen analog	$C_8H_{19}O_4PS$
0.41	Chlorpropham (CIPC)	$C_{10}H_{12}ClNO_2$
0.42	Methyl ester, 2,4-D	$C_9H_8Cl_2O_3$
0.42	Hexachlorobenzene	C_6Cl_6
0.45	Acephate (Orthene)	$C_4H_{10}NO_3PS$
0.45	Phorate (Thimet)	$C_7H_{17}O_2PS_3$
0.46	CDEC (Vegedex)	$C_8H_{14}ClNS_2$
0.46[c]	BHC, α	$C_6H_6Cl_6$
0.46	Pentachloroanisole	$C_7H_3Cl_5O$
0.47	Phorate oxygen analog	$C_7H_{17}O_3PS_2$
0.47	Sulfotep	$C_8H_{20}O_5P_2S_2$
0.50[c,d]	TEPP (tetraethyl pyrophosphate)	$C_8H_{20}O_7P_2$
0.50	Propachlor (Ramrod)	$C_{11}H_{14}ClNO$
0.51	Tetraiodoethylene	C_2I_4
0.53[c]	Chlordane	$C_{10}H_6Cl_8$
0.54[c]	Simazine	$C_7H_{12}ClN_5$
0.54[c]	Thiometon	$C_6H_{15}O_2PS_3$
0.54	Atrazine	$C_8H_{14}ClN_5$
0.54[c]	Propazine	$C_9H_{16}ClN_5$
0.55	Isopropyl ester, 2,4-D	$C_{11}H_{12}Cl_2O_3$
0.56	Diazinon	$C_{12}H_{21}N_2O_3PS$
0.56	Chlordene	$C_{10}H_6Cl_6$

Appendix E Retention Values for a Gas Chromatographic Column Containing a 1:1 Mixture of 10% DC-200 and 15% QF-1 (Continued)

RRT[a]	Compound	M.F.[b]
0.57	Benfluralin (benefin)	$C_{13}H_{16}F_3N_3O_4$
0.57	Methyl ester, silvex	$C_{10}H_9Cl_3O_3$
0.58[c]	BHC, Γ (lindane)	$C_6H_6Cl_6$
0.60	Trifluralin	$C_{13}H_{16}F_3N_3O_4$
0.60[c]	BHC, β	$C_6H_6Cl_6$
0.61	Quintozene (PCNB)	$C_6Cl_5NO_2$
0.63	Nitroanisole, 2,3,4,5-tetrachloro-	$C_7H_3Cl_4NO_2$
0.63	Terbuthylazine	$C_9H_{16}N_5Cl$
0.63	Terbufos	$C_9H_{21}O_2PS_3$
0.64	Anisidine, 2,3,5,6-tetrachloro-	$C_7H_5Cl_4NO$
0.64	Fonofos oxygen analog	$C_{10}H_{15}O_2PS$
0.65[c,d]	TEPP (tetraethyl pyrophosphate)	$C_8H_{20}O_7P_2$
0.66	Pentachlorobenzonitrile	C_7Cl_5N
0.66	Fonofos (Dyfonate)	$C_{10}H_{15}OPS_2$
0.66	Pronamide (Kerb)	$C_{12}H_{11}Cl_2NO$
0.66	Disulfoton (Disyston)	$C_8H_{19}O_2PS_3$
0.67	Methyl ester, 2,4,5-T	$C_9H_7Cl_3O_3$
0.68	Anisidine, 2,3,4,6-tetrachloro-	$C_7H_5Cl_4NO$
0.68	Demeton-S (Systox thiol isomer)	$C_8H_{19}O_3PS_2$
0.68	Dioxathion (Delnav)	$C_{12}H_{26}O_6P_2S_4$
0.68[c]	BHC, δ	$C_6H_6Cl_6$
0.69	Nitroanisole, 2,3,4,6-tetrachloro-	$C_7H_3Cl_4NO_2$
0.70	Dichloran (Botran)	$C_6H_4Cl_2N_2O_2$
0.70	Amiben methyl ester	$C_8H_7Cl_2NO_2$
0.70	Pentachloroaniline	$C_6H_2Cl_5N$
0.71	Nitroanisole, 2,3,5,6-tetrachloro-	$C_7H_3Cl_4NO_2$
0.74	Anisidine, 2,3,4,5-tetrachloro-	$C_7H_5Cl_4NO$

Appendix E Retention Values for a Gas Chromatographic Column Containing a 1:1 Mixture of 10% DC-200 and 15% QF-1 (Continued)

RRT[a]	Compound	M.F.[b]
0.76	Diazinon oxygen analog	$C_{12}H_{21}N_2O_4P$
0.78	Isobutyl ester, 2,4-D	$C_{12}H_{14}Cl_2O_3$
0.78	Dichlofenthion (VC-13 Nemacide)	$C_{10}H_{13}Cl_2O_3PS$
0.81	Heptachlor	$C_{10}H_5Cl_7$
0.82[c]	Chlordane	$C_{10}H_6Cl_8$
0.82[c]	BEP ester, 2,4,5-T	$C_{17}H_{23}Cl_3O_3$
0.82[c]	Chlorfenethol (Dimite)	$C_{14}H_{12}Cl_2O$
0.83	Dimethoate oxygen analog	$C_5H_{12}NO_4PS$
0.84	Isopropyl ester, 2,4,5-T	$C_{11}H_{11}Cl_3O_3$
0.85	Dichlone	$C_{10}H_4Cl_2O_2$
0.85	Methyl ester, 4- (2,4-DB)	$C_{11}H_{12}Cl_2O_3$
0.85	Prometryn	$C_{10}H_{19}N_5S$
0.85[c]	Chlordene, α	$C_{10}H_6Cl_6$
0.86[c]	Chlordane (Compound K)	$C_{10}H_6Cl_8$
0.87	Sirmate, 2,3 isomer	$C_9H_9Cl_2NO_2$
0.88	Phthalate, diisobutyl	$C_{16}H_{22}O_4$
0.90[c]	Thiometon	$C_6H_{15}O_2PS_3$
0.90	Dichlormate (Sirmate, 3,4 isomer)	$C_9H_9Cl_2NO_2$
0.90[c,d]	BEP ester, 2,4-D	$C_{17}H_{24}Cl_2O_4$
0.93	Pentachlorophenyl methyl sulfide	$C_7H_3Cl_5S$
0.94	Diphenamid	$C_{16}H_{17}NO$
0.95	Butyl ester, (n-), 2,4-D	$C_{12}H_{14}Cl_2O_3$
0.97	Dimethoate	$C_5H_{12}NO_3PS_2$
0.97	Ronnel (fenchlorphos)	$C_8H_8Cl_3O_3PS$
1.00[d]	Terbacil	$C_9H_{13}ClN_2O_2$
1.00	Aldrin	$C_{12}H_8Cl_6$
1.03	Dicrotophos (Bidrin)	$C_8H_{16}NO_5P$

Appendix E Retention Values for a Gas Chromatographic Column Containing a 1:1 Mixture of 10% DC-200 and 15% QF-1 (Continued)

RRT[a]	Compound	M.F.[b]
1.03	Dinitramine	$C_{11}H_{13}F_3N_4O_4$
1.04[c]	Chlordene, Γ	$C_{10}H_6Cl_6$
1.05[c]	Chlordene, β	$C_{10}H_6Cl_6$
1.07	Monocrotophos (Azodrin)	$C_7H_{14}NO_5S$
1.09	Chlorothalonil (Daconil 2787)	$C_8Cl_4N_2$
1.10[c]	Dicofol, o,p- (Kelthane, o,p-)	$C_4H_9Cl_5O$
1.10	Dichlorbenzophenon, o,p-	$C_{13}H_8Cl_2O$
1.10	Alachlor (Lasso)	$C_{14}H_{20}ClNO_2$
1.11[c]	Hydroxychlordene, 1-	$C_{10}H_6Cl_6O$
1.13	Ronnel oxygen analog	$C_8H_8Cl_3O_4P$
1.14	Zytron	$C_{10}H_{14}Cl_2NO_2PS$
1.14	Isobenzan (Telodrin)	$C_9H_4Cl_8O$
1.15	Propanil (Stam F-34)	$C_9H_9Cl_2NO$
1.15[c,d]	Diamidafos (Nellite)	$C_8H_{13}N_2O_2P$
1.17	Chlorpyrifos (Dursban)	$C_9H_{11}Cl_3NO_3PS$
1.18[c]	Phthalate, diisooctyl	$C_{24}H_{38}O_4$
1.20	Phthalate, di-n-butyl	$C_{16}H_{22}O_4$
1.21	TDE, o,p-, olefin	$C_{14}H_9Cl_3$
1.22	Aspon	$C_{12}H_{28}O_5P_2S_2$
1.24[c]	Chlordane	$C_{10}H_5Cl_8$
1.24	Fenthion	$C_{10}H_{15}O_3PS_2$
1.25	Isodrin	$C_{12}H_8Cl_6$
1.26	Picloram methyl ester	$C_7H_5Cl_3N_2O_2$
1.26	Isobutyl ester, 2,4,5-T	$C_{12}H_{13}Cl_3O_3$
1.28	Bromophos	$C_8H_8BrCl_2O_3PS$
1.30[c,d]	Dicofol, p,p'- (Kelthane)	$C_{14}H_9Cl_5O$
1.30	Dichlorbenzophenone, p,p'-	$C_{13}H_8Cl_2O$

Appendix E Retention Values for a Gas Chromatographic Column Containing a 1:1 Mixture of 10% DC-200 and 15% QF-1 (Continued)

RRT[a]	Compound	M.F.[b]
1.31[c]	Chlorfenethol (Dimite)	$C_{14}H_{12}Cl_2O$
1.31	Perthane olefin	$C_{18}H_{19}Cl$
1.32[c]	BEP ester, 2,4,5-T	$C_{17}H_{23}Cl_3O_3$
1.34[c]	Chlordane	$C_{10}H_6Cl_8$
1.35[c]	Chlorthion	$C_8H_9ClNO_5PS$
1.38	Octachlor epoxide	$C_{10}H_4Cl_8O$
1.40	Methyl ester, 4- (2,4,5-TB)	$C_{11}H_{11}Cl_3O_3$
1.40	Butyl ester, n-, 2,4,5-T	$C_{12}H_{13}Cl_3O_3$
1.42	Parathion-methyl	$C_8H_{10}NO_5PS$
1.43[d]	Anilazine (Dyrene)	$C_9H_5Cl_3N_4$
1.45[c]	Chlordane	$C_{10}H_6Cl_8$
1.45	Pirimiphos-ethyl	$C_{13}H_{24}N_3O_3PS$
1.46	DDE, o,p-	$C_{14}H_8Cl_4$
1.47	Heptachlor epoxide	$C_{10}H_5Cl_7O$
1.48	Malathion	$C_{10}H_{19}O_6PS_2$
1.50[d]	Linuron	$C_9H_{10}Cl_2N_2O_2$
1.50	Parathion, amino	$C_{10}H_{16}NO_3PS$
1.50	TDE, p,p-, olefin	$C_{14}H_9Cl_3$
1.51	Chlorbenside	$C_{13}H_{10}Cl_2S$
1.52	Dacthal	$C_{10}H_6Cl_4O_4$
1.52	Dacthal monoacid	$C_9H_4Cl_4O_4$
1.56	Carbaryl	$C_{12}H_{11}NO_2$
1.57[c]	Chlordane, trans	$C_{10}H_6Cl_8$
1.58[c]	Chlordane	$C_{10}H_6Cl_8$
1.62	Malathion oxygen analog	$C_{10}H_{19}O_7PS$
1.62	Fenitrothion (Sumithion)	$C_9H_{12}NO_5PS$
1.62	Desmethyl diphenamid	$C_{15}H_{15}NO$

Appendix E Retention Values for a Gas Chromatographic Column Containing a 1:1 Mixture of 10% DC-200 and 15% QF-1 (Continued)

RRT[a]	Compound	M.F.[b]
1.66[c]	Propylene glycol butyl ether ester, 2,4-D	$C_{15}H_{20}Cl_2O_4$
1.66[c]	Ethyl hexyl ester, 2,4-D	$C_{16}H_{22}Cl_2O_3$
1.66	BEP ester, 2,4,5-T	$C_{17}H_{23}Cl_3O_3$
1.67	Thiabendazole	$C_{10}H_7N_3S$
1.69	Isopropalin	$C_{15}H_{23}Cl_3O_3$
1.70	Demeton-methyl	$C_6H_{15}O_3PS_2$
1.70	Nonachlor, trans	$C_{10}H_5Cl_9$
1.72	Chlorfenvinphos, α	$C_{12}H_{14}Cl_3O_4P$
1.73	Chlorpyrifos oxygen analog	$C_9H_{11}Cl_3NO_4P$
1.73[c]	Chlordane, cis	$C_{10}H_6Cl_8$
1.8	Bromacil	$C_9H_{13}BrN_2O_2$
1.8	Cypromid	$C_{10}H_9Cl_2NO$
1.82[c]	Chlorthion	$C_8H_9ClNO_5PS$
1.82[c]	Chlordane	$C_{10}H_6Cl_8$
1.84	DDA, p,p'-, methyl ester	$C_{15}H_{12}Cl_2O_2$
1.86	Dicapthon	$C_8H_9ClNO_5PS$
1.86	Phenthoate	$C_{12}H_{17}O_4PS_2$
1.86	Photodieldrin B	$C_{13}H_9Cl_5O$
1.87	Chlorfenvinphos, β	$C_{12}H_{14}Cl_3O_4P$
1.88	Parathion-methyl oxygen analog	$C_8H_{10}NO_6P$
1.88	Cyanazine (Bladex)	$C_9H_{12}ClN_6$
1.88	Parathion	$C_{10}H_{14}NO_5PS$
1.88	DDE, p,p'-	$C_{14}H_8Cl_4$
1.89[c]	Endosulfan I (Thiodan I)	$C_9H_6Cl_6O_3S$
1.89[c]	Isooctyl ester, 2,4-D	$C_{16}H_{22}Cl_2O_3$
1.9[c,d]	TEPP (tetraethyl pyprophosphate)	$C_8H_{20}O_7P_2$

Appendix E Retention Values for a Gas Chromatographic Column Containing a 1:1 Mixture of 10% DC-200 and 15% QF-1 (Continued)

RRT[a]	Compound	M.F.[b]
1.92[c]	Propylene glycol butyl ether ester, 2,4-D	$C_{15}H_{20}Cl_2O_4$
1.92[c]	Chlordane	$C_{10}H_6Cl_8$
1.94[c]	Ethyl hexyl ester, 2,4-D	$C_{16}H_{22}Cl_2O_3$
1.97	Crufomate (Ruelene)	$C_{12}H_{19}ClNO_3P$
1.98[c]	Butoxy ethanol ester, 2,4-D	$C_{14}H_{18}Cl_2O_4$
1.99	Dihydromirex, 5,10-	$C_{10}H_2Cl_{10}$
2.02	Perthane	$C_{18}H_{20}Cl_2$
2.03	Phorate sulfoxide	$C_7H_{17}O_3PS_3$
2.03	Folpet (Phaltan)	$C_9H_4Cl_3O_2NS$
2.04	TDE, o,p-	$C_{14}H_{10}Cl_4$
2.07	Phosphamidon	$C_{10}H_{19}ClNO_5P$
2.10	Parathion oxygen analog	$C_{10}H_{14}NO_6P$
2.10	Captan	$C_9H_8Cl_3NO_2S$
2.10[c]	BEP ester, 2,4-D	$C_{17}H_{24}Cl_2O_4$
2.11[c]	Isooctyl ester, 2,4-D	$C_{16}H_{22}Cl_2O_3$
2.14	Merphos	$C_{12}H_{27}PS_3$
2.14	DEF	$C_{12}H_{27}OPS_3$
2.18[c]	Ethyl hexyl ester, 2,4-D	$C_{16}H_{22}Cl_2O_3$
2.18	Demeton-O sulfone	$C_8H_{19}O_5PS_2$
2.20	Dihydromirex, 5,10-	$C_{10}H_2Cl_{10}$
2.22	Dieldrin	$C_{12}H_8Cl_6O$
2.27[c]	Chlorthion	$C_8H_9ClNO_5PS$
2.29	Phorate oxygen analog sulfone	$C_7H_{17}O_5PS_2$
2.29	Phoxim oxygen analog	$C_{12}H_{15}N_2O_4P$
2.32[c]	Butoxy ethanol ester, 2,4-D	$C_{14}H_{18}Cl_2O_4$
2.32	Dihydromirex, 2,8-	$C_{10}H_2Cl_{10}$

Appendix E Retention Values for a Gas Chromatographic Column Containing a 1:1 Mixture of 10% DC-200 and 15% QF-1 (Continued)

RRT[a]	Compound	M.F.[b]
2.33	Phorate sulfone	$C_7H_{17}O_4PS_3$
2.33	Methidathion (Supracide)	$C_6H_{11}N_2O_4PS_3$
2.34	Methyl Trithion oxygen analog	$C_9H_{12}ClO_3PS_2$
2.36[c]	Chlordane	$C_{10}H_6Cl_8$
2.40[c]	BEP ester, 2, 4-D	$C_{17}H_{24}Cl_2O_4$
2.41	Genite	$C_{12}H_8Cl_2O_3S$
2.44	Schradan	$C_8H_{24}N_4O_3P_2$
2.46	Tetrachlorvinphos (Gardona)	$C_{10}H_9Cl_4O_4P$
2.48[c]	Isooctyl ester, 2,4-D	$C_{16}H_{22}Cl_2O_3$
2.48	Nonachlor, cis	$C_{10}H_5Cl_9$
2.48	DDT, o,p-	$C_{14}H_9Cl_5$
2.50	Profenofos (Curacron)	$C_{11}H_{15}ClBrO_3PS$
2.54[c]	Aramite	$C_{15}H_{23}ClO_4S$
2.55	Endrin	$C_{12}H_8Cl_6O$
2.57	Dihydromirex, 10,10-	$C_{10}H_2Cl_{10}$
2.59	Crotoxyphos (Ciodrin)	$C_{14}H_{19}O_6P$
2.62	Sulphenone	$C_{12}H_9ClO_2S$
2.62	Tetrasul	$C_{12}H_6Cl_4S$
2.64[c]	Chlordane (Compound K)	$C_{10}H_6Cl_8$
2.66[c]	Phthalate, diisohexyl	$C_{20}H_{30}O_4$
2.67	Chlordecone (Kepone)	$C_{10}H_8Cl_{10}O_5$
2.70	TDE, p,p'-	$C_{14}H_{10}Cl_4$
2.70	Dihydromirex, 5,10-	$C_{10}H_2Cl_{10}$
2.73	Methyl Trithion	$C_9H_{12}ClO_2PS_3$
2.73	Chlorobenzilate	$C_{16}H_{14}Cl_2O_3$
2.73[d]	Chlorpropylate	$C_{17}H_{16}Cl_2O_3$
2.74[c]	Aramite	$C_{15}H_{23}ClO_4S$

Appendix E Retention Values for a Gas Chromatographic Column Containing a 1:1 Mixture of 10% DC-200 and 15% QF-1 (Continued)

RRT[a]	Compound	M.F.[b]
2.78	Ovex (Chlorfenson)	$C_{12}H_8Cl_2O_3S$
2.78[c]	Isooctyl ester, 2,4,5-T	$C_{16}H_{21}Cl_3O_3$
2.80[c]	Phthalate, diisooctyl	$C_{24}H_{38}O_4$
2.87[c]	Phthalate, diisohexyl	$C_{20}H_{30}O_4$
2.90[c,d]	TEPP (tetraethyl pyrophosphate)	$C_8H_{20}O_7P_2$
2.92[c]	Endosulfan II (Thiodan II)	$C_9H_6Cl_6O_3S$
2.92[c]	BEP ester, 2,4,5-T	$C_{17}H_{23}Cl_3O_3$
2.97	Nemacur	$C_{13}H_{22}NO_3PS$
3.00	Methoxychlor olefin	$C_{16}H_{14}Cl_2O_2$
3.04	Leptophos photo product	$C_{13}H_{11}Cl_2O_2PS$
3.05	Dihydromirex, 5,10-	$C_{10}H_2Cl_{10}$
3.08[c]	Butoxy ethanol ester, 2,4,5-T	$C_{14}H_{17}Cl_3O_4$
3.11	Isooctyl ester, 2,4,5-T	$C_{16}H_{21}Cl_3O_3$
3.13[c]	Phthalate, diisohexyl	$C_{20}H_{30}O_4$
3.18	Dihydromirex, 5,10-	$C_{10}H_2Cl_{10}$
3.2	Nitrofen (TOK)	$C_{12}H_7Cl_2NO_3$
3.23	Ethion	$C_9H_{22}O_4P_2S_4$
3.25[c]	Propargite	$C_{19}H_{26}O_4S$
3.26	Dioxin, 2,3,7,8-tetrachloro dibenzo-p-	$C_{12}H_4Cl_4O_2$
3.28[c]	DDT, p,p'-	$C_{14}H_9Cl_5$
3.28[c]	BEP ester, 2,4,5-T	$C_{17}H_{23}Cl_3O_3$
3.31	Carbophenothion oxygen analog	$C_{11}H_{16}ClO_3PS_2$
3.33	Carbophenothion (Trithion)	$C_{11}H_{16}ClO_2PS_3$
3.33	Chlorthiophos	$C_{11}H_{15}Cl_2O_3PS$
3.40	Methoxychlor, o,p-	$C_{16}H_{15}Cl_3O_2$
3.42[c]	Phthalate, diisohexyl	$C_{20}H_{30}O_4$

Appendix E Retention Values for a Gas Chromatographic Column Containing a 1:1 Mixture of 10% DC-200 and 15% QF-1 (Continued)

RRT[a]	Compound	M.F.[b]
3.45	Endrin alcohol	$C_{12}H_8Cl_6O$
3.50[c]	BEP ester, 2,4-D	$C_{17}H_{24}Cl_2O_4$
3.52	Monohydromirex, 8-	$C_{10}HCl_{11}$
3.58	MO	$C_{12}H_{16}Cl_3NO_3$
3.6[c]	Butoxy ethanol ester, 2,4,5-T	$C_{14}H_{17}Cl_3O_4$
3.6[c]	Dilan	$C_{15}H_{14}Cl_2NO_2$
3.6[c]	Propargite	$C_{19}H_{26}O_4S$
3.7[c]	Isooctyl ester, 2,4,5-T	$C_{16}H_{21}Cl_3O_3$
3.8[c]	Phthalate, diisohexyl	$C_{20}H_{30}O_4$
3.95	Monohydromirex, 10-	$C_{10}HCl_{11}$
3.95	Mephofolan (Cytrolane)	$C_8H_{16}NPS_2$
4.0	Endrin aldehyde	$C_{12}H_8Cl_6O$
4.0	Phthalate, butylbenzyl	$C_{19}H_{20}O_4$
4.0	Dieldrin chlorohydrin	$C_{12}H_9Cl_7O$
4.03	Dihydromirex, 5,10-	$C_{10}H_2Cl_{10}$
4.1	Demeton-S sulfone	$C_8H_{19}O_5PS_2$
4.1	Disulfoton sulfone	$C_8H_{19}O_4PS_3$
4.3	Triazophos (Hostathion)	$C_{12}H_{16}N_3O_3PS$
4.3[c]	Dicofol, o,p- (Kelthane, o,p-)	$C_{14}H_9Cl_5O$
4.3[c]	Propargite	$C_{19}H_{26}O_4S$
4.4[c]	Propylene glycol butyl ether ester, 2,4-D	$C_{15}H_{20}Cl_2O_4$
4.4[c]	Dilan	$C_{15}H_{14}Cl_2NO_2$
4.5[c]	Propargite	$C_{19}H_{26}O_4S$
4.6	Binapacryl	$C_{15}H_{18}N_2O_6$
4.6[c]	Dicofol, p,p'- (Kelthane)	$C_{14}H_9Cl_5O$
4.7[c]	Dilan	$C_{15}H_{14}Cl_2NO_2$

Appendix E Retention Values for a Gas Chromatographic Column Containing a 1:1 Mixture of 10% DC-200 and 15% QF-1 (Continued)

RRT[a]	Compound	M.F.[b]
4.8	Methoxychlor, p,p'-	$C_{16}H_{15}Cl_3O_2$
5.0[c]	BEP ester, 2,4-D	$C_{17}H_{24}Cl_2O_4$
5.0	Acarol	$C_{17}H_{16}Br_2O_3$
5.1	Captafol (Difolatan)	$C_{10}H_9Cl_4NO_2S$
5.1	Mirex	$C_{10}Cl_{12}$
5.1[c]	Phthalate, diisooctyl	$C_{24}H_{38}O_4$
5.3	Phenkapton	$C_{11}H_{15}Cl_2O_2PS_3$
5.4[c]	Dilan	$C_{15}H_{14}Cl_2NO_2$
5.4[c]	Endosulfan sulfate	$C_9H_6Cl_6O_4S$
5.4	Bulan	$C_{16}H_{15}Cl_2NO_2$
5.6	Chlornidine (Torpedo)	$C_{11}H_{13}Cl_2N_3O_4$
5.9	Leptophos oxygen analog	$C_{13}H_{10}BrCl_2O_3P$
6.0	Endrin ketone	$C_{12}H_8Cl_6O$
6.1	Leptophos (Phosvel)	$C_{13}H_{10}BrCl_2O_2PS$
6.2	Fensulfothion (Dasanit)	$C_{11}H_{17}O_4PS_2$
6.4[c]	BEP ester, 2,4,5-T	$C_{17}H_{23}Cl_3O_3$
6.5	Suffix (benzoylprop-ethyl)	$C_{18}H_{17}Cl_2NO_3$
6.6[c]	Propargite	$C_{19}H_{26}O_4S$
6.6[c]	Dinocap (Karathane)	$C_{18}H_{24}N_2O_6$
6.6	Phthalate, di-2-ethylhexyl	$C_{24}H_{38}O_4$
6.8[c]	Phthalate, diisooctyl	$C_{24}H_{38}O_4$
7.0	Tetrasul sulfoxide	$C_{12}H_6Cl_4OS$
7.2[c]	Dinocap (Karathane)	$C_{18}H_{24}N_2O_6$
7.3	EPN	$C_{14}H_{14}NO_4PS$
7.5	Phosmet (Imidan)	$C_{11}H_{12}O_4NPS_2$
7.5	Photodieldrin A	$C_{12}H_8Cl_6O$
7.6	SD 7438	$C_{11}H_{18}O_4P_2S_4$

Appendix E Retention Values for a Gas Chromatographic Column Containing a 1:1 Mixture of 10% DC-200 and 15% QF-1 (Continued)

RRT[a]	Compound	M.F.[b]
8.0[c]	Phthalate, diisooctyl	$C_{24}H_{38}O_4$
8.1	Fensulfothion oxygen analog	$C_{11}H_{17}O_5PS$
8.1	Phosmet oxygen analog	$C_{11}H_{12}NO_5PS$
8.3	Fensulfothion sulfone	$C_{11}H_{17}O_6PS_2$
8.4[c]	Dinocap (Karathane)	$C_{18}H_{24}N_2O_6$
8.5	Tetradifon (Tedion)	$C_{12}H_6Cl_4O_2S$
8.8[c]	Propargite	$C_{19}H_{26}O_4S$
9.3	Azinphos-methyl (Guthion)	$C_{10}H_{12}N_3O_3PS_2$
9.5[c]	Phthalate, diisooctyl	$C_{24}H_{38}O_4$
9.5	Hexachlorphene dimethyl ether	$C_{15}H_{10}Cl_6O_2$
10.0	Carbophenothion sulfoxide	$C_{11}H_{16}ClO_3PS_3$
10.2	Fensulfothion oxygen analog sulfone	$C_{11}H_{17}O_7PS_2$
10.2	Carbophenothion sulfone	$C_{11}H_{16}ClO_4PS_3$
10.3	Cythioate	$C_8H_{12}NO_5PS_2$
10.3	Dialifor	$C_{14}H_{17}ClNO_4PS_2$
10.5	Phosalone	$C_{12}H_{15}ClNO_4PS_2$
11.6	Azinphos-ethyl (Ethyl Guthion)	$C_{12}H_{16}N_3O_3PS_2$
11.9	Phthalate, di-n-octyl	$C_{24}H_{30}O_4$
12.0[c]	BEP ester, 2,4-D	$C_{17}H_{24}Cl_2O_4$
12.4	Pyrazophos	$C_{14}H_{20}O_5N_3PS$

Appendix E Retention Values for a Gas Chromatographic Column Containing a 1:1 Mixture of 10% DC-200 and 15% QF-1 (Continued)

RRT[a]	Compound	M.F.[b]
13.8	Planavin	$C_{13}H_{19}N_3O_6S$
14[c]	Hexachlorophene	$C_{13}H_6Cl_6O_2$
20[c]	Hexachlorophene	$C_{13}H_6Cl_6O_2$
20	Bensulide (Prefar)	$C_{14}H_{24}NO_4PS_3$
25	Coumaphos	$C_{14}H_{16}ClO_5PS$
28	Coumaphos oxygen analog	$C_{14}H_{16}ClO_6P$
28	Dioxin, octachloro-dibenzo-p-	$C_{12}Cl_8O_2$

[a]Retention time relative to aldrin at 200°.

[b]Molecular formula.

[c]One of two or more related peaks.

[d]Peak height response varies.

Source: Ref. 12.

Appendix F Alphabetical Listing of Retention Data for the DC-200 and the DC-200/QF-1 Columns

Compound	DC-200[a]	DC-200/QF-1[b]
Acarol	4.3	5.0
Acephate	0.24	0.45
Alachlor	0.74	1.10
Allidochlor	0.09	0.17
Amiben methyl ester	0.43	0.70
Anilazine	1.21	1.43
Anisidine, 2,3,4,5-tetrachloro-		0.74
Anisidine, 2,3,4,6-tetrachloro-		0.68
Anisidine, 2,3,5,6-tetrachloro-		0.64
Anisole, 2,3,4,5-tetrachloro-		0.38
Anisole, 2,3,4,6-tetrachloro-		0.24
Anisole, 2,3,5,6-tetrachloro-		0.24
Aramite	1.96	2.54
Aramite	2.10	2.74
Aspon	0.95	1.22
Atrazine	0.41	0.54
Azinphos-ethyl	6.2	11.6
Azinphos-methyl	5.0	9.3
Benfluralin	0.34	0.57
Bensulide	9.3	20
BEP ester, 2,4-D	0.68	0.90
BEP ester, 2,4-D	1.63	2.10
BEP ester, 2,4-D	1.96	2.40
BEP ester, 2,4-D	3.16	3.5
BEP ester, 2,4-D	4.0	5.0
BEP ester, 2,4-D	10.0	12
BEP ester, 2,4,5-T	0.16	0.25

Appendix F Alphabetical Listing of Retention Data for the DC-200 and the DC-200/QF-1 Columns (Continued)

Compound	DC-200[a]	DC-200/QF-1[b]
BEP ester, 2,4,5-T	0.67	0.82
BEP ester, 2,4,5-T	1.06	1.32
BEP ester, 2,4,5-T	2.79	1.66
BEP ester, 2,4,5-T	3.24	2.92
BEP ester, 2,4,5-T	5.2	3.28
BEP ester, 2,4,5-T	6.9	6.4
BHC, α	0.38	0.46
BHC, β	0.42	0.60
BHC, Γ	0.47	0.58
BHC, δ	0.49	0.68
Binapacryl	2.15	4.6
Bis(trichloromethyl disulfide)	0.19	
Bomyl	0.36	
Bromacil	0.90	1.8
Bromophos	1.09	1.28
Bromophos-ethyl	1.48	
Bulan	3.32	5.4
Butoxy ethanol ester, 2,4-D		2.32
Butoxy ethanol ester, 2,4-D	1.78	1.98
Butoxy ethanol ester, 2,4,5-T		3.6
Butoxy ethanol ester, 2,4,5-T	2.85	3.08
Butyl ester, (n-), 2,4-D	0.71	0.95
Butyl ester, n-, 2,4,5-T	1.08	1.40
Captafol	3.05	5.1
Captan	1.17	2.10
Carbaryl	0.68	1.56
Carbophenothion	2.83	3.33

Appendix F Alphabetical Listing of Retention Data for the DC-200 and the DC-200/QF-1 Columns (Continued)

Compound	DC-200[a]	DC-200/QF-1[b]
Carbophenothion oxygen analog	2.09	3.31
Carbophenothion oxygen analog sulfone	3.7	
Carbophenothion oxygen analog sulfoxide	4.1	
Carbophenothion sulfone	5.0	10.2
Carbophenothion sulfoxide	5.3	10.0
CDEC	0.37	0.46
Chloranil	0.29	0.40
Chlorbenside	1.36	1.51
Chlordane (technical)	0.44	0.53
Chlordane (technical)	0.62	0.82
Chlordane (technical)	0.72	1.24
Chlordane (technical)	0.79	1.34
Chlordane (technical)	0.95	1.45
Chlordane (technical)	1.14	1.58
Chlordane (technical)	1.42	1.82
Chlordane (technical)	1.59	1.92
Chlordane (technical)	2.56	2.36
Chlordane, cis	1.60	1.73
Chlordane, trans	1.43	1.57
Chlordecone	2.70	2.67
Chlordene	0.55	0.56
Chlordene, α	0.80	0.86
Chlordene, β	0.96	1.05
Chlordene, Γ	0.94	1.04
Chlorfenethol	0.78	0.82
Chlorfenethol	0.95	1.31

Appendix F Alphabetical Listing of Retention Data for the DC-200 and the DC-200/QF-1 Columns (Continued)

Compound	DC-200[a]	DC-200/QF-1[b]
Chlorfenvinphos	1.26	
Chlorfenvinphos, α	1.15	1.72
Chlorfenvinphos, β	1.24	1.87
Chlornidine	2.34	5.6
Chlorobenzilate	2.26	2.73
Chloroneb	0.19	0.23
Chlorothalonil	0.52	1.09
Chlorpropham	0.31	0.41
Chlorpropylate	2.28	2.73
Chlorpyrifos	0.98	1.17
Chlorpyrifos, oxygen analog	0.92	1.73
Chlorthion		1.82
Chlorthion		2.27
Chlorthion	1.05	1.35
Chlorthiophos	2.5	3.33
Compound K	0.81	0.86
Compound K	2.48	2.64
Coumaphos	9.5	25
Coumaphos oxygen analog	7.3	28
Crotoxyphos	1.34	2.59
Crufomate	1.06	1.97
Cyanazine	0.87	1.88
Cypromid	1.10	1.8
Cythioate	3.09	10.3
Dacthal	0.99	1.52
Dacthal monoacid	1.03	1.52
DBCP	0.04	0.06

Appendix F Alphabetical Listing of Retention Data for the DC-200 and the DC-200/QF-1 Columns (Continued)

Compound	DC-200[a]	DC-200/QF-1[b]
DDA, p,p'-, methyl ester	1.57	1.84
DDE, o,p-	1.48	1.46
DDE, p,p'-	1.81	1.88
DDT, o,p-	2.44	2.48
DDT, p,p'-	3.03	3.28
DEF	1.85	2.14
Demeton-methyl		1.70
Demeton-O	0.27	0.36
Demeton-O oxygen analog	0.22	0.41
Demeton-O sulfone	0.70	2.18
Demeton-S	0.39	0.68
Demeton-S sulfone	1.04	4.1
Desmethyl diphenamid	0.96	1.62
Dialifor	6.4	10.3
Diamidafos	0.70	1.15
Diazinon	0.50	0.56
Diazinon oxygen analog	0.43	0.76
Dicapthon	0.98	1.86
Dichlobenil	0.11	0.20
Dichlofenthion	0.66	0.78
Dichlone	0.54	0.85
Dichlormate	0.56	0.90
Dichlorobenzene, p-	0.03	0.06
Dichlorobenzophenone, o,p-	0.80	1.1
Dichlorobenzophenone, p,p'-	0.97	1.30
Dichlorvos	0.07	0.13
Dicloran	0.40	0.70

Appendix F Alphabetical Listing of Retention Data for the DC-200 and the DC-200/QF-1 Columns (Continued)

Compound	DC-200[a]	DC-200/QF-1[b]
Dicofol	0.80	1.1
Dicofol, o,p-	4.0	4.3
Dicofol, p,p'-	0.97	1.30
Dicofol, p,p'-	4.3	4.6
Dicrotophos	0.33	1.03
Dieldrin	1.83	2.22
Dieldrin chlorohydrin	3.7	4.0
Dihydromirex, 10,10-	2.62	2.57
Dihydromirex, 2,8-	2.36	2.32
Dihydromirex, 5,10-		3.18
Dihydromirex, 5,10-		4.03
Dihydromirex, 5,10-	2.10	1.99
Dihydromirex, 5,10-	2.42	2.20
Dihydromirex, 5,10-	3.15	2.70
Dihydromirex, 5,10-	4.22	3.05
Dilan		5.4
Dilan	2.28	3.6
Dilan	2.75	4.4
Dilan	3.32	4.7
Dimethoate	0.40	0.97
Dimethoate oxygen analog	0.30	0.83
Dinitramine	0.51	1.03
Dinocap	3.9	6.6
Dinocap	4.2	7.2
Dinocap	4.7	8.4
Dinocap	5.0	
Dioxathion	0.46	0.68

Appendix F Alphabetical Listing of Retention Data for the DC-200 and the DC-200/QF-1 Columns (Continued)

Compound	DC-200[a]	DC-200/QF-1[b]
Dioxin, octachlorodibenzo-p-	30	28
Dioxin, 2,3,7,8-tetrachloro-dibenzo-p-	3.10	3.26
Diphenamid	1.08	0.94
Disulfoton	0.53	0.66
Disulfoton sulfone	1.37	4.1
Diuron	0.11	0.14
Endosulfan I	1.58	1.89
Endosulfan II	2.08	2.92
Endosulfan sulfate	2.67	5.4
Endrin	2.05	2.55
Endrin alcohol	2.50	3.45
Endrin aldehyde	2.30	4.0
Endrin ketone	3.5	6.0
EPN	4.2	7.3
EPTC	0.12	0.11
Ethion	2.46	3.23
Ethoprop	0.32	
Ethyl hexyl ester, 2,4-D		1.94
Ethyl hexyl ester, 2,4-D		2.18
Ethyl hexyl ester, 2,4-D	2.07	1.66
Famphur	2.60	
Fenitrothion	0.81	1.62
Fensulfothion	2.35	6.2
Fensulfothion oxygen analog	2.44	8.1
Fensulfothion oxygen analog sulfone	1.95	10.2
Fensulfothion sulfone	1.86	8.3

Appendix F Alphabetical Listing of Retention Data for the DC-200 and the DC-200/QF-1 Columns (Continued)

Compound	DC-200[a]	DC-200/QF-1[b]
Fenthion	0.94	1.24
Folpet	1.21	2.03
Fonofos	0.50	0.66
Fonofos oxygen analog	0.38	0.64
Genite	1.47	2.41
Heptachlor	0.79	0.81
Heptachlor expoxide	1.24	1.47
Hexachlorobenzene	0.43	0.42
Hexachlorophene		20
Hexachlorophene	13	14
Hexachlorophene dimethyl ether	9.5	9.5
Hydroxy chloroneb	0.15	0.18
Hydroxychlordene, 1-	0.97	1.11
Isobenzan	1.10	1.14
Isobutyl ester, 2,4-D	0.61	0.78
Isobutyl ester, 2,4,5-T	0.92	1.26
Isodrin	1.15	1.25
Isooctyl ester, 2,4-D	1.71	1.89
Isooctyl ester, 2,4-D	1.84	2.11
Isooctyl ester, 2,4-D	2.09	2.48
Isooctyl ester, 2,4,5-T	2.51	2.78
Isooctyl ester, 2,4,5-T	2.90	3.11
Isooctyl ester, 2,4,5-T	3.19	3.7
Isopropalin	1.12	1.69
Isopropyl ester, 2,4-D	0.41	0.55
Isopropyl ester, 2,4,5-T	0.66	0.84
Leptophos	5.6	6.1

Appendix F Alphabetical Listing of Retention Data for the DC-200 and the DC-200/QF-1 Columns (Continued)

Compound	DC-200[a]	DC-200/QF-1[b]
Leptophos oxygen analog	4.1	5.9
Leptophos photo product	2.33	3.04
Linuron	0.83	1.50
Malathion	0.87	1.48
Malathion oxygen analog	0.67	1.62
Mephofolan	1.32	3.95
Merphos	1.82	2.14
Methidathion	1.38	2.33
Methoxychlor, o,p-	3.2	3.4
Methoxychlor, p,p'-	4.5	4.8
Methoxychlor olefin	2.91	3.00
Methyl ester, silvex	0.44	0.57
Methyl ester, 2,4-D	0.29	0.42
Methyl ester, 2,4,5-T	0.48	0.67
Methyl ester, 4- (2,4-DB)	0.61	0.85
Methyl ester, 4- (2,4,5-TB)	1.05	1.40
Methyl trichlorobenzoate, 2,3,6-	0.23	0.31
Methyl Trithion	2.12	2.73
Methyl Trithion oxygen analog	1.52	2.34
Mevinphos	0.13	0.31
Mirex	5.7	5.1
MO	2.79	3.58
Monocrotophos	0.39	1.07
Monohydromirex, 10-	4.18	3.95
Monohydromirex, 8-	3.67	3.52
Monuron	0.10	0.10
Naled	0.33	0.19

Appendix F Alphabetical Listing of Retention Data for the DC-200 and the DC-200/QF-1 Columns (Continued)

Compound	DC-200[a]	DC-200/QF-1[b]
Neburon	0.11	0.14
Nemacur	1.63	2.97
Nitroanisole, 2,3,4,5-tetrachloro-		0.63
Nitroanisole, 2,3,4,6-tetrachloro-		0.69
Nitroanisole, 2,3,5,6-tetrachloro-		0.71
Nitrofen	1.99	3.2
Nitrofen, amino	1.41	
Nitrofen, N-acetyl	6.5	
Nonachlor, cis	2.37	2.48
Nonachlor, trans	1.67	1.70
Oxtachlor epoxide	1.26	1.38
Ovex	1.58	2.78
Ozadiazon	1.93	
Parathion	0.96	1.88
Parathion oxygen analog	0.76	2.10
Parathion-methyl	0.68	1.42
Parathion-methyl oxygen analog	0.54	1.88
Parathion, amino	1.03	1.50
Pentachloroaniline	0.66	0.70
Pentachloroanisole	0.44	0.46
Pentachlorobenzene	0.24	0.24
Pentachlorobenzonitrile	0.50	0.66
Pentachlorophenyl methyl sulfide	0.90	0.93
Perthane	2.13	2.02
Perthane olefin	1.47	1.31
Penkapton	4.6	5.3
Phenthoate	1.23	1.86

Appendix F Alphabetical Listing of Retention Data for the DC-200 and the DC-200/QF-1 Columns (Continued)

Compound	DC-200[a]	DC-200/QF-1[b]
Phorate	0.35	0.45
Phorate oxygen analog	0.28	0.47
Phorate oxygen analog sulfone	0.65	2.29
Phorate sulfone	0.88	2.33
Phorate sulfoxide	0.87	2.03
Phosalone	5.3	10.5
Phosmet	3.9	7.5
Phosmet oxygen analog	2.81	8.1
Phosphamidon	0.52	2.07
Phosphamidon	0.66	
Phostex	0.80	
Phostex	0.89	
Phostex	0.96	
Phostex	4.2	
Phostex	4.3	
Photodieldrin A	4.3	7.5
Photodieldrin B	1.4	1.86
Phoxim oxygen analog	0.83	2.29
Phthalate, butylbenzyl	3.00	4.0
Phthalate, di-n-butyl	0.85	1.20
Phthalate, di-n-octyl	11.8	11.9
Phthalate, di-2-ethylhexyl	6.4	6.6
Phthalate, diisobutyl	0.62	0.88
Phthalate, diisohexyl		3.8
Phthalate, diisohexyl	2.40	2.66
Phthalate, diisohexyl	2.61	2.87
Phthalate, diisohexyl	2.84	3.13

Appendix F Alphabetical Listing of Retention Data for the DC-200 and the DC-200/QF-1 Columns (Continued)

Compound	DC-200[a]	DC-200/QF-1[b]
Phthalate, diisohexyl	3.21	3.42
Phthalate, diisooctyl	0.89	1.18
Phthalate, diisooctyl	5.4	2.80
Phthalate, diisooctyl	6.1	5.1
Phthalate, diisooctyl	6.6	6.8
Phthalate, diisooctyl	7.4	8.0
Phthalate, diisooctyl	8.8	9.5
Phthalate, diisooctyl	10.3	
Phthalate, dimethyl	0.14	0.26
Picloram methyl ester	0.74	1.26
Pirimiphos-ethyl	1.12	1.45
Planavin	3.7	13.8
Profenophos	1.78	2.5
Promecarb	1.55	
Prometryn	0.75	0.85
Pronamide	0.50	0.66
Propachlor	0.28	0.50
Propanil	0.65	1.15
Propargite		4.5
Propargite		6.6
Propargite		8.8
Propargite	3.0	3.25
Propargite	3.6	3.6
Propargite	5.8	4.3
Propazine	0.18	0.26
Propazine	0.43	0.54
Propylene glycol butyl ether ester, 2,4-D		1.92

Appendix F Alphabetical Listing of Retention Data for the DC-200 and the DC-200/QF-1 Columns (Continued)

Compound	DC-200[a]	DC-200/QF-1[b]
Propylene glycol butyl ether ester, 2,4-D		4.4
Propylene glycol butyl ether ester, 2,4-D	1.51	1.66
Pyrazophos	7.5	12.4
Quintozene	0.50	0.61
Ronnel	0.78	0.97
Ronnel oxygen analog	0.63	1.13
Schradan	0.49	2.44
SD 7438	5.8	7.6
Sencor	0.56	
Simazine	0.18	0.26
Simazine	0.39	0.54
Sirmate, 2,3 isomer	0.56	0.87
Suffix	4.2	6.5
Sulfotep	0.33	0.47
Sulphenone	1.24	2.62
TDE, o,p-	1.86	2.04
TDE, o,p-, olefin	1.17	1.21
Triazophos	2.51	4.3
Vinclozolin	0.68	

[a]Retention relative to aldrin for a 10% DC-200 column.

[b]Retention relative to aldrin for a GC column containing a 1:1 mixture of 10% DC-200 and 15% QF-1.

Source: Ref. 12.

Appendix G Relative Retention Data for a 2% DEGS Gas Chromatographic Column at 180°

RRT[a]	Compound	M.F.[b]
0.08	Tributyl phosphate	$C_{12}H_{27}PO_4$
0.10	Ethoprop (Mocap)	$C_8H_{19}O_2PS_2$
0.14	Diazinon	$C_{12}H_{21}N_2O_3PS$
0.14	Sulfotepp	$C_8H_{20}O_5P_2S_2$
0.14[c]	Demeton-O	$C_8H_{19}O_3PS_2$
0.15	Phorate	$C_7H_{17}O_2PS_3$
0.15	Terbufos (Counter)	$C_9H_{21}O_2PS_3$
0.15[c]	Mevinphos, α (Phosdrin)	$C_7H_{13}O_6P$
0.19[c]	Mevinphos, β (Phosdrin)	$C_7H_{13}O_6P$
0.19	Merphos	$C_{12}H_{27}PS_3$
0.21	Fonofos (Dyfonate)	$C_{10}H_{15}OPS_2$
0.23	Disulfoton (Disystox)	$C_8H_{19}O_2PS_3$
0.23	Diazinon oxygen analog	$C_{12}H_{21}N_2O_4P$
0.24	TEPP (tetraethyl pyrophosphate)	$C_8H_{20}O_7P_2$
0.24[c]	Demeton-O	$C_8H_{19}O_3PS_2$
0.24	Demeton-S	$C_8H_{19}O_3PS_2$
0.26	Etrimfos	$C_{10}H_{17}N_2O_4PS$
0.26	Dichlofenthion	$C_{10}H_{13}Cl_2O_3PS$
0.27	Naled	$C_4H_7Br_2Cl_2O_4P$
0.29	Methamidophos (Monitor)	$C_2H_8NO_3PS$
0.31	Aspon	$C_{12}H_{28}O_5P_2S_2$
0.38[d]	Dioxathion	$C_{12}H_{26}O_6P_2S_4$
0.39	Pirimiphos-methyl	$C_{11}H_{20}N_3O_3PS$
0.40	Ronnel	$C_8H_8Cl_3O_3PS$
0.40	Chlorpyrifos (Dursban)	$C_9H_{11}Cl_3NO_3PS$
0.40	Dowco 214	$C_7H_7Cl_3NO_3PS$
0.40	Salithion	$C_8H_9O_3PS$

Appendix G Relative Retention Data for a 2% DEGS Gas Chromatographic Column at 180° (Continued)

RRT[a]	Compound	M.F.[b]
0.41	Pirimiphos-ethyl	$C_{13}H_{24}N_3O_3PS$
0.44	Tris(chloropropyl)phosphate	$C_9H_{18}Cl_3O_4P$
0.50	Schraden	$C_8H_{24}N_4O_3P$
0.50	DEF	$C_{12}H_{27}OPS_3$
0.53	Bromophos-ethyl	$C_{10}H_{12}BrCl_2O_3PS$
0.54	Ronnel oxygen analog	$C_8H_8Cl_3O_4P$
0.57	Trichlorfon	$C_4H_8Cl_3O_4P$
0.58[c]	Phosphamidon	$C_{10}H_9ClNO_5P$
0.60	Bromophos	$C_8H_8BrCl_2O_3PS$
0.61	Dicrotophos (Bidrin)	$C_8H_{16}NO_5P$
0.61	Phoxim	$C_{12}H_{15}N_2O_3PS$
0.64	Acephate (Orthene)	$C_4H_{10}NO_3PS$
0.76	Malathion	$C_{10}H_{19}O_6PS_2$
0.82	Fenthion	$C_{10}H_{15}O_3PS_2$
0.91[c]	Phosphamidon	$C_8H_9ClNO_5P$
0.92	Malathion oxygen analog	$C_{10}H_{19}O_7PS$
1.00	Parathion	$C_{10}H_{14}NO_5PS$
1.03	Tris(2-chloroethyl)phosphate	$C_6H_{12}Cl_3O_4P$
1.07	Profenofos (Curacron)	$C_{11}H_{15}BrClO_3PS$
1.09	Dimethoate oxygen analog	$C_5H_{12}NO_4PS$
1.10	Fenitrothion (Sumithion)	$C_9H_{12}NO_5PS$
1.17	Phenthoate	$C_{12}H_{17}O_4PS_2$
1.17	Iodofenphos	$C_8H_8Cl_2IO_3PS$
1.18	Methyl parathion	$C_8H_{10}NO_5PS$
1.22	Phoxim oxygen analog	$C_{12}H_{15}N_2O_4P$
1.23	Parathion oxygen analog	$C_{10}H_{14}NO_6P$
1.23	Mecarbam	$C_9H_{20}NO_5PS$

Appendix G Relative Retention Data for a 2% DEGS Gas Chromatographic Column at 180° (Continued)

RRT[a]	Compound	M.F.[b]
1.23[c]	Chlorthiophos	$C_{11}H_{12}Cl_2O_3PS_2$
1.32	Phorate sulfoxide	$C_7H_{17}O_3PS_3$
1.34[c]	Chlorthiophos	$C_{11}H_{12}Cl_2O_3PS_2$
1.36	Dimethoate	$C_5H_{12}NO_3PS_2$
1.37	Ethion	$C_9H_{22}O_4P_2S_4$
1.41	Methyl parathion oxygen analog	$C_8H_{10}NO_6P$
1.48	Crufomate (Ruelene)	$C_{12}H_{19}NClO_3P$
1.61[c]	Chlorthiophos	$C_{11}H_{12}Cl_2O_3PS_2$
1.63	Monocrotophos (Azodrin)	$C_7H_{14}NO_5P$
1.66	Diamidfos (Nellite)	$C_8H_{13}N_2O_2P$
1.75	Tetrachlorvinphos (Gardona)	$C_{10}H_9Cl_4O_4P$
1.78	Sulprofos (Bolstar)	$C_{12}H_{19}O_2PS_2$
1.81	Crotoxyphos (Ciodrin)	$C_{12}H_{19}O_6P$
1.86	Carbophenothion (Trithion)	$C_{11}H_{16}ClO_2PS_3$
1.89	Demeton-O sulfone	$C_8H_{19}O_5PS_2$
2.18	Carbophenothion oxygen analog	$C_{11}H_{16}ClO_3PS_2$
2.25	Methyl carbophenothion	$C_9H_{12}ClO_2PS_3$
2.43	Methidathion (Supracide)	$C_6H_{11}O_3N_2PS_3$
2.95	Phenkapton	$C_{11}H_{15}Cl_2O_2PS_3$
3.49	Mephosfolan (Cytrolane)	$C_8H_{16}O_3NPS_2$
3.62	Oxydemeton-methyl (Metasystox R)	$C_7H_{17}O_4PS$
4.43	Phosfolan (Cyolane)	$C_7H_{14}NO_3PS_2$
5.14	Cyanofenphos (Surecide)	$C_{15}H_{14}NO_2PS$
5.26	Triphenylphosphate	$C_{18}H_{15}O_4P$
5.42	Oxydemeton-methyl sufone	$C_7H_{17}O_6PS$
5.92	Tris(dichloropropyl)phosphate	$C_9H_{15}ClO_4P$
6.53	Fensulfothion	$C_{11}H_{17}O_4PS_2$

Appendix G Relative Retention Data for a 2% DEGS Gas Chromatographic Column at 180° (Continued)

RRT[a]	Compound	M.F.[b]
7.18	EPN	$C_{14}H_{14}NO_4PS$
7.18	Triazophos (Hostathion)	$C_{12}H_{16}N_3O_3PS$
10.7	Phosalone	$C_{12}H_{15}ClNO_4PS_2$
11.9	Famphur	$C_{10}H_{16}O_5NPS_2$
14	Phosmet (Imidan)	$C_{11}H_{12}O_4NPS_2$
16.4	Sulprofos sulfoxide	$C_{12}H_{19}O_3PS_2$
17.5	Azinphos-ethyl (Ethyl Guthion)	$C_{12}H_{16}N_3O_3PS_2$
20	Azinphos-methyl (Guthion)	$C_{10}H_{12}N_3O_3PS_2$
29	Sulprofos sulfone	$C_{12}H_{19}O_4PS_2$

[a]Retention time relative to parathion at 180°.

[b]Molecular formula.

[c]One of two or more related peaks.

[d]Peak height response varies with injections.

REFERENCES

1. Subcommittee on Oversight and Investigation, Environmental Protection Agency III. Case studies B. Pesticide regulations. In Federal Regulations and Regulatory Reform, U.S. Government Printing Office, Washington, D.C., Oct. 1976, pp. 134-145.
2. R. L. Ridgway, J. C. Tinney, J. T. MacGregor, and N. J. Starler, Pesticides in argiculture. Environ. Health Perspect. *27*, 103-112 (1978).
3. T. H. Maugh II, Chemicals: how many are there? Science *199*, 162 (1978).
4. R. A. Mills, J. H. Onley, and R. A. Gaither, Rapid method for chlorinated pesticide residues in nonfatty foods, J. Assoc. Off. Anal. Chem. *46*, 186-191 (1963).
5. R. C. Hall, A highly sensitive and selective microelectrolytic conductivity detector for gas chromatography, J. Chromatogr. Sci. *12*, 152-160 (1974).
6. R. J. Anderson and R. C. Hall, Hall bipolar pulse; differential electrolytic conductivity detector for GC, Amer. Lab. *12*(2), 108-124 (1980).
7. A. K. Klein, Report on extraction procedures for chloro-organic pesticides, J. Assoc. Off. Anal. Chem. *41*, 551-555 (1958).
8. A. K. Klein, Report on extraction procedures for chloro-organic insecticides, J. Assoc. Off. Anal. Chem. *42*, 539-544 (1959).
9. L. J. Hardin and C. T. Sarten, Comparison of five extraction procedures for the removal of DDT residues in field-treated collards, J. Assoc. Off. Anal. Chem. *45*, 988-990 (1962).
10. F. A. Gunther and R. C. Blinn, Sample processing, In Analysis of Insecticides and Acaricides. Interscience, New York, 1955, pp. 41-53.
11. R. E. J. Moddes and J. W. Cook, The extraction and identification of parathion and diazinon from lettuce, J. Assoc. Off. Anal. Chem. *42*, 208-211 (1959).
12. Pesticide Analytical Manual, Vol. 1, Food and Drug Administration, Washington, D.C., 1980.
13. Multiresidue methods, In Official Methods of Analysis, 13th ed. Association of Official Analytical Chemists, Washington, D.C., Secs. 29.001-29.049.
14. R. W. Storherr, P. Ott, and R. R. Watts, A general method for organophosphorus pesticide residues in nonfatty foods, J. Assoc. Off. Anal. Chem. *54*, 513-516 (1971).
15. M. A. Luke, J. F. Forberg, and H. T. Masumoto, Extraction and cleanup of organochlorine, organophosphate, organonitrogen and hydrocarbon pesticides in produce for determination by gas-liquid chromatography, J. Assoc. Off. Anal. Chem. *58*, 1020-1026 (1975).

16. R. O. Mumma, W. B. Wheeler, and D. E. H. Frear, Dieldrin: extraction of accumulations by root uptake, Science *152*, 530-531 (1966).
17. J. G. Saha, Comparison of several methods for extracting dieldrin-^{14}C from soil, Bull. Environ. Contam. Toxicol. *3*, 26-36 (1968).
18. P. F. Bertuzzi, L. Kamps, and C. I. Miles, Extraction of pesticide residues from nonfatty samples of low moisture content, J. Assoc. Off. Anal. Chem. *50*, 623-627 (1967).
19. J. A. Burke and M. L. Porter, A study of the effectiveness of some extraction procedures for pesticide residues in vegetables, J. Assoc. Off. Anal. Chem. *49*, 1157-1162 (1966).
20. L. R. Snyder, Individual adsorbents, In Principles of Adsorption Chromatography, Marcel Dekker, New York, 1968, pp. 155-184.
21. R. A. Moffitt, Residue analysis in the dairy industry, In Analytical Methods for Pesticides, Plant Growth Regulators, and Food Additives, Vol. 1 (G. Zweig, Ed.), Academic Press, New York, 1963, pp. 545-570.
22. W. B. Wheeler, N. P. Thompson, P. Andrade, and R. T. Krause, Extraction efficiencies for pesticides in crops. 1. [^{14}C]Carbaryl extraction from mustard greens and radishes, J. Agric. Food Chem. *26*, 1333-1337 (1978).
23. M. Beroza and M. C. Bowman, Correlation of pesticide polarities with efficiencies of milk extraction procedures, J. Assoc. Off. Anal. Chem. *49*, 1007-1012 (1966).
24. P. A. Mills, Detection and semiquantitative estimation of chlorinated organic pesticide residues in foods by paper chromatography, J. Assoc. Off. Anal. Chem. *42*, 734-740 (1959).
25. G. M. Doose and M. A. Luke, Private communication.
26. J. E. Lovelock, Electron absorption detectors and technique for use in quantitative and qualitative analysis by gas chromatography, Anal. Chem. *35*, 474-481 (1963).
27. M. A. Luke, J. E. Froberg, G. M. Doose, and H. T. Masumoto, Improved multiresidue gas chromatographic determination of organophosphorus, organonitrogen, and organohalogen pesticides in produce, using flame photometric and electrolytic conductivity detectors, J. Assoc. Off. Anal. Chem. *64*, 1187-1195 (1981).
28. L. R. Jones and J. A. Riddick, Separation of organic insecticides from plant and animal tissues, Anal. Chem. *24*, 569-571 (1952).
29. L. Johnson, Separation of dieldrin and endrin from other chlorinated pesticide residues, J. Assoc. Off. Anal. Chem. *45*, 363-365 (1962).

30. P. A. Mills, B. A. Bong, L. R. Kamps, and J. A. Burke, Elution solvent system for florisil column cleanup in organochlorine pesticide residue analysis, J. Assoc. Off. Anal. Chem. *55*, 39-43 (1972).

31. D. C. Holmes and N. F. Wood, Removal of interferring substances from vegetable extracts prior to the determination of organochlorine pesticide residues, J. Chromatogr. *67*, 173-174 (1972).

32. H. A. McLeod and P. J. Wales, A low temperature cleanup procedure for pesticides and their metabolites in biological samples, J. Agric. Food Chem. *20*, 624-631 (1972).

33. Analytical Methods for Pesticide Residues in Foods, rev. ed. Health Protection Branch, Information Canada, Ottawa, 1973.

34. E. R. Holden, Gas chromatographic determination of residues of methylcarbamate insecticides in crops as their 2,4-dinitrophenyl ether derivative, J. Assoc. Off. Anal. Chem. *56*, 713-717 (1973).

35. K. Remsteiner, W. D. Howmann, and D. O. Eberle, Multiresidue method for the determination of trizaine herbicides in field-grown agricultural crops, water, and soils, J. Assoc. Off. Anal. Chem. *57*, 192-201 (1974).

36. J. R. Mann and S. T. Preston, Selection of preferred liquid phases, J. Chromatog. Sci. *11*, 216-220 (1973).

8
Polynuclear Aromatic Hydrocarbons

PETER W. JONES* Electric Power Research Institute, Palo Alto, California

I. INTRODUCTION

The objectives of this chapter is to critically review the state-of-the-art knowledge relating to the measurement of polycyclic aromatic hydrocarbons (PAHs). Other aspects are addressed only to the extent to which they affect measurement.

Concern regarding environmental contamination by PAHs arises since many of these species have been demonstrated to be carcinogenic to animals and are probably carcinogenic to humans. Furthermore, the adverse occupational health risk associated with high-PAH-exposure industries, such as coking and asphalt production, has been well established. A large number of PAHs were included in the Federal Water Pollution Control Act, and the World Health Organization has recommended maximum levels of PAHs for drinking water, further emphasizing the significance attached to this class of compounds.

II. NOMENCLATURE

Earlier literature concerning PAHs frequently contains ambiguities of nomenclature. These primarily arise because of lack of a consistent ring-carbon numbering system. The currently accepted numbering system is based on International Union of Pure and Applied Chemistry (IUPAC) 1957 nomenclature rules, which state that:

**Present affiliation*: President, Peter Jones & Associates, Morgan Hill, California.

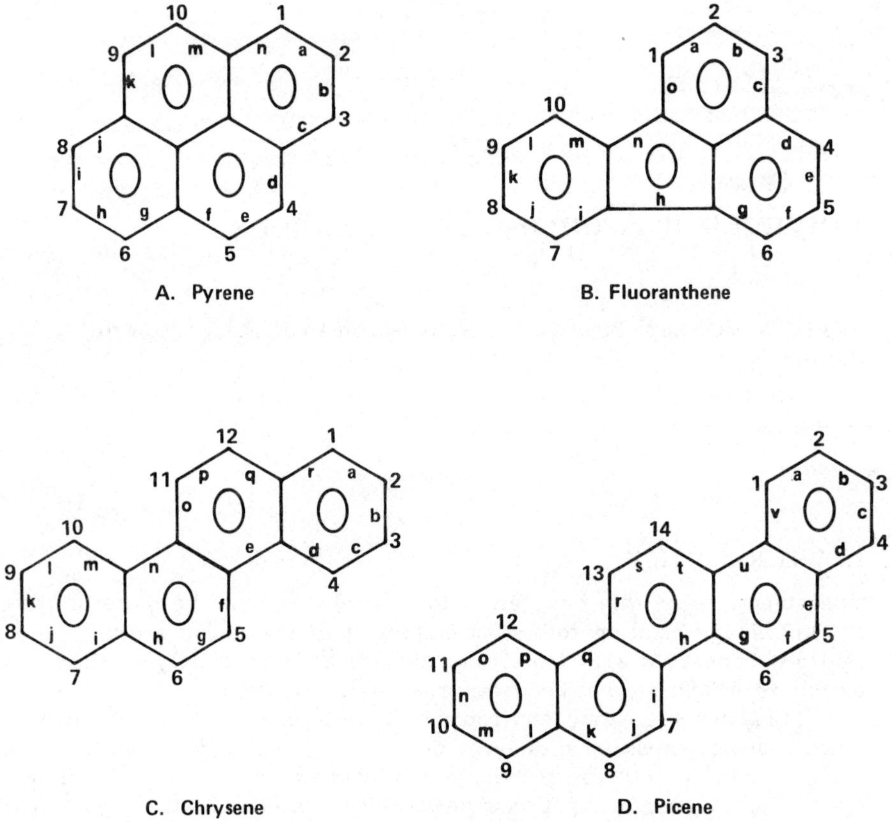

Figure 1 Examples of numbering and lettering for PAHs. (From *Polycyclic Aromatic Hydrocarbons*, NAS Washington, D.C., 1972.)

1. The maximum number of aromatic rings are in a horizontal row.
2. The maximum number of aromatic rings are in the upper right quadrant with respect to the horizontal row.
3. If more than one orientation meets the first two conditions, or more than one horizontal row has the maximum number of rings, the orientation with the minimum number of rings in the lower left quadrant is selected.

The PAH compound is then numbered (Fig. 1) in a clockwise direction beginning with the carbon atom not engaged in ring fusion in the most counterclockwise position of the uppermost ring, or the uppermost ring that is a farthest to the right. Carbon atoms engaged in ring

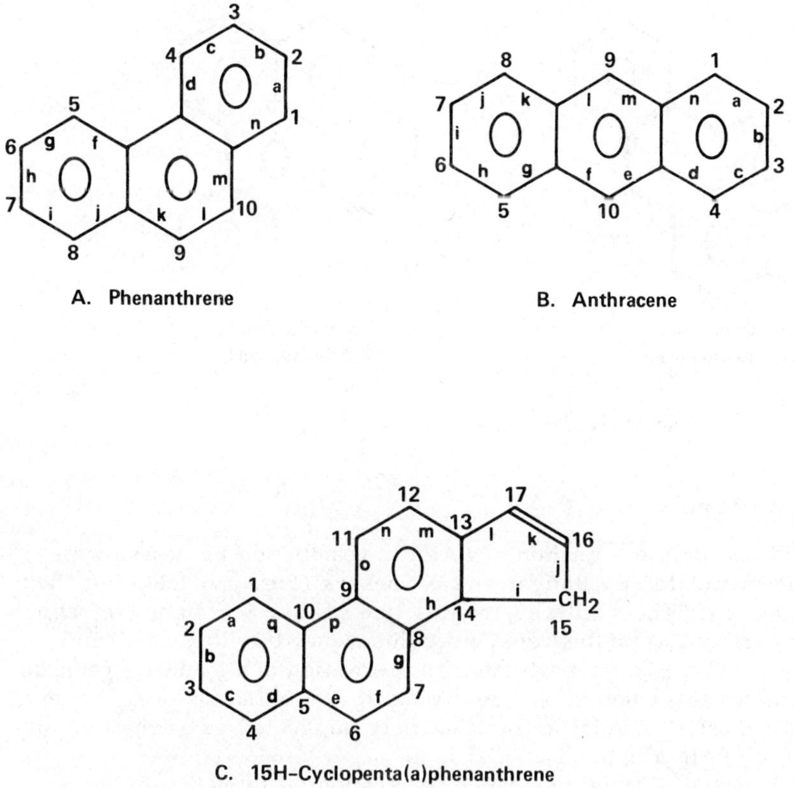

Figure 2 Exceptions to IUPAC nomenclature for PAHs. (From Ref. 1.)

fusion are not numbered. All external sides are numbered clockwise, beginning at the 1,2 side.

There appear [1] to be only three accepted exceptions to the IUPAC nomenclature system for PAHs (Fig. 2), two of the most abundant species, phenanthrene and anthracene, being included in this category.

The names of PAHs that do not have trivial names are obtained by prefixing the name of a component ring system. The component ring system selected must of necessity be part of the compound to be named and must have the maximum number of rings possible. For example, from Figure 1, the benzpyrene isomers are named benz[a]pyrene and benz[e]pyrene (Fig. 3). PAHs whose names are derived in this manner are then numbered and lettered as described above. For substituted PAHs, the point of substitution is indicated by the carbon number preceding the substituted group.

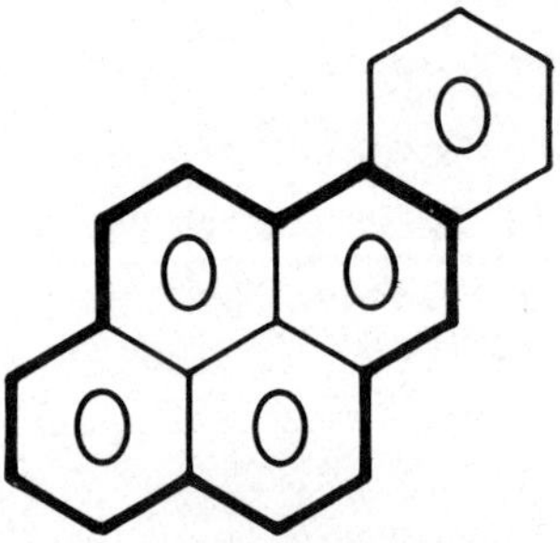

Benz(a)pyrene
(1,2-Benzpyrene)

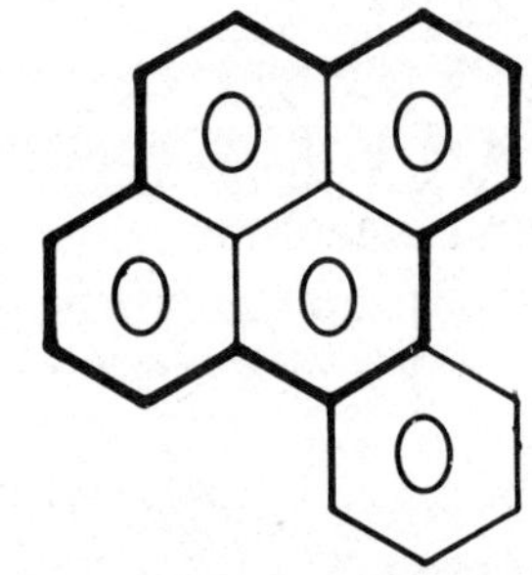

Benz(e)pyrene
(4,5-Benzpyrene)

Figure 3 Nomenclature for benzpyrenes.

III. FORMATION

Mechanisms for the formation of PAHs in combustion processes were initially postulated by Badger and coworkers (Fig. 4A) following their pyrolitic experiments with styrene, 1-phenylbuta-1,3-diene, tetralin, indene, toluene, ethylbenzene, propylbenzene, butylbenzene, and acetylene [2]. Badger postulated the formation of C_2 and C_4 radicals (or diradicals), which subsequently led to the formation of C_6-C_2 and C_6-C_4 radicals. The latter radicals were suggested to be the building blocks for PAH compounds.

Reasonable kinetic evidence for sequential formation of large PAHs from smaller compounds may be derived from the quantitative data reported by Commins [3]. In this work, results for the formation of naphthalene, pyrene, benzpyrenes, and coronene from the pyrolysis of acetylene between 1022 and 1132°F are reported. If graphs of experimentally measured changes in concentration against 1/T are made for these compounds, essentially parallel plots are obtained, exhibiting maxima at about 1440°F. This parallelism implies that the kinetics of formation and disappearance are virtually the same for each PAH, regardless of molecular size. Furthermore, the magnitude of the temperature effect on the rising portion of the plots corresponds to an activation energy of approximately 35 kcal. For the disappearance reaction the activation energy appears to be somewhat higher, so that the disappearance process dominates at higher temperatures. The significance of this interpretation of Commins's data is that despite the range of different PAHs considered, they appear to be formed and destroyed by reactions having similar rate constants. The suggestion by Badger that PAHs may be formed by a recurring additive mechanism is clearly in accord with such kinetics. Phenylacetylene and styrene have been detected in all hydrocarbon flames studied [4] (Fig. 4B), which

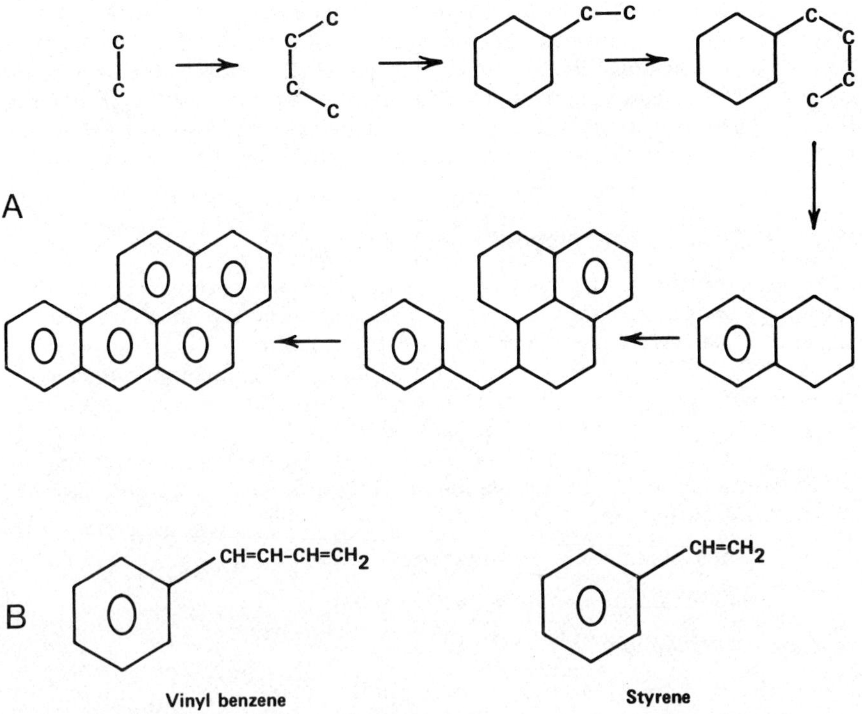

Figure 4 Suggested pathways and known intermediates for PAH formation during combustion. (A) Hypothesis for benz[a]pyrene formation during combustion. (B) Intermediates observed in hydrocarbon flames. (A from Ref. 2.)

further supports the importance of C_6-C_2 and C_6-C_4 species in the Badger mechanism.

In other work with acetylene flames [5], it has been found that two zones of the flame are important to PAH production. The first of these, which may be analogous to the pyrolitic conditions examined by Commins, lies in the rapidly rising temperature portion of the preflame zone, near the end of the blue tip of the flame. The other portion lies in the falling-temperature region of the flame, where temperatures fall from 1650 to 1200°F. Between these two zones, PAH concentration passes through a minimum.

PAH formation in the falling temperature zone may depend upon the persistence of radicals in the combustion gases that can reinitiate a formation process similar to that on the initial pyrolysis zone. If this analogy is valid, the temperature range below 1440 down to 1000°F might be expected to be the range in which most PAH is produced.

On this basis, the PAH content of combustion gases will be constant by the time they have cooled below about 1000°F. Continued cooling will ultimately lead to adsorption of PAH vapors onto particulate matter. The measurement of the PAH content of combustion gases must thus address questions relating to the physical state of the PAH species at the temperature at which they are sampled.

IV. PHYSICAL PROPERTIES

Rather limited data on physical properties are presently available for PAHs, as shown in Table 1. Vapor pressure data appear to be available for only nine PAHs, and varies from $6 \cdot 8 \times 10^{-4}$ to $1 \cdot 5 \times 10^{-12}$ torr [6-8]. Although few quantitative ultraviolet (UV) spectral data have been reported [9], some descriptions of UV and flourescence spectra are included in the section "Analysis of PAHs."

Available relative carcinogenicity ratings are included for convenience in Table 1. These values are taken from Ref. 10 and may be summarized as follows:

-, not carcinogenic, or unknown

±, uncertain or weakly carcinogenic

+, carcinogenic

++, +++, ++++, strongly carcinogenic

V. CHEMICAL REACTIVITY

Chemical reactions of PAHs are important, primarily for their impact in two areas. First, atmospheric reactions such as photooxidation are presumed to be the major route for removal of these species. Second, to achieve reliable measurement of PAHs, it is important to avoid or take into account any reactions that are a function of the measurement system, which may lead to their loss. The low vapor pressure of PAHs has, with few exceptions, restricted reaction studies to the liquid phase. This section makes no attempt to cover all aspects of PAH chemical reactivity but rather will address primarily those reactions that are most likely to affect PAH measurement. Detailed reviews of PAH chemistry have appeared elsewhere [9,11].

A. Photooxidation

Most workers have attempted to simulate atmospheric solar radiation (>300 nm) in laboratory studies of PAH photooxidation. Kuratsune and Hirohata [12] photolyzed 13 PAHs in both cyclohexane and dichloromethane with sunlight and with fluorescent lamps filtered to provide wavelengths longer than 300 nm. They found that naphthacene was the most unstable of the PAHs examined, and that benz[a]pyrene and alkyl benz[a]anthracenes were photoreactive. The following compounds were apparently stable under the experimental conditions: phenanthrene, fluorene, pyrene, fluoranthene, chrysene, benz[a] anthracene, and benz[k]fluoranthene. Subsequent photooxidation of benz[a]pyrene in benzene (>280 nm) [13] allowed the isolation of 6,12-, 1,6-, and 3,6-quinones.

Environmental PAHs are frequently adsorbed on particulate materials; several studies of photolysis of PAHs on substrates have been made. Inscoe [14] examined photooxidation of PAHs during thin layer chromatography by exposing PAHs adsorbed on four different adsorbents (silica gel G, aluminum oxide G, cellulose powder, and acetylated cellulose) to ultraviolet light and ordinary room light. No changes were noted for phenanthrene, chrysene, triphenylene, and picene, but pronounced changes were detected for other compounds when silica gel and aluminum oxide were used; less dramatic changes were found with the other two adsorbents. Exposure to ordinary room light gave slower but similar results. Photosensitive PAHs were anthracene, naphthacene, benz[a]anthracene, dibenz[a,c]anthracene, dibenz[a,h]anthracene, pyrene, benz[a]pyrene, benz[e]pyrene, perylene, benz[ghi]perylene, and coronene. 1,6-Pyrenedione and 1,8-pyrenedione were identified as photoproducts of pyrene.

Tebbens [15] deposited benz[a]pyrene on various filters from ether solution, and examined the results of photooxidation by real or simulated sunlight. Significant losses of this compound were noted. The reactivity of benz[a]pyrene and perylene in smoke passed through a 22 ft Pyrex flow chamber was examined in the presence and absence of light. It was found that irradiation caused the disappearance of 35 to 65% of the original PAH content, and that oxygen increased the rate of PAH disappearance.

Thomas et al. demonstrated the importance of high surface area for the photooxidation of benz[a]pyrene [16]. Using a light source which was estimated to have one-fourth of the intensity of the noon July sun, benz[a]pyrene in emissions from a furnace was significantly reduced following residence on an illuminated flow chamber. However, benz[a]pyrene adsorbed on 220 and 28 μm glass beads exposed in agitated flasks was insignificantly photooxidized.

Lane and Katz have pointed out that many earlier experiments were not truly representative of atmospheric photochemistry, since ozone concentrations were too high and the light sources used were poor simulations of sunlight [17]. They studied the reactivity of 500 ng aliquots of benz[a]pyrene, benz[b]fluoranthene, and benz[k] fluoranthene distributed as thin films on a petri dish, exposed to a few ppm of ozone and irradiated by a Quartzline lamp. The results showed that benz[a]pyrene was by far the most reactive, having a half life of less than an hour in various ozone concentrations in both dark

Table 1 Physical Properties of PAHs, Carcinogenicity Rating

Compound	Molecular weight	M.P./B.P. (°C)	Vapor pressure (torr STP)	λ_{max} (nm)/ log e (solvent)	Carcinogenicity
Fluorene	166	115/294	-	309/2.40, 314/2.48, 323/2.54, 330/2.52, 337/3.40, 345/3.46 (ethanol/methanol)	-
Acenaphthene	154	96/278	-	-	-
Anthracene	178	217/340	1.95×10^{-4}	-	-
Phenanthrene	178	100/340	6.8×10^{-4}	308/3.15, 323/3.47, 338/3.75, 355/3.86, 375/3.87 (ethanol/methanol)	-
2-Methylfluorene	180	85/318	-	-	-
3-Methylfluorene	180	104/318	-	-	-
2-Methylanthracene	192	207/360	-	-	-
1-Methylphenanthrene	192	119/354	-	-	-
3-Methylphenanthrene	192	65/350	-	-	-
9-Methylphenanthrene	192	92/354	-	-	-
2,7-Dimethylanthracene	206	225/-	-	-	-
Fluoranthrene	202	109/382	-	-	-
Pyrene	202	149/393	6.85×10^{-7}	-	-

Chrysene	228	250/440	-	344/2.88, 351/2.62, 360/3.00 (ethanol)	±
Benz[a]anthracene	228	159/400	1.10×10^{-7}	314/3.67, 327/3.81, 341/3.87, 359/3.72, 376/3.73, 386/3.86 (ethanol)	+
7,12-Dimethylbenz[a] anthracene	256	122/-	-	296/4.90, 345/3.83, 364/394, 384/3.83 (ethanol)	++++
Naphthacene	228	350/-	-	-	-
Triphenylene	228	199/-	-	-	-
Benz[c]phenanthrene	228	68/-	-	296/4.13, 303/4.07, 315/4.06, 325/3.07, 353/2.63, 372/2.38 (ethanol)	+++
Benz[a]fluorene	216	189/-	-	-	-
Benz[b]fluorene	216	208/415	-	-	-
Benz[c]fluorene	216	188/413	-	-	-
Aceanthrylene	204	113/-	-	-	-
Perylene	252	265/500	-	-	-
Benz[a]pyrene	252	179/-	5.49×10^{-9}	296/4.76, 330/3.76, 347/4.12, 364/4.38, 384/4.48, 403/3.60 (ethanol)	+++
Benz[e]pyrene	252	179/-	5.54×10^{-9}	-	-
Picene	278	364/520	-	-	-
Benz[a]naphthacene	278	425/-	-	-	-

Table 1 (Continued)

Compound	Molecular weight	M.P./B.P. (°C)	Vapor pressure (torr STP)	λ_{max} (nm)/ log e (solvent)	Carcinogenicity
Dibenz[a,j]anthracene	278	-	-	-	-
Dibenz[a,h]anthracene	278	266/-	-	299/5.2, 322/4.28, 335/4.23, 350/4.16, 374/3.00, 384/2.61 (dioxane)	+++
Dibenz[a,c]anthracene	278	-	-	-	+
Dibenz[a,h]fluorane	266	-	-	-	±
Dibenz[a,g]fluorene	266	-	-	-	+
Dibenz[a,c]fluorene	266	-	-	-	-
Dibenz[a,c]fluorene	266	-	-	-	±
Benz[b]fluoranthene	252	167/-	-	-	++
Benz[j]fluoranthene	252	166/-	-	-	-

Benz[k]fluoranthene	252	215/-	9.59×10^{-11}	-	-
Benz[g,h,i]fluoranthene	250	-	-	-	-
Cholanthrene	254	-	-	-	++
3-Methylcholanthrene	268	179/-	-	-	++++
Dibenz[a,l]pyrene	302	-	-	-	±
Dibenz[a,h]pyrene	302	320/-	-	290/4.54, 301/694, 313/5.23, 379/3.60, 401/4.03, 424/4.40, 451/4.59 (benzene)	+++
Dibenz[a,i]pyrene	302	281/-	-	-	+++
Dibenz[cd,jk]pyrene	276	257/-	-	-	-
Indeno[1,2,3-cd]pyrene	276	-	-	-	+
Benz[ghi]perylene	276	273/-	1.01×10^{-10}	-	-
Coronene	300	438/525	1.47×10^{-12}	-	-

Source: *Health Assessment for Polycyclic Organic Matter*, EPA, May 1978.

and illuminated experiments. Illumination caused a significant decrease in the half lives for all the PAHs.

Very few useful data are available on the oxidation of PAHs; some studies which attempted to examine storage lives in air, and attribute losses to oxidation, were more likely subject to loss of PAH through volatilization [18]. The recent work by Lane and Katz [17] does, however, demonstrate the susceptibility of PAHs to oxidation in the absence of light, as noted earlier.

Thus while the photooxidative data are somewhat fragmentary and have been reported for widely differing experimental conditions, photooxidation of PAHs is clearly important. Degradation in the atmosphere is expected to be substantial, but probably ranges widely for different PAH compounds. Although this generalization appears to be in conflict with the finding of Lunde and Bjørseth [19], who reported on long-range atmospheric transport of PAHs, the experimental uncertainity associated with such studies may be large, while selected PAHs may in fact have greater stability. Notwithstanding, the physical state of atmospheric PAHs, which may depend on the nature of the substrate on which they are adsorbed, may profoundly affect ambient photooxidation.

One of the most critical aspects of PAH photooxidation seems to be often overlooked. True, photooxidation is probably the primary mechanism for removal of PAHs from the atmosphere, but concern regarding the nature of the photoproducts is seldom raised. The most likely photooxidation products from PAHs are known to include quinones, expoxides, phenols, and dihydrodiols, yet some of these are the very species that are implicated as the true carcinogens in PAH carcinogenisis; all of these species are produced from the incubation of PAH with human lymphocytes [20]. Thus the photooxidative destruction of PAH may simply be producing vast quantities of true carcinogens. This aspect of PAH reactivity should clearly be the subject of further research.

Finally, the implications of photooxidation for the measurement of PAHs indicate that stringent care must be taken to store, handle, and analyze all samples for PAHs in the absence of UV light. Experience has shown that the use of gold fluorescent lighting adequately meets this requirement in the laboratory.

B. Chlorination

Chlorination is commonly used at water treatment facilities for the production of drinking water. There is thus considerable interest in the effect of chlorination on PAHs present in untreated drinking water and in any effects this may have on attempts to measure PAHs in treated drinking water.

When chlorine gas is dissolved in water, the following equilibrium is established, hypochlorous acid being the effective chlorinating agent:

$$Cl_2 + H_2O \rightleftharpoons HOCl + HCl$$

The further dissociation of HOCl is clearly pH dependent.

Measurements of 12 PAH compounds (fluoranthene, pyrene, benz[a]anthracene, chrysene, benz[b]fluoranthene, benz[j]fluoranthene, benz[k]fluoranthene, benz[a]pyrene, benz[e]pyrene, perylene, indeno[1,2,3-cd]pyrene, and benz[ghi]perylene) through each stage of a water treatment facility, where effective chlorine was reported to be about 10 ppm [21], shows the effective reaction of PAHs to be about 50 to 75%. For example, benz[a]pyrene was reduced from 0.03 to 0.009 μg 1 liter, and chrysene was reduced from 0.033 to 0.012 μg 1 liter. Laboratory studies by Harrison et al. [21] show slightly higher reaction rates for PAHs; the typical PAH concentration used was about 0.1 ppb, chlorine concentration was varied from zero to about 12 ppm, and reaction times were up to 25 min.

A recent sample preservation study [22] for 16 PAHs (including all compounds studied by Harrison et al. [21], in which approximately 0.4 ppb of each PAH was exposed to about 2 ppm chlorine for 7 days, gave somewhat different results. This work showed significant (>50%) reaction only for benz[a]pyrene, aceanthrylene, anthracene, and benz[a]anthracene, at both pH 2 and 7; other PAHs shown less clear or insignificant reduction with chlorine exposure.

Thus, while both the specific PAHs reaction to chlorine and the extent of the reaction are not precisely delineated, chlorination does appear to react significantly with PAH compounds in water. Thus, in designing programs for the measurement of PAHs in chlorinated water, appropriate precautions must be taken to avoid further reaction of the samples collected.

C. Action of Nitrogen and Sulfur Oxides

PAHs are particularly sensitive to both oxidation and electrophilic substitution. Nitrogen oxides or dilute nitric acid react with anthracene to form anthraquinone [23] (Fig. 5A), while sulfur dioxide in the presence of oxygen and UV light (>300 nm) has been shown to oxidize 9-methylanthracene to 9-anthraldehyde [24] (Fig. 5B). Nitrogen dioxide substitutes in anthracene to yield 9-nitroanthracene [25] (Fig. 5C), while benz[a]pyrene has been shown to react in high yield with 2 ppm of nitrogen dioxide on a filter to yield 6-nitrobenz[a]pyrene [26] (Fig. 5D). Pyrene is readily sulfonated by concentrated sulfonic acid to give a mixture of disulfonic acids [27] (Fig. 5E).

The main significance of such reactions when attempting to measure PAH in liquids, as vapors, or as particulates, is that nitrogen

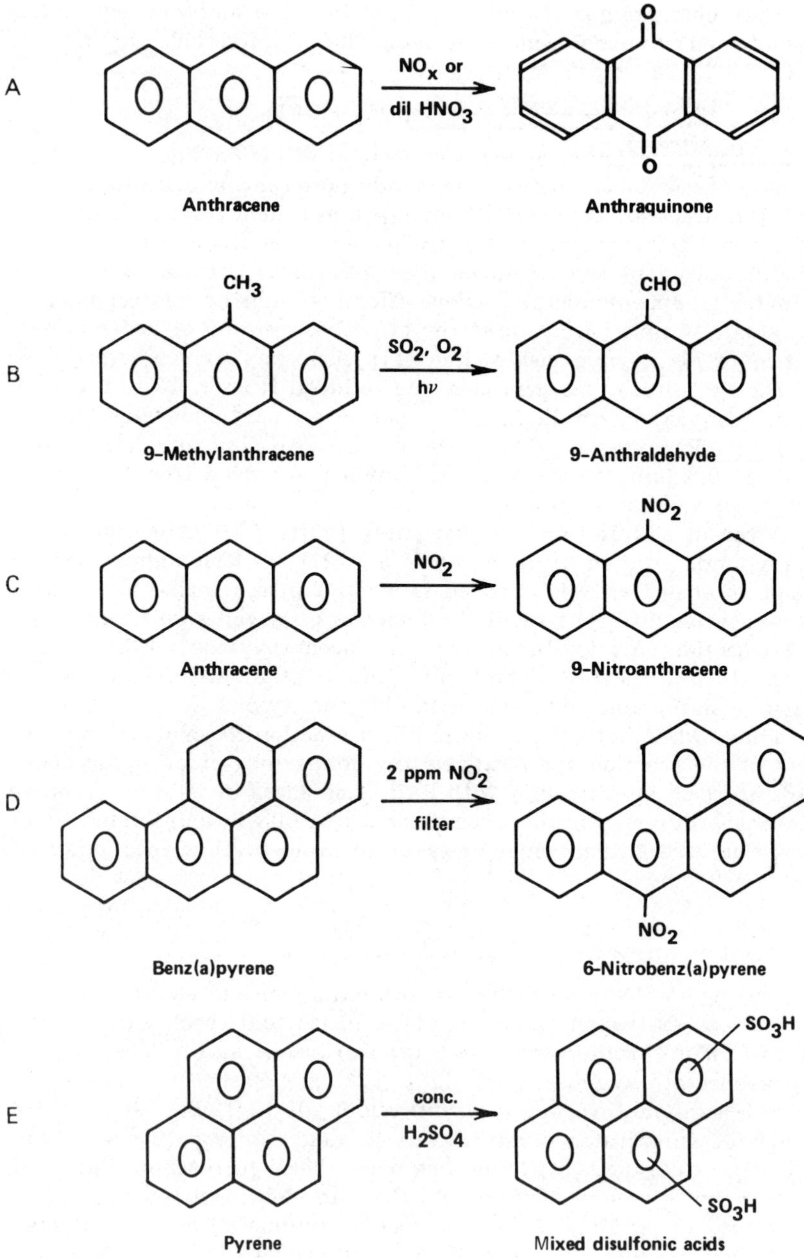

Figure 5 Reactions of PAHs with nitrogen and sulfur oxides. (A, C-E from *Polycyclic Aromatic Hydrocarbons*, NAS, Washington, D.C., 1972.)

and sulfur oxides occur very widely and may readily interfere with truly representative sample collection.

VI. SAMPLING FOR PAHs

PAHs occur widely throughout the environment, both as a result of human technological activities and as a result of natural production [28]. The PAH load resulting from natural production is difficult to assess; however, assuming that emission of benz[a]pyrene represents 1% of the total environmental PAH load, worldwide PAH production may be estimated as follows (tons per year) [28]:

Heating and power generation	260,000
Industrial processes	105,000
Incineration and open burning	135,000
Vehicular transportation	4,500
Total PAH emissions	504,500

As a result, occasions for PAH measurement arise from all environmental media and under a variety of industrial and other technological conditions. Consequently consideration of sampling parameters is most usefully broken into several categories: stack gases, ambient air, automobile exhaust, and aqueous systems.

A. Stack Gases

Sampling is perhaps the most critical stage in the measurement of organic species in stack gases; in the absence of a reproducible and quantitative sampling procedure, sophisticated and sensitive analytical procedures are of no value. The objective of this section is to examine the parameters necessary for the efficient collection of PAHs from stack gases.

There are several fundamental requirements of any sampling system for organic materials present in stack gases if the subsequent analytical data are to be meaningful.

1. Organic compounds of interest must be quantitatively collected.
2. The integrity of the sample must be preserved.
3. The sampling system must be amenable to quantitative sample recovery in a manner appropriate for subsequent analysis.
4. The capacity of the sampling system must enable sufficient sample to be quantitatively collected for whatever analytical technique is to be applied.

Either through lack of concern, or an inability to overcome technical difficulties, little progress has been made until recently toward the development of a sampling system that would satisfactorily meet these requirements.

Early sampling methods

Among the earliest collection methods employed were those which made use of filtration combined with impinger systems. Although such techniques may give efficient collection of particulate, losses of organic vapors would appear to be inevitable. This feature was highlighted by Stenberg [29], who made use of a filter, impingers containing xylene, and cold traps for the collection of combustion effluents, with special concern for benz[a]pyrene. At high filter temperatures (>300°F) significant losses of benzo[a]pyrene were reported, but at cooler filter temperatures (<95°F) more efficient collection was reported. At the higher temperature range a substantial portion of the benz[a]pyrene would be present on the vapor phase, while at the lower temperature particulate formation would be favored; accordingly, much of the benz[a]pyrene would be retained on the filter at low temperature, but at the higher temperatures, both filter and the impingers were unable to trap the vapor effectively.

The most widely used impinger method for the collection of PAHs from stack gases used to be EPA Method 5 [30,31], a technique designed for the collection of particulate material which was first published in the Federal Register in 1971. Unfortunately, Method 5 was never intended for the collection of organics; it has poor efficiency for collection of vapors, and sample recovery is at best difficult. Nevertheless, a large number of PAH measurement programs have been carried out on stack gases using this method; all of the data from these must unfortunately be regarded as questionable.

A more recent program for the development of a method for sampling PAHs and polychlorinated biphenyls (PCBs) from combustion effluent led to a modified Method 5 utilizing xylene impinger cooled with dry ice [32]. The prescribed technique for sample recovery from the impingers and filters extract would preclude accurate quantification, since this involved evaporation of the sample to dryness followed by redissolution in xylene. While removal of excess solvent from a sample extract always presents the risk of sample loss, evaporation of a sample solution to dryness will lead to significant loss of PAH materials. This sampling system was used on a study of the emissions of PCBs from incineration of domestic refuse [33]; although other experimental difficulties prevented meaningful data from being obtained, no attempt was made to validate the sampling system.

Attempts have been made to collect stack gas samples by using evacuated containers or collapsible bags [34]. Such methods will undoubtedly provide quantitative collection, but are characterized by

Table 2 PAH Emissions from Coke Oven Doors[a]

Compound	Filter	Adsorber
Indene	-	100.0
Naphthalene	-	350.0
Methyl naphthalene	-	200.0
Acenaphthalene	-	120.0
Biphenyl	-	60.0
Methyl biphenyl	-	60.0
Anthracene	7.0	30.0
Fluoranthene	22.0	10.0
Pyrene	15.0	10.0
Methyl pyrenes/fluoranthenes	6.0	1.0
Benzphenanthrenes	6.0	0.5
Chrysene	31.0	0.7
Methyl chrysene	6.0	-
Dibenzanthracenes	3.0	-
Benzfluoranthenes	22.0	-
Benzpyrenes	16.0	-
Methyl benzpyrenes/fluoranthenes	1.5	-
Indenopyrenes	6.0	-
Benzperylenes	6.0	-
Coronene	1.5	-

[a]mg/hr; 120°F sample collection.

large sample losses to the container walls. Another major drawback is the small volume of gas collected in this manner, which would result in very low analytical sensitivity.

Within the last three years, a new concept in stack sampling for organic materials has come into increasingly common use. A combination of conventional filtration with collection of organic vapors by means of a high-surface-area polymetric adsorbent has proved highly efficient for collection of all but the more volatile organic species. The necessity for sampling systems of this type, where both particulate and vapor phase PAHs are collected, may be illustrated by early sampling experiments of this nature.

A filter and a Tenax GC adsorbent sampler were used in series to collect volatile emission from coke oven doors [35]. In this program the filter temperature was approximately 120°F; the analytical data for one experiment are shown in Table 2. Since the filter temperature was relatively low, the majority of the PAH species, particularly the higher molecular weight compounds, were collected on the filter. However, the more volatile two- and three-ring species were predominantly collected as vapor.

In a further study where a similar sampling system was used to collect PAHs from simulated forest fire conditions [36] and the filter temperature was about 80°F, over 95% of the PAHs were collected on the filter.

Thus, in view of the clear importance attached to filter temperature on the distribution of PAHs between the filter and the adsorber, a semiquantitative series of experiments to examine the distribution of PAHs in the sampling system was carried out during the sampling of an asphalt production facility [37]. The data derived from this work are illustrated schematically in Figure 6 and clearly highlight the importance of considering both the particulate and vapor-phase PAHs in any sampling program.

These data are in entire agreement with the theoretical considerations explored by Natusch and Tomkins [38]. Calculations indicate that PAHs would almost certainly exist as vapors at temperatures above 300°F in stack gases, and that at ambient temperatures (up to 80°F) essentially quantitative adsorbtion to particulates would be expected.

Appropriate selection of filter temperature will permit sample to be collected so as to represent the state of PAHs in the source sampled. For example, if a 400°F stack is sampled with a probe and filter temperature of 400°F, the distribution of PAH collected should reasonably approximate the state of PAHs existing in the stack at that temperature.

The earliest sampling systems making use of both particulate filtration and vapor adsorbtion by polymeric resins were modifications of EPA Method 5 in which the polymeric adsorbent was located between the heated filter and the conventional impingers. The first reported sampler of this type was developed at Battelle Columbus Laboratories [39] and is shown in Figure 7. The stack gases are sampled isokinetically by a sampling probe and passed through a heated filter, as described in EPA Method 5. Immediately after leaving the hot filter, the emissions pass into the cooling coil (120×0.8 cm) of the adsorbent sampler and then pass through a Pyrex frit and into a cylindrical (7×3 cm) column of adsorbent. The flow rate through this first adsorbent sampler was typically 14 liters/min. The cooling coil and

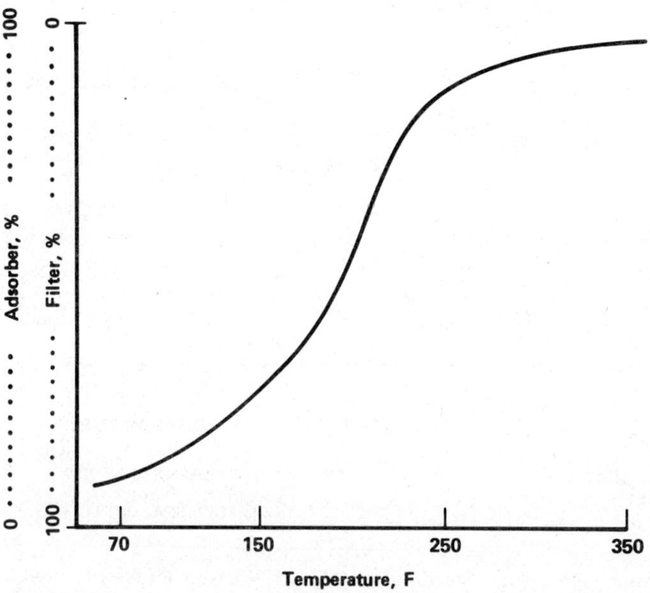

Figure 6 PAH distribution between particulates and vapor (schematic).

Tenax adsorbent are maintained at a constant known temperature by means of a thermostated circulating water bath. The incoming gases are cooled to maintain adsorbent efficiency, yet the adsorbent is maintained above ambient temperature to preclude condensation of the large quantities of water vapor present in all combustion effluents. The gases leaving the sampler are drawn through an aqueous impinger, Drierite trap, and dry gas meter by a Gast-0522 vacuum pump (as in Method 5 sampling). Thus this adsorbent sampling system consisted of the standard EPA train with the adsorbent sampler located between the filter and the impingers. With this system, filterable particulates can be determined from the filter catch and the probe wash according to Method 5, whereas the PAHs and organic materials present can be determined from analysis of the filterable particulates and the adsorbent sampler catch. The impingers are used only to cool the stream and protect the dry gas meter, and their contents are discarded. A schematic diagram illustrating the use of such a sampling system is shown in Figure 8. The adsorbent sampler was designed to collect sufficient sample for organic analysis; quantification of known species from stack gases may routinely be carried out at the ppt level, or lower, through use of an appropriate analytical technique.

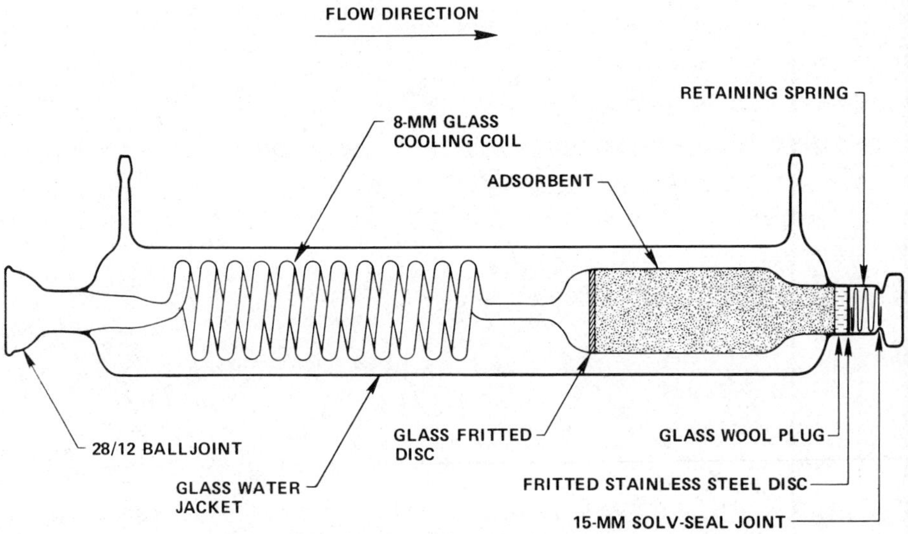

Figure 7 Adsorbent sampling system for PAHs. [From Ref. 39, reprinted with permission from P. W. Jones, R. D. Giammar, P. E. Strup, and T. B. Stanford, Environ. Sci. Technol. *10*, 806 (1976).]

Adsorbent sampler laboratory validation studies

Preliminary laboratory validation studies involved setting up a Battelle Adsorbent Sampler to collect air drawn through a 500°F tube furnace. A precisely measured quantity of polynuclear compounds in a few microliters of methylene chloride solution was then injected into the inlet of the adsorbent sampler, and heated air was passed through the system for at least 1 hr. Following solvent extraction of the sampler, a suitable internal standard was added, and analysis for the spiked PAHs were made by gas chromatography-mass spectrometry (GC-MS).

Preliminary experiments were carried out to determine the most suitable solvent for extraction of the adsorbent sampler. Extraction was attempted with methylene chloride, acetone, methyl alcohol, p-dioxane, pentane, cyclohexane, benzene, and toluene. Only saturated hydrocarbons proved entirely suitable for Tenax because of its partial solubility in more polar solvents; and pentane was selected because of its high volatility, which minimizes sample loss during solvent concentration. Methylene chloride was selected for use with XAD-2; both resins may be extracted with methyl alcohol for recovery of polar species.

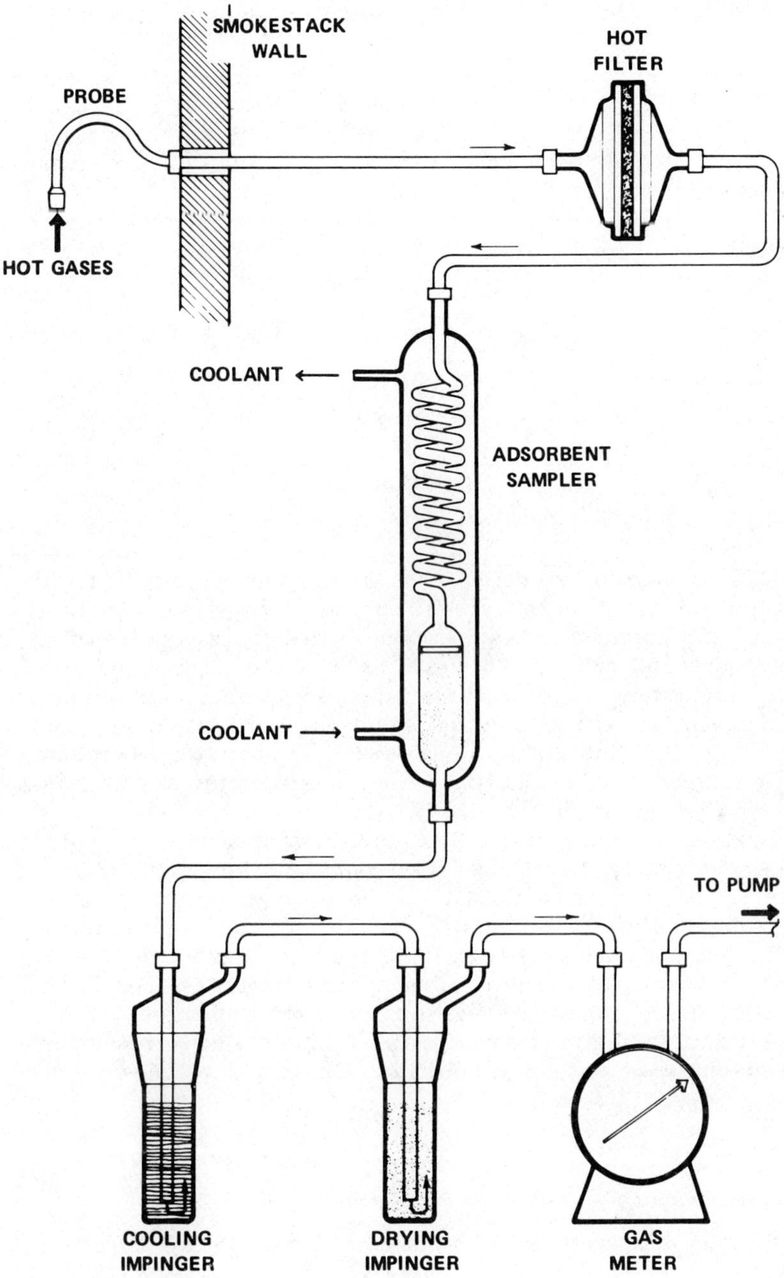

Figure 8 Schematic of combustion effluent sampling system.

Table 3 Recovery of PAH from Adsorbent Sampler as Determined by GC-MS

Compound	Spiked (μg)	Sample 1 average recovery (%)	Sample 2 average recovery (%)	Sample 3 average recovery (%)
Pyrene	10	91 ± 3	98 ± 4	104 ± 4
Chrysene	10	90 ± 5	92 ± 5	106 ± 5
Perylene	10	91 ± 4	105 ± 5	102 ± 6
Benz[ghi]perylene	10	101 ± 10	106 ± 10	103 ± 7
Coronene	10	80 ± 7	92 ± 8	100 ± 14

Source: Ref. 46.

The subsequent validation experiments were carried out with the sampler at 130°F using pyrene, chrysene, perylene, benz[ghi] perylene, and coronene; these compounds are representative of commonly encountered PAH species. Each of these compounds (10 μg) was separately sampled over a 2 hr period; following pentane extraction and addition of internal standard, the PAHs were quantified by GC-MS. The results of several representative laboratory validation experiments demonstrate the validity of the sampling technique, and are given in Table 3.

Further laboratory validation studies were carried out, which more closely simulated real stack gas conditions [40]. In this study, prepurified air was heated to 400°F; precisely known quantities of nitric oxide, sulfur dioxide, water vapor, and PAHs and other organic compounds were added; and the resultant gases were passed through an adsorbent sampler. The specific variables used in this study were chosen to reflect extremes normally encountered under actual stack sampling, to challenge the sampling system realistically under precisely measurable conditions. The variables chosen were:

Sulfur dioxide	200 and 2000 ppm
Nitric oxide	150, 500, and 1500 ppm
Water vapor	2, 4, and 8% by volume
Sampler temperature	80, 105, 130, 155, and 180°F
Organic compound level	10 and 50 μg

To elucidate the effects, if any, of both individual variables and combinations of variables, two fractional factorial statistical experimental designs were selected. The results demonstrated that none of the variables listed were statistically significant for the sampling of PAHs, and quantitative recoveries were achieved within the limits of uncertainty.

A parallel laboratory validation study of the Adsorbent Sampler has been carried out by the IIT Research Institute [41]. In this work, constant concentration atmospheres of anthracene and benz[a] pyrene were generated and subsequently sampled. Recoveries of these compounds from the sampler averaged 90%; any minor losses were attributed to the sample recovery step.

Field validation experiment—analysis of PAH effluent from a secondary leader smelter

The objectives of this field validation study was to investigate the reproducibility of the adsorbent sampling system. A normal Method 5 sampling probe and filter were used, following which the gas stream was split in two and identical gas volumes were drawn through two separate samplers [42]. The results of separate PAH analyses from two separate experiments (run 1 and run 2) are given in Table 4. The close agreement between 1A and 1B, and between 2A and 2B, demonstrates the very good reproducibility of the entire sampling and analytical procedures.

Table 4 PAH Emissions from a Secondary Lead Smelter (ng)

Compound	1A	1B	2A	2B
Anthracene-phenanthrene	1900	2400	2100	2600
Methyl anthracenes	80	110	110	90
Fluoranthene	500	560	900	850
Pyrene	100	72	77	82
Methyl pyrenes-fluoranthenes	5	7	8	6
Benzo[c]phenanthrene	33	36	47	37
Chrysene-benz[a]anthracene	78	76	77	69
Benz[a]pyrene	3	4	3	3

Source: Ref. 46.

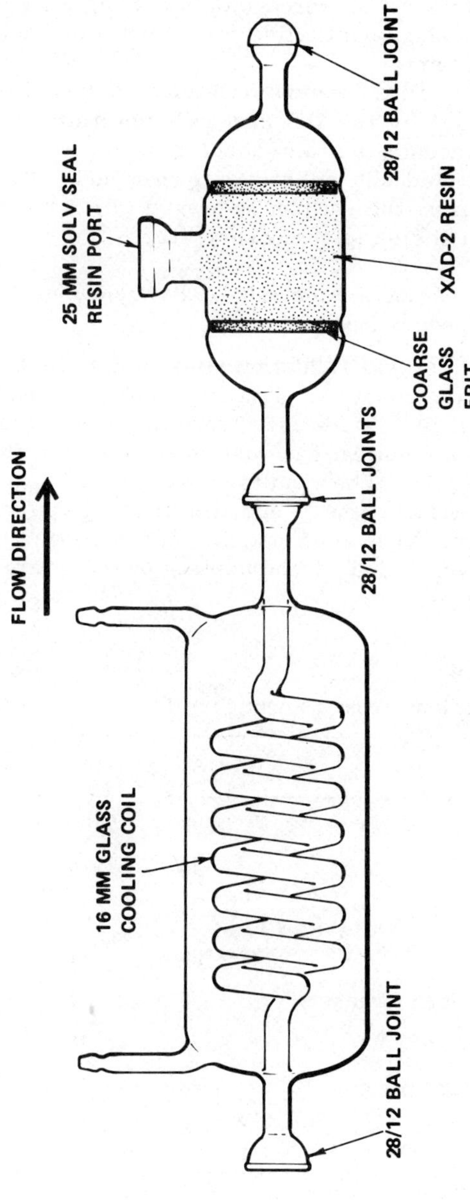

Figure 9 High capacity adsorbent sampling system for PAHs.

High-capacity stack gas sampling systems for PAHs

A high-capacity version of the adsorbent sampling system described above has been developed, which is capable of flow rates up to 6 scfm for at least 8 hr at 130°F. This sampling system, which is shown in Figure 9, was subjected to field and laboratory validation studies in a program for the Electric Power Research Institute. Results have demonstrated reasonable recovery of internal standards which are added through a probe-tip injector during a stack sampling experiment [43].

In view of the apparent success of filtration-adsorbtion sampling systems for organic materials in stack gases, the Environmental Protection Agency (EPA) developed the Source Assessment Sampling System (SASS) for the collection of particulate and volatile materials. This sampling system described in detail in two EPA reports [44,45], is summarized here.

The SASS train consists of a stainless steel probe which enters a thermostated oven containing three series cyclones and a filter holder. The cyclones facilitate collection of particulates in the following size fractions: >10 μm, 3 to 10 μm, 1 to 3 μm; a 142 mm filter collects the <1 μm particulate size fraction. Following the oven containing the cyclones and filter, volatile organic materials are collected in a sorbent trap containing XAD-2 resin; a vessel for the collection of any condensate is provided directly below the XAD-2 trap. After exiting the sorbent trap, the gases pass through an oxidative impinger system for the collection of volatile inorganic materials, before exiting the system through a 10 scfm pump and dry gas meter. The EPA SASS train has a nominal flow rate of 3 to 5 scfm. A schematic diagram of the EPA SASS train is shown in Figure 10.

The EPA SASS train promises to be a particularly effective sampling system for source assessment studies in view of the relatively large amount of material that may be obtained for both chemical analysis and bioassay studies; it has been proposed that an acceptable sample size for the SASS train will be 30 scfm [44,45], which is equivalent to approximately 6 to 8 hr of sampling. Additionally, the size fractionation of the particulate material may permit the association of hazardous materials with a particular size range, which could provide valuable input to emission control strategies.

It should, however, be borne in mind that the entire SASS train must be subjected to laboratory and field validation for collection of hazardous materials of concern. Validation data and acceptable operating parameters which have been obtained for the 0.5 and 5 scfm Battelle Adsorbent Samplers [39,40,43] may serve as a guide for the operation of the SASS XAD-2 sorbent trap.

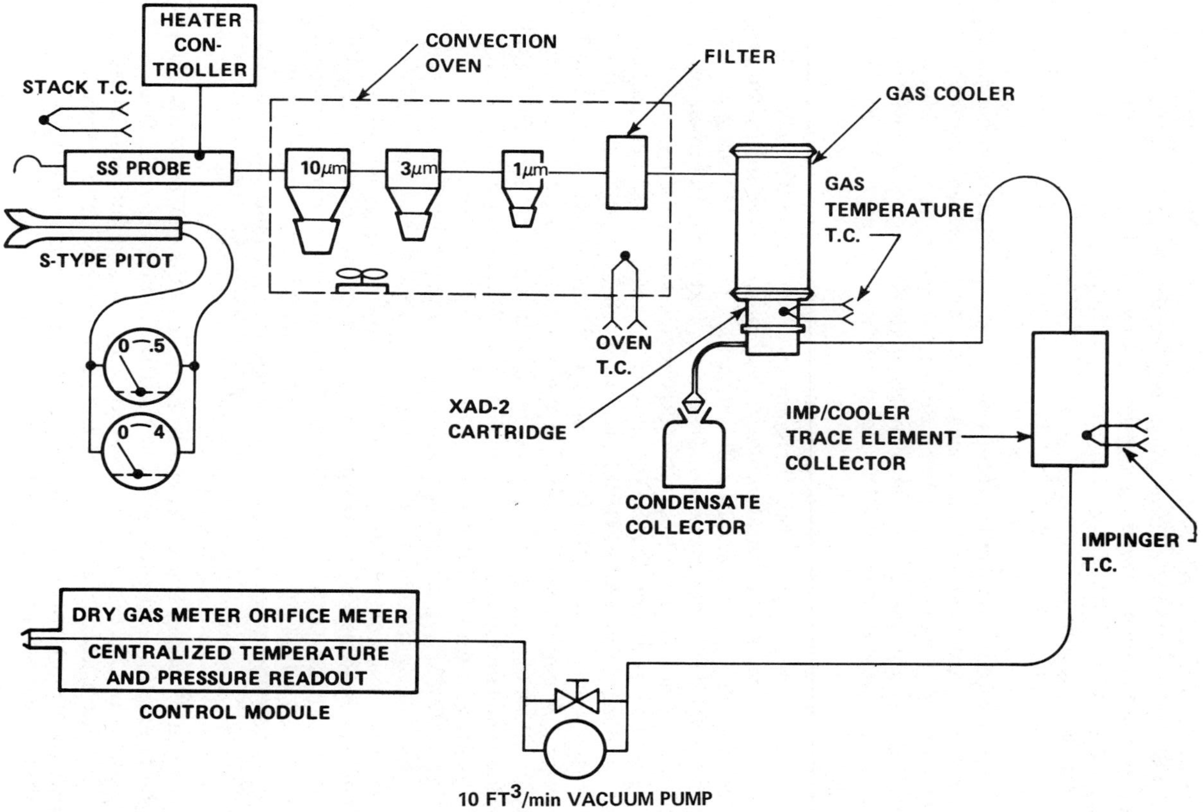

Figure 10 Source assessment sampling schematic. (From Refs. 45 and 46.)

Selection of substrate for adsorbent sampling

Adsorbtion of organic materials present in gaseous and aqueous media on macroreticular resins, and subsequently eluting the trapped material with solvent, is the subject of increasing study. The resins most widely used have been Tenax [46-48], XAD resins [49,50], and polyurethane foam [51,52]. The appropriate choice of resin has very often been made from an empirical standpoint, experimental parameters being verified by laboratory simulation studies prior to in-field analyses.

A recent study [53] to characterize the behavior of different resins used in adsorbent samplers showed that XAD-2 has a greater volumetric and weight capacity than Tenax GC resin. XAD-2 appears to have been efficiency than Tenax GC for lower-boiling organic species, but their efficiency in regard to PAH collection was found to be similar.

The most important considerations in the selection of a resin material are:

1. The capacity of the resin, breakthrough volume
2. The selectivity of the resin toward compounds sought
3. The possibility of contamination from the resin
4. The compatibility of the resin with eluting solvents, or thermal stability during thermal desorbtion
5. The resin must be amenable to quantitative sample recovery in a manner compatible with subsequent analytical techniques
6. Particle size and permissible flow rate

A combination of two or more different resins may prove desirable for efficient collection of a wider polarity range of organic species than for PAHs, which are considered in this chapter. In designing appropriate adsorbent traps for water sampling, it has been pointed out that a predictive model for adsorbtion may be based upon the aqueous solubility of the organic compounds sought [50].

XAD-2 and Tenax have been among the most widely used resins. Tenax has several disadvantages, including its incompatibility (soluble) with most nonhydrocarbon solvents and the difficulty of eliminating background contamination. Studies [54] using Fourier transform infrared spectroscopy (FT-IR) and GC-MS have shown that a much cleaner blank may be obtained upon the extraction of XAD-2 than with Tenax, which persistently degrades into diphenyl quinones [55], for example. XAD-2, on the other hand, may be conveniently cleaned up with a multisolvent sequence ranging from water through methanol, acetone, diethyl ether, methylene chloride, and pentane. The uniformity and mechanical ruggedness of XAD-2 also gives more reproducible flow characteristics than Tenax, which is somewhat brittle and tends to produce fines which impair flow.

B. Ambient Air

PAH compounds in ambient air exist primarily as adsorbed particulate matter, as is clear from the earlier discussion on stack gases. Many considerations, such as vapor/particulate equilibria and selection of adsorbent materials for PAHs, have been discussed earlier and will not be addressed at length in this section.

Thus, since the ambient PAH problem is concerned primarily with particulate matter, this section concerns mainly the collection of particulate matter for PAH measurement. The use of adsorbent sampling techniques will be addressed briefly, since although ambient PAHs are largely in the particulate phase, PAHs are seldom sought to the complete exclusion of other more volatile organic species.

In addition to the selection of a preferred sampling method, other factors must be adequately taken into consideration during ambient sampling. The height of the sampler intake above ground level, the local topography, and the climate all affect the data obtained. For example, the influence of temperature on losses of benz[a]pyrene from airborne particles has been studied during atmospheric sampling [56]. The seasonal variation in specific surface areas and densities of suspended particulate matters has been reported [57]. The effects of local meteorology on the collection efficiencies of particulate matter has been demonstrated by Ogden and Wood [58]. Sampling rate is important since the vapor/particulate equilibrium will inevitably lead to some PAH losses, which may be most efficiently accounted for by passing a portion of the filtered air through an adsorbent sampler.

The method for collection of PAHs from ambient air and the quantity of sample collected will naturally depend upon the sensitivity of the quantitative technique to be used.

Collection of ambient particulate matter

One of the more common and useful particulate sampling devices for PAH and other materials from ambient air is the Anderson Hi-Vol cascade impactor [59-61]. The first four stages of the sampler comprise the fractionating head, while the fifth stage is a glass fiber backup filter positioned between the fractionating head and a standard High-Volume Air Sampler. At a flow rate of 20 scfm the sampler fractionates particulate matter into five size ranges, with calculated cutoff diameters shown in Table 5. For measuring airflow through the sampling unit, a calibrated rotometer must be used [62].

One of the problems associated with sampling for PAHs in ambient particulate matter is the very low concentration of these species normally encountered. On the average a High-Volume Air Sampler in an urban area will collect approximately 250 mg of particulate matter in a 25 hr period. This weight is distributed among five size ranges, and only about 10% of this will be organic material [63]. In practice, this

Table 5 Size Ranges of Suspended Particulate Matter Collected by an Anderson Hi-Vol Cascade Impactor (50% cutpoint diameter)

Stage number	Size range (μm)
1	>7.0
2	3.3-7.0
3	2.0-3.3
4	1.1-2.0
5 (filter)	<1.0

Source: Ref. 61.

is found to be up to a factor of 10 too small for comprehensive PAH analysis, and pooling of samples is often necessary.

A major advance in the collection of ambient particulate matter in quantities ideally suited for PAH analysis was made with the advent of the Massive Volume Air Sampler [64]. The three-stage Massive Volume Air Sampler was designed to provide for the rapid collection of gram quantities of ambient aerosols in three cutoff size ranges: >3.5, 3.5 to 1.7, and <1.7 μm. The latter two ranges are regarded as the sizes respirable by humans. The samplers are unique in their capability to provide respirable-size particulates in sufficient masses for both bioassay screening and, when indicated, detailed chemical characterization of the collections.

The sampler design utilizes two impactor stages (Teflon-coated steel) followed by a high-efficiency electrostatic precipitator (55 steel plates coated with conductive Teflon) to effect the three-stage size separation. [A scalping stage before the first impactor removes the very large (>20 μm diameter) particles.] A flow rate of 600 scfm (compared to a nominal 40 scfm High-Vol sampling rate) is obtained which, with a particulate loading of 100 μg/m^3, gives a total 24 hr collection of about 2.5 g. The collection efficiency of the sampler has been determined to be better than 90% for submicron particles, and the precision between two side-by-side samplers better than 5%.

A comparison of the ACGIH (American Conference of Governmental Industrial Hygienists) curve (theoretical deposition characteristics of the human lung, plot of percent retained against particle size) and the collection efficiency of the first stage of the Massive Volume Air Sampler [64] shows a very close similarity. This finding highlights the utility of the sampler in the assessment of the threat of PAH and other hazardous materials to humans.

With the exception of the Anderson Hi-Vol cascade impactor, and particularly the Massive Volume Air Sampler, no other particulate sampling devices presently appear to have a sufficiently high capacity for ambient PAH measurement.

Collection of ambient PAH vapors

As previously discussed, the great majority of ambient PAH will be present as particulate matter. Nevertheless, some PAH vapors, particularly of the lower molecular weight compounds, will be present. Furthermore, as mentioned earlier, it is important to sample a small portion of the High Volume or Massive Volume Air Samplers' exhaust, in order to measure the volatilization of collected PAHs, plus noncollected vapors.

It is important to appreciate that techniques using adsorbent samplers for collection of PAH vapors from stack gases are entirely applicable to ambient sampling. Similar configuration and flow rates of the adsorbent samplers may be used, whether operating simply with a filter, or sampling the exhaust from a large-volume particulate sampler.

Finally, a number of studies have incorporated small, low-flow-rate, modular sampling systems for PAHs and other organic species. These systems used a wide range of adsorbents, but their small capacity makes them unsuitable for source/environmental assessment on detailed PAH studies [52,65-71].

C. Automobile Exhaust

As we have seen earlier, the fractional load of PAHs in the environment contributed by emissions from vehicular transportation is scarcely significant compared to worldwide emission totals. Nevertheless, such emissions tend to be concentrated in the more densely populated urban centers, and thus their potential significance as a health hazard cannot be ignored.

The fuel, air/fuel ratio, operating temperature, and engine condition all contribute to the nature of exhaust emission and thus may modify the PAH emissions [72]. Several studies have demonstrated the influence of fuel aromaticity on PAH emissions [73-77].

The state of the art in the collection of PAHs from automotive exhaust appears to have lagged behind ambient and stack gas methods; in one study only 10% recovery of PAHs was obtained in some experiments [72]. However, more recent studies on a CRC project at Battelle Columbus Laboratories appear to demonstrate significantly better PAH recovery.

Several programs addressed PAH collection by simply condensing all the organic materials in the exhaust [78,79], while others have used a solvent exhaust scrubbing system [80]. A recent study with a promising approach but disappointing results [72] involved passing raw exhaust into a dilution tunnel, followed by various filtration steps and finally a Chromosorb 102 adsorbent sampler. The sample workup scheme employed was very complex, and full advantage was not taken of the internal standard that was incorporated into the emissions. Sample measurement of total ^{13}C activity in the collected sample negates the advantages of incorporating a ^{13}C internal standard. It would have been more appropriate to incorporate deuterium-labeled PAH internal standards and then to perform precision analysis using GC-MS techniques (see later).

Clearly, there is much room for improvement in this area. One suggestion would be to utilize a dilution tunnel, followed by stack gas sampling techniques, but to maintain the temperature of the tunnel and front end of the sampling system above 300°F to minimize tar formation and condensation losses. The thermal injection of internal standards (deuterium-labeled PAHs) into the beginning of the dilution tunnel would greatly facilitate analytical precision.

D. Aqueous Systems

PAH compounds are ideally suitable for extraction from water through use of macroreticular resins. Only the lower molecular weight members are sufficiently volatile to be partially removed by purge and trap techniques; the relatively low polarity and lyphophobic nature of PAHs thus makes them ideal candidates for sampling by resin adsorbtion. Much of the work carried out so far has emphasized the use of XAD resins, particularly XAD-2. Contrary to the significant work being accomplished by resin adsorbtion, a recently initiated EPA program [22] is reevaluating the technique of solvent extraction.

One of the more comprehensive evaluations of XAD resins for a variety of common water pollutants, including a few lower molecular weight PAHs, has recently been reported [81]. In this work organic compounds were spiked into distilled water and then passed through small columns of resin at 20 liter/min. Analysis down to 1/liter ng was accomplished by GC-MS. For acenaphthene, naphthalene, and methyl naphthalenes, XAD-2 gave marginally better recoveries, although XAD-4 was almost as good. XAD-7 and XAD-8 were generally less effective. This study showed that no breakthrough occurred for a 3 × 1.5 cm XAD-2 resin column for 1 liter of water, but small losses to the reservoir walls were noted. The XAD columns were eluted with 10 ml of acetone followed by 40 ml of chloroform.

A similar study using a slightly higher capacity XAD-2 resin column examined a range of PAHs which are more typical of environmental samples [82]. Figure 11 shows a schematic diagram of the macroreticular resin sampling module, which is based essentially on a commercial 400 × 25 mm liquid chromatography column (Fischer Porter

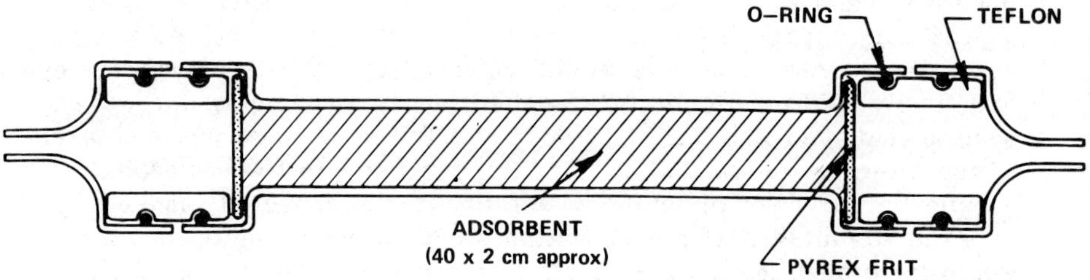

Figure 11 Adsorbent sampler for aqueous effluents. (From Ref. 82.)

Co.) with appropriate modification; XAD-2 resin was slurry-packed into the module using methanol. For laboratory validation studies, water was drawn through the sampling module using an aspirator pump.

The advantages of a pumping system, as opposed to gravity flow, are that substantially lower detection limits may be achieved from the greater water volumes sampled. With the described sampling module, up to 20 liters/hr may be readily achieved, which provides sufficient sample for qualitative and quantitative capillary column GC-MS (Cap-GC-MS) analysis substantially below 1 ppt.

Elution of PAHs from XAD-2 resin in this study was accomplished by means of 8 hr Soxhlet extraction in cellulose thimbles, using methylene chloride, followed by volume reduction using Kuderna-Danish evaporation after addition of internal standards. Preparation of commercial XAD-2 resin was routinely carried out as shown in Table 6. The initial water washes were tested with silver nitrate solution to ensure freedom from sodium chloride; all solvents were distilled-in-glass (Burdick and Jackson) quality.

Table 6 XAD-2 Cleanup Solvent Scheme

Solvent	Soxhlet extraction time
Water	5-6 washes
Methanol	24 hr
Diethyl ether	24 hr
Pentane	24 hr
Methylene chloride	24 hr

Source: Ref. 82.

Table 7 PAH Recovery Methylene Chloride Extraction

Compound	Average recovery (%)
Anthracene	95
Pyrene	91
Chrysene	89
Benz[a]pyrene	88
Indeno[1,2,3-cd]pyrene	78

Source: Ref. 82.

Laboratory studies were carried out to examine the selectivity of XAD-2 toward PAHs. One microgram each of five representative PAHs dissolved in acetone were spiked directly into the sampling module inlet, while 4 liters of distilled water was drawn through the module. Reasonably good recoveries were achieved (Table 7): losses with higher molecular weight compounds may be partly attributable to chromatographic inefficiency. In a subsequent experiment, 4 liters of distilled water was spiked with the PAHs in a glass reservoir, and significantly poorer recoveries were obtained. The losses were attributed to PAH adsorbtion on the container walls. The results of this study demonstrate that excellent sampling/recovery for PAHs from aqueous systems may be accomplished using XAD-2 resin, and that apparent losses through adsorbtion on glass containers and connective tubing demand in-field sampling of aqueous systems.

Breakthrough studies using a series backup sampling module were conducted in which 5 μg of anthracene was spiked onto the main sampling module. Forty liters of water was drawn through the system; GC-MS analyses indicated that no breakthrough occurred in these experiments.

XAD-2 resin prepared and cleaned up as described earlier was subject to two modes of storage/sampler packing. First, XAD-2 resin was dried and stored under nitrogen and was then dry packed. Second, XAD-2 resin was washed with methanol, stored under methanol, and slurry packed with methanol. Following each mode of sampler preparation, 4 liters each of an identical batch of distilled water was passed through the sampler, after which the usual extraction and analytical procedure was carried out; corresponding GC traces are shown in Figures 12 and 13. Clearly, the XAD-2 which was stored

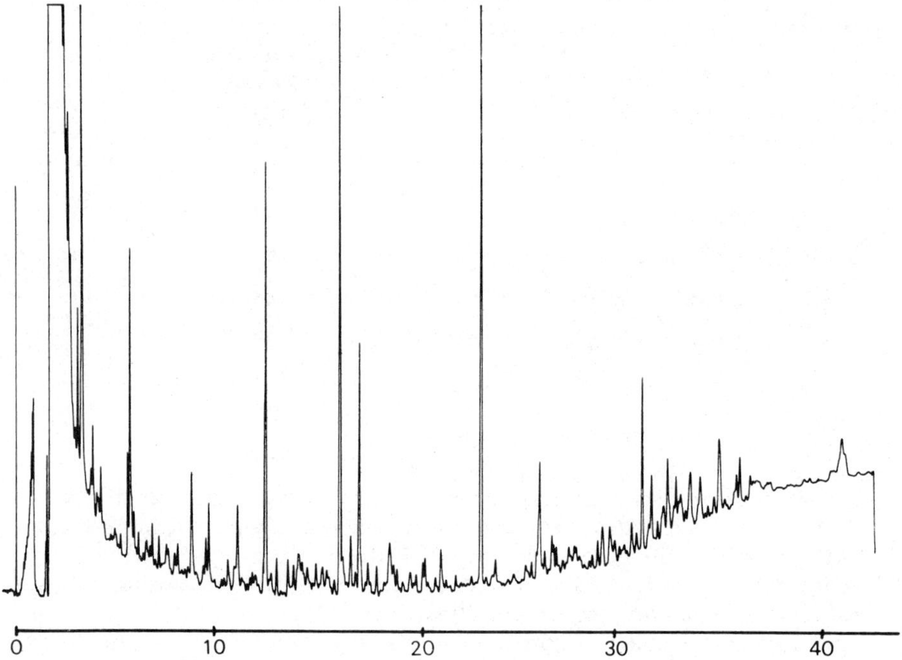

Figure 12 GC of XAD-2 blank after dry storage. (From Ref. 82.)

under methanol and slurry packed (Fig. 13) gave a much more satisfactory blank; this was found to be true consistently. The possibility that some of the minor remaining contaminants may originate from the sample of distilled water which was used was not precluded [82].

A combination of head space analysis and coupled-column (precolumn) PAH analysis using both Tenax GC and μBondapak C_{18} precolumns has been reported [83,84]. The earlier studies with volatile PAHs [81] achieved good recoveries using resin adsorbtion techniques, which suggests that the coupled-column methods would probably be applicable to all PAHs without preanalysis of the more volatile species by head space analysis.

Two further studies [49,50] have evaluated the utility of XAD resins and again demonstrated their efficiency on PAH sampling.

Solvent extraction of PAHs from water using methylenes chloride [22] and hexane [85] has been shown to result in outstanding recoveries of PAH compounds from freshly prepared PAH solutions on water. However, sample preservation studies [22] have demonstrated that some sample deterioration with time (up to 7 days) occurs even

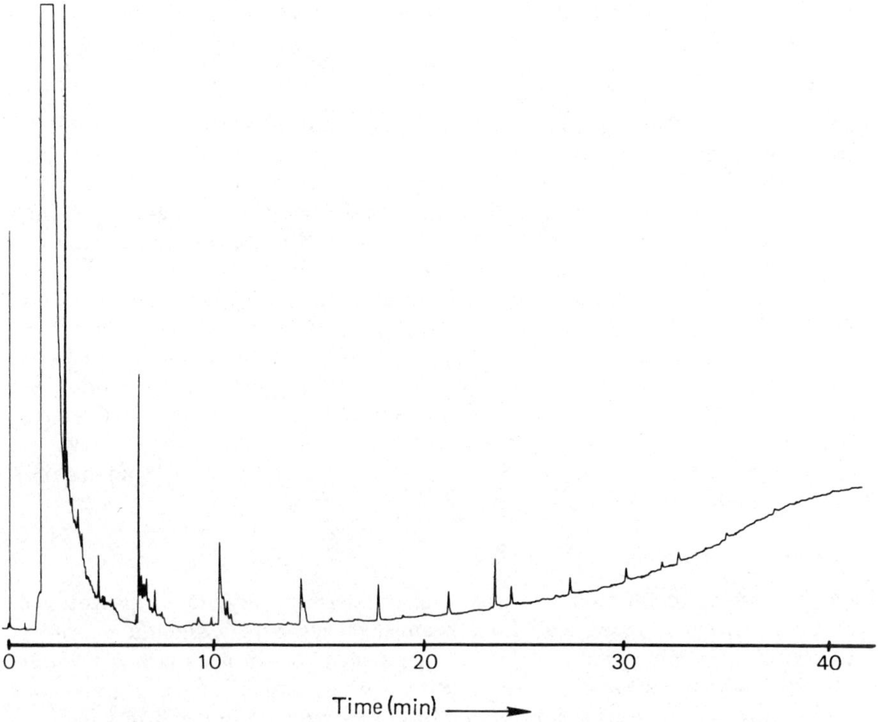

Figure 13 GC of XAD-2 blank after methanol storage. (From Ref. 82.)

under favorable conditions (dark, 4°C, chlorine free). Solvent extraction techniques impose an artificial limit on analytical sensitivity, since large volumes of water may not be conveniently transported.

In conclusion, the use of XAD-2 resins for in-field sampling of water is recommended. The resin columns may then be eluted conventionally or subject to handling-free coupled-column analysis [83, 84]. The transportation of large water volumes followed by solvent extraction in the laboratory is not recommended, in view of sample loss and lower sensitivity.

VII. RECOVERY OF PAHs FROM COLLECTION MEDIA

Sampling handling, which includes recovery and preservation, is probably the major source of analytical error. Very high sample concentration is generally sought, with the attendant high risk of sample loss. For simplicity the elements of various sampling systems are addressed separately.

A. Recovery of PAHs from Stack Gas and Ambient Trains [86]

Filters

Extraction of filter material may be conveniently carried out initially with methylene chloride followed by a reextraction of the residue and filter with methyl alcohol to ensure that all polar and nonpolar organic material is efficiently recovered. Extraction may be carried out using a Soxhlet apparatus for 24 hr or by ultrasonic agitation of the filter with solvent in a sealed glass container for 1 hr, followed by conventional filtration of the shredded filter and insoluble particulate matter. A variety of solvents have been used for extraction of PAHs from filtered particulate matter, including acetone [87-90], benzene [63, 76,90-92], cyclohexane [90,92-95], methanol [90,92], methylene chloride [63,90,96,97], tetrahydrofuran [52,53,90], chloroform [98], pentane [39], and mixed methanol-benzene [99,100]. Comparative studies of several solvents [90,92] recommend the use of benzene or carbon disulfide.

Cyclones, impactors, and probe rinse

Particulate material that has been removed from a cyclone, impactor, or rinsed from a probe may be solvent-extracted in a similar manner to a filter. Soxhlet extraction being carried out in a cellulose thimble plugged with glass wool, or in a fritted glass thimble with a glass wool plug. Ultrasonic extraction of particulates may be carried out by agitation with solvent in a sealed glass container followed by conventional filtration to remove the insoluble material.

Porous polymer adsorbent traps

Recovery of sample may be carried out by either solvent extraction or thermal desorbtion.

Solvent extraction. The preferred method of solvent extraction involves continuous solvent extraction of the adsorbent for a period of 24 hr by transferring the adsorbent resin to a Soxhlet extractor.

The choice of solvent for extracting a porous polymer adsorbent trap depends partly on the nature of the adsorbent. It is important that the solvent chosen does not affect the adsorbent in any way, yet is still an effective solvent for the removal of collected material. For porous polymer adsorbent traps utilizing Tenax, extracting with a hydrocarbon such as pentane is recommended [39], since more polar solvents readily dissolve the adsorbent. For XAD-2 traps, methylene chloride is efficient for PAHs [82].

Thermal Desorbtion. Thermal desorbtion has proved useful for qualitative and semiquantitative analyses of low-capacity adsorbent samplers used for stack gas and ambient sampling, and several approaches have been described [66,67,70]. However, data demonstrating efficient sample recovery by this technique are lacking, and high temperatures may cause decomposition of the collected sample and/or adsorbent substrate. All studies to date have met serious difficulties through contamination from artifacts from the adsorbent. The addition of internal standards for quantitative analysis is very difficult to accomplish, and finally, there is only one opportunity to analyze each collected sample.

Preparation of extracts for analysis

The manner in which the various sample extracts are combined depends on the information that is required. It is possible that particulates and vapor may need to be analyzed separately because of data required for an emission control strategy, for example. In any case, each extract or combination of extracts should be reduced in volume by Kuderna-Danish evaporation, the sample is then ready for analysis or separation by liquid chromatography. Although it is true that some more volatile species may be partly lost during this procedure, representative PAHs have been shown to be efficiently recovered [39].

B. Recovery of Volatile PAHs from Aqueous Media

Volatile organic compounds, broadly defined as those purgeable from aqueous solution, may be recovered from aqueous media to a greater or lesser extent by several techniques. It is appropriate at this point to review a few of the most promising recovery techniques for purgeable volatile organics, and to point out the important advantages and limitations of each. Some of the more volatile PAHs have been efficiently recovered by these techniques.

Liquid-liquid extraction

Various liquid-liquid extraction techniques are commonly used, the efficiency of all of which depend on the partition coefficient and volatility of the sought compounds. Volatility is an important consideration since the more volatile species are more easily lost during volume reduction of extracting solvents.

The simplest form of liquid-liquid extraction involves shaking the water sample repeatedly with a water-immiscible solvent such as methylene chloride [22]. Although this method can achieve very good recoveries initially, the reduction of the solvent volume by techniques such as rotary evaporation, Kuderna-Danish evaporation, and vortex evaporation can lead to serious losses of more volatile species. For PAHs, however, good recoveries may be achieved [39].

A liquid-liquid technique that utilizes very small solvent volumes, and thus overcomes solvent volume reduction difficulties, has been described by Grob et al. [101]. This method suffers from incomplete recovery of organics, in view of the unfavorable volume ratios even for species with a high partition coefficient. It is a useful and rapid qualitative method but is not likely to have value in a comprehensive quantitative analytical protocol.

A promising liquid-liquid technique is continuous extraction. There are a variety of apparatus which are commonly used, but all involve a Soxhlet-type cyclic distillation, agitated liquid-liquid contact, and return of the solvent plus recovered organics to the warmed solvent reservoir. For solvents less dense than water, the distillate passes through a funnel-shaped tube to the bottom of the water reservoir and then percolates through a fritted disk through the stirrer-agitated reservoir; after collection at the top of the reservoir, the solvent returns to the heated solvent reservoir. Alternatively, the liquid-liquid interface may be vigorously stirred to achieve extraction. For solvents more dense than water, an apparatus more nearly like a Soxhlet extractor is used, with solvent return from the bottom of the aqueous reservoir.

Continuous extraction can offer the advantage of reasonably small solvent volumes, even with large aqueous volumes. An efficient solvent-return condenser is nevertheless essential to minimize losses of recovered organic species. Low-boiling-point solvents are preferred for the same reason.

The question of drying small volume extracts must also be considered, since it is essential that this step does not lead to losses of the compounds sought. Numerous drying agents, such as magnesium perchlorate or phosphorus pentoxide, have been used for either direct drying or by vapor transfer under partial vacuum. When a drying agent is used, there is an increased risk of adsorption losses, although a 3A molecular seive minimizes this problem both in vapor drying and direct liquid contact [102].

Treatment of emulsions. One of the major problems often encountered in solvent extraction of aqueous solutions is that of emulsion formation. To achieve a complete phase separation necessary for good recovery, either emulsion formation must be avoided or emulsion must be broken. Some emulsions are much more difficult to break than others. Although various techniques to break emulsions are available, the techniques that will work best for a given situation can usually only be determined empirically. In some cases the addition of salt or methanol will help avoid emulsion or help to break it after formation. In trace component analysis work the introduction of interferring contaminants must be avoided; commercial defoamers are generally unsatisfactory. Centrifugation is frequently effective in breaking emulsions, and in some cases, vacuum filtration of the mixture is effective. In many cases, too vigorous an agitation causes emulsion formation; the use of stirring (e.g., with a magnetic stirrer instead of shaking) sometimes permits coagulation to be achieved without emulsion formation. Emulsions are caused by the presence of traces of certain materials that stabilize the air in water, oil in water, or water in oil phases. The proper choice of extracting solvents is often the best approach to solving emulsion problems; for any specific emulsion problem, the techniques mentioned above need to be tried on a primarily empirical basis.

Purge and trap techniques

Most organic compounds with boiling points below about 150°C can be purged from aqueous solution by an inert gas stream such as helium or nitrogen. The completeness of removal depends on the distribution coefficient of the compound between the water and gas phases and on the volume ratio of gas to water. Nonpolar compounds (e.g., saturated hydrocarbons and halocarbons) actually distribute in favor of the gas phase and are more than half removed from water when incorporated with an equal volume of gas. Aromatic hydrocarbons and halocarbons have somewhat lower distribution coefficients, about 0.1 to 0.2, which is still high enough to permit them to be purged from water; some lower molecular weight PAHs have been quantitatively purged from water [83,84]. More polar and hydrated organic compounds, such as alcohols, amines, acids, and certain aldehydes, are much less readily purged. For any given compound, the flow rate time and temperature of purging need to be determined experimentally.

One of the main problems involved in purge and trap work is that of getting the material onto the GC column as a sharp plug to permit good GC resolution; several approaches have been used. One approach involves the use of a cold trap to condense out the components, followed by rapid heating of the trap to flash the components onto the GC column. A drying agent (e.g., magnesium perchlorate) may be used in front of the cold trap to remove water vapor which may be detrimental to the GC column or detector system. A more common approach involves the use of an adsorbent precolumn (e.g., Tenax or XAD-2), followed by rapid thermal desorption [103-106]. The maximum temperatures and flow rates that can be used are limiting factors which affect the desorption time required. If a desorption time greater than a few seconds is necessary, the head of the GC column can be cooled to -50°C or lower to obtain a sharp plug of sample and good GC resolution. The design of the GC injector system can be very critical in this case since a sharp transition from hot to cold is required.

Another approach involves a combination of the polymer adsorption-thermal desorption approach with cold trapping [105]. If an appreciable desorption time is required, the desorbed components can be collected in a cold trap and subsequently flashed onto the GC column by heating. This approach is particularly useful for GC-MS studies. In addition to polymer adsorbents, materials such as charcoal and silica gel can be used. Since it is usually more difficult to thermally desorb components from these latter adsorbents, they are mainly used for highly volatile materials such as vinyl chloride, which breaks through polymer adsorbents too quickly. Flow rates, times, temperatures, and adsorbent conditioning parameters which give satisfactory recoveries, sensitivities, reproducibilities, and levels of interferences must be established.

There are a number of variations of the purge and trap method in use, varying between the open flow systems originally described by Bellar and Lichtenberg [106], which used subsequent thermal desorbtion, and the closed-loop technique described by Grob and Zurcher [107], which utilized recovery from the adsorbent filter by solvent extraction. It is more difficult to accurately add internal standards to a sample using thermal desorbtion than when using solvent extraction, but sample handling losses are potentially much lower when using thermal desorbtion. The Grob closed-loop system is claimed to have very high efficiency for recovery of most purgeable organics from aqueous media. The adsorbents used in purge and trap systems vary from Tenax, Chromosorbs, and XAD resins for the Bellat type, to activated charcoal micro filters in the Grob closed-loop system.

Recovery of PAHs adsorbed by resins

Adsorbtion of organic materials present in aqueous media on macroreticular resins was described earlier; the most common method of subsequent recovery involves solvent elution. XAD resins have been eluted with methylene chloride and methanol [82], acetone and chloroform [81], and diethyl ether [49,50].

Although most laboratories have made use of solvent elution for the recovery of organic materials stripped from aqueous media by macroreticular resins, the utility of thermal desorbtion, more commonly used for air samples, has been described [103-105]. One study involved trapping on a mixture of Tenax and glass beads to improve flow characteristics, and then drying the resin over phosphorus pentoxide under partial vacuum prior to conventional thermal desorbtion onto the head of a cooled capillary column [103]. The reported recovery of more polar compounds was less satisfactory since a real potential for losses must exist during the water removal step.

VIII. ANALYSIS OF PAHs

Following recovery of the collected sample, it is first necessary to determine whether its complexity is amenable to the technique selected for quantitative analysis. High-resolution, high-specificity techniques such as Cap-GC-MS can achieve facile analysis of PAHs in relatively gross mixtures of organic species. Low-resolution, low-specificity techniques, such as liquid chromatography (LC), thin layer chromatography (TLC), flame ionization detection, and UV detection, require proportionately higher degrees of sample cleanup and prefractionation.

Initially, techniques for enrichment and fractionation will be discussed, followed by a description of high-resolution separation techniques.

A. Solvent Partitioning

Using this technique, PAHs in one solvent are allowed to exchange to another immiscible solvent which has either significantly higher or lower distribution coefficient for the PAHs than the original solvent. In the first instance, PAHs are extracted by the second solvent, and in the latter instance, the undesirable species present accumulate in the second solvent, leaving the first solvent relatively enriched in PAHs. A number of solvents have been used for solvent partitioning.

Methanol-water

This solvent partitioning scheme permits the PAHs in cyclohexane solution to partition with methanol-water solution. The polar species present in cyclohexane solution preferentially distribute themselves in the more polar methanol-water, leaving the cyclohexane phase containing the PAHs relatively free of other species. The methanol-water system has been used by a number of authors as a preliminary step for removing the polar components from the PAH fraction [108-110].

Dimethyl formamide

This solvent was found to be very efficient for the removal of PAHs from heptane [111], and has subsequently been used [110] for extracting PAHs from cyclohexane.

Nitromethane

The partition coefficients of PAHs between nitromethane and cyclohexane were determined [112] to vary between 4.4 and 1.65 for a number of PAHs tested. Similar partition coefficients were determined between nitromethane and other aliphatic solvents [111,113], and the system has been used by a number of authors, particularly for cleaning up samples of automobile exhaust [95,96,104,114].

Dimethyl sulfoxide

The first evaluation of this solvent as a partitioning medium for PAHs involved a comparison of acetonitrile, mitromethane, dimethyl formamide, and dimethyl sulfoxide, and showed that the last solvent was much more suitable on the basis of distribution coefficients and selectivity for PAH compounds [111,115].

Acid, base, and neutral fractionation

The analysis of complex mixtures is often facilitated by the inclusion of an acid, base, and neutral separation step, prior to chromatography [96,102,114]. Extraction with dilute base removes acidic components, and extraction with dilute acid removes basic components. For recovery of PAHs, successive extraction with dilute sodium hydroxide and hydrochloric acid has demonstrated that over 90% remains in the neutral fraction [116].

B. Thin Layer Chromatography

The resolution of thin layer chromatography (TLC) is too low to have realistic applicability to measurement of large numbers of individual PAHs in complex environmental mixtures. Single PAH compounds, such as benz[a]pyrene, may frequently be amenable to simple and rapid separation by TLC. However, in view of the limited applicability of TLC to comprehensive PAH analysis, it will only be summarized here.

Numerous studies of PAHs by TLC have been undertaken, including the use of silica [113,117,118], alumina [119,120], and cellulose acetate [119,121-123]. With the advent of in situ scanning techniques [122], reasonably reproducible and accurate results have been obtained. Highest resolution has been achieved using two-dimensional development on 2:1 alumina-40% acetylated cellulose [124,125], when the majority of PAHs have had recoveries of 85 to 95%.

Lack of resolution is a major disadvantage with TLC; the ease of PAH photodecomposition on large surface areas may lead to serious quantitation errors.

C. Liquid Chromatography

Liquid chromatography (LC) is a valuable technique for sample cleanup prior to high-resolution quantitative separation. Like TLC, columns should be protected from light during separations, to avoid photochemical decomposition of PAHs. The most useful and commonly used adsorbents for LC separation of PAHs are alumina silica gel and Porasil.

Alumina is available in various size ranges and activities; neutral alumina is generally used for PAH separation. The recommended sample adsorbent ratio is between 1:100 and 1:1000; the alumina is partly deactivated with water prior to use [126]. Elution is achieved by gradually increasing the polarity of the eluting solvent, generally by stepwise polarity changes [86]. Solvent systems that have been found useful for PAH elution are pentane-ether [127], cyclohexane-ether [128], cyclohexane-benzene [109,129], and benzene-methanol [130].

The most commonly used grade of silica gel for LC is 100-200 mesh, the usual sample/adsorbent ratio is similar to alumina. Silica gel is found useful in activities ranging from dried [120,129] to 5% moisture content [90,98]. Elution of PAHs is most commonly accomplished by using benzene [98,120,129], or hexane-benzene [90]. A general LC separation scheme developed for the EPA (level 1 analysis) makes use of deactivated silica gel (>200 mesh), and achieves elution through a stepwise solvent gradient beginning with pentane through methylene chloride to methanol [86,130]. The recovery of PAHs from silica gel has been reported to average about 80% [90].

An advantage of Porasil is relatively rapid elution times compared to alumina and silica gel; good resolution of PAHs has been reported however. Activated 60-100 mesh is commonly used [112,130], and elution is generally carried out with benzene [131] or hexane-benzene [130].

D. High-Performance Liquid Chromatography

High-performance liquid chromatography (HPLC) is a very powerful separation technique whose application is essential to the separation of very complex mixtures. HPLC is often used as a sole measurement technique since resolution of more than 10,000 theoretical plates may now be accomplished. Most useful detector systems are presently fluorescence, UV, and refractive index, although mass spectrometer interfaces are now commercially available; the efficiency of HPLC-MS transfer is commonly poor for PAHs (5 to 10%) but is expected to improve with experience.

However, since the resolution attainable by HPLC is still about an order of magnitude lower then may be achieved with the very best capillary gas chromatographic columns (Cap-GC), the most useful role of HPLC in the analysis of very complex mixtures (coal conversion liquids, crude oil, shale oil, combustion products) at the present time is as a high-resolution prefractionation technique for Cap-GC separation. Of course, this presupposes sufficient volatility of the collected fractions for GC; when mixtures (or fractions) of very highly polar species are to be separated, HPLC is the only analytical technique available. For the analysis of PAHs, HPLC alone only begins to be superior to Cap-GC for compounds of approximately higher molecular weight than coronene, when low volatility causes significant loss of GC efficiency.

The true potential of HPLC is frequently not realized or is poorly understood; there are three primary modes of HPLC which are commonly used, depending on the system under study. All three are applicable to PAH separation when circumstances warrant, and will thus be briefly addressed here.

Gel permeation chromatography

Gel permeation chromatography (GPC) is an exclusion technique in which retention is based on the ability to penetrate the pores of the chromatographic substrate (or support); large molecules elute more quickly, closer to the solvent front, while smaller molecules will more fully permeate the chromatographic substrate and have an appropriately delayed elution from the column. The relative degree of permeation of the chromatographic substrate dictates the relative separation of compounds by virtue of differences in elution volume (or time).

There are advantages in using GPC as an initial separation method for very complex mixtures. GPC is a fast fractionation step which results in excellent molecular size separations, and subsequent knowledge of the molecule size range of individual fractions can dictate the choice of further separation techniques (HPLC or GC) that may be desirable. Narrow molecular size ranges also aid in the subsequent qualitative analysis. Once GPC fractions of a complex mixture have been obtained, they can be further separated into classes according to functional groups by adsorption chromatography or by reverse-phase chromatography. Either chromatographic mode can be used after GPC, depending on the complexity of the fraction. It is possible that GPC separation may not prove necessary and that the sample can be directly separated by adsorption chromatography.

Adsorption chromatography

Adsorbtion chromatography is the most commonly encountered mode of HPLC (or LC), and is often used to the exclusion of GPC and reverse-phase chromatography. Adsorbtion chromatography, as the name implies, achieves separation on the basis of the adsorbtion equilibrium of the sample between the chromatographic substrate (frequently silica) and the eluting mobile phase. Separation is thus achieved primarily on the basis of the polarity of function groups present, or on the basis of molecular charge separation for hydrocarbons. Thus adsorption chromatography separates mixtures broadly into classes with little regard for aliphatic or aromatic character. For this reason adsorbtion chromatography (HPLC or LC) is an ideal cleanup procedure for PAHs present in complex mixtures; other classes of compounds are readily separated from them. Further advantages of adsorbtion chromatography are that it presently permits the highest resolution obtainable by HPLC, and the fractions are obtained in a relatively low boiling point solvent, which minimizes sample loss on volume reduction. The main disadvantage of adsorbtion chromatography is that highly polar compounds may be retained indefinitely.

Reverse-phase liquid chromatography

Reverse-phase LC, silica gel with bound octadecyl or other groups, is an extremely important separation mode in HPLC. Its two main advantages over silica gel are its ability to elute both highly polar and non-polar compounds from a mixture and its ease of equilibration. The disadvantage of reverse-phase chromatography is that it is not as chromatographically efficient as adsorption. Despite this limitation, reverse-phase LC is an excellent complement to adsorption when optimizing selectivity. Reverse-phase LC, on the other hand, separates on the basis of water solubility and is therefore selective for aliphatic and aromatic differences within a given class of compounds. It demonstrates significant selectivity for length and branching of aliphatic side chains, for example.

Thus the use of appropriate combination of GPC, adsorbtion chromatography, and reverse-phase LC will provide the best opportunity for reducing very complex mixtures to manageable fractions to permit quantitative analysis by the last applied technique, or GC-MS. Simpler mixtures are generally amenable to quantitative analysis by adsorbtion chromatography or reverse-phase LC alone.

Quantitative HPLC analysis

A good description of the analysis of a complex mixture [132] involving sequential solvent partition, gel permeation, reverse-phase LC and Cap-GC was included in a study of PAHs on ambient particulate matter. This work demonstrated the utility of HPLC on the sequential fractionation of a complex sample, into simple fractions amenable to quantitative analysis by HPLC or Cap-GC.

A comparison of a number of adsorbtion chromatography materials with μBondapak C_{18} (reverse-phase) for the separation of over 40 PAHs has been made in a recent study [95]. This work demonstrates very clearly the value of normal-phase HPLC in the initial fractionation of very complex mixture of PAH and methyl-PAH compounds. The study shows that groups of one, two, three, four, and five ring aromatic compounds may be collected separately, and the fractions could then be ideally subject to reverse-phase LC for maximum PAH resolution. The extract of a sediment sample is subjected to sequential μBondapak NH_2 (normal phase) and μBondapak C_{18} (reverse-phase) separation; both UV and fluorescence detection are demonstrated, and stopped-flow fluorescence scans are made on each peak in the reverse-phase analysis.

Further examples of quantitative fluorescence detection for many PAHs are given in earlier studies [52,133]. A study of the analysis of 16 PAHs in water achieved their partial separation on Sperisorb ODS and demonstrated the utility of UV and fluorescence detection [22]; representative chromatograms are shown in Figures 14A and

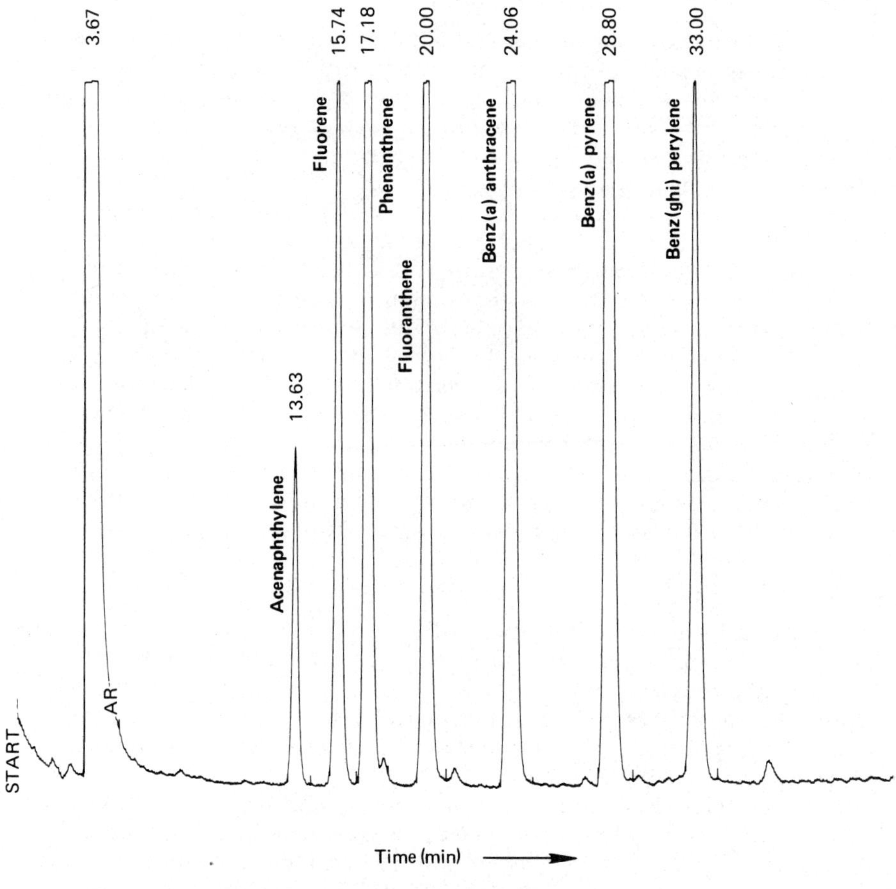

Figure 14A HPLC separation of standard PAHs (250 × 4.6 mm, 5 μm Sperisorb ODS. 50/50% acetonitrile-water linear gradient to 100% acetronitrile in 50 min. UV monitoring at 254 nm). (From Ref. 22.)

14B. Superior resolution was achieved in this study using a Perkin-Elmer HC-ODS column when all 16 compounds were well resolved at one time (Fig. 14C). However, the direct application of such single-pass separation schemes to very complex samples would appear to be unrealistic.

HPLC analysis schemes that achieve separation of the benzpyrene isomers have been described [134-136]. Using an HPLC-Sorb polyamide-6 column with various polar solvents, good separations were obtained [134]; the detection limit with a 45% acetylated column was rather poor, around 200 ng of benz[a]pyrene [135]. Cross-linked

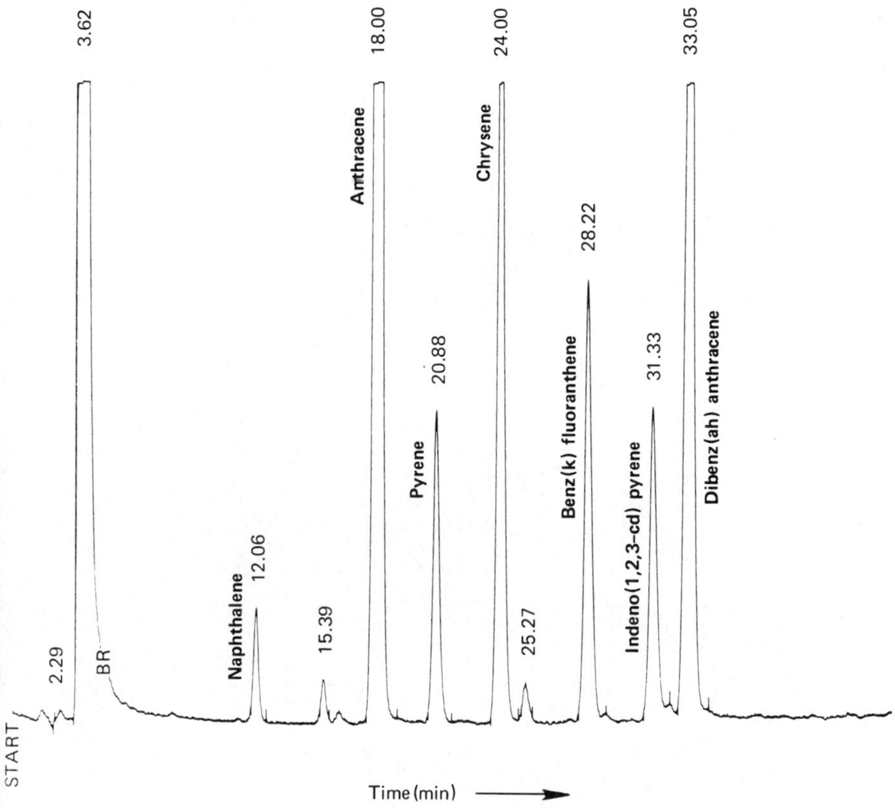

Figure 14B HPLC separation of standard PAHs (250 × 4.6 mm, 5 μm Sperisorb ODS. 50/50% acetonitrile-water linear gradient to 100% acetonitrile in 50 min. UV monitoring at 254 nm). (From Ref. 22.)

cellulose acetate was found to be a better column packing since it is granular and possesses a lower swelling capacity than that of regular cellulose acetate [136]. The structure is more uniform and thus has as greater permeability with lower pressure than the previously described system. The UV detection limit measured at 297 nm was 30 ng of benz[a]pyrene/5 μl injection by the use of a fluorescence detector with a 326 to 380 nm exitation filter and a 377 nm emission filter. It was necessary to clean up the sample on an aluminum oxide LC column prior to the HPLC procedures to remove anthracene, which would interfere with the benzpyrene detection.

The comparison of three HPLC column-solvent systems using a UV detector set at 383 nm for quantitation of benz[a]pyrene and at 275 nm for less selective measurements has been described [137]. The

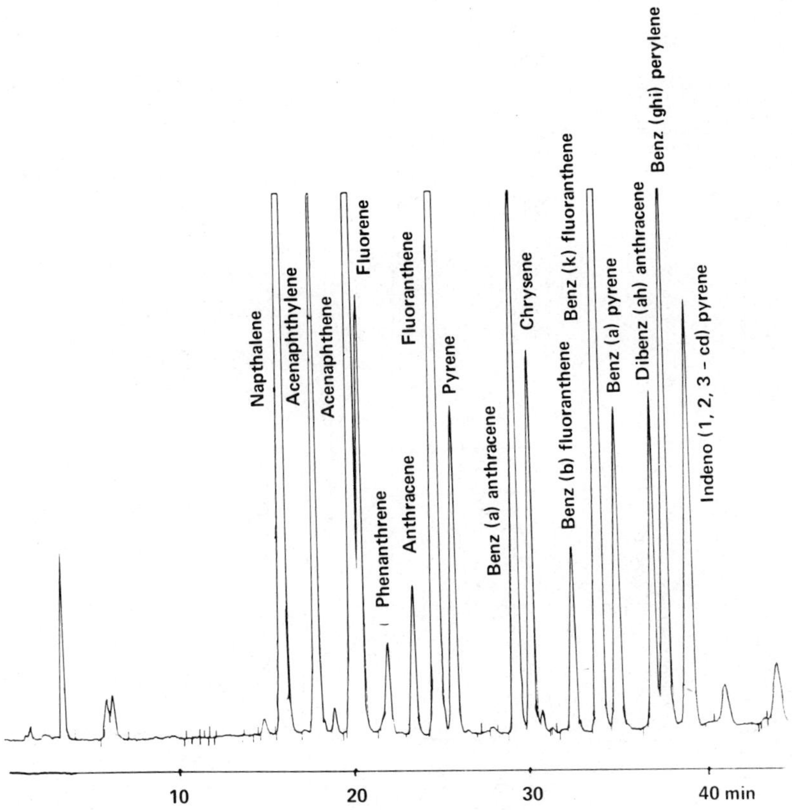

Figure 14C HPLC separation of standard PAHs (250 × 2.6 mm, Perkin-Elmer HC-ODS, water-acetonitrile, 60-40 isocratic for 5 min, then linear gradient to 100% acetonitrile over 25 min). (From Ref. 22.)

three systems are: (a) 24 cm Lichrosorb column eluted with cyclohexane at a flow rate of 0.2 to 0.6 ml/min, which achieved a detection limit of 0.1 ng; (b) 30 cm μBondapak C_{18} eluted with 60:40 acetonitrile-H_2O at a flow rate of 1.5/4 ml/min, which achieved a detection limit of 1 ng; (c) 30 cm Porasil eluted with cyclohexane at 1 to 4 ml/min, which achieved a detection limit of 1 ng. Although system (a) was the most sensitive, system (c) achieved the best separation of benz[a]pyrene from interfering compounds.

A routine analysis for PAHs from filtered particulates using HPLC has been described [138]. After extracting particulate-containing filters in cyclohexane, the sample was prefractionated on silica gel TLC plates using cyclohexane-benzene (1.5:1.0) as the mobile phase. Separation by HPLC was subsequently achieved on an ODS Zorbax column using MeOH-H_2O (65:35) as the eluting solvent. A fixed-wavelength (254 nm) UV detector was used for quantification and identification, the method is sensitive for submicrogram quantities, with a detection limit of 10 ng of benz[a]pyrene routinely achieved.

A sensitive HPLC method using a fluorimetric detector for PAH analyses has also been described [139]. Separation was carried out on a Jascopack SV-02 packed column using a (30:70) water-methanol eluent. The detector was a spectrofluorometer equipped with a 3 μl volume flow cell; wavelengths were optimized for specific PAHs. At an exitation wavelengths of 280 nm and an emission wavelength of 430 nm, a detection limit of 1 ng was achieved for benz[a]pyrene.

Further studies have demonstrated the use of UV detection [63, 87,89,112,126,127,129,140-142], and fluorescence detection [68,93, 109,120,121,126,132,142-148] for monitoring PAHs in HPLC eluate.

E. Gas Chromatography and Mass Spectrometry

At the time of writing, gas chromatography (GC) offers the highest reported resolution of complex PAH mixtures attainable in a single pass. Mass spectrometry (MS) presently offers the greatest selectivity for PAHs in complex organic mixtures, although it fails to distinguish between PAH structural isomers. MS demonstrates excellent sensitivity (subnanogram) for PAHs, similar to that exhibited by fluorescence detection for HPLC. In consequence, GC-MS presently offers the highest resolution, selectivity, and sensitivity that is attainable in a single pass for PAHs in complex organic mixtures.

Gas chromatography

Several years ago the satisfactory separation of PAHs was widely considered to be beyond the foreseeable future, and statements that the benzpyrene isomers would never be resolved by GC [149] were not uncommon or surprising. However, the gradual appearance of higher-thermal-stability GC column packing materials permitted reasonably good separation to be achieved on packed GC columns. A much referenced study reported the partial or complete resolution of 124 PAH compounds on a Dexsil 300 packed column [150]. The next few years saw a great deal of significant work in this area, and the highest resolution that appears to have been reported to date [19,82,151,152] facilitates the simultaneous resolution of the previously problematic isomer pairs: phenanthrene-anthracene, chrysene-benz[a]anthracene, and benz[a]pyrene-benz[e]pyrene. A typical chromatogram [82] is shown in Figure 15.

A number of relatively nonpolar stationary phases have been used for the analysis of PAHs in packed columns, the better of which include OV-1 [143,153], OV-25 [154], SE-30 [129,155,156], SE-52 [98,157], Dexsil 300 [39,92,143,150,153,158,159], Dexsil 400 [153,160],

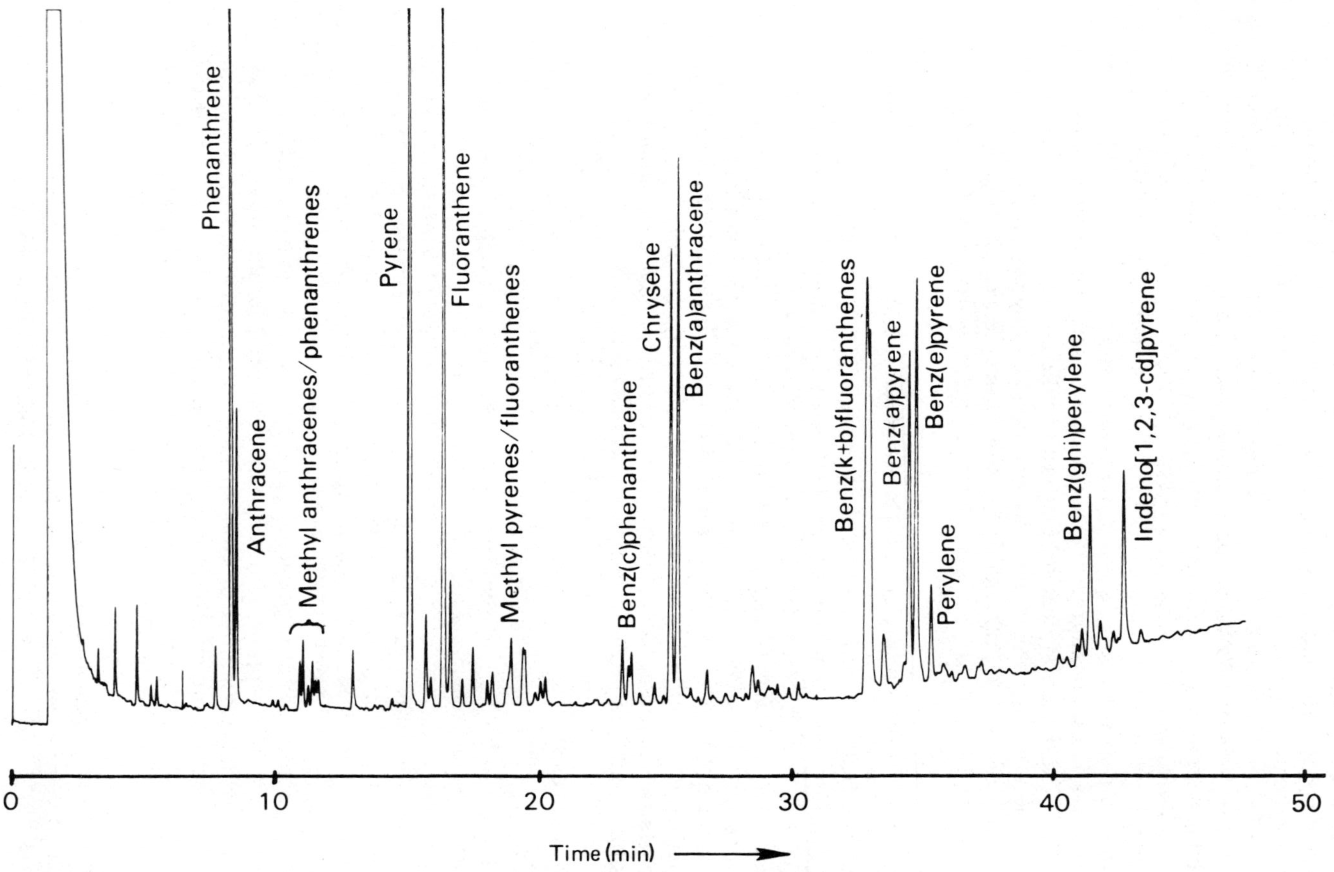

Figure 15 PAH separation on industrial effluent sample (20 m × 0.25 mm SE-54, programmed from 150 to 275°C at 3°C/min). (From Ref. 82.)

Dexsil 410 [153], and nematic liquid crystals [39,161,162]. Dexsil 300 and 400 are perhaps the more satisfactory, both in terms of resolution and low column bleed; the latter is particularly important for GC-MS application. Nematic liquid crystals exhibit extraordinarily good resolution, and it appears that conditions may be established for the separation of any specific group of PAH isomers. Although these materials suffer from chronic column bleed, they have been found useful for the routine separation of benzpyrene isomers [39].

With the widespread application of capillary columns to PAH separation problems, significant gains in resolution of structurally similar isomers have been achieved. The resolution of capillary columns used to date has ranged from about 20,000 to 50,000 theoretical plates for columns between 20 and 50 m in length, although substantially higher resolution is feasible. The most commonly used stationary phases for wall-coated glass capillary columns in PAH analysis have been SE-30 [83,163], SE-52 [95,97,132,163-165], SE-54 [82], OV-1 [19,151,167], OV-17 [152,166], OV-25 [160], OV-101 [141,166,167], and SP-2100 [168]. In general, the efficiency of support-coated open tubular (SCOT) columns does not appear to approach that of wall-coated glass capillary columns [150], although excellent resolution is reported occasionally [152].

The advantages of glass capillary columns over conventional packed columns are particularly relevant to the separation of complex organic mixtures. In addition to much better resolution, glass capillary columns are less likely to cause loss of organic compounds due to adsorption on active sites [169]. The significantly sharper peaks obtained can provide at least a tenfold gain in sensitivity during quantitative analysis. Furthermore, compounds can be chromatographed on glass capillary columns at significantly lower temperatures than those required by packed columns. Finally, the carrier gas flow rates used in capillary column chromatography are more compatible with coupling to a mass spectrometer; whether electron impact (EI) or chemical ionization (CI) is used, no separator is required to enrich the GC effluent.

The major disadvantages of capillary column GC have been largely overcome, injector designs such as the Grob injector [170] and the "dropping-needle injector" [171] permit introduction of relatively large quantities of sample directly onto the column without requiring a splitter. Improved liquid phases and methods of coating have raised the maximum temperatures at which the columns can be used and have thereby increased the molecular weight of compounds that can be separated efficiently.

An example of superior resolution attainable by capillary column GC is shown in Figure 15. This demonstrates the separation of polynuclear aromatic hydrocarbons in a sample of ferroalloy industry effluent. Many of the important compounds, such as benz[a]pyrene and benz[a]anthracene, are quite well resolved; this resolution cannot be achieved using packed columns.

Mass spectrometry

Mass spectrometry affords sensitive and relatively selective detection of PAH compounds. Four techniques are available for introducing samples to the mass spectrometer [172]: direct insertion probe, controlled leak inlet, gas chromatographic interface, and liquid chromatographic interface. The latter method has not proved useful for PAHs, because of their relatively high volatility.

Direct Insertion Probe. Relatively involatile organic compounds, including PAHs, are readily amenable to this mode of inlet. The sample is deposited in a small glass capillary, either as crystals or as a thin-film residue from solvent evaporation, and placed in the cavity at the tip of a thermally programmable probe. The probe is admitted to the mass spectrometer via a vacuum lock and heated sufficiently to volatilize the sample ($\sim 10^{-5}$ to 10^{-6} torr). Sample fractionation may sometimes be achieved by carefully controlling the rate of heating [173], mass spectra being continuously recorded. MS analyses of TLC bands have been obtained by transfering adsorbent containing the band of interest directly into the glass capillary [174]; however, it is usually preferable to elute the adsorbed material prior to MS analysis [172].

Controlled Leak Inlet. This type of inlet is more commonly used for organic materials of higher volatility than most PAHs, and generally requires several milligrams of sample. A reservoir at room temperature is usually connected to the ion source of the mass spectrometer through a controlled leak. However, application to less volatile materials may be accomplished readily by heating the reservoir and transfer lines; GC inlets have been satisfactorily used for this purpose when the reservoir is situated in the GC oven.

Gas Chromatographic Inlet. The objective of the GC inlet is to permit compounds eluted from the GC column to be separated as efficiently as possible from the 1 to 30 ml/min flow of carrier gas, and to allow the pressure in the ion source to be maintained at less than 10^{-5} torr. Separators such as the Watson-Bieman, Becker-Ryhage, and Llewellyn [175-177] have been designed in an attempt to accomplish this task, and are not discussed further here.

Mass spectra may be obtained by electron impact ionization or by chemical ionization; in the latter mode, sample ionization is accomplished by means of an ionized reagent gas such as methane [178], isobutane [179], or ammonia [180]. The MS source pressure for CI with methane, for example, is typically as high as 1 torr, and the far higher concentration of methane than sample in the source assures that sample ionization will occur exclusively by collision with ionized methane. Chemical ionization results in a mass spectrum that is rather different to electron impact, in view of its being a much lower energy process; CI spectra are characterized by less extensive fragmentation of the molecular ion, and the fragmentation that does occur generally proceeds through loss of neutral molecules and appreciably more stable fragments than is the case with EI. It is usual to observe a protonated molecular ion in CI; this is frequently accompanied by two adduct ions at M + 29 and M + 41, in the case of methane CI, caused by the addition of $\overset{+}{C}_2H_5$ and $\overset{+}{C}_3H_5$ ions in the source of the mass spectrometer. Such adduct ions are generally diagnostic for the protonated molecular ion, and thus it is frequently possible to quickly assign a molecular weight during CI GC-MS analysis.

CI (methane) mass spectra of PAHs are dominated by the protonated molecular ion; although the EI mass spectra are almost equally devoid of fragmentation, CI may provide slightly greater sensitivity by reducing interference from fragments due to co-eluting aliphatic hydrocarbons.

The use of argon to ionize PAHs primarily by charge exchange has been reported to result in significant specificity between isomeric PAHs [181,182]. It has been established that spectra of PAHs have characteristic ratios of protonated molecular ions to the molecular ion when 5 to 10% of methane in argon is used as the reagent gas. This finding may prove particularly valuable in the analysis of very complex PAH mixtures.

Quantitative GC-MS analysis of PAHs

A desirable objective of any analytical approach is to provide simultaneous qualitative and quantitative analysis. Quantitative analyses may be carried out by GC or specific ion monitoring (SIM) GC-MS (see later), but these techniques cannot easily assist with qualitative analysis. When ion current integration (specific or total) from the mass spectral reconstructed gas chromatograms (RGC) is used for quantification, qualitative analyses can be achieved simultaneously and thus optimize cost-and information-effectiveness. In some instances this is less desirable, since it is not then possible to use the high sensitivity and precision of SIM quantification. The more sensitive and highly specific mode of SIM GC-MS analysis is most appropriately utilized when specific compounds are sought in a particular sample and maximum sensitivity is required.

Internal Standards. Internal standards are used to minimize errors due to losses in the sample handling and analytical procedures, since they are carried through the entire analytical scheme with the compounds sought. Compounds are quantified by adding known quantities of internal standards, and calculating the ratio of response factors (MS ion currents) for the two compounds. Calibration factors (see later) are applied, which take peak shapes and differing ionization efficiencies into account to obtain absolute quantitative data.

In selecting internal standards, it is important to choose compounds that are similar to the compounds sought, to ensure that they will follow a similar fate in the extraction/separation scheme and will elute close to the sought species in the final chromatogram. Consequently, the final selection of internal standards will be the result of an iterative procedure, since only when an analytical protocol is finally developed will it be known how many individual analytical measurements are necessary and thus how many standards are required. Clearly, ideal internal standards for any compound are deuterium-substituted analogs, and this is also true for PAHs. However, in view of the large numbers of PAHs that are commonly sought, this would be impractical.

However, the most important single requirement of any internal standard is that it should not already be present in the sample to be analyzed. The appropriate selection requires great care; structurally unique or ideally isotopically labeled compounds are preferred. Deuterium-labeled standards should preferably contain a minimum of four deuterium atoms to avoid confusion between respective M - 1, M, M + 1, and M + 2 ions. For environmental samples, 9,10-disubstituted anthracenes have been used with success [39,65,82,86]. Since it is impossible to predict the level of PAH compounds that may be present, and because the quantity of internal standards present should be within a factor of 10 of the concentration of the compounds sought, several different internal standards may need to be incorporated into each chromatographic analysis. Different quantities of each of the standards may need to be added, so that whatever multiplier gain and attenuation is subsequently required, there will be an internal standard present at similar concentrations to the PAHs sought.

Total Ion and Selected Ion Quantification. The recommended quantification procedure when highest sensitivity is not required and very complex mixtures of PAHs are present is specific ion current integration, where specific ion currents are extracted from the total ion RGC and quantified by computer program. An exception to this occurs when specifically known species are sought or when highest sensitivity is required; in this event, SIM GC-MS should be utilized.

The basic routines available with all commercial minicomputers for GC-MS are RGC and a mass spectrum printing routine. Modifications of the RGC routine are invaluable for the location of minor chromatographic peaks and for performing rapid quantitative analyses. The normal RGC plot consists of a reconstructed chromatogram which contains ions of all mass numbers; see, for example, the total ion chromatogram in Figure 16. To locate the GC peak for a compound whose mass spectrum is known, RGC plots containing prominant ions in the

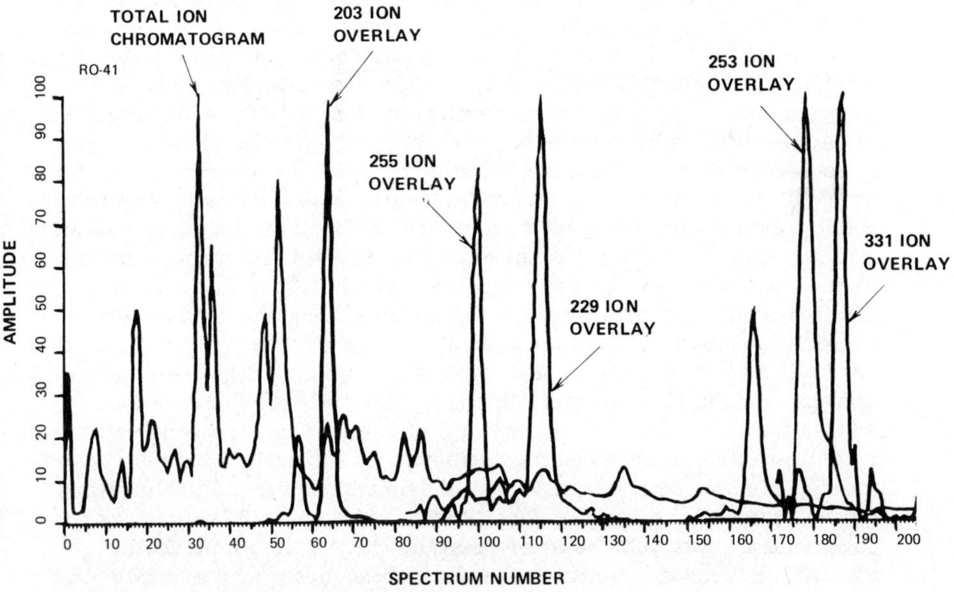

Figure 16 Reconstructed ion chromatograms for combustion effluent sample (14 ft × 2 mm, 2.5% Dexsil 300 programmed from 170 to 350°C at 4°C/min). (From Ref. 46.)

mass spectrum of this compound should be overlaid on the original total ion RGC. Maxima in the RGC specific ion overlays will occur at the spectrum number corresponding to the compound of interest in the total ion RGC.

For example, Figure 16 shows a portion of the RGC for a low-resolution separation GC-MS analysis of a sample of combustion effluent. Several individual ion overlays are shown superimposed on the total ion chromatogram. The 253 ion overlay shows maxima at spectrum numbers 166 and 179, although it is apparent that no peaks are visible on the original total ion chromatogram. If the spectra at spectrum numbers 166 and 179 are displayed or printed out, it is evident that these two peaks are benzfluoroanthene or benzpyrene isomers; the spectra are both characterized by a base peak at m/e = 253 (M + 1) and adduct ions (M + 29, M + 41) at m/e = 281 and 293. It is important that the presence of the compound sought should be confirmed by printing out its mass spectrum in this manner, since spurious "hits" sometimes occur due to interfering fragments from other compounds.

Specific ion current integration is the basis for a very rapid quantification routine. To obtain the specific ion currents due to minor peaks which are confused and overlaid by other major peaks, the precise position of the minor peak is first determined by means of the RGC overlay technique. For example, in Figure 16, the location of pyrene (spectrum 64) and fluoranthene (spectrum 56) is established by overlaying the 203 ion on the total ion chromatogram; 203 is the mass number for the protonated molecular ion of both of these compounds. Peak width limits are then read off from the chromatogram, or located with a CRT cursor, and in this case are seen to be spectra 54 to 61 and spectra 61 to 69 for fluoranthene and pyrene, respectively. Having established the peak's width limits, another computer routine may be used to sum the ion currents due to all of the prominent ions in the mass spectrum of the compounds of interest. The ion integration procedure is then repeated for an internal standard that was previously added in a known quantity to the complex mixture. In this example, the internal standard used was 9-phenylanthracene, whose position is indicated by the 255 ion overlay in Figure 16, as spectrum 100. Quantification of the compound of interest is then achieved by ratioing the ion current of the compound of interest to that of the internal standard, and applying a previously determined calibration factor which allows for the difference in ionization efficiencies of the compound sought and the internal standard. This quantification procedure has been demonstrated to have an accuracy and reproducibility of rather better than ±10%.

SIM quantification is applicable when known compounds are being sought in a complex mixture and when highest sensitivity is required. In the SIM quantification mode, up to eight single ion intensities are usually measured simultaneously unless a sequential SIM mode is employed. In sequential SIM, the group of ions being monitored are changed every few minutes, to coincide with the compounds sought, which are eluting from the GC column. In this manner, large numbers of preselected compounds can be quantified with very high sensitivity. This quantification procedure typically requires the incorporation of known quantities of three unique internal standards into the sample of industrial effluent to be analyzed. 9-Methylanthracene, 9-phenylanthraceee, and 9,10-diphenylanthracene have been used in several studies since these PAH species have not apparently been observed in combustion or other industrial effluent samples [39,65,82,86]. Clearly, for samples such as those from coal conversion processes, where very complex PAH mixtures are expected, great care must be taken in the selection of internal standards to ensure their uniqueness; isotopically labelled compounds are preferred. Quantification may be achieved by integrating the molecular ions in the mass spectrum of each individual PAH species present, including internal standards, and then ratioing the ion current for each individual PAH compound to the ion current for an appropriate internal standard. Allowance must be made for the various ionization efficiencies for each PAH compound; the appropriate factors are previously determined in a calibration experiment.

More than one internal standard is added, since experience has shown that it is usually necessary to increase the mass spectrometer sensitivity to detect trace quantities of high molecular weight species, and it is essential to have at least one internal standard detected at each sensitivity setting. Control experiments with prepared mixtures have demonstrated that reproducibility and accuracy of this technique are appreciably better than ±2%.

Calibration and Response Factors. To carry out quantitative analyses by any technique, it is necessary to calibrate the chosen detector with both of the compounds sought and internal standards, and thus determine the response ratio between each compound and the standard. Using the response factors thus obtained, it is only necessary to multiply them by the ratio of peak (or height) areas of compound to internal standard to obtain the quantitative value for the compounds sought. Response factors automatically take into account such factors as peak shape and detector response; it is usual to calibrate the detector with six to eight concentrations of both the compounds sought and internal standards.

Sample Recovery. The sample recovery is that portion of the original sample which is ultimately analyzed by the detector. Sample recoveries must necessarily be factored into the quantification response ratios and must be determined for as many individual PAH compounds as is necessary. Recovery involves the determination of an absolute quantity, rather than a relative quantity, and may be calculated by adding an additional standard to a sample immediately prior to GC or GC-MS analysis, provided that it may be assumed that no preferential chromatographic losses of the compound sought or standard occurs. Lowest recoveries usually originate in the sample extraction and solvent reduction operations; great care is necessary during these steps.

Detection Limits. Detection limits are a function of both the detector response and the sharpness of the chromatographic separation. The greatest sensitivity is obtained by capillary column SIM GC-MS, when a few picograms of PAHs may be routinely measured. The specific (or total) ion integration technique can generally achieve a sensitivity of a few nanograms under favorable conditions. The use of capillary columns is clearly important to achieve good detection limits, as discussed earlier.

REFERENCES

1. A. Dipple. Chemical Carcinogens, Am. Chem. Soc. 173 (C. E. Searle, Ed.), American Chemical Society, Washington, D.C., 1976, p. 245.

2. G. M. Badger and T. M. Spotswood, J. Chem. Soc., 4431 (1960).
3. B. T. Commins, Atmos. Environ. *3*, 565 (1969).
4. B. D. Crittenden and R. Long. Carcinogenesis, Vol. 1: Polynuclear Aromatic Hydrocarbons: Chemistry, Metabolism, and Carcinogenesis (R. I. Freudenthal and P. W. Jones, Eds.), Raven Press, New York, 1976.
5. E. E. Thomplins and R. Long. Presented at the 12th International Symposium on Combustion, 1969, p. 625.
6. S. B. Radding, T. Mill, C. W. Gould, D. H. Liu, H. L. Johnson, D. C. Bomberger, and C. V. Fojo. The Environmental Fate of Selected Polynuclear Aromatic Hydrocarbons, Stanford Research Institute, Report to EPA (Washington) on Contract No. EPA-68-01-2681. NTIS PB-250 948, 1976.
7. J. J. Murray, R. F. Pottie, and C. Pupp. Can. J. Chem. *52*, 557 (1974).
8. C. Pupp, R. C. Lao, J. J. Murray, and R. F. Pottie. Atmos. Environ. *8*, 915 (1974).
9. E. Clar. Polycyclic Hydrocarbons. Academic Press, New York, 1964.
10. Particulate Polycyclic Organic Matter. National Academy of Sciences, Washington, D.C., 1972.
11. R. S. Tipson, National Bureau of Standards Report No. 8363. U.S. Government Printing Office, Washington, D.C., 1964.
12. M. Kuratsune and T. Hirohata. Natl. Cancer Inst. Monogr. No. 9, 117 (1962).
13. Y. Masuda and M. Kuratsune. Int. J. Air Water Pollut. *10*, 805 (1966).
14. M. N. Inscoe. Anal. Chem. *36*, 2505 (1964).
15. B. D. Tebbens, J. F. Thomas, and M. Mukai. J. Am. Ind. Hyg. Assoc. *27*, 415 (1966).
16. J. F. Thomas, M. Mukai, and B. D. Tebbens. Environ. Sci. Technol. *2*, 33 (1968).
17. D. A. Lane and M. Katz. Fate of Pollutants in Air and Water Environments, Part 2 (I. A. Suffet, Ed.). Wiley-Interscience, New York, 1977.
18. B. T. Commins. Natl. Cancer Inst. Monogr. No. 9, 225 (1962).
19. G. Lunde and A. Bjørseth. Nature (Lond.) *268*, 518 (1977).
20. Carcinogenesis: A Comprehensive Survey, Vol. 1 and 3, Proceedings of the First and Second International Symposia on Polynuclear Aromatic Hydrocarbons (P. W. Jones and R. I. Freudenthal, Eds.), Raven Press, New York, 1976 and 1978.

21. R. M. Harrison, R. Perry, and R. A. Wellings. Environ. Sci. Technol. *10*, 1151 (1976).
22. P. E. Strup, F. R. Moore, and P. W. Jones. Phase I Report of Development of Methods for Analysis of PAHs in Industrial Wastewater. Contract No. 68-03-2624. EPA, Cincinnati, Ohio, May 1978.
23. P. S. Varma and J. L. Das Gupta. J. Indian. Chem. Soc. *4*, 297 (1927).
24. P. W. Jones. Unpublished results, (1972).
25. E. de B. Barnett, J. W. Cook, and H. H. Grainger. J. Chem. Soc. *121*, 2059 (1922).
26. J. N. Pitts, Jr., W. L. Belser, Jr., K. A. Van Cauwenberghe, D. Grosjean, J. P. Schmid, D. R. Fritz, G. B. Knudson, and P. M. Hynds. Chemical and microbiological studies of mutagenic pollutants in real and simulated atmospheres. Presented at the Symposium on the Application of Short-Term Bioassays in the Fractionation and Analysis of Complex Environmental Mixtures, Williamsburg, Va., Feb. 1978.
27. H. Vollman, H. Becker, M. Corell, and H. Streeck. Justus Liebigs Ann. Chem. *531*, 1 (1937).
28. M. J. Suess. Sci. Total Environ. *6*, 239 (1976).
29. R. L. Stenberg. Sample Collection Techniques for Combustion Sources--Benzpyrene Determination. NTIS PB-214 953, 1961.
30. Fed. Reg. *36*(247) 24888 (Dec. 23, 1971).
31. Fed. Reg. *41*(111), 23076 (June 8, 1976).
32. T. S. Herman. Development of Sampling Procedures for Polycyclic Organic Matter and Polychlorinated Biphenyls. NTIS PB-243 362, 1974.
33. Sampling Survey Related to Possible Emission of PCBs from the Incineration of Domestic Refuse. EPA, Chicago. NTIS PB-251 285, 1975.
34. D. Scheutzle, T. J. Prater, and S. R. Ruddell. J. Air Pollut. Control Assoc. *25*, 925 (1975).
35. R. E. Barrett, W. L. Margard, J. B. Purdy, P. W. Jones, and P. E. Strup. Sampling and Analysis of Coke Oven Door Emissions. EPA-600/2-77-213. NTIS No. PB-276 485, 1977.
36. P. W. Jones and P. E. Strup. Final Report to EPA (North Carolina) on Contract No. 68-02-1409 (Task 28), 9175.
37. R. E. Barrett, P. E. Strup, and P. W. Jones. Final Report to EPA (North Carolina) on Contract No. 68-02-1409 (Tasks 32, 35, 36, 37), 1976.
38. D. F. S. Natusch and B. A. Tomkins. Theoretical considerations of the adsorbtion of PAH vapor onto flyash in a coal-fired power plant. In Carcinogenesis, Vol. 3: Polynuclear Aromatic Hydrocarbons (P. W. Jones and R. I. Freudenthal, Eds.). Raven Press, New York, 1978, p. 145.

39. P. W. Jones, R. D. Giammar, P. E. Strup, and T. B. Stanford. Environ. Sci. Technol. *10*, 806 (1976).
40. M. B. Neher, P. J. Perry, and P. W. Jones. Validation of the Battelle Sorbent Sampling System. Final Report to EPRI on Contract No. RP383-2, Jan. 1977.
41. J. T. Veal. Evaluation of a Polycyclic Organic Material Sampling System. Final Report to EPRI on Contract No. RP800-1, Sept. 1977.
42. P. W. Jones, J. E. Wilkinson, and P. E. Strup. Measurement of PAH Emissions from Secondary Lead Smelters, Interim Report to EPA, Contract No. 68-02-2457, 1977.
43. K. L. Maloney and T. W. Sonnichsen. Progress Report No. 3 on EPRI Contract No. RP1075-1, 1978.
44. W. Feairheller, P. J. Mann, D. H. Harris, and D. L. Harris. Technical Manual for Process Sampling Strategies for Organic Materials. EPA-600/2-76-122 (North Carolina), 1976.
45. J. W. Hamersma, S. L. Reynolds, and R. F. Maddalone. IERL-RTP Procedures Manual: Level I Environmental Assessment. EPA-600/2-76-106a (North Carolina), 1976.
46. P. W. Jones, J. E. Wilkinson, and P. E. Strup. Measurement of Polycyclic Organic Materials and Other Hazardous Organic Compounds in Stack Gases, State-of-the-art, EPA-600/2-77-202, 1977.
47. S. F. Stepan and J. F. Smith. Water Res. *11*, 339 (1977).
48. V. Leoni, G. Puccetti, R. J. Columbo, and A. M. D'Ovidio. J. Chromatogr. *125*, 339 (1976).
49. G. A. Junk, J. J. Richard, D. Witiak, M. D. Arguello, R. Vick, H. Svec, J. S. Fritz, and G. V. Calder. J. Chromatogr. *99*, 745 (1974).
50. R. L. Malcolm, E. M. Thurman, and G. R. Aiken. Proceedings of the 11th Annual Conference on Trace Substances in Environmental Health, Columbia, Mo. 1977.
51. J. Saxena, J. Mozuchowski, and D. K. Basu. Environ. Sci. Technol. *11*, 682 (1977).
52. A. M. Krstulovic, D. M. Rosie, and P. R. Brown. Am. Lab. *11* (July 1977).
53. J. Adams, K. Menzies, and P. Levins. Selection and Evaluation of Sorbent Resins for Collection of Organic Compounds. NTIS No. PB-268 559, 1977.
54. P. W. Jones and R. J. Jakobsen. A critique of organic level-1 analysis. Presented at Process Measurements for Environmental Assessment Symposium, Atlanta, Ga., Feb. 13-15, 1978 (in press--IERL, EPA, North Carolina).
55. M. B. Neher and P. W. Jones. Anal. Chem. *49*, 513 (1977).
56. F. DeWiest and D. Ronia. Atmos. Environ. *10*, 487 (1976).
57. M. Corn, T. L. Montgomery, and N. A. Esmen. Environ. Sci. Technol. *5*, 155 (1971).

58. T. L. Ogden and J. D. Wood. Ann. Occup. Hyg. *17*, 187 (1975).
59. M. Katz and R. C. Pierce. Quantitative distribution of PAHs on relation to particle size of urban particulate. In Carcinogenesis, Vol. 1: Polynuclear Aromatic Hydrocarbons (R. I. Freudenthal and P. W. Jones, Eds.), Raven Press, New York, 1976, p. 413.
60. R. C. Pierce and M. Katz. Environ. Sci. Technol. *9*, 347 (1975).
61. R. M. Burton, J. N. Howard, R. L. Penley, P. A. Ramsey, and T. A. Clark. J. Air Pollut. Control Assoc. *23*, 277 (1973).
62. R. S. Sholtes, R. B. Engdahl, R. A. Herrick, C. Phillips, E. Stein, J. Wagman, and P. R. Woolrich. Health Lab. Sci. *7*, 279 (1970).
63. E. Sawicki, R. C. Corey, A. E. Dooley, J. R. Gisclard, J. L. Monkman, R. G. Neligon, and L. A. Ripperton. Health Lab. Sci. *7* (Suppl.), 31 (1970).
64. R. I. Mitchell, W. M. Henry, and N. C. Henderson. Final Report to EPA (North Carolina) on Contract No. 68-02-2281, 1977.
65. P. W. Jones. Analysis of nonparticulate organic compounds in ambient atmospheres. Presented at the 67th Annual Meeting of the Air Pollution Control Association, Denver, June 9-13, 1974. EPA-600/9-76-007a, June 1976.
66. A. Zlatkis, H. A. Lichtenstein, and A. Tishbee. Chromatographia *6*(2), 67 (1973).
67. A. Dravnieks, B. K. Krotaszynski, J. Burton, A. O'Donnel, and T. Burgwald. High speed collection of organic vapors from the atmosphere. Presented at the 11th Conference on Methods in Air Pollution and Industrial Hygiene Studies, Berkeley, Calif., Apr. 1970.
68. M. A. Fox and S. W. Staley. Anal. Chem. *48*, 992 (1976).
69. D. Scheutzle, A. L. Crittenden, and R. J. Charlson. J. Air Pollut. Control Assoc. *23*, 704 (1973).
70. W. Bertsch, R. C. Chang, and A. Zlatkis. J. Chromatogr. Sci. *12*, 175 (1974).
71. G. D. Mendenhall, P. W. Jones, P. E. Strup, and W. L. Margard. Organic Characterization of Aerosols and Vapor Phase Compounds in Urban Atmospheres. EPA-600/3-78-031, 1978.
72. R. A. Spindt. Polynuclear Aromatic Content of Heavy Duty Diesel Engine Exhaust Gases. NTIS PB-267 774, 1977.
73. C. R. Bergman and J. M. Calucci. Polynuclear aromatic hydrocarbon emissions from automotive engines. SAE Trans. *79*, 1682 (1970).
74. M. E. Griffing, A. R. Maler, J. E. Borland, and R. R. Decker. Applying a new method for the measuring of benz[a]pyrene in

vehicle exhaust to the study of fuel factors. Presented at the Symposium on Current Approaches to Automotive Emission Control, ACS, Los Angeles, Calif., 1971, p. 13.
75. A. Candeli, V. Mastrandrea, G. Morozzi, and S. Toccaceli, Atmos. Environ. *8*, 693 (1974).
76. W. E. Rinehart, S. A. Gendermalik, and L. F. Gilbert. Fuel factors in automotive tailpipe emissions. Presented at the American Industrial Hygiene Conference, Detroit, Mich., 1970, Paper No. 127, p. 15.
77. Strichting Concawe. Effect of Gasoline Aromatic Content on Polynuclear Aromatic Exhaust Emissions. Report No. 6-74, Sept. 1974, 60 Van Hagenhonckleaan, The Hague 2018.
78. C. R. Begeman and J. M. Calucci. Natl. Cancer Inst. Monogr. No. 9, 17 (1962).
79. A. Condeli, G. Morozzi, A. Paolacci, and L. Zoccolillo. Atmos. Environ. *9*, 843 (1975).
80. H. K. Newhall, R. E. Jentoft, and P. R. Ballinger. SAE No. 730834, Sept. 1973.
81. P. Van Rossum and R. G. Webb. J. Chromatogr. *150*, 381 (1978).
82. P. E. Strup, J. E. Wilkinson, and P. W. Jones, Trace analysis of PAHs in aqueous systems using XAD-2 resin and capillary column gas chromatography-mass spectrometry analysis. In Carcinogenesis, Vol. 3: Polynuclear Aromatic Hydrocarbons (P. W. Jones and R. I. Freudenthal, Eds.), Raven Press, New York, 1978, p. 131.
83. W. E. May, S. N. Chesler, S. P. Cram, B. H. Gump, H. S. Hertz, D. P. Enagonio, and S. M. Dyszel. J. Chromatogr. Sci. *13*, 535 (1975).
84. S. A. Wise, S. N. Chesler, H. S. Hertz, L. R. Hilpert, and W. E. May. Methods for PAH analysis in the marine environment. Carcinogenesis, Vol. 3: Polynuclear Aromatic Hydrocarbons (P. W. Jones and R. I. Freudenthal, Eds.), Raven Press, New York, 1978, p. 175.
85. D. W. Ellis. The Analysis of Aromatic Compounds in Water Using Fluorescence and Phosphorescence. NTIS PB-212 268, 1972.
86. P. W. Jones, A. P. Graffeo, R. Detrick, P. A. Clarke, and R. J. Jakobsen. Technical Manual for Analysis of Organic Materials on Process Streams. EPA-600/2-76-072 (1976). Revised under Contract No. 68-02-2156 (in press), June 1978.
87. B. T. Commins, Int. J. Air Pollut. *1*, 14 17, (1958).
88. T. W. Stanley, D. F. Bender, and W. C. Elbert. Quantitative aspects of thin-layer chromatography in air pollution measurements. Quantitative Thin-Layer Chromatography. Wiley, New York, 1973, pp. 305-322.

89. G. J. Cleary. J. Chromatogr. *9*, 204 (1962).
90. A. Liberti, G. Morozzi, and L. Zoccolillo. Ann. Chem. *65*, 573 (1975).
91. M. Kertesz-Saringer and Z. Morlin. Atmos. Environ. *9*, 831 (1975).
92. W. Cautreels and K. Van Cauwenberghe. Water Air Soil Pollut. *6*, 103 (1976).
93. E. Sawicki, R. C. Corey, A. E. Dooley, J. B. Gisclard, J. L. Monkman, R. E. Neligan, and L. A. Ripperton. Health Lab. Sci. *7*, 45 (1970).
94. C. Golden, and E. Sawicki. Int. J. Environ. Anal. Chem. *4*, 9 (1975).
95. K. D. Bartle, M. L. Lee, and M. Novotny. Int. J. Environ. Anal. Chem. *3*, 349 (1974).
96. M. Novotny, M. L. Lee, and K. D. Bartle. J. Chromatogr. Sci. *12*, 606 (1974).
97. M. L. Lee, M. Novotny, and K. D. Bartle. Anal. Chem. *48*, 1566 (1976).
98. B. B. Chakraborty and R. Long. Environ. Sci. Technol. *1*, 828 (1967).
99. J. M. Colucci and C. R. Begeman. In Polynuclear Aromatic Hydrocarbons and Other Pollutants in Los Angeles Air, Proceedings of the 2nd International Clean Air Congress, 1970, (H. M. Englund, Eds.). Academic Press, New York, 1971, pp. 28-35.
100. W. Cautreels and K. Van Cauwenberghe. J. Chromatogr. *131*, 253 (1977).
101. K. Grob, K. Grob, Jr., and G. Grob. J. Chromatogr. *106*, 299 (1975).
102. W. E. Schwartz, G. D. Mendenhall, P. W. Jones, C. J. Riggle, A. P. Graffeo, and D. F. Miller. Chemical Characterization of Model Aersols. EPA-600/3-76-085, 1976.
103. B. Versino, H. Knoppel, M. DeGroot, A. Peil, J. Poelman, H. Schuuenburg, H. Vissers, and F. Geiss. J. Chromatogr. *122*, 373 (1976).
104. W. Bertsch, E. Anderson, and G. Holzer. J. Chromatogr. *112*, 701 (1975).
105. R. E. Seivers, R. M. Barkley, G. A. Eiceman, R. H. Shapiro, H. F. Walton, K. J. Kolonko, and L. R. Field. J. Chromatogr. *142*, 745 (1977).
106. T. A. Bellar and J. J. Lichtenberg. J. Am. Water Works Assoc. *66*, 739 (1974).
107. K. Grob and F. Zurcher. J. Chromatogr. *117*, 285 (1976).
108. D. Hoffman and E. L. Wynder. Cancer *13*, 1062 (1960).
109. C. J. Ledford, G. P. Morie, and C. A. Glover. Tob. Sci. *14*, 158 (1970).

110. H. P. Harke, D. Schuller, H. J. Klimisch, and K. Meisner. Z. Lebensm. Unters. Forsch. *162*, 291 (1976).
111. E. O. Haenni, J. W. Howard, and F. L. Joe, Jr. J. Assoc. Off. Agric. Chem. *45*, 67 (1962).
112. D. Hoffman and E. L. Wynder. Anal. Chem. *32*, 295 (1960).
113. A. Candeli, G. Morozzi, A. Paolacci, and L. Zoccolillo. Atmos. Environ. *9*, 843 (1975).
114. D. Hoffman and E. L. Wynder. Respiratory carcinogens: their nature and precursors. Presented at the Identification and Measurement of Environmental Pollutants Symposium (B. Westley, Ed.), Ottawa, Canada, June 14-17, 1971, pp. 9-16.
115. M. A. Acheson, R. M. Harrison, R. Perry, and R. A. Wellings. Water Res. *10*, 207 (1976).
116. W. Cautreels and K. Van Cauwenberghe. Water Air Soil Pollut. *6*, 103 (1976).
117. A. Liberti, G. Morozzi, and L. Zoccolillo. Ann. Chem. *65*, 573 (1975).
118. L. Hunter, Environ. Sci. Technol. *9*, 241 (1975).
119. H. Wordich, W. Piannhauser, G. Blaicher, and K. Tiefenbacher. Chromatographia *10*, 140 (1977).
120. E. Sawicki, R. C. Corey, A. E. Dooley, J. B. Gisclard, and J. L. Monkman. Health Lab. Sci. *7*, 56, 68 (1970).
121. M. J. Schultz, R. M. Orheim, and H. H. Boree. Am. Ind. Hyg. Assoc. J. *34*, 404 (1973).
122. R. Tomingas, G. Voltmer, and R. Bednarik. Sci. Total Environ. *7*, 261 (1977).
123. E. K. Harrison and C. I. B. Powell. Ann. Occup. Hyg. *18*, 194 (1975).
124. G. Chatnot, R. Dougy-Cage, and R. Fontages. Chromatographia *5*, 460 (1972).
125. R. C. Pierce and M. Katz. Anal. Chem. *67*, 1743 (1975).
126. E. Sawicki, W. Elbert, T. W. Stanley, T. R. Hauser, and F. T. Fox, Anal. Chem. *32*, 810 (1960).
127. E. Sawicki, J. L. Meeker, and M. J. Morgan. Int. J. Air Water Pollut. *9*, 291 (1965).
128. C. J. Clearly. J. Chromatogr. *9*, 204 (1962).
129. E. Sawicki, P. R. Atkins, T. Belsky, F. A. Friedel, D. L. Hyde, J. L. Monkman, R. A. Rasmussen, L. A. Ripperton, J. E. Sigsby, and L. D. White. Health Lab. Sci. *11*, 228 (1974).
130. H. J. Brass, W. C. Elbert, M. A. Feige, E. M. Gliek, and A. W. Lington. United States Steel, Lorain, Ohio, Black River Survey: Analysis for Hexane Organic Extractables and Polynuclear Aromatic Hydrocarbons. Office of Enforcement and General Counsel, EPA, Cincinnati, Ohio, Oct. 1974.

131. D. K. Basu and J. Saxens. Environ. Sci. Technol., in press (1978).
132. M. Novotny, M. L. Lee, and K. D. Bartle. J. Chromatogr. Sci. *12*, 606 (1974).
133. B. B. Wheals, C. G. Vaughan, and M. J. Whitehouse. J. Chromatogr. *106*, 109 (1975).
134. J. J. Klimisch. J. Chromatogr. *83*, 11 (1973).
135. H. J. Klimisch. Anal. Chem. *45*, 11 (1973).
136. H. J. Klimisch and D. Ambrosius. J. Chromatogr. *120*, 299 (1976).
137. H. J. Boden. J. Chromatogr. Sci. *14*, 391 (1976).
138. M. Dong, D. C. Locke, and E. Ferrand. Anal. Chem. *48*, 368 (1976).
139. H. Hatano, Y. Yamamoto, M. Saito, E. Mochida, and S. Watanabe. J. Chromatogr. *120*, 482 (1976).
140. V. G. Grimmer and J. G. Burgan. Analyst *85*, 723 (1960).
141. T. Panalaks. J. Environ. Sci. Health *B11*, 299 (1976).
142. A. H. Qazi, C. A. Nau, H. Turner, and G. T. Taylor. J. Am. Ind. Hyg. Assoc. *34*, 554 (1973).
143. H. P. Burchfield, E. E. Green, R. J. Wheller, and S. M. Billedeau. J. Chromatogr. *99*, 697 (1974).
144. H. Matsushita, K. Arashidani, and H. Hayashi. Bunseki Kagaku *25*, 412 (1976).
145. H. Shirayama. Nippon Kagaku Kaishi *1*, 118 (1977).
146. W. Strubert. Chromatographia *4*, 205 (1975).
147. D. A. Skoog and D. M. West. Principles of Instrumental Analysis. Holt, Rienhart and Winston, New York, 1971, p. 222.
148. H. Hellmann. Anal. Chem. *278*, 263 (1976).
149. E. Sawicki. EPA (North Carolina), 1972.
150. R. C. Lao, R. S. Thomas, H. Oja, and L. Dubois. Anal. Chem. *45*, 908 (1973).
151. A. Bjørseth. Analysis of PAHs in environmental samples by glass capillary gas chromatography. In Carcinogenesis, Vol. 3: Polynuclear Aromatic Hydrocarbons (P. W. Jones and R. I. Freudenthal, Eds.), Raven Press, New York, 1978, p. 75.
152. P. Burchill, A. A. Herod, and R. G. James. A comparison of some methods for estimation of PAHs in pollutants. In Carcinogenesis, Vol. 3: Polynuclear Aromatic Hydrocarbons (P. W. Jones and R. I. Freudenthal, Eds.), Raven Press, New York, 1978, p. 35.
153. R. C. Lao, R. S. Thomas, and J. L. Monkman. J. Chromatogr. *112*, 681 (1975).
154. W. H. Griest, H. Kubota, and M. R. Guerin. Anal. Lett. *8*, 949 (1975).
155. L. DeMaio and M. Corn. Anal. Chem. *38*, 131 (1966).

156. A. F. Shushunova, P. E. Shkodich, N. G. Shkanakin, and L. Z. H. Lembik. Gig. Sanit. *8*, 61 (1975).
157. G. Chatot, R. Dangy-Caye, and R. Fontanges. J. Chromatogr. *72*, 202 (1972).
158. K. A. Schulte, D. J. Larsen, R. W. Hornung, and J. V. Crable. J. Am. Ind. Hyg. Assoc. *36*, 131 (1975).
159. R. C. Lao, H. Oja, R. S. Thomas, and J. L. Monkman. Sci. Total Environ. *2*, 223 (1973).
160. M. R. Guerin, J. L. Epler, W. H. Griest, B. R. Clarke, and T K. Rao. PAHs from fossil fuel conversion processes. In Carcinogenesis, Vol. 3: Polynuclear Aromatic Hydrocarbons (P. W. Jones and R. I. Freudenthal, Eds.), Raven Press, New York, 1978, p. 21.
161. G. M. Janini, K. Johnston, and W. L. Zielinski, Jr. Anal. Chem. *47*, 670 (1975).
162. G. M. Janini, G. M. Muschik, J. A. Schroer, and W. L. Zielinski, Jr. Anal. Chem. *48*, 1879 (1976).
163. V. Cantuti, G. P. Cartoni, A. Liberti, and A. G. Torri. J. Chromatogr. *17*, 60 (1965).
164. K. Grob, Jr., and K. Grob. Chromatographia *10*, 250 (1977).
165. N. Carungo and S. Rossi. J. Gas Chromatogr. *5*, 103 (1967).
166. V. G. Grimmer, A. Hildebrandt, and H. Bohnke. Erdoel Vnd Kohle, Erdgas, Petrochem. Ver. Brennst. Chem. *25*, 442, 531 (1972).
167. H. P. Harke, D. Schuller, H. J. Klimisch, and K. Meisner. Z. Lebensm. Unters Forsch. *162*, 291 (1976).
168. P. Van Rossum and R. G. Webb. J. Chromatogr. *150*, 381 (1978).
169. M. Novotny, M. L. McConnell, M. L. Lee, and R. Farlow. Clin. Chem. *20*, 1105 (1974).
170. K. Grob and G. Grob. Chromatographia 5, (1972).
171. R. M. J. Van den Berg and T. P. H. Cox. Chromatographia *5*, 301 (1972).
172. R. L. Foltz. Guidelines for Analytical Toxicology Programs, Organization-Instrumentation-Technique (J. J. Thoma and I. Sunshine, Eds.). CRC Press, Cleveland, Ohio, 1977.
173. D. Scheutzle, A. L. Crittenden, and R. J. Charlson. J. Air Pollut. Control Assoc. *23*, 704 (1973).
174. G. J. Down and S. A. Gwyn. J. Chromatogr. *102*, 208 (1975).
175. W. McFadden (Ed.). Techniques of Combined Gas Chromatography/Mass Spectrometry. Wiley-Interscience, New York, 1973.
176. G. A. Junk. Int. J. Mass Spectrom. Ion Phys. *8*, 1 (1972).
177. R. Ryhage. Quant. Rev. Biophys. *6*, 311 (1973).
178. M. S. B. Munson and F. H. Field. J. Am. Chem. Soc. *88*, 2621 (1966).

179. R. Saferstein, J. M. Chao, and J. Monura. J. Forensic Sci. *19*, 463 (1974).
180. D. Horton, J. D. Wonder, and R. L. Foltz. Carbohydr. Res. *36*, 75 (1975).
181. R. A. Hites and G. R. Dubay. Charge exchange-chemical ionization of polycyclic aromatic compounds. In Carcinogenesis, Vol. 3: Polynuclear Aromatic Hydrocarbons (P. W. Jones and R. I. Freudenthal, Eds.), Raven Press, New York, 1078, p. 85.
182. M. L. Lee and R. A. Hites. J. Am. Chem. Soc. *99*, 2008 (1977).

9
Toxic Metals and Metalloids

WILLIAM M. BLAKEMORE National Center for Toxicological Research, U.S. Food and Drug Administration, Jefferson, Arkansas

I. INTRODUCTION

This chapter addresses only those elements known to have toxic effects upon overexposure; however, it should be noted that many of these elements, in lower concentrations, are essential to biological processes in humans. Certain elements, although present in minute amounts in the tissues, are essential nutrients. Their presence was long overlooked, and even after their identification, shortcomings of the methods available for analysis, together with a failure to recognize their importance, led to their being reported present in traces and their somewhat depreciatory designation as the trace elements. They perform functions indispensable to maintenance of life, growth, and reproduction. On the other hand, other elements also present in low concentrations may interfere with vital functions.

The subject of trace elements in health and disease has received relatively little attention until recent years. The availability of refined instrumentation and of new methods of analysis for traces of atomic constituents has changed this. New emphasis is being placed on trace elemental analysis and interpretation of these data, whether the problems are excesses (toxicology) or deficiency (malnutrition).

Most imbalances of trace element nutrition are characterized by the absence of acute, easily recognizable disease. To diagnose marginal deficiencies or excesses of trace elements, the analyst must use rather sophisticated procedures, and even where an imbalance of trace element nutrition can be proven, the implications for health are not always evident. There are conspicuous gaps in our knowledge of deviations in trace element nutrition and their effect on health and disease. Etiologic factors for many chronic disease processes are unknown, resulting in hypotheses that may be one sided. To date, the biological roles of many trace elements are hypothetical at best. Although the short-term consequences of extreme under- or overexposures are reasonably well known, it is very difficult to investigate the marginal imbalances and their long-term consequences, which are most likely related to existing health problems in humans.

The rapid development of analytical methodology in the past decade has created powerful tools for trace element research. However, these tools can be dangerous if their technical and general limitations are not clearly understood. It is necessary to appreciate these limitations, not only in technology, but also with regard to the interpretation of the results, in view of the ever-increasing demands on the analytical chemist.

The three criteria that the analysis must meet if results are to be meaningful are specificity, precision, and sensitivity, in that order. The determination of one element in a mixture of many others is a very complex procedure, influenced by a wide variety of factors. These factors become more and more dominant as the concentration of the element to be determined decreases. These influences are termed matrix effects for the substrate to be analyzed. The printout from even the most sophisticated instrument is only a number, which may or may not be related to the amount of the trace element that was fed into the instrument. The validity of analytical results rests on the utmost effort of the chemist to establish a strong cause-and-effect relationship between the element to be analyzed and the final signal. Additional separation techniques, such as ion exchange columns, or chelation and extraction, may be used to isolate one element from an interfering matrix. Sample contamination is extremely important in trace analysis and demands the constant attention of the analyst. Glassware must be scrupulously cleansed, and clean areas, utilizing laminar flow hoods and benches, must be provided for sample handling and analysis. To develop an analysis, more than one method should be used and the results compared. Even if any given analytical method is well controlled, the results should not be regarded as factual until they have been found to agree with those obtained by a basically different procedure. If a sample requires digestion or ashing, all three common methods should be used: wet digestion, high-temperature ashing, and low-temperature ashing in an oxygen plasma. These should all be determined by different techniques. Upon comparing all the results, the investigator should be aware of the potential errors in any particular method. Certified standards of the same or a similar matrix should be analyzed, spiked with standard additions before analyzing, and the results checked for precision and accuracy.

There are many techniques available for trace elemental analysis, including x-ray fluorescence, emission spectrometry with the inductively coupled argon plasma, atomic absorption spectrometry, neutron activation analysis, gas chromatography, and electrochemical analysis. No one instrument is ideal for every analysis to be performed, but they tend to complement each other.

All forms of the ecological system are affected to varying extents by metals, which are the most insidious pollutants because of their nonbiodegradable nature. Metals in the environment are from natural and man-made sources, with natural pollution accounting for 82% of the total emission (natural dusts and forest fires) [1]. Ultratrace levels of metals in soil and water can result in accumulations by both flora and fauna through their various food chains; and humans being at the top of the food chain, consume foods representative of the total environment. Studies have correlated geographical location to varying levels of dental caries [2]. This correlation shows dependence between type of food consumed and where it was grown with respect to the metal content of the soil and potable water.

II. OCCURRENCE, TOXICITY, AND ANALYSIS OF METALS AND METALLOIDS

A. Beryllium

Beryllium, one of the lightest of metals, although widely distributed, exists in relatively small quantities, comprising less than 0.006% of the earth's crust. Beryl ($3BeO \cdot Al_2O_3 \cdot 6SiO_2$) is the only one of the more than 30 recognized minerals of beryllium that is of any commercial importance. Theoretically, beryl contains 14% BeO, 19% Al_2O_3, and 67% SiO_2. Gem beryl (emerald or aquamarine) approaches this composition, but the commercial ore is contaminated with quartz, feldspar, granite, and mica, with which it is usually associated.

Beryllium is the only stable light metal of high melting point. It possesses fair strength, good electrical conductivity, and excellent sound transmission. It is extremely penetrable to x-rays, has a low neutron capture, high neutron scatter cross section, and provides a good source of neutrons. Beryllium-copper alloys are known for forming qualities prior to heat treating, followed by a remarkable increase in physical properties after simple precipitation hardening, for their antisparking properties, and unusual resistance to fatigue.

Almost all the presently known beryllium compounds are acknowledged to be toxic in both the soluble and insoluble forms, depending on the amount of material inhaled and the length of exposure [2]. Soluble beryllium compounds commonly produce acute pneumonitis, while insoluble compounds such as beryllium and beryllium oxide can produce berylliosis.

Beryllium can be analyzed by atomic absorption spectrophotometry, in an acetylene nitrous oxide flame, at a wavelength of 234.9 nm, with a sensitivity of 30 μg/liter. It can be chelated with 8-hydroxyquinoline at pH 10 and extracted with methyl isobutyl ketone, concentrating 10 times. The methyl isobutyl ketone chelate solution is aspirated directly into the acetylene nitrous oxide flame for analysis, with a sensitivity of 3 μg/liter.

Owens and Gladney [3] determined beryllium in environmental and biological samples using direct injection into a graphite furnace for analysis by flameless atomic absorption spectroscopy with deuterium lamp background correction. Operating parameters for the graphite furnace were 60 seconds drying time at 100°, 60 sec charring time at 1700°, and 7 sec atomization time at 2700°.* Extreme care must be taken when analyzing solid samples in the graphite furnace, as position within the tube and charring conditions affect the results.

One method of introducing solid samples into a graphite furnace is weighing the sample in a tantalum boat and placing the boat inside the furnace tube. However, the presence of tantalum within the furnace causes wide variations in the beryllium signal. Weighing the sample in a tantalum boat, dumping the sample inside the furnace, and removing the boat greatly enhances the precision. With finely powdered samples, the analyst must take the precaution of shutting off the flow of gas to the furnace before inserting the boat, to prevent loss of sample.

Beryllium can be quantitatively determined by chelating with acetylacetone, extracting with chloroform, and spectrophotometric determination at 295 nm. A very selective method for the isolation and determination of beryllium is based on the extraction of beryllium acetylacetonate in the presence of ethylenediaminetetraacetic acid.

To a 50 ml aqueous sample (pH 0.5 to 1.5) containing up to 50 μg of beryllium, add 2 ml of 10% EDTA and adjust to pH 6.0 to 7.0. Add 5 ml of 5% aqueous acetylacetone and readjust to pH 6.0 to 8.0. Allow the solution to stand 5 min and extract with three 10 ml portions of chloroform. Chloroform is preferable to carbon tetrachloride, as it absorbs less light in the ultraviolet region, and the solution of beryllium acetylacetonate is more resistant to washing with aqueous alkali. Before the spectrophotometric determination of the beryllium chelate at 295 nm, the excess reagent, which also absorbs at this wavelength, must be removed by washing with two 4 ml portions of 0.1 N sodium hydroxide.

Wolf and Taylor [4] determined beryllium at picogram levels in biological samples by first chelating with trifluoroacetyl-acetate and analyzing the extracted chelate, using a gas chromatograph-mass spectrometer. There have been several methods reported for the

---

*All temperature data are in degrees Celsius.

analysis of beryllium trifluoro-acetylacetate by gas-liquid chromatography with electron capture detection [5].

B. Chromium

Chromium occurs in nature in the combined state, more generally in rocks of high magnesia and low silica content. The principal source is chrome iron ore (chromite) ($FeOCr_2O_3$) found mainly in the USSR, southern Rhodesia, South Africa, and Turkey. Soils have been found to contain from a trace to 2.4% chromium. Vegetables of 25 botanical families contain 10 to 1000 μg of chromium/kg of dry matter, with most plants falling within the range 100 to 500 μg/kg.

The industrial uses of chromium include stainless steel, corrosion-resisting steels, plating industry, production of catalysts, chrome tanning, paint and primer pigments, as mordants in the textile industry, and graphic arts. Sodium chromate and complex chromate salts are widely used in cooling tower recirculating water systems as rust inhibitors as well as wood preservatives. The circulating water usually contains from 15 to 300 ppm chromate ion, and such systems continuously discharge about 1% of their flow to wastewater and some is lost to the atmosphere. Chromates are also used for the oxidation of organic materials in the production of synthetic dyes, saccharin, benzoic acid, anthraquinone, hydroquinone, camphor, and synthetic fibers. The chromates are used extensively as cleaning agents, in the purification of chemicals, and in organic oxidation.

Chromium was first identified as an essential trace nutrient for mammals in 1959. Trivalent chromium is an essential ingredient of the "glucose tolerance factor," the term given to a yet unidentified water-soluble chromium complex of low molecular weight which occurs naturally in brewer's yeast and mammalian tissues. It is a necessary dietary constituent for optimal glucose utilization, as shown by Jeejeebhoy et al. in a patient receiving long-term total parenteral nutrition [6].

The majority of elderly patients over 70 years of age show evidence of impaired glucose tolerance. In one study, 40% of these cases of mild glucose intolerance in elderly patients were corrected following dietary chromium supplementation. Chromium deficiencies were shown to occur in children with diabetes mellitus [7].

Chromium(III) is less toxic than chromium(VI), whose toxicity has been noted in humans exposed to industrial dichromates. The principal toxic effects of chromium are exerted on the skin, the nasal membrane, and the lungs. It causes perforation of the nasal septum, congestion, hyperemia, emphesema, tracheitis, bronchitis, pharyngitis, broncho-pneumonia, cancer of the respiratory tract, and dermatitis.

Chromium can be determined by atomic absorption spectrophotometry in an air-acetylene flame, at a wavelength of 357.9 nm, with a sensitivity of 100 μg/liter. Sensitivities as low as 1 μg/liter have been achieved using the graphite furnace flameless atomic absorption technique, drying the sample for 15 sec at 15°, charring for 30 sec at 1000° and atomizing at 2700° for 10 sec. Chromium in biological samples can be determined by flameless atomic absorption after enrichment by chelation and extraction [8].

Chromium(VI) can be determined colorimetrically by reaction with diphenylcarbazide in acid solution, with a sensitivity of 20 μg/liter. If total chromium is to be determined, Cr(III) may be oxidized to Cr(VI) with potassium permanganate before reacting with diphenylcarbazide to form the red-violet color. Read absorbance against a blank determination at 540 nm.

Chromium was determined at the picogram level by gas chromatography-mass spectrometry [4]. The chromium is chelated with trifluoracetylacetate and extracted with benzene. The benzene extract is then injected into the gas chromatograph-mass spectrometer.

Chromium has also been analyzed in the low-nanogram range by first chelating with hexafluoroacetyl acetone, extracting the chelate with hexane, and injecting into a coupled gas chromatograph-atomic absorption spectrometer [9].

Chromium(III) is inert to chelate formation with acetylacetone and solvent extraction at ambient temperature. This fact can be used for the selective separation of chromium from most other metals as follows. Adjust the sample solution to pH 3 to 4 and extract with 50% (v/v) acetylacetone in chloroform to remove other metals. Separate the aqueous phase, which still contains all the chromium, adjust to pH 6, add 10 ml of acetylacetone, and heat under reflux for 1 hr to ensure that the formation of the chromium acetylacetonate proceeds to completion. Cool and acidify to between 1 and 3 N sulfuric acid, and extract with a 50% solution (v/v) of acetylacetone in chloroform. Measure the absorption of the red-violet extract at 560 nm.

C. Manganese

Manganese is widely distributed in the combined state, ranking twelfth in abundance among the elements in the earth's crust. The more important minerals are: pyrolusite, black oxide of manganese, MnO_2, the chief source; manganite, $Mn_2O_3 \cdot H_2O$; psilomelane, a hydrous manganese manganate; rhodochrosite, $MnCO_3$; rhodenite, $MnSiO_3$; and spessarite, $Mn_3Al_2(SiO_4)_3$. The metal is used mainly in the production of steel alloys. Manganese bronze is an alloy of manganese and copper; manganin is an alloy of copper, nickel, and manganese.

Manganese is listed as an essential nutrient. There is a scarcity of research on the nutritional role of manganese in nucleic acid synthesis, glucose utilization and gluconeogenesis, intermediary metabolism, and endocrine gland function. The manganese concentration of the earth's crust and most plants is relatively higher than that of other trace metals, but the animal body is greatly selective as to what minerals it retains, and contains much less manganese than other elements that are present in lesser concentration in the environment. The mechanism of absorption of manganese from the gastrointestinal tract is unknown. Absorbed manganese rapidly appears in the bile and is excreted almost exclusively in the feces, almost none appearing in the urine.

Manganese is one of the least toxic of the trace metals, and toxicity occurs only after long, continuous inhalation of large quantities of the element. Symptoms of chronic poisoning in manganese ore miners are seen after exposures ranging from 7 months to 20 years, and sometimes are not seen at all. The clinical manifestations of the disease are both psychiatric and neurologic. The disease progresses to a permanent crippling neurological disorder of the extrapyramidal system and is, in some ways, clinically similar to Parkinson's disease and Wilson's disease.

Manganese can be determined by atomic absorption spectrometry at a wavelength of 279.5 nm, in an air-acetylene flame, with a sensitivity of 50 μg/liter. Suitable background corrections should be made for the sample substrate, and where possible a deuterium lamp background correction should be employed.

Manganese can be oxidized to the permanganate ion with either ammonium persulfate [$(NH_4)_2S_2O_3$] or potassium metaperiodate (KIO_4), in the presence of silver nitrate ($AgNO_3$). Absorbance from the violet permanganate ion can be measured with a spectrophotometer at 525 nm. All organic material in the sample must be completely oxidized before formation of the permanganate ion.

D'Amico and Klawans [10] determined manganese in 50 μl samples of normal serum and cerebrospinal fluid, in the 1 ng/ml range, by flameless atomic absorption spectrometry, with a graphite furnace. Deuterium lamp background correction allowed the samples to be analyzed directly without pretreatment or dilution. The parameters employed were, drying for 120 sec at 125°, charring for 60 sec at 800°, and atomization at 2300° for 8 sec. Lower detectable limits are achieved with enrichment by extraction [11].

Manganese can be selectively determined by solvent extraction as a complex with 8-hydroxyquinaldine. The interfering metals are masked by cyanide or removed from the organic phase by washing with ethylenediaminetetraacetic acid as follows: to 50 ml of the slightly acid solution containing 2 to 60 μg of manganese, add 5 ml of 30% ammonium citrate solution and 3 ml of a 2% solution of 8-hydroxyquinaldine. Add 1 ml of 5% potassium cyanide and dilute to 100 ml. Transfer the solution to a separatory funnel, add exactly 10.0 ml of chloroform and shake vigorously for 1 min. Transfer the chloroform extract to another separatory funnel containing about 10 ml of EDTA wash solution (0.1% EDTA, adjusted to pH 11 to 12 before use). Although EDTA completely prevents the extraction of manganese, the complex once extracted is not affected by shaking with EDTA solution. After shaking for 1 min, manganese is determined by measuring the absorbance of the chloroform extract at 395 nm.

D. Cobalt

Cobalt is found chiefly in the cooper-cobalt area of Zaire and also as smalite (FeNiCo)(As_2), cobalt bloom [$Co(AsO_4)_4 \cdot 2.8H_2XO_4$], and cobalite or cobalt glance [(CoFe)AsS]. Cobalt is an important constituent of many high-speed steels, magnets, cemented carbides, and high-temperature alloys. It is also used as a catalyst, for electroplating, to impart color in the glass and ceramic industries, in enamelware, and as a drier in paints and varnishes.

Cobalt is believed to be physiologically active only in the form of vitamin B_{12} (cobamide and its derivatives), and humans are dependent on absorption of this vitamin for metabolically effective cobalt. Nutritional cobalt deficiency may occur when strict vegetarianism, with total abstinence from B_{12}-containing foods of animal origin, is practiced. Pernicious anemia, the familiar form of vitamin B_{12} deficiency, results from defective absorption of vitamin B_{12} as a consequence of failure to secrete intrinsic factor. As little as 1 μg of cobalamin, administered parenterally, can cause remission of pernicious anemia.

The toxic effects of cobalt in humans have included both lung affection and skin lesions following exposures in the tungsten carbide industry.

Cobalt is determined by atomic absorption spectrophotometry in an air-acetylene flame, at a wavelength of 240.7 nm, with a sensitivity of 150 μg/liter. Matrix interferences can be eliminated, and the sample concentrated, by chelating with ammonium pyrrolidine dithiocarbamate at pH 2 and extracting with methyl isobutyl ketone. The extract is aspirated directly into the flame, and pure methyl isobutyl ketone is used as the blank.

Cobalt can also be determined directly in a graphite furnace by flameless atomic absorption spectrometry, at a wavelength of 240.7 nm, with a sensitivity of 2 μg/liter. Nitric acid is added to the sample in sufficient quantity that the final concentration is 0.5%, and the temperatures for drying, charring, and atomization are 125°, 1000°, and 2200°, respectively.

Both 1-nitroso-2-napthol and 2 nitroso-1-napthol yield strongly colored complexes which can be extracted by nonpolar solvents. Once formed, the cobalt(III) complex is very stable, and is not destroyed even on being shaken with relatively concentrated acids or alkalis. Under these conditions the excess of the reagent and most interfering metals are stripped into the aqueous phase. Make the sample acid with hydrochloric acid and add 10 ml of a 40% aqueous solution of citric acid to complex ferric ions present. Dilute to 50 to 75 ml and adjust the pH to 3 to 4. Add 10 ml of 3% hydrogen peroxide and after a short interval, 2 ml of 2-nitroso-1-napthol solution (1 g dissolved in 100 ml of glacial acetic acid). Allow to stand for 30 min and extract with one 25 ml, and two 10 ml portions of chloroform. Combine the chloroform extracts and wash first with 20 ml of 2 N hydrochloric acid and then with 20 ml of 2 N sodium hydroxide. Transfer the chloroform extract to a 50 ml volumetric flask, make up to volume, and read the absorbance at 530 nm.

E. Nickel

Nickel occurs naturally in meteoric iron and in the minerals josephinite ($FeNi_3$) and awaurite ($FeNi_2$). It occurs in arsentates, antimonates, silicates, sulfides, and phosphates, together with cobalt, copper, iron, zinc, and chromium. It is widely distributed and accounts for 0.016% of the earth's crust. Nickel is used as the metal and in alloys with copper, manganese, iron, zinc, chromium, molybdenum, and other compounds. It is widely used in the electroplating industry. It is used in finely divided particles as a catalyst for hydrogenation of hyrdrocarbons.

There is indirect evidence suggesting that nickel has physiological functions in higher animals and humans. It is present in all human tissues and is one of the metals found firmly associated with DNA and RNA. Experimental confirmation of its essential role has been obtained in chicks and rats by means of diets low in nickel, fed in controlled environments.

Although nickel metal itself is relatively nontoxic, most nickel salts are highly toxic and nickel carbonyl [$Ni(CO)_4$] is extremely toxic. Inhalation causes dermatitis, respiratory disorders, and cancer of the respiratory system. It also reduces activities of cytochrome oxidase, isocitrate dehydrogenase of the liver, and maleic dehydrogenase of the kidney.

Nickel may be determined by atomic absorption spectrophotometry in an air-acetylene flame, at 232.0 nm, with a sensitivity of 100 μg/liter. Matrix interferences can be reduced and the sample concentrated by chelating with ammonium pyrrolidine dithiocarbamate at pH 2 and extraction with methyl isobutyl ketone. The extract is aspirated directly into the flame, using pure methyl isobutyl ketone as the blank.

Nickel can also be determined in the graphite furnace by flameless atomic absorption at a wavelength of 232.0 nm, with a sensitivity of 2 μg/liter. Nitric acid should be added to the sample in sufficient amount that the final concentration is 0.5%, and the optimum temperatures for drying, charring, and atomization are 125°, 1000°, and 2000°, respectively.

One very selective method for extracting nickel from a sample solution is by chelating with dimethylgloxime and extracting with chloroform. To 25 ml of sample solution add 5 ml of 10% sodium citrate solution. Neutralize with concentrated ammonium hydroxide and add a few drops excess. Add 2 ml of dimethylglyoxime solution (1% reagent in ethanol) and extract with three 3 ml portions of chloroform. Wash the combined chloroform extracts with two 5 ml portions of 0.5 N ammonium hydroxide, then wash the ammonium hydroxide portions with 2 ml of chloroform and add the latter to the chloroform extracts. Return the nickel into the aqueous phase by shaking with two 5 ml portions of 0.5 N hydrochloric acid. Combine the acid portions and analyze by atomic absorption spectrophotometry.

F. Cadmium

Cadmium occurs in nature as the mineral greenockite (CdS), in sparingly mineable amounts of sufficiently high cadmium content. It occurs in small amounts in practically all zinc ores, and is obtained largely as a by-product from zinc smelting. Cadmium is used in plating processes for corrosion resistance, in pigments (CdS), in alloys, and as dimethyl and diethyl cadmium for polymerization catalysts.

Cadmium toxicity arises from its possible presence in the diet and its occurrence as an industrial and environmental chemical. Occupational cadmium poisoning has been studied extensively and involvement of the lungs and kidneys seem to be of primary importance. Acute cadmium poisoning also includes the development of bronchitis pneumonitis, pulmonary edema, and in cases of severe exposure, renal cortical necrosis.

Cadmium can be determined by atomic absorption spectrophotometry at a wavelength of 228.8 nm, in an air-acetylene flame, with a sensitivity of 25 μg/liter. Matrix interferences can be reduced and the sample concentrated by chelating with ammonium pyrrolidine at pH 2 and extraction with methyl isobutyl ketone. The extract is aspirated directly into the flame, using pure methyl isobutyl ketone as the blank.

Cadmium may also be determined in the graphite furnace by flameless atomic absorption, at a wavelength of 228.8 nm, provided that the sample is pretreated to contain 0.2% ammonium dichromate and 1% nitric acid. The optimum temperatures for drying, charring, and atomization are 125°, 75°, and 1800°, respectively.

Evanson and Anderson [12] analyzed 5 to 15 mg samples of liver tissue for cadmium by first digesting in nitric acid and injection into a graphite furnace for flameless atomic absorption analysis. Matrix interferences are reduced by the use of a zirconium-coated graphite tube [13].

G. Tin

The natural occurrence of tin is limited. The mineral cassiterite or tin stone (SnO_2) is the chief source of tin and the mineral stannite or tin pyrites ($Cu_2S \cdot FeS \cdot SnS_2$) is of lesser commercial importance. It is also found in small amounts of soils, silicic rocks, feldspars, niobates, ilmenite, and tantalate. Tin is used in the manufacture of tin plate and for electrodeposited coatings. Tin is a constituent in a number of alloys, such as brass, bronze, Babbit metal, pewter, solder, and type metal.

Tin is an essential nutrient that has reportedly produced accelerated growth when included in highly purified diets of rats in a controlled environment. The association of tin with lipids makes dietary fats potentially important as sources of tin.

The toxicity of tin is due almost exclusively to its organic compounds, more specifically to the alkyl derivatives. The lower alkyl derivitives, especially triethyl tin, have a specific effect on the central nervous system, producing cerebral edema. The conversion of tetraalkyltins to trialkyltins in vivo accounts for the latent toxicity of the tetraalkyltins, the site of the conversion being the liver. The trialkyltin ion is a stable entity which is toxic per se and persists for some time in the tissues.

Tin can be determined by atomic absorption spectrophotometry in a nitrous oxide-acetylene flame, using the 286.3 resonance line, with a sensitivity of 3 mg/liter. In a fuel-rich air-hydrogen flame, at the 224.6 nm line, a sensitivity of 150 μg/liter has been reported; however, this analytical wavelength is subject to interferences. Another means to determine tin is by emission spectroscopy, using an inductively coupled argon plasma source, at the wavelength of 189.9 nm, with a sensitivity of 10 μg/liter.

Tin has also been determined in a graphite furnace by flameless atomic absorption spectrophotometry, at the wavelength of 286.3 nm, with a sensitivity of 1 μg/liter [14]. The method entails the use of an electrodeless discharge lamp for tin with deuterium arc background correction. The temperature cycles were: drying, 100° for 30 sec; charring, 700° for 30 sec; and atomization, 2700° for 8 sec.

A selective method for the isolation and determination of tin is its chelation with 8-hydroxyquinoline and subsequent extraction from acid solution with chloroform. Adjust the pH of a 50 ml sample to 9.85 with sulfuric acid. Add 5 ml of 20% ammonium chloride and 25 ml of oxine (4% solution in dilute sulfuric acid, pH 0.85). Extract the tin (IV) oxinate with exactly 20 ml of chloroform. Wash the extract with 10 ml of dilute sulfuric acid (pH 0.85), filter the organic phase, and measure the absorbance at 385 nm.

H. Lead

The natural occurrence of lead is relatively rare and it is found in comparatively small amounts, principally as the sulfide in galenite (PbS). Some of the more common minerals are cerussite ($PbCO_3$), anglesite ($PbSO_4$), pyromorphite [$PbCl_2 \cdot 3Pb_3(PO_4)_2$], minium ($Pb_3O_4$), wulfenite ($PbMoO_4$), and crocoite ($PbCrO_4$). Lead ores are widely found in the United States, England, Mexico, Spain, Germany, South America, and Australia.

Lead has been used by man for many centuries and objects made from this metal have been found in ancient ruins. It is used in alloys such as pewter, type metal, Babbit, and solder. Lead is used for the manufacture of pipe, as radiation shielding, in storage batteries, and as vibration pads for high-speed machinery. Compounds of lead are used in paint pigments, as drying agents for oils, lead glass, plumber's cement, and gasoline additives.

All lead compounds are cumulative poisons that accumulate in bones and soft tissues, particularly in the brain, resulting in reduced functioning. Lead complexes with S—H groups, inhibits the biosynthesis of heme, and causes loss of amino acids, glucose, and phosphate in urine by structural damage to the mitochondria of the kidneys. It has been linked to increased dental caries and is poorly excreted.

Lead can be determined by atomic absorption spectrometry in an air-acetylene flame, at a wavelength of 283.3 nm, with a sensitivity of 500 μg/liter. Matrix interferences can be reduced and the sample concentrated by chelating with ammonium pyrrolidine at pH 2 and extracting with methyl isobutyl ketone. The extract is aspirated directly into the flame using pure methyl isobutyl ketone as the blank.

Fernandez [15] describes a method for determining lead in whole blood in a graphite furnace by flameless atomic absorption spectrophotometry, with a sensitivity of 1 μg/liter. The wavelength used was 283.3 nm with a slit width of 0.7 nm. The optimum temperature program selected was: dry at 100° for 25 sec, ash at 525° for 50 sec, and atomize at 2300° for 9 sec. Baily et al. used a tungsten-coated graphite tube to reduce matrix interferences [16].

It has been suggested that pretreating samples with nitric acid and phosphoric acid (0.5% nitric acid and 1.0% phosphoric acid) will greatly enhance the thermal stability of lead by forming lead phosphide (PbP). This would allow ashing temperatures up to 900° without loss of analyte. However, there are no data to support this.

Lead can be determined by dithizone extraction. From a slightly ammoniacal cyanide solution, only lead, bismuth, thallium(I), indium(III), and tin(II) can be extracted with dithizone solution. Lead can be separated from bismuth by shaking the organic extract with dilute nitric acid (1:100). Bismuth remains in the organic phase. Adjust the pH to 8 to 10 with ammonium hydroxide and extract with a 0.006% solution of dithizone in carbon tetrachloride and read the absorbance at 250 nm.

I. Arsenic

Arsenic is present in small amounts on the earth's crust (2 to 5 ppm) and is found chiefly combined with minerals such as arsenolite (As_2O_3), realgar (As_2S_2), orpiment (As_2S_3), arsenopyrites ($FeAs_2$), and mispickel (FeAsS). Virtually all of the arsenic produced, however, is as a by-product in the smelting of lead, copper, and gold ores (containing up to 4% arsenic). Arsenic is used in alloys to increase hardness and heat resistance, in the manufacture of glass, Paris green, enamels, textile mordants, colored glass, and weed killers.

Two forms of arsenic exist, pentavalent and trivalent. Pentavalent arsenic, as arsenate, is nontoxic in normal concentrations, is excreted rapidly through the kidneys, and probably does not accumulate in human tissues. Trivalent arsenic, the principal form produced commercially, is toxic and accumulates in the mammalian body. It is an accumulative, general system poison, causing dermatitis and bronchitis. It is also carcinogenic in the mouth, esophogus, larynx, and bladder.

Arsenic can be determined by atomic absorption spectrophotometry at the resonance band of 193.7 nm, in an air -acetylene flame; however, the background interference is great and the sensitivity is poor. A more acceptable method is to generate the hydride (AsH_3) into a hydrogen-argon flame, using an electrodeless discharge lamp and deuterium arc background correction. This method gives sensitivities in the low-ppb range. There are several types of apparatus offered for the generation of arsine and then sweeping the arsine into the flame with the argon flow. Some are offered commercially; others can be made in the laboratory. The analyst can decide which best suits his or her needs. The various methods are discussed by Siemer and Koteel [17]. Feldman [18] describes an arsine accumulation-helium glow detector for determining traces of arsenic.

Andreae [19] describes a method to reduce sequentially the various forms of arsenic for analysis by gas chromatography or atomic absorption spectrophotometry. He was able to differentiate among arsine, arsenic(III), arsenic(V), monomethylarsenic acid, dimethylarsenic acid, and trimethylarsine oxide.

Much work has been done on matrix modification for arsenic determinations in the graphite furnace by flameless atomic absorption spectrophotometry [20,21]. The sample should be prepared so that the solution contains 1% nitric acid and 200 μg/ml nickel ion. This will allow a charring temperature of 1000° without loss of arsenic. One proposed set of parameters is: wavelength, 193.7 nm; slit width, 0.7 nm; drying, 125° for 60 sec; charring, 1000° for 40 sec; and atomization, 2700° for 5 sec. This analysis would require an electrodeless discharge lamp for arsenic and deuterium arc background correction.

Silver diethyldithiocarbamate method for arsenic in animal feed [22]

General Description of Method. This modification of the method of Hundley and Underwood [23] involves the very careful ashing of a 20 g sample, evolution of arsine, development of a colored complex with silver diethyldithiocarbamate, and subsequent colorimetric analysis at 540 nm.

Preparation of Sample. Mix 20 g of the sample with 3 g of MgO and 10 ml of cellulose powder in a porcelain dish, then add 50 ml of deionized water and stir to form a slurry. Rinse the stirring rod with water and heat the dish in a 110° oven overnight or until the contents are dry. Next, prechar the sample in a muffle furnace at 300° until evolution of smoke ceases. Allow the dish to cool and overlay the contents with 3 g of $Mg(NO_3)_2 \cdot 6H_2O$. Place the dish in a cool furnace and slowly increase the heat to 550°, then ash the sample at that temperature for 2 hr. Again, allow the dish to cool, moisten the residue with deionized water, and dissolve it with 50 ml of 6 N HCl. Transfer the solution and any residue to a 250 ml flask used for evolution of arsine. Use two 20 ml portions of 6 N HCl and several small portions of deionized water to rinse the contents of the dish into the flask. The total volume added to the flask should be 90 ml of 6 N HCl plus 85 ml of water.

Apparatus for Arsine Evolution. Use a 250 ml flask with a ground glass neck (24/40 joint) for an evolution flask. Saturate glass wool with a saturated aqueous solution of lead acetate and dry just to touch in a 110° oven. Use a delivery tube with a 24/40 joint to connect to the flask, with an open end to dip into the trapping solution contained in a 15 ml conical tube. Plug the 24/40 joint with lead acetate-saturated glass wool and wrap the other end of the delivery tube with unimpregnated glass wool to diffuse the bubbles of gas.

Evolution of Arsine. Pipet 5 ml of Ag-DDC solution (0.5% silver diethyldithiocarbamate in pyridine) into a 15 ml conical receiving tube. Add 2 ml of KI solution (15% potassium iodide in deionized water) and 1 ml of $SnCl_2$ solution (40% $SnCl_2 \cdot 2H_2O$ in HCl) separately to the evolution flask and swirl the contents after each addition. Finally, add 6 g of zinc to the flask and quickly connect the delivery tube to the evolution flask and place the receiving tube to allow the evolved arsine and hydrogen to pass through the Ag-DDC solution. Analyze the Ag-DDC solution colorimetrically for arsine content.

Analysis of Arsenic. Prepare a series of standards for use in constructing a calibration curve (absorbance versus concentration) by spiking evolution flasks containing 90 ml of 6 N HCl and 85 ml of water with various amounts of arsenic up to a total of 10 μg. Proceed with the generation of arsine and the trapping of the vapors from each flask in Ag-DDC solution. Determine the absorbance of the Ag-DDC solutions by using a spectrophotometer set at 540 nm employing pyridine as a reference. Prepare a reagent blank in the same manner and subtract its absorbance from that of each sample. Calculate the arsenic content of the samples for analysis by relating their absorbance to the standard curve.

Typical Results

1. Five reagent blanks carried through the procedure gave 0.033 ± 0.009 ppm As.
2. Five samples of Laboratory Chow 5010-C (Ralston Purina Co., St. Louis, MO) unspiked and spiked with 0.1 ppm of arsenic gave 0.090 ± 0.004 and 0.167 ± 0.009 ppm As, respectively; therefore, the recovery of arsenic at the 0.100 ppm level was about 77%.
3. Triplicate samples of laboratory chow 5010-C assayed before and after being autoclaved gave results of 0.114 ± 0.009 and 0.115 ± 0.005 ppm as As corrected for 77% recovery.

J. Phosphorus

Phosphorus is the twelfth most abundant element and is widely distributed in both igneous and sedimentary rocks. It is commonly mined from secondary deposits of marine origin. Phosphorus is essential to all living matter and is found in high concentration in bones and teeth.

Over a half billion tons of elemental phosphorus are produced in the United States each year, the majority of which is converted to phosphoric acid. Sodium tripolyphosphate and tetrasodium pyrophosphate are used in detergents. Calcium phosphates are the most important source for fertilizers.

There are three different types of elemental phosphorus: white or yellow, red, and black. Each possesses different physiochemical and biological properties. Elemental white phosphorus is an extremely toxic substance and a protoplasmic poison. Chronic exposure to small quantities of phosphorus can result in epthelial damage of bone capillaries with thrombosis and bone necrosis, and heart damage has resulted from acute phosphorus poisoning. Phosphorus vapor is believed to be the chief industrial cause of poisoning, although phosphorus can be absorbed through the skin or by ingestion. Red phosphorus is considered relatively nontoxic unless it contains white phosphorus as an impurity.

White phosphorus is soluble in benzene and insoluble in water. Water sludge and biological samples can be extracted with benzene and the extract analyzed for white phosphorus by gas liquid chromatography using a flame photometric detector. Addison and Ackman [24] reported determinations of white phosphorus at low-picogram levels. Organophosphorus compounds can be determined by gas-liquid chromatography with the selective flame photometric detector.

Phosphorus has also been determined by x-ray fluorescence, neutron activation analysis, and emission spectrometry. With the inductively coupled argon plasma source for emission spectrometry, a sensitivity of 30 μg/liter has been reported [25].

Phosphorus can be determined in the graphite furnace by flameless atomic absorption spectrophotometry if the sample is prepared to contain 0.2% nitric acid and 200 μg/ml nickel before introduction into the furnace. The wavelength setting is 213.6 nm and temperatures for drying, charring, and atomization are 125°, 1100°, and 2600°, respectively, with a sensitivity of 100 μg/liter.

Orthophosphate can be determined colorimetrically by the formation of vanadomolybdophosphoric acid in 0.5 N acid solution. Hunt and Hargis [26] have studied reaction rates versus pH for this reaction. Orthophosphate can be determined by forming molybdophosphoric acid and then reduction to the intensely colored molybdenum blue. This reduction is accomplished by using either stannous chloride or ascorbic acid.

K. Selenium

Selenium is widely distributed in the earth's crust at a concentration of about 0.09 ppm. It is concentrated mainly in sulfide minerals and in the soils of dry plains; some plants can absorb and accumulate selenium in large amounts from the soil (e.g., varieties of astragalus or milk weed, woody aster, and golden weed). These plants contain large quantities of selenium, generally 1000 to 10,000 ppm. The consumption of these plants by livestock produces the disease syndrome of blind staggers or acute selenium poisoning.

Selenium is an essential trace element to certain biological processes in humans. It complexes with plasma proteins, is related to vitamin E, and is distributed to all tissues. Overexposure to selenium causes irritation of the eyes, noise, throat, and respiratory tract. It causes cancer of the liver, pneumonia, degeneration of the liver and kidneys, and gastrointestinal disturbances.

Selenium can be determined by atomic absorption spectrophotometry at the resonance band of 196.0 nm, in an air-acetylene flame; however, the background interference is great and the sensitivity is poor. A more acceptable method is to generate the hydride into a hydrogen-argon flame, using an electrodeless discharge lamp and deuterium background correction. There are several types of apparatus offered for the generation of selenium hydride and then sweeping the generated gas into the flame with the argon flow. Some are offered commercially; others can be made in the laboratory. The analyst can decide which best suits his or her needs. The various methods have been compared by Siemer and Koteel [17] and evaluated by McDaniel and Shendrikar [27].

Matrix modifications for selenium determinations in the graphite furnace by flameless atomic absorption spectrophotometry have been studied extensively [20,21]. The sample should be prepared so that the solution contains 200 μg/ml of nickel ion to allow a charring temperature of 1000° without loss of selenium. One proposed set of parameters is: wavelength, 196.0 nm; slit width, 0.7 nm; drying, 125° for 60 sec; charring, 1000° for 40 sec; and atomization, 2700° for 3 sec. The analysis requires an electrodeless discharge lamp for selenium and deuterium arc background correction. Enhancement of sensitivity by solvent extraction of the diethyldithiocarbamate chelate and back-extraction with 50 ppm of CN^- was reported [28].

Diaminonaphthalene method for selenium in animal feed [22,29]

General Description of Method. The sample is prepared by wet digestion with $HClO_4$-H_2SO_4-HNO_3 and treatment with H_2O_2. A complex is then formed by using NH_4OH, 2,3-diaminonaphthalene (DAN), and ethylenedinitrilotetraacetate (EDTA) reagents. The complex is extracted with hexane and selenium determined by spectrophotofluorescence.

Special Reagents

DAN reagent. Add 50 mg of 2,3-diaminonaphthalene (DAN) to a 125 ml separatory funnel containing 50 ml of sulfuric acid solution (140 ml of concentrated H_2SO_4 added to water, then diluted to 1 liter with water). Shake the contents for 15 min, add 50 ml of hexane, and shake for an additional 15 min. After the layers have separated, place a plug of glass wool in the stem of the funnel and draw off the bottom layer for immediate use.

EDTA reagent. Prepare a 0.02 M solution by dissolving 7.445 g of disodium ethylenedinitrilotetraacetate in water and diluting to 1 liter.

Procedure. Accurately weigh 1 g or less of the sample, containing up to 0.5 μg of selenium, and place it into a 100 ml Kjeldahl flask. Sequentially add 6 ml of concentrated HNO_3, 2 ml of 70% $HClO_4$, and 5 ml of concentrated H_2SO_4. Use a micro Kjeldahl digestion unit to heat slowly in initial stages to avoid any loss, and slowly increase the heat to a vigorous boil. Add small amounts of HNO_3 at the first signs of charring. The solution will turn yellow and then water-white. Remove the flask and swirl the contents to contact the bulb area and the lower neck; the yellow color may reappear. Continue heating until the contents are water-white and white fumes appear. In some instances the solution may remain pale yellow, and in those cases a heating time of about 2.5 hr is considered sufficient.

Remove the flask, add 1 ml of 30% H_2O_2, and swirl the contents; after all action ceases, return to heating until the contents are boiling briskly and white fumes appear. Add H_2O_2 twice more and continue final boiling for 5 min after the appearance of white fumes. Cool the flask, carefully add 30 ml of water, and quantitatively transfer the contents to a 250 ml Erlenmeyer flask by using two 10 ml portions and one 5 ml portion of water. Prepare DAN reagent as time permits. Add to the flask, with mixing, 10 ml of EDTA reagent, 25 ml of aqueous NH_4OH (40 ml of concentrated NH_4OH diluted to 100 ml), and 5 ml of DAN reagent. Bring the mixture rapidly to a vigorous boil by using a burner and place the flask on a preheated hot plate to continue boiling. Boil the mixture for exactly 2 min, then set it aside for 1 hr. Add 6 ml of hexane, shake the contents for 5 min, then transfer the mixture to a separatory funnel and allow the phases to separate. Discard the aqueous phase (bottom), collect the hexane layer in a tube, and centrifuge the contents at about 1000 rpm for 5 min. Measure the relative fluorescent intensity of the hexane extract by using a spectrophotofluorometer set with approximate excitation and emission wavelengths of 374 and 520 nm, respectively. Calculate the selenium content of the sample by relating the relative intensity (corrected for the reagent blank) to a standard curve prepared from known amounts of selenium analyzed in the same manner.

Typical Results

1. Quaduplicate reagent blanks yielded 180 ± 8 ppb of selenium.
2. Quaduplicate samples of unspiked laboratory chow 5010-C analyzed versus samples spiked with 200 ppb of selenium gave recoveries of 104 ± 6%.
3. Quadruplicate samples of laboratory chow 5010-C (unspiked), analyzed before and after being autoclaved, contained 420 ± 16 and 388 ± 2 ppb of selenium, respectively.
4. Triplicate samples of NIH rat and mouse ration were found to contain 383 ± 35 ppb of selenium.

L. Tellurium

Tellurium occurs in tellurides and arsenical iron pyrites, and is frequently associated with gold, silver, lead, bismuth, and iron. It has also been found as the native metal. Almost all of the commercially produced tellurium is received from electrolytic copper refinery slimes. The main industrial uses of tellurium include alloys with copper, lead, and steel for increased resistance to corrosion and stress; as a vulcanizing agent for natural rubber and styrene-butadiene; in the form tellurium diethyldithiocarbamate as an accelerating agent for butyl rubber; and as a catalyst in diverse industrial chemical processes. Industrial poisoning due to tellurium exposure and poisoning due to ingestion of sodium telluride were reported [2]. Tellurium has no known nutrient requirements and reportedly is not involved in enzyme systems. It is complexed by plasma proteins and causes renal and hepatic degeneration.

The chemical behavior of tellurium is very similar to that of selenium and can be determined in much the same manner. Tellurium can be determined in the graphite furnace, by flameless atomic absorption spectrophotometry, if the sample is prepared to contain 1% nitric acid and 200 μg/ml of nickel ion [20]. Instrumental settings for the determination of tellurium are: wavelength, 214.3 nm; slit width, 0.7 nm; drying, 125° for 60 sec; charring, 700° for 40 sec; and atomization, 2700° for 5 sec.

The applicability of the iodotellurite complex to the estimation of small amounts of tellurium is indicated by the fact that at 335 nm the complex obeys Berris's law over the concentration range 0.2 to 2 mg/liter. Since selenite is reduced to elemental selenium by iodide, a prior separation of selenium is necessary, for example, by repeated sulfuric acid-bisulfate fuming to dryness. Precautions must be taken to prevent the oxidation of iodide to free iodine.

Tellurium can be determined by emission spectroscopy, using the inductively coupled argon plasma source, with a reported sensitivity of 20 μg/liter.

M. Mercury

Mercury is a comparatively rare element and is not widely distributed. The metal is found in the upper portions of cinnabar deposits, as HgS, the chief source of the element. Important deposits are located in Spain, Italy, the United States, Canada, Mexico, Brazil, Peru, China, Japan, the USSR, Hungary, Yugoslavia, and Germany. A less common ore is the mercurous chloride found in Texas. The ore found in Spain has the highest mercury content, with an average of 0.5 to 1.2% mercury, with values occasionally as high as 10% mercury.

There is evidence that the knowledge of metallic mercury dates back to 1600 B.C. Aristotle refers to mercury as "fluid silver." Mercury was used by the ancients in guilding; the sulfide was employed as a pigment. Today there are over 3000 recognized applications for mercury and its inorganic and organic derivitives. The world production of mercury amounts to about 10,000 tons per year, of which about 3000 tons is used in the United States. The main areas of utility of mercury include the electrolytic preparation of chlorine and caustic soda, agricultural chemicals, pharmaceuticals (diuretics, cathartics, antibacterial agents), hair dressings and preservatives in cosmetics, pulp and paper making (slimicides and algicides), paint (antifouling pigment), electrical apparatus, catalyst, dental preparations, and amalgamations. The element is used extensively in the extraction of gold from its ores by formation of gold amalgam.

Mercury salts, if at all soluble, are poisonous, as is the vapor of mercury. Mercurous salts are oxidized by tissues and ethrocytes to the highly toxic mercuric ion. Mercury is retained by the liver, kidney, brain, heart, lung, and muscle tissues. It inhibits s-aminoleulinic acid dehydratase and cholinesterase activity. Mercury is a protoplasmic poison and damages the central nervous system. Elimination of mercury from brain, thyroid, and testes is slow, permitting accumulation in these organs. Mercury is excreted by the kidney, by the liver via bile, by the intestinal mucosa, sweat glands, and salivary glands; urinary and fecal routes are the most important for elimination.

Mercury can be determined by atomic absorption spectrophotometry in the graphite furnace, with a charring temperature of 300° [21]. This procedure requires that the sample solution contain 1% nitric acid and 5% ammonium sulfide. There are several methods for reducing mercury to elemental mercury with stannous chloride and measuring the vapor by atomic absorption in a quartz tube. Toffaletti and Savory reported a method for reducing inorganic and organic mercury to the element, using sodium borohydride as the reducing agent, with subsequent analysis of the vapor in a quartz tube by atomic absorption [30].

Cappon and Smith developed a method for the extraction, cleanup, and gas chromatographic determination of organic (alkyl and aryl) and inorganic mercury in biological materials by gas-liquid chromatography [31]. Methyl, ethyl, and phenyl mercury are first extracted as the chloride derivatives. Inorganic mercury is then isolated as methyl mercury upon reaction with tetramethyltin. The initial extracts are subjected to thiosulfate cleanup, and the organomercury species are isolated as the bromide derivatives. Longbottom reported an inexpensive mercury specific detector for gas chromatography [32].

Muscat et al. reported a flameless atomic fluorescence system for mercury which makes use of either reduction-aeration or combustion techniques for the generation of mercury vapor and a silver amalgamator for collection of mercury prior to the final measurement [33]. The system is capable of measuring as little as 0.6 ng of mercury.

Mercury in animal feed [22]

General Description of Method. This modified method of Hatch and Ott [34] is based on wet digestion of the sample, acid oxidation for dissolution, reduction of mercury to the elemental state, and analysis of the vapors by flameless atomic absorption spectrometry.

Procedure. Accurately weigh 1 g of sample and transfer it to a 100 ml Kjeldahl flask containing three glass beads. Add, in sequence, 6 ml of concentrated HNO_3, 2 ml of $HClO_4$, 5 ml of concentrated H_2SO_4 and 1 ml of 2% sodium molybdate. Using a micro Kjeldahl digestion unit, slowly heat the flask in the initial stage to avoid any loss and gradually increase the heat to a vigorous boil. If charring occurs, add a few drops of concentrated HNO_3. The solution will turn yellow and then to water-white . Remove the flask from the digestion unit and swirl the contents; the yellow color may reappear. Continue heating until the contents are water-white and white fumes appear. The total digestion time should be almost 2 hr. Remove the flask, swirl the contents, cool, and add 1 ml of 30% hydrogen peroxide; the contents will turn yellow. Heat the flask until white fumes again appear, then swirl and cool the contents. Repeat the hydrogen peroxide additions twice more and continue final boiling for 5 min after the appearance of white fumes.

Quantitatively transfer the sample to a 100 ml volumetric flask using several rinses of deionized water; adjust the solution to 100 ml. Use a Coleman Model MAS-50 Mercury Analyzer System (Coleman Instruments Division, Perkin-Elmer Corp., Maywood, Illinois) to determine residue of mercury in the sample as described.

Pour the 100 ml sample solution into a BOD bottle and add 2 drops of 5% potassium permanganate solution. Next, add 5 ml of 5.6 N HNO_3, swirl the contents, and after 15 sec add 5 ml of 18 N H_2SO_4, swirl the contents, and wait for 45 sec. Add 5 ml of 1.5% hydroxylamine hydrochloride and swirl the contents; the sample should turn clear in about 15 sec. Finally, add 5 ml of 10% stannous chloride and immediately insert the bubbler of the mercury analyzer into the BOD bottle and make sure that the stopper is tightly sealed. Record the highest meter reading and then place the bubbler into a BOD bottle containing 100 ml of 1 N HNO_3 and purge for several minutes to clean the system. (Note: The various reagents used in this procedure are available in a Mercury Analysis Reagent Kit; Coleman No. 50-050.)

Although the instrument is designed to read total micrograms of mercury directly from the meter, it is suggested that a standard curve be prepared as follows. Prepare a series of BOD bottles containing 0.1 to 2.0 μg of mercury in a volume of 100 ml. Follow the procedure previously described beginning with the addition of 2 drops of potassium permanganate solution. Plot micrograms of mercury versus the the meter reading. Calculate the mercury content in the samples for analysis by relating their meter readings to the standard curve.

Typical Results

1. Quadruplicate reagent blanks yielded 0.0435 ± 0.005 ppm of mercury.
2. Triplicate samples of unautoclaved laboratory chow 5010-C spiked with 0.2 and 0.5 ppm of mercury gave recoveries of 71.7 ± 2.6 and 87.3 ± 4.4%, respectively.
3. Triplicate samples of unspiked laboratory chow 5010-C analyzed before and after being autoclaved gave values essentially identical to the reagent blanks. Therefore, based on the criterion of twice background (reagent blank), all samples contained less than 0.1 ppm of mercury.

N. Thallium

Thallium occurs in quantity in a few rare minerals, such as crookesite [$(CuTlAg)_2Se$], lorandite ($TlAsS_2$), and orboite ($TlAs_2SbS_5$). Commercial sources of thallium, however, are generally flue dusts, either from pyrites burners or from lead and zinc smelters and refiners. It is also recovered as a by-product in the production of cadmium. The chief use of thallium appears to be in the manufacture of rat and vermin poison, because the metal and its compounds are extremely toxic. It is also used in the preparation of artificial stones and optical glass of very high refracting power.

Thallium is one of the most toxic elements both acutely and chronically in both humans and animals, regardless of the route of entry, or of the valence state (Tl^+ or Tl^{3+}). It accumulates in erythrocytes, agglutinates, kidneys, bones, and soft tissues.

Thallium has two valence states, thallous (Tl^+) and thallic (Tl^{3+}). Thallous sulfate, hydroxide, and carbonate are soluble in water, whereas the cobalnitrite, chloroplatinate, and perrhenate are only very slightly soluble. These salts resemble the corresponding potassium compounds. The halides and chromate have slight solubilities, similar to the corresponding lead compounds. Thallous sulfide is insoluble in alkaline solution but dissolves readily in acids.

Thallic salts are formed by the oxidation of thallous salts with permanganate or some other oxidizing agent. Thallic salts resemble ferric salts in being readily hydrolyzed and yielding a brown flocculent precipitate with ammonia.

Thallium can be determined by atomic absorption spectrophotometry in an air-acetylene flame, with a sensitivity of 0.5 ppm, at the wavelength 276.8 nm. In the graphite furnace the volatility of thallium limits the charring temperature to a maximum of 400°. In sample matrixes that are amenable to this charring temperature, a sensitivity of 10.0 μg/liter can be achieved.

Thallium can also be selectively determined as dithizonate after its extraction from a strongly alkaline solution. The interfering metals can easily be removed by a preliminary dithizone extraction at pH < 6. The extractions are made with a 100 μM solution of dithizone in chloroform and the absorbance of thallium dithizonate is measured at 505 nm.

O. Vanadium

Vanadium, ranking twenty-second among the elements of the earth's crust, is widely distributed in nature in ores, hard coal, igneous rocks, limestones, and sandstones. The principal source of vanadium is patronite, a sulfide of vanadium (28 to 34% V_2O_5), associated with pyrites and carbonaceous matter. Other minerals include vanadinite [$(PbCl)Pb_4(NO_4)_3$], roscoelite, a vanadium mica with variable composition, carnotite ($K_2O \cdot 2UO_3 \cdot V_2O_5 \cdot 3H_2$), and other minerals in which vanadium is associated with lead, zinc, copper, aluminum, manganese, bismuth, calcium, and barium.

Vanadium is used in many special steels, either alone or in combination with other elements. All American high-speed tool steels contain vanadium associated with tungsten and chromium and sometimes other elements; in these products the proportions are generally from 0.75 to 2.5%. Vanadium oxide (V_2O_5) is widely used as a catalyst for primary oxidation reactions such as in the oxidation of SO_2 to SO_3 in the contact process for the manufacture of sulfuric acid, the oxidation of ammonia in nitric acid manufacture, and in the production of phthalic anhydride from naphthalene. Other catalytic uses are in the control of motor vehicle exhaust gas and in petroleum refining.

Vanadium is moderately toxic to humans and animals, and when inhaled, the chief damage is to the respiratory tract. Other effects may include fatty degeneration of the liver and tubules of the kidneys. Vanadium is also an essential nutrient to humans and animals. The oral intake by humans is approximately 2 mg daily, of which more than half is constantly present in circulating serum. Vanadium inhibits the synthesis of cholesterol, lipids, phospholipids, and amino acids (theotic acid, uric acid); and mobilizes iron to the liver and calcium to the bones.

Vanadium can be determined by atomic absorption spectrophotometry in a nitrous oxide-acetylene flame, at 318.4 nm wavelength, with a sensitivity of 1.5 mg/liter. Using the graphite furnace for flameless atomic absorption, with a charring temperature of 1700° and an atomizing temperature of 2900°, at the wavelength 318.4 nm, vanadium can be determined at a sensitivity of 5 μg/liter.

Vanadium can also be selectively determined as vanadium(V) oxinate, by chelating with 8-hydroxyquinoline at pH 3 to 5. Interfering metals may be removed by extraction at pH 9 to 10. To the aqueous solution containing vanadium(V), add 2 ml of 0.1 M sodium tartrate and dilute sodium hydroxide to adjust the pH to 9 to 10. Dilute with distilled water to 20 ml and extract the interfering metals with several portions of 0.1 M 8-hydroxyquinoline in chloroform until the organic phase is colorless. Discard the organic portions and adjust to pH 3 to 5 with dilute hydrochloric acid. Extract with two 20 ml portions of 0.1 M 8-hydroxyquinoline combining the organic phases. Measure the absorbance of the vanadium(V) oxinate at 550 nm. Molybdenum, tungsten, and zirconium oxinates are extracted with vanadium, but do not interfere at this wavelength.

P. Copper

Copper is found in nature as the free metal, and combined, principally as sulfide, oxide, and carbonate. It is less commonly found as antimonides, arsenates, phosphates, silicates, and sulfates. Among the more common minerals are chalcopyrite ($CuFeS_2$), chalcocite (Cu_2S), bornite (Cu_5FeS_4), tetrahedrite ($Cu_8Sb_2S_7$), cuprite (Cu_2O), malachite [$CuCO_3 \cdot Cu(OH)_2$], and azurite [$2CuCO_3 \cdot Cu(OH)_2$]. Copper is widely distributed throughout the world, being found in seawater, mineral water, plants, and many animal organisms. Pure copper is a salmon-pink ductile metal. The reddish cast usually associated with the metal is due to a surface film of Cu_2O, which may be stripped with a dilute cyanide solution. Copper forms two oxides: red cuprous oxide and black cupric oxide. Both are basic anhydrides, forming cuprous (univalent) and cupric (divalent) salts, respectively.

Copper is toxic to humans and animals in high concentration (LD_{50} for mice, 50 mg/kg), causing hemolysis. Copper is an essential nutrient in trace amounts, and copper deficiencies have been noted in infants, manifested as moderate to severe anemia. Other symptoms linked to copper deficiency in infants are chronic diarrhea, retardation of growth, defective keratinization and pigmentation of hair, hypothermia, degenerative changes in aortic elastin, scurvy-like changes in the skeleton, and progressive mental retardation.

Copper can be determined by atomic absorption spectrophotometry in an air-acetylene flame, at 324.7 nm wavelength, with a sensitivity of 100 μg/liter. With the use of the graphite furnace for flameless atomic absorption, a charring temperature of 1000°, and an atomization temperature of 2700°, copper can be determined with a sensitivity of 1 μg/liter.

Jan and Young [35] have determined copper in seawater with a detection limit of 0.05 μg/liter. The procedure entails chelation of the copper with ammonium pyrrolidine dithiocarbamate, extraction into methyl isobutyl ketone, and back-extraction into 4 N nitric acid, resulting in a 20-fold concentration of the original sample. The nitric acid solution is then analyzed by flameless atomic absorption spectrophotometry in the graphite furnace.

Copper can be extracted from slightly acid solutions (pH 2) with diphenylthiocarbazone (dithizone). Under these conditions, dithizonates of silver, mercury, and bismuth, which are co-extracted, can be destroyed by shaking with potassium iodide solution as follows: Adjust the sample solution to pH 2 with dilute hydrochloric acid and extract with portions of a 0.0015% solution of dithizone in carbon tetrachloride until the organic phase after extraction remains green, and note the volume used. Then shake the combined extracts with a 2% solution of potassium iodide in 0.01 N hydrochloric acid to decompose the dithizonates of silver, mercury, and bismuth. Copper is left alone in the organic phase, in which it can be determined by the mixed color method. Only palladium and gold will interfere.

Copper in animal feed [22]

General Description of Method. The sample is ashed, dissolved in HCl, reacted with tetraethylenepentamine, and the copper content determined spectrophotometrically at 620 nm.

Preparation of Sample. Ash 8 g of sample at 600° for 2 hr and transfer the residue to a 200 ml volumetric flask by using 20 ml of HCl and 50 ml of water. Boil the contents for 5 min, allow it to cool, and adjust the volume to 200 ml with water. Transfer a 50 ml aliquot to a 100 ml volumetric flask for color development and subsequent analysis.

Prepare standard solutions of copper in 100 ml volumetric flasks by using 1 to 10 ml of aqueous copper sulfate (1 mg of Cu/ml). Next, add 4 ml of HCl, dilute to 50 ml with water, then add 5 ml of tetraethylenepentamine. Finally, adjust the volume to 100 ml with water and mix thoroughly; also, prepare a reagent blank using all the reagents except the copper sulfate solution.

Add 5 ml of tetraethylenepentamine to the 50 ml aliquots of samples of unknown copper content, adjust the volume to 100 ml with water, mix thoroughly, and filter the mixture prior to analysis.

Analysis of Copper. Prepare a calibration curve (absorbance versus concentration) for copper by using a spectrophotometer set at 620 nm to measure the standard solutions. Correct all absorbance readings by subtracting the value obtained for the reagent blank. Determine the absorbance of the samples for analysis and calculate their copper content using the following relationship:

$$\text{Cu (ppm)} = \frac{\mu\text{g Cu/ml in unknown (from curve)}}{\text{g/ml of sample analyzed}}$$

Q. Silver

Silver occurs as the native metal, but more commonly in combination as silver glance or argentite (Ag_2S). It is found as antimonide, arsenide, bismuthide, bromide, chloride, iodide, selenide, sulfide, telluride, and in thio salts. It is found associated with sulfide of lead, gold, copper, antimony, mercury, bismuth, and platinum. The more important minerals include native silver, argentite, hessite prousite, pyrargyrite, and cerargyrite. Silver is found in trace amounts in seawater.

Silver has been known to humans since prehistoric times. It was employed as a standard of value in coins many centuries before the Christian era and still continues in the currency of all civilized countries of the world. The element is used in silver plating, the making of mirrors, table silverware, jewelry, and ornaments. The nitrate of silver and various colloidal preparations are used in medicine; the chloride and bromide salts are used in photography.

Silver is not an essential nutrient. Silver salts absorb poorly and remain impregnated in tissue, causing argyria, a permanent blue-gray discoloration of the skin and eyes that imparts a ghostly appearance. Concentrations in the range 0.4 to 1 mg/kg have caused pathologic changes in the kidneys, liver, and spleen of rats. The LD_{50} for rabbits is 8 mg/kg [1].

Silver can be determined by atomic absorption spectrophotometry in an air-acetylene flame, at 328.1 nm wavelength, with a detection limit of 60 μg/ml using the graphite furnace for flameless atomic absorption at the same wavelength, with a charring temperature of 700° and an atomizing temperature of 2700°, a sensitivity of 1 μg/liter can be achieved. Jan and Young [35] achieved a detection limit of 0.02 μg/liter in seawater by first chelating with ammonium pyrrolidine dithiocarbamate, extracting into methyl isobutyl ketone and back-extracting into 4 N nitric acid, with a 20-fold concentration prior to analysis in the graphite furnace by flameless atomic absorption. Sheaffer et al. [36] were able to achieve a detection limit of 1×10^{-6} μg/ml with evaporative preconcentration in the graphite tube prior to analysis by flameless atomic absorption. The tubes were placed on a hot plate at 40°, and sequential aliquots of 50 μl were injected into the tubes and dried. The individual tubes were placed in the furnace for analysis.

III. CONCLUSIONS

New instrumentation is available for multielement analysis, including x-ray fluorescence, neutron activation analysis, and emission spectroscopy using an inductively coupled argon plasma source. Zander and O'Haver [37] reported a continuum source for multielement analysis by atomic absorption spectrometry. Capar et al. [38] gave results on multielement analysis of animal feed, animal wastes, and sewage sludge using the inductively coupled argon plasma source for emission spectrometry. Horlick [39] explained the spectral characteristics of the inductively coupled argon plasma, and Ward [25] listed minimum detectable levels for this instrument. Kahn reported on an automatic sampler to improve the precision of analyses, in the graphite furnace, by flameless atomic absorption spectrophotometry [40].

Even with all the new and sophisticated instruments available, the analyst must remember that the analytical value obtained is not necessarily specific or accurate. Any analytical result may be questioned, and the chemist should maintain some skepticism to ensure accuracy of analyses. Samples should be taken with care to ensure that they are representative and that no contamination results from the sampling procedure or the container. Samples must be handled and stored in a manner that ensures their integrity until the final determination is made.

Errors affecting an experimental result may be classified as either systematic or random. The former, occasionally referred to as determinate errors, are due to causes over which the analyst has control; these undesirable effects on the accuracy and precision can be avoided or corrected. Random errors are not subject to control and are manifested even in the absence of systematic errors, by variations in the result. The magnitude of random errors can be reduced by carefully keeping all steps in the procedure identical; however, they can never be completely eliminated.

The analyst must prove that the method is applicable to a particular substrate by analyzing similar standard reference materials, performing recovery assays with spiked samples, and obtaining comparable results by using a different method of analysis.

REFERENCES

1. J. J. Dulka and T. H. Risby. Ultratrace metals in some environmental biological systems. Anal. Chem. *48*, 640-653 (1976).
2. L. Fishbein. *Chromatography of Environmental Hazards*, Vol. 2. Elsevier, New York, 1973.
3. J. W. Owens and E. S. Gladney. Determination of beryllium in environmental materials by flameless atomic absorption spectroscopy. At. Absorpt. Newsl. *14*, 76-77 (1975).
4. W. R. Wolf and M. L. Taylor. Determination of chromium and beryllium at the picogram level by gas chromatography-mass spectrometry. Anal. Chem. *44*, 616-618 (1972).
5. M. L. Taylor and E. L. Arnold. Ultratrace determination of metals in biological specimens. Anal. Chem. *43*, 1328-1331 (1971).
6. K. N. Jeejeebhoy, R. C. Chu, E. B. Marliss, G. R. Greenberg, and A. Bruch-Robertson. Chromium deficiency, glucose intolerance, and neuropathy reversed by chromium supplementation, in a patient receiving long-term total parenteral nutrition. Am. J. Clin. Nutr. *30*, 531-538 (1977).
7. K. M. Hambridge and D. O. Rogerson. Concentration of chromium in the hair of normal children and children with diabetes mellitus. Diabetes *17*, 517-519 (1968).
8. S. S. Chao and E. E. Pickett. Trace chromium determination by furnace atomic absorption spectrometry following enrichment by extraction. Anal. Chem. *52*, 335-339 (1980).
9. W. R. Wolf. Coupled gas chromatography-atomic absorption spectrometry for the nanogram determination of chromium. Anal. Chem. *48*, 1717-1720 (1976).
10. D. J. D'Amico and H. L. Klawans. Direct determination of manganese in normal serum and cerebrospinal fluid by flameless atomic absorption spectrophotometry. Anal. Chem. *48*, 1469-1472 (1976).
11. G. P. Klinkhammer. Determination of manganese in seawater by flameless atomic absorption spectrometry after preconcentration with 8-hydroxyquinoline in chloroform. Anal. Chem. *52*, 117-120 (1980).
12. M. A. Evenson and C. T. Anderson. Ultramicro analysis for copper, cadmium, and zinc in human liver by use of atomic

absorption spectrophotometry and the heated graphite tube analyzer. Clin. Chem. *21*, 537-543 (1975).

13. W. Schmidt and F. Dietl. Determination of cadmium in digested soils and sediments, resp. in soil and sediment extracts by means of flameless atomic absorption with zirconium coated graphite tubes. Analytische Chemie *295*, 110-115 (1979).
14. H. L. Trachman and A. J. Tyberg. Atomic absorption spectrometric determination of sub-part-per-million quantities of tin in extracts and biological materials with a graphite furnace. Anal. Chem. *49*, 1090-1093 (1977).
15. F. J. Fernandez. Micromethod for lead determination in whole blood by atomic absorption with use of the graphite furnace. Clin. Chem. *21*, 558-561 (1975).
16. P. Baily, E. Norval, T. A. Kilroe-Smith, M. L. Skikue, and H. B. Rollin. The application of metal-coated graphite tubes to the determination of trace metals in biological materials. Microchem. J. *24*, 107-116 (1979).
17. D. D. Siemer and P. Koteel. Comparisons of methods of hydride generation atomic absorption spectrometric arsenic and selenium determination. Anal. Chem. *49*, 1096-1199 (1977).
18. C. Feldman. Improvements in the arsine accumulation-helium glow detector procedure for determining traces of arsenic. Anal. Chem. *51*, 664-669 (1979).
19. M. O. Andreae. Determination of arsenic species in natural waters. Anal. Chem. *49*, 820-823 (1977).
20. G. C. Kunselman and E. A. Huff. The determination of arsenic, antimony, selenium, and tellurium in environmental water samples by flameless atomic absorption. At. Absorpt. Newsl. *15*, 29-32 (1976).
21. R. D. Ediger. Atomic absorption analysis with the graphite furnace using matrix modification. At. Absorpt. Newsl. *14*, 127-130 (1975).
22. M. C. Bowman. *Carcinogens and Related Substances*. Marcel Dekker, New York, 1979.
23. H. K. Hundley and J. C. Underwood. Determination of total arsenic in total diet samples. J. Assoc. Off. Anal. Chem. *53*, 1176-1178 (1970).
24. R. F. Addison and R. G. Ackman. Direct determination of elemental phosphorus by gas liquid chromatography. J. Chromatogr. *47*, 421-426 (1970).
25. A. F. Ward. Inductively coupled argon plasma spectroscopy. Am. Lab., 79-87 (Nov. 1978).
26. R. W. Hunt and L. G. Hargis. Spectrophotometric and stopped-flow reaction-rate study of the formation of 10-molybdo-2-vanadophosphoric acid. Anal. Chem. *49*, 779-784 (1977).

27. M. McDaniel and A. D. Shendrikar. Concentration and determination of selenium from environmental samples. Anal. Chem. *48*, 2240-2242 (1976).
28. J. C. Chambers and B. E. McClellan. Enhancement of atomic absorption sensitivity for copper, cadmium, antimony, arsenic, and selenium by means of solvent extraction. Anal. Chem. *48*, 2061-2066 (1976).
29. I. Hoffman, R. J. Westerby, and M. Hidiroglou. Precise fluorometric microdetermination of selenium in agricultural materials. J. Assoc. Off. Anal. Chem. *51*, 1039-1042 (1968).
30. J. Toffaletti and J. Savory. Use of sodium borohydride for determination of total mercury in urine by atomic absorption spectrometry. Anal. Chem. *47*, 2091-2096 (1975).
31. C. J. Cappon and J. C. Smith. Gas chromatographic determination of inorganic mercury and organomercurials in biological materials. Anal. Chem. *49*, 365-369 (1977).
32. J. E. Longbottom. Inexpensive mercury-specific gas chromatographic detector. Anal. Chem. *44*, 1111-1112 (1972).
33. W. I. Muscat, T. J. Vickers, and A. Andren. Simple and versatile atomic fluorescence system for determination of nanogram quantities of mercury. Anal. Chem. *44*, 218-221 (1972).
34. W. R. Hatch and W. L. Ott. Determination of submicrogram quantities of mercury by atomic absorption spectrophotometry. Anal. Chem. *40*, 2085-2087 (1968).
35. T. K. Jan and D. R. Young. Determination of microgram amounts of some transition metals in seawater by methyl isobutyl ketone-nitric acid successive extraction and flameless atomic absorption spectrophotometry. Anal. Chem. *50*, 1250-1253 (1978).
36. J. D. Sheaffer, G. Mulvey, and R. K. Skogerboe. Determination of silver in precipitation by furnace atomic absorption spectrometry. Anal. Chem. *50*, 1239-1242 (1978).
37. A. T. Zander and T. C. O'Haver. Continuum source atomic absorption spectrometry with high resolution and wavelength modulation. Anal. Chem. *48*, 1166-1174 (1976).
38. S. G. Capar, J. T. Tanner, M. H. Friedman, and K. G. Boyer. Multielement analysis of animal feed, animal wastes, and sewage sludge. Environ. Sci. Technol. *12*, 785-790 (1978).
39. G. Horlick. Spectral characteristics of the inductively coupled argon plasma. Ind. Res./Dev. *20*(8), 70-73 (1978).
40. H. L. Kahn, R. G. Schleicher, and S. B. Smith. Control of AA sensitivity. Ind. Res./Dev. *20*(2), 101-104 (1978).

10

Halogenated Contaminants: Dibenzo-p-Dioxins and Dibenzofurans

LAWRENCE FISHBEIN National Center for Toxicological Research, U.S. Food and Drug Administration, Jefferson, Arkansas

I. INTRODUCTION

It is generally acknowledged that there is a continuing need to assess the status of existing potentially hazardous chemicals and strategies as well as those that may be introduced in the future that may affect human beings and the environment. This assessment is needed primarily from the predictive view of avoiding or ameliorating potentially catastrophic episodes similar to those that have occurred in the past.

In recent years, there has been recognized concern over the environmental and toxicological effects of a spectrum of halogenated hydrocarbons, primarily the organochlorine pesticides and related derivatives: for example, DDT, dieldrin, mirex, kepone, hexachlorobenzene (HCB), dibromochloropropane (DBCP), polychlorinated biphenyls (PCBs), and polybrominated biphenyls (PBBs).

This concern has now been extended to practically all of the major commercial halogenated saturated and unsaturated derivatives, numerous members of which have extensive utility as solvents, aerosol propellants, degreasing agents, dry-cleaning agents, refrigerants, flame retardants, synthetic feedstocks, cuttng fluids, monomers in the production of textiles and plastics, and so on, and hence are manufactured on a large scale (e.g., vinyl chloride, trichloroethylene, perchloroethylene, chloroform, and carbon tetrachloride).

The halogenated aliphatic and aromatic hydrocarbons represent one of the most important categories of industrial chemicals from a consideration of volume, use categories, environmental and toxicological considerations, and hence most important, potential populations at risk.

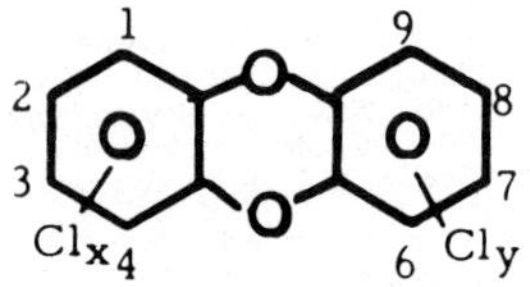

PCDD

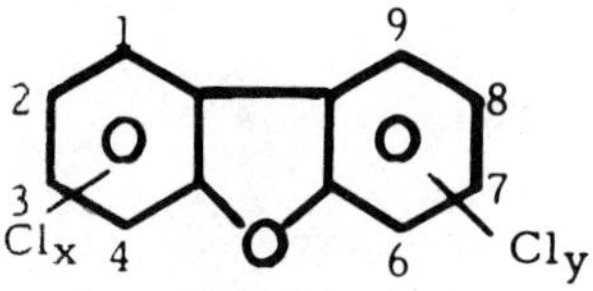

PCDF

Figure 1 Structures of polychlorinated dibenzo-p-dioxins (PCDDs) and dibenzofurans (PCDFs).

The findings of extremely toxic and environmentally persistent trace quantities of synthetic impurities (e.g., chlorodioxins and chlorodibenzofurans) in a number of halogenated industrial chemicals and pesticides of broad utility illustrates the need to acquire additional knowledge of the synthetic routes of organic compounds that will enter the market in quantity and for which there can exist potential human risk via occupational and environmental exposure. Concomitantly, information regarding refinement and development of sensitive submicrogram analysis, knowledge of stability and transport, and toxicity of potential hazardous trace organic impurities is of course vital.

Two major classes of hazardous trace organic contaminants are the chlorodioxins and chlorodibenzofurans, which can be formed as a consequence of a number of synthetic processes and hence can be present in a variety of products (Fig. 1). The importance of discerning the hazards to human health from dioxin compounds was dramatized after an accidental release of TCDD from a chemical plant contaminated the Seveso, Italy, area in July 1976. This accident revealed that insufficient data were available to properly evaluate the long-term health risks posed by dioxin compounds. It also became apparent that development and refinement of analytical methodology was required to permit the monitoring of extremely low levels of this toxicant.

Before discussing aspects of cleanup procedures and analytical methodology for their determination, it is germane to consider their formation and occurrence as well as toxicity.

II. CHLORODIOXINS

Chlorinated dibenzo-p-dioxins are a group of chemical compounds which are chemically persistent and are among the most toxic and hazardous pollutants in the environment. The lethal dose and toxic manifestations are structure and species dependent.

Although a number of the simple chlorodioxins have been known to chemists for three to four decades [1,2], major concern for the whole chemical group of chlorodioxins arose only when the extremely toxic and teratogenic properties of 2,3,7,8-tetrachlorodibenzo-p-dioxin (TCDD) became apparent in widely distributed pesticides such as the herbicide 2,4,5-trichlorophenoxy acetic acid (2,4,5-T) [3-5]. TCDD is perhaps the most potent small molecule toxin and teratogen known. The oral LD_{50} for many animal species is in the microgram per kilogram range, although there is considerable variability in different animal species. As little as 1 to 10 μg/kg TCDD has been found to be lethal for rabbits [4]; the LD_{50} of 2,4,5-T containing less than 0.05 to 0.1 ppm of TCDD administered to mice at 35 to 130 mg/kg caused both embryotoxic and teratogenic effects (primarily cleft palate).

The potential for human exposure to TCDD occurs (1) in the workplace when dioxins are formed during the industrial synthesis of 2,4,5-trichlorophenol (TCP), 2,4,5-T, pentachlorophenol, and hexachlorophene; (2) environmental contamination may also result from manufacturing processes, and from exposure to herbicides and other materials containing TCDD; and (3) exposure to the agent in the laboratory. Although chloroacne is perhaps the best known toxic effect of TCDD, exposed individuals have been found to develop a wide variety of lesion and symptoms, as shown in Table 1.

Clinically, therapy for TCDD exposure is limited to symptomatic treatment. There is no known agent, for example, that will accelerate the excretion of TCDD from the body, and patients who develop liver or kidney abnormalities after exposure can be given only supportive measures [6].

There is a presumption that adverse effects may result from long-term exposure to very small doses of TCDD as well as from a heavy single exposure of the sort sustained in a factory accident, such as that in Seveso, Italy. This has serious implications for the inhabitants of Seveso, for example, if significant traces of TCDD linger in the environment.

Although a number of cases of cancer have been reported in workers exposed to TCDD [7], adequate epidemiological studies were not available. An increased proportion of liver cancers have been reported in Hanoi after the spraying of herbicides (2,4-D and 2,4,5-T) containing TCDD in South Vietnam. The International Agency for Research on Cancer concluded that the significance of these observations cannot be assessed because of the inadequacy of details. It was suggested that more details of the reported cases, in addition to more

Table 1 Toxic Effects of TCDD in Humans

Dermatological	
	Chloroacne
	Porphyria cutanea tarda
	Hyperpigmentation and hirsutism
Internal	
	Liver damage[a]
	Raised serum hepatic enzyme levels
	Disorders of carbohydrate metabolism
	Cardiovascular disorders
	Urinary tract disorders
	Respiratory disorders
	Pancreatic disorders
Neurological	
	Polyneuropathies
	Lower extremity weakness
	Sensorial impairments (sight, hearing, smell, taste)
Psychiatric	
	Neurasthenic or depressive syndromes

[a]Mild fibrosis, fatty changes, haemofuscin deposition, and parenchymal cell degeneration were observed in a few cases.

extensive observations of the exposed people, are required before an evaluation of the carcinogenicity of chlorinated dibenzodioxins to humans could be made [7]. Hence, at present, the scientific picture remains unclear concerning the carcinogenic as well as mutagenic potential of TCDD in humans. It has been suggested that TCDD may be a promoter of neoplastic changes rather than an inducer of a particular kind of tumor [6]. However, it should also be noted that Van Miller et al. [8] recently reported carcinomas in the ear duct, kidney, liver, and ductal epithelium (lung, sebaceous gland) in male Sprague-Dawley rats fed ground chow containing 5, 50, or 500 parts per trillion and 1 or 5 ppb TCDD in a 2 year study.

While 2,3,7,8-TCDD has been the isomer of major research interest to date, as noted earlier, other chlorinated dibenzo-p-dioxins may occur in the environment, but they are less toxic than TCDD. McConnell et al. [9] recently described the comparative toxicity of chlorinated dibenzo-p-dioxins in mice and guinea pigs. It was found that the 2,3,7, and 8 positions must be chlorinated to achieve the

Table 2 Possible Number of Positional PCDD and PCDF Isomers

Chlorine substitution	Number of isomers	
	PCDDs	PCDFs
Mono-	2	4
Di-	10	16
Tri-	14	28
Tetra-	22	38
Penta-	14	28
Hexa-	10	16
Hepta-	2	4
Octa-	1	1
	75	135

greatest degree of toxicity. Additional chlorine atoms at an ortho position reduced toxicity, but not nearly to the degree caused by deletion of a chlorine atom at one of the lateral positions. At the toxic dose, the spectrum and severity of lesions and organ weight effects were similar for all homologs and isomers within the same animal species, although there were interspecies differences.

A variety of polychlorinated dibenzo-p-dioxins (PCDDs) and polychlorinated dibenzofurans (PCDFs) can occur as impurities from the manufacture of many industrial and agricultural chemicals based on chlorophenols and certain chlorinated aromatic hydrocarbons. In the case of the PCDDs, 75 isomers exist, ranging from the mono- to the octachloro compound; the corresponding number of isomers of the PCDFs is 135 (Table 2).

Dioxins found in 2,4,5-T, pentachlorophenol (PCP), and hexachlorophene are formed during the manufacturing processes used to produce chlorophenols [7-13]. Chlorophenols can contain a variety of contaminants and by-products. In addition to other chlorophenols, they may contain up to several percent of polychlorinated phenoxyphenols (predioxins) [12] in addition to polychlorinated dibenzo-p-dioxins, dibenzofurans, and diphenyl ethers, which are often present in the range of tens to hundreds of parts per million [14].

Production statistics [15] suggest that at least 50 million pounds of 2,4,5-trichlorophenol and its derivatives are manufactured in the United States each year, almost all of which contains low but detectable levels of TCDD.

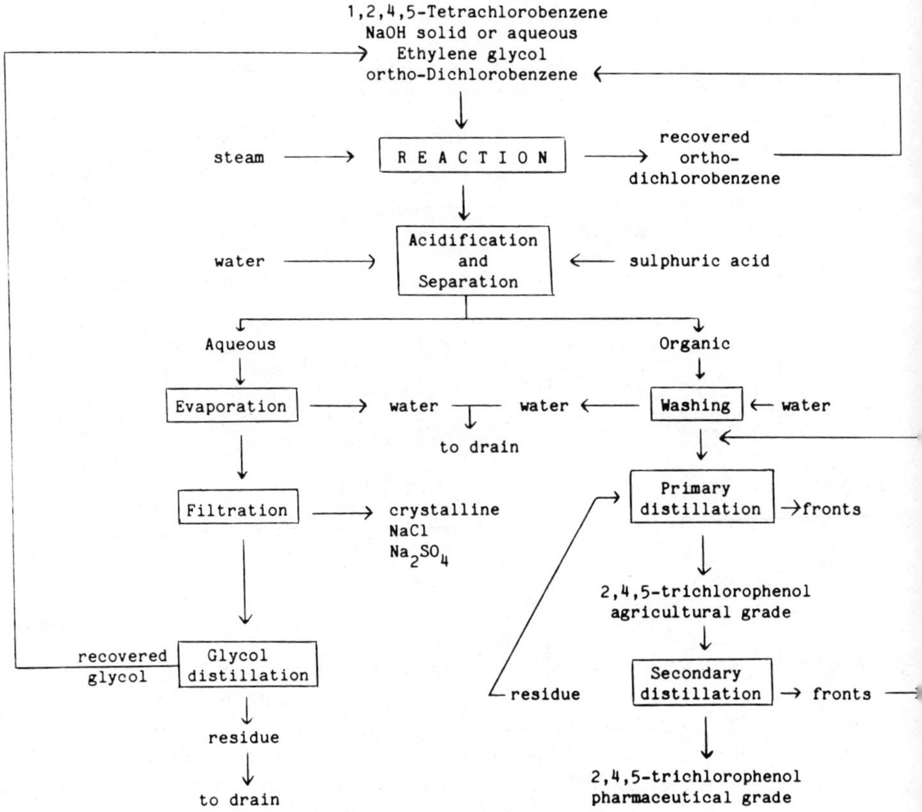

Figure 2 Schematic representation of the reaction involved in 2,4,5-trichlorophenol production. (From Ref. 16.)

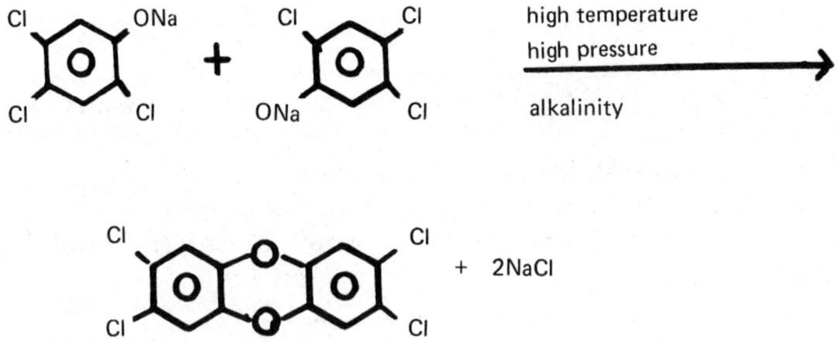

Figure 3 Formation of TCDD by condensation of sodium trichlorophenate. (From Ref. 16.)

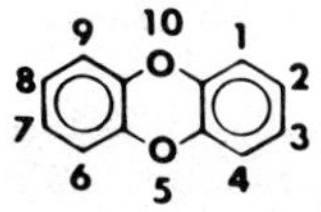

Basic structure of dibenzo-dioxin (dioxin). Chlorine may be attached, in various combinations, at the 1,2, 3,4,5,6,7,8 or 9 positions.

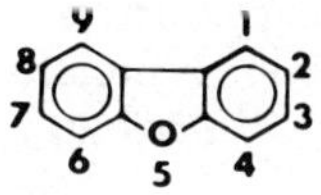

Basic structure of Dibenzofuran (furan)

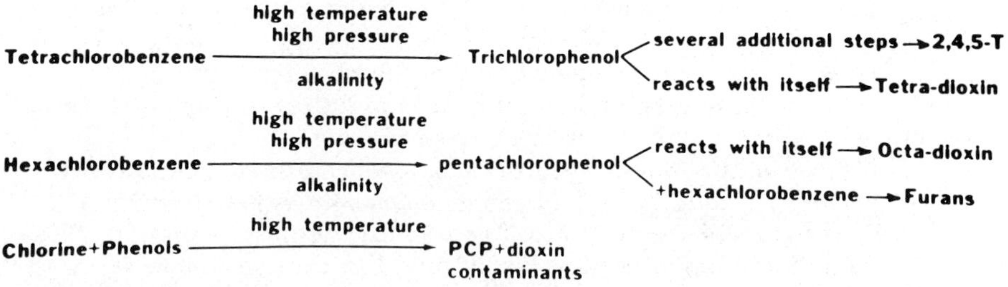

Figure 4 Formation of dioxins and furans.

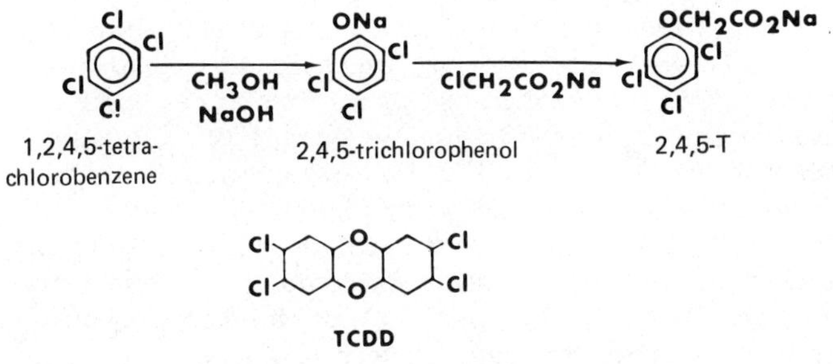

Figure 5 Formation of 2,3,7,8-tetrachlorodibenzo-p-dioxin (TCDD) as a by-product in the synthesis of 2,4,5-T.

TCDD can be formed as a by-product during the synthesis of 2,4,5-trichlorophenol, which involves the hydrolysis of 1,2,4,5-tetrachlorobenzene using methanol and caustic soda at elevated pressure or ethylene glycol and caustic soda at atmospheric pressure [7,16-20] (Figs. 2 to 5). If the reaction proceeds at temperatures higher than the normal 180°,* ethylene glycol is distilled off or polymerized, and an exothermic reaction starts at about 230° and proceeds rapidly and uncontrollably to about 410° [7]. TCDD is then formed in the distillate via the condensation of two molecules of sodium trichlorophenate under the influence of the highly exothermic decomposition of sodium 2-hydroxyethanol. When the mixture is heated at the normal temperature (180°) even for long periods, 2,4,5-trichlorophenol contains less than 1 mg/kg TCDD [7]. Much larger amounts of TCDD (e.g., 1600 mg/kg) have been reported when sodium 2,4,5-trichlorophenate was heated at 230 to 260° for 2 hr [7].

Since 2,4,5-trichlorophenol is also the precursor of 2,4,5-T (Figs. 4 and 5), another potential source of TCDD is during the manufacture of 2,4,5-T and its esters per se [7,10,16,20].

A facet of the dioxin problem was observed in connection with the employment of Agent Orange (Herbicide Orange, a 1:1 mixture of butyl esters of 2,4-D and 2,4,5-T) in South Vietnam in the late 1960s [21]. The formulation employed was found to contain 0.1 to 47 μg/g TCDD [22].

Although efforts were made in the 1970s to check and minimize the formation of TCDD during the preparation of 2,4,5-T, there is a paucity of information available on the levels of impurities in formulations used prior to the late 1960s.

Samples of 2,4,5-T produced in the United States by one manufacturer during the period 1966 to 1968 often contained 10 ppm TCDD. Eight additional samples of technical 2,4,5-T were found to contain 0.1 to 55 mg/kg TCDD [23]. Recent U.S. samples of 2,4,5-T have been reported to contain 0.5 ppm TCDD [24].

Rappe et al. [25] recently described the identification and quantification of isomers present in a select number of 2,4,5-T preparations of European origin from the 1960s and samples of Herbicide Orange. Table 3 lists the amounts of polychlorinated dibenzo-p-dioxins and polychlorinated dibenzofurans (ppm formulation) in five 2,4,5-T ester formulations and three Herbicide Orange formulations. The 2,3,7,8-TCDD was in all cases by far the most abundant isomer, found at levels ranging from 0.1 to 0.95 μg/g in four of the five 2,4,5-T esters analyzed. Only in sample 5, with the highest level of 2,3,7,8-TCDD, were traces of other PCDDs detected (e.g., 2,3,7-tri- and 1,3,7,8-tetrachlorodibenzo-p-dioxins. Two of the samples containing 2,3,7,8-tetrachlorodibenzodioxins showed the presence of a

---

*All temperature data are in degrees Celsius.

Table 3 Amounts of PCDDs and PCDFs (μg/g Formation) in 2,4,5-T Ester Formulations and Herbicide Orange

Sample description[a] and production date	PCDDs[b]					PCDFs[b]				
	Di-	Tri-	Tetra-	Penta-	Hexa-	Di-	Tri-	Tetra-	Penta-	Hexa-
1. 2,4,5-T ester, 1967	nd	nd	nd	nd	nd	nd	nd	nd	nd	nd
2. 2,4,5-T ester, 1966	nd	nd	0.10	nd	nd	nd	nd	nd	nd	nd
3. 2,4,5-T ester, 1967	nd	nd	0.22	nd	nd	nd	nd	0.11	nd	nd
4. 2,4,5-T ester, 1967	nd	nd	0.18	nd	nd	nd	nd	0.15	nd	nd
5. 2,4,5-T ester, 1962	ns	0.01	0.95	nd	nd	nd	nd	nd	nd	nd
6. Herbicide Orange[c]	0.15	0.02	0.12	nd	nd	-	nd	nd	nd	-
7. Herbicide Orange[c]	0.15	0.50	1.1	0.05	nd	-	0.10	0.40	0.20	nd
8. Herbicide Orange[c]	nd	0.02	5.1	nd	nd	nd	nd	nd	nd	nd

[a]Sample description: 1, isooctyl ester, 240 g/liter; 2, butyoxyethyl ester, 500 g/liter; 3, butoxyethyl ester, 165 g/liter; 4, isooctyl ester, 750 g/liter; 5, butyl ester, 865 g/liter; 6-8, butyl esters, 450-500 g/liter.
[b]nd, not detected.
[c]Production dates unknown.
Source: Ref. 25.

tetrachlorodibenzofuran isomer of unknown substitution. All the samples of the series showed the presence of tri-, tetra-, and/or pentachlorodiphenylethers.

All three samples of Herbicide Orange contained trace amounts of 1,3,7,8-tetrachlorodibenzo-p-dioxin (1 to 2% relative to the 2,3,7,8-isomer). It should be noted that the same isomer at the level of 4 to 5% relative to 2,3,7,8-tetrachlorodibenzo-p-dioxin was also found in the soil after an accidental discharge from a 2,4,5-trichlorophenol production plant near Seveso, Italy [25]. In addition, two samples of Herbicide Orange (samples 1 and 2, Table 3) contained 1,3,6,8- and 1,3,7,9-tetrachlorodibenzo-p-dioxin (2 and 10% relative to the 2,3,7,8-isomer). These two isomers are the normal and the Smiles-rearranged dimerization products of 2,4,6-trichlorophenol, the expected overchlorination product in the synthesis of 2,4-dichlorophenol. Significant levels of 2,7- or 2,8-substituted isomer (the normal and the Smiles-rearranged dimerization product of 2,4-dichlorophenol) were also found in samples 6 and 7. The major trichlorinated dibenzo-p-dioxin found in these samples was the 1,3,7-isomer, an expected condensation product of 2,4-di- and 2,4,6-trichlorophenol. Polychlorinated dibenzofurans were detected in only one of the Herbicide Orange samples (number 7, Table 3) (e.g., one tri-, four tetra-, and one penta-chlorinated dibenzofuran isomer at a total level of 0.7 $\mu g/g$). The results obtained in the above study of Rappe et al. [25] differ somewhat from those reported previously by Huckins et al. [26] and Ahling et al. [27] and seems to emphasize that significant variations between individual samples exist and that for a rigorous identification of PCDDs and PCDFs, a careful inspection of all the mass spectra is required and that for accurate isomer assignments high-resolution gas chromatography should be used [28].

The conditions that enhance TCDD formation are high temperature, high pressure, and alkalinity. The same types of conditions are necessary for the production of pentachlorophenol (PCP) when hexachlorobenzene is used as the starting material (Fig. 4, reaction 2). Under these conditions, both chlorinated dioxins and the chlorinated dibenzofurans may be formed [12]. Thus a reaction between two molecules of pentachlorophenol may occur, resulting in the formation of octachlorodibenzo-p-dioxin (OCDD). The more highly chlorinated dibenzo-p-dioxin may also be formed if too much heat is applied when the chlorophenols are produced by the reaction of chlorine with phenol, especially during the manufacture of tetra- and pentachlorophenols. Since chlorinated dioxins are formed by the condensation of chlorinated phenols under conditions of heat and alkalinity [7-13,16-20,29-31], and although the precise conditions in all cases have not been experimentally determined, it is theoretically possible for any ortho-chlorinated phenol to undergo this reaction. For example, any pesticide with a chlorinated phenoxy nucleus or which is derived from a chlorinated phenol precursor could contain chlorinated dioxin.

Table 4 Chlorinated Dibenzo-p-Dioxins Found in Commercial Pesticides

Pesticide	Chlorodibenzo-p-dioxin detected				Sample		
	Tetra-	Hexa-	Hepta-	Octa-	Contaminated	Tested	Date of manufacture
Phenoxyalkanoates							
2,4,5-T	++[a]	++	-	-	23	42	1950-1970
Silvex	+	-	-	-	1	7	1965-1970
2,4-D	-	a	-	-	1	24	1964-1970
2,4-DB	-	-	-	-	0	3	1967-1970
2,4-DEP	-	-	-	-	0	2	1967
Dichloroprop	-	-	-	-	0	1	1967
Erbon	-	-	-	++	1	1	1967
Sesone	-	+	-	-	1	1	1970
Dicamba	-	-	-	-	0	8	1968-1970
Chlorophenols							
Tri-	-	+	+	-	4	6	1950-1970
Tetra-	-	++	++	++	3	3	1953-1970
Penta- (PCP)	-	++	++	++	10	11	1953-1970
Others[b]	-	++	++	+	5	22	

[a]Concentration of at least one sample was >10 ppm (++), 0.5 to 10 ppm (+), or <0.5 ppm (-).
[b]DMPA, ronnel, and tetrafidon had chlorodioxin residues; chloroneb, hexachlorophene, nematoxide, and nitrofen had none.
Source: Reprinted with permission from Ref. 32, E. A. Woolson, R. F. Thomas, and P. D. J. Ensor, Survey of polychlorinated dibenzo-p-dioxin in selected pesticides, J. Agric. Food Chem. 20, 351-354; © 1972 American Chemical Society.

Woolson et al. [32] surveyed the polychlorodibenzo-p-dioxin content in 129 samples of 17 different pesticides derived from chlorophenols. Seventy-six percent of the samples analyzed contained less than 0.1 μg/g of TCDD in the technical material, whereas 7% contained less than 0.1 μg/g and 9% contained more than 10 μg/g of TCDD. While no TCDD was detected in the 20 tri-, tetra-, or pentachlorophenol samples examined, high levels of other dioxins were found (e.g., hexa-, hepta-, and octachlorodibenzo-p-dioxins) (Table 4).

Analysis of 21 mono-, di-, tetra-, and pentachlorophenols for the presence of polychlorodibenzo-p-dioxins was reported by Firestone et al. [33]. No PCDDs were found in samples of 2-chlorophenol, 2,4-dichloro, or 2,6-dichlorophenol obtained from laboratory chemical suppliers. TCDD in the range 0.07 to 6.2 mg/kg was found in three of six samples of 2,4,5-trichlorophenol (or its sodium salt). The isomeric 1,3,6,8-tetrachlorodibenzo-p-dioxin was found at a level of 49 mg/kg in a sample of 2,4,6-trichlorophenol. Although tetrachlorodibenzo-p-dioxins were not found in the tetrachlorophenols examined, hexachlorodibenzo-p-dioxins were found in two of three samples of 2,3,4,6-tetrachlorophenol. In addition, one of the tetrachlorophenol samples contained 29, 5.1, and 0.17 mg/kg hexa-, hepta-, and octachlorodibenzo-p-dioxins, respectively. Although no tetrachlorodibenzo-p-dioxins were found in eight commercial samples of pentachlorophenol (received during the period 1967-1970), heptachlorodibenzo-p-dioxins were found in the range 0.5 to 39 mg/kg in seven samples, and 3.3 to 15 mg/kg was found in five samples. Hexachlorodibenzo-p-dioxins were present in all eight of the pentachloro samples at levels ranging from 0.03 to 38 mg/kg [33].

Buser [34], utilizing mass fragmentography, reported that commercial samples of 2,3,4,6-tetrachlorophenol (TCP) and of technical pentachlorophenol (PCP) contained less than 0.2 mg/kg of tetra- and pentachlorodibenz-p-dioxins, respectively. The TCP contained 6 mg/kg hexachlorodibenzo-p-dioxins, 55 mg/kg heptaachlorodibenzo-p-dioxins and 39 mg/kg octachlorodibenz-p-dioxins. The PCP contained 9 mg/kg hexachloro-, 235 mg/kg heptachloro-, and 250 mg/kg octachlorodibenzo-p-dioxins. The positional isomers of the dioxins were not identified [34].

Villaneuva et al. [35], utilizing gas chromatographic techniques, detected hexa-, hepta-, and octachlorodibenzo-p-dioxins in both technical and analytical grades of commercial pentachlorophenol. With electron capture detection, the technical grade material was found to contain 42, 24, and 10 mg/kg of the respective dioxins. The positional isomers of the various dioxins were not specified in this study [35].

It has been suggested that the combustion or burning of vegetation sprayed with 2,4,5-T could result in formation of TCDD [36]. Stehl and Lamparski [37] reported the formation of small amounts of TCDD when grass and paper coated with several compounds containing the 2,4,5-trichlorophenoxy moiety (e.g., Esteron 245, a formation of 2,4,5-T esters) were subjected to combustion at 350 to 600° and 600 to 800°. Although the experiments did not duplicate all possible burning conditions, they did strongly suggest that only a very small fraction of 2,4,5-T (or other 2,4,5-trichlorophenoxy species) is converted to TCDD, as determined by a multiple cleanup procedure followed by gas chromatography-mass spectrometry [37]. When these data are combined with other observations on the degradation of both large and small amounts of 2,4,5-T and TCDD [38,39], the TCDD burden added to the environment by the combustion of natural materials treated with 2,4,5-trichlorophenoxy species is no larger than 1 part per trillion of TCDD per ppm of 2,4,5-T residue burned [37].

Anderson et al. [40] reported that no TCDD could be found (at a detection limit of 4 μg TCDD/g 2,4,5-T burned) by burning various samples of vegetation sprayed or spiked with 2,4,5-T ester or salts.

Ahling et al. [27] described the formation of PCDDs and PCDFs during the combustion of a 2,4,5-T formulation (containing 500 g/liter of 2-butoxyethyl 2,4,5-trichlorophenoxyacetate) under controlled experimental conditions. Under normal combustion temperatures (>500°) the 2,4,5-T ester was destroyed to the extent of 99.995%. The emission of PCDDs decreased with increased temperature and transit time; the highest emitted amount was 4 mg of tetrachlorinated dibenzo-p-dioxins per kilogram of formulation at a temperature of 500°. The concentration of 2,4,5-T ester in the burnt material (about 10^{-2} g/g of wood chips) was higher than the concentrations found after normal use in the environment (10^{-4} to 10^{-3} g/g of dry leaves) [41]. A high concentration will favor the formation of dimers and smaller amounts of PCDDs are to be expected from sources such as forest fires. The largest formation of tetrachlorodibenzo-p-dioxins found in the study of Ahling et al. [27] would correspond to a formation of about 1 μg of tetrachlorodioxin/m^2 in a forest fire directly after application of the herbicide formulation.

Polychlorinated dibenzo-p-dioxins can be formed by dimerization of chlorophenates during pyrolysis. Large quantities of chlorophenols are used as fungicides in the wood industry. Prior to the final use, the top layers with the applied chlorophenate are removed and the wood shavings burned for heating purposes or used in the production of plywood. During this burning, it is possible that PCDDs could be formed [29]. Rappe et al. [29] identified and quantified PCDDs and PCDFs formed during the uncontrolled open burning of leaves and wood wool impregnated with commercial and purified chlorophenates (e.g., chlorophenol formulations consisting of a mixture of 2,4,6-tri-, 2,3,4,6-tetra-, and pentachlorophenate). (Tables 5 and 6 illustrate the amounts of PCDDs found in burning experiments of commercial chlorophenates and of purified chlorphenates, respectively. In the case of the major isomer, more information concerning discrete PCDDs

Table 5 Amounts of PCDDs Found in Burning Experiments of Commercial Chlorophenates[a]

Compound	Servarex						KY-5	
	Original sample	Birch leaves			Wood wool		Original Sample	Birch leaves: charcoal
		Charcoal	Ash	XAD-2	Charcoal	XAD-2		
Tetra-CDDs	0.7	35	17	26	95	210	0.4	30
Penta-CDDs	5.2	90	58	59	120	357	3.5	84
Hexa-CDDs	9.5	80	74	57	110	347	5.3	82
Hepta-CDDs	5.6	8	18	8	65	29	2.1	8.2
Octa-CDD	0.7	0.3	6.4	0.2	1.2	1.2	0.3	0.4

[a] μg PCDDs/g chlorophenate.

Source: Ref. 29.

Table 6 Amounts of PCDDs Found in Burning Experiments of Purified Chlorophenates[a]

Compound	2,4,6-Trichlorophenate		Pentachlorophenate	
	Original sample	Birch leaves: charcoal	Original sample	Birch leaves: charcoal
Tetra-CDDs	<0.02	2100	<0.02	5.2
Penta-CDDs	<0.03	5.0	<0.03	14
Hexa-CDDs	<0.03	1.0	<0.03	56
Hepta-CDDs	<0.1	3.0	0.3	172
Octa-CDDs	<0.1	6.0	0.9	710

[a] μg PCDDs/g chlorophenate.
Source: Ref. 29.

and PCDFs was obtained by running complete EI mass spectra.) Among the tetrachlorinated dibenzo-p-dioxins found, the main isomers were the 1,3,6,8- and 1,3,7,9-tetrachloro derivatives, both of which are found to possess minor biological activity [42,43]. These two isomers are the normal dimerization [44,45] and the Smiles-rearrangement [46,47] products from 2,4,6-trichlorophenate. TCDD was found in extremely minor amounts. Among the pentachlorodibenzo-p-dioxins, 9 of the 14 theoretically possible 14 isomers were found, while 5 isomeric hexachlorodibenzo-p-dioxins in medium to higher concentrations were detected of the possible 10 theoretically possible isomers.

Fly ash and flue gases of municipal incinerators and of an industrial heating facility have been shown to contain polychlorinated dibenzo-p-dioxins and polychlorinated dibenzofurans in addition to other chlorinated compounds [48,49]. The fly ash from two different facilities in Switzerland showed a remarkably similar distribution of the PCDD isomers [45]. The major PCDD isomers found from both facilities were those formed in the pyrolytic dimerization of the most common chlorophenates (e.g., the 2,4-di-, and 2,4,6-tri-, 2,3,4,6-tetra-, and pentachlorophenate), suggesting that these commonly used products as precursors of the polychlorinated dibenzo-p-dioxins. The known toxic PCDD isomers, such as 2,3,7,8-tetra-, 1,2,3,7,8-penta-, 1,2,3,6,7,8-, and 1,2,3,7,8,9-hexa derivatives were present as minor components. In addition to PCDDs, the fly ash from both facilities showed the presence of PCDFs at a similar level as the PCDDs [49].

In the studies of Olie et al. [48] of trace components of fly ash and flue gas of three municipal incinerators in the Netherlands, the most abundant chlorine-containing compounds found in the condensate from flue gas were chlorophenols, but smaller quantities of chlorodibenzodioxins (e.g., tetra-, penta-, hepta-, and octaisomers), as well as tetra-, penta-, hexa-, hepta-, and octachlorodibenzofurans, could also be detected by single ion monitoring. It is important to note that the composition of fly ash and flue gas at any given incineration plant varies considerably with time due to such factors as composition of waste and operating conditions. These variations, in addition to the difficulty of representative sampling of flue gases generally and variations in the effectiveness of electrostatic precipitators, make it extremely difficult to obtain accurate quantitative data [48]. The presence of relatively large amounts of chlorophenols in flue gas condensate in the study of Olie et al. [48] strongly suggests that these compounds are the most likely precursors of chlorodibenzo-p-dioxins in the incineration process. The thermal synthesis of chlorophenols is considered possible since relatively large quantities of hexachlorobenzene and other highly chlorinated benzenes were found in all fly ash samples examined in this study [48].

Although no quantitative data on the release of PCDDs or PCDFs into the environment via municipal incinerators are available at present, the amount of these agents entering the atmosphere via flue gases is considered to be probably quite small [48]. However, owing to the extreme toxicity of some of these agents and the fact that a large number of incineration plants are located in the proximity of heavily populated areas, extensive monitoring of such facilities might be advisable. In addition, since the origin of PCDDs and PCDFs in fly ash and flue gases of municipal incinerators is largely unknown and since conditions of high temperature are thought likely to be importants fly ash and flue gases of other installations from industry and energy production should be investigated [48].

TCDD has been identified as the major PCDD formed in a number of accidental contamination episodes [7,13,18]. An explosion in 1963 at the Philips Duphar 2,4,5-trichlorophenol and 2,4,5-T plant in the Netherlands released between 30 and 200 g of TCDD [7,18,50,51]. The factory was subsequently dismantled, embedded in concrete, and dumped at a deep point into the Atlantic Ocean [7]. TCDD was identified as a product of an explosion at the Coalite and Chemical Products 2,4,5-trichlorophenol plant in the United Kingdom in 1968 [7,16,17]. The manufacturing process at this plant involved the hydrolysis of 1,2,4,5-tetrachlorobenzene using ethylene glycol and caustic soda at atmospheric pressure.

In July 1976, an accident occurred at the ICMESA 2,4,5-trichlorophenol plant in northern Italy, resulting in the contamination of a large populated area [7,15,21,51-54]. In this plant, in which the ethylene glycol manufacturing process was used, a malfunction occurred in thermal regulation, resulting in the rupture of a safety valve. The subsequent release of 2 to 3 kg of TCDD, as well as trichlorophenol and other substances, spread from the factory into a triangular area approximately 3 to 5 km long and 600 to 700 m wide.

Accidental TCDD contamination has also occurred in several other factories: in Ludwigshaven, Federal Republic of German, in 1953 [55]; in Hamburg, Federal Republic of Germany, in 1954 [56]; in Newark, New Jersey, in 1964 [57]; in France in 1966]58]; and in Czeckoslovakia in 1965-1968 [59]. However, no data were available on either the amount of TCDD produced or on the concentrations in the work places or environment. Thus far the only factory that emitted detectable levels of TCDD into the environment as a result of accidental contamination was that described in the Italian episode.

Polychlorinated dibenzo-p-dioxins can also theoretically be formed via the photolysis of chlorophenols. Although the irradiation of aqueous solutions of dioxin-free sodium salt of pentachlorophenol has been found to generate the octachloro isomer in very small amounts, repeated attempts to produce TCDD from the irradiation of 2,4,5-T, 2,4,5-trichlorophenol or sodium 2,4,5-trichlorophenate solution have been unsuccessful [24].

The failure to detect TCDD as a photolysis product of 2,4,5-trichlorophenol can be attributed to the extreme instability of the lower chlorinated dioxins to light in the presence of organic substrates

[18,60]. Although the PCDDs can theoretically be generated under environmental conditions, light provides a mechanism for their destruction [18,60]. Neither microbial or chemical condensation of 2,4,5-trichlorophenol in soil has yielded TCDD [11].

III. ANALYTICAL CONSIDERATIONS

In the previous discussion, we considered germane aspects of the toxicity and occurrence primarily of the chlorinated dioxins, with the greatest emphasis placed on the most toxic member, TCDD. We can readily recognize that there are a number of major problem areas in the separation and analysis of the chlorodioxins as well as the chlorodibenzofurans. First, there is the problem of separation of these compounds, not only from each other but from related compounds, such as the polychlorinated biphenyls (PCBs), DDT, DDE, polychlorinated

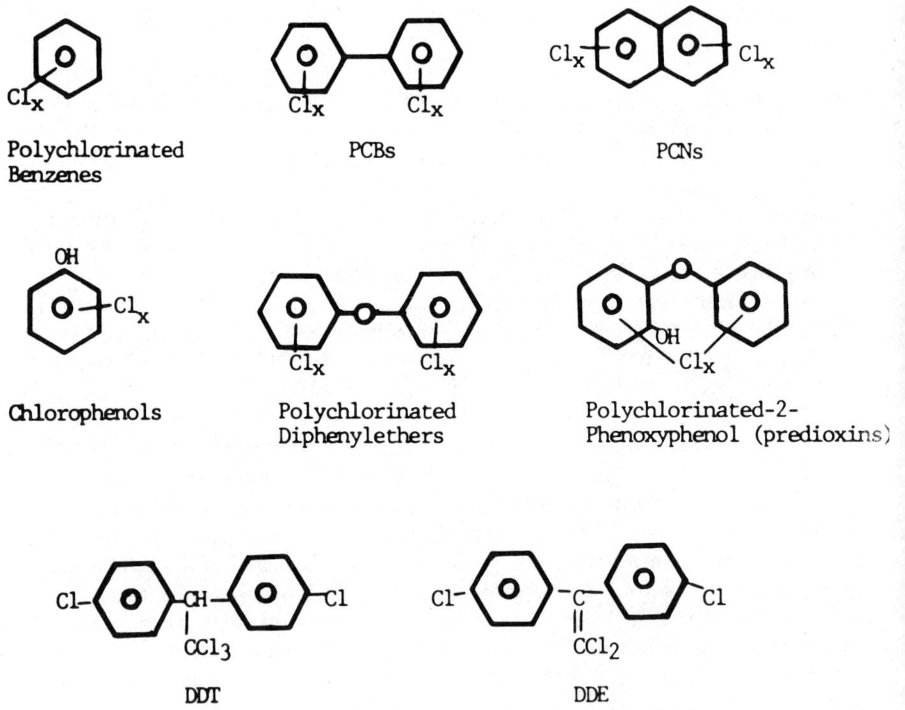

Figure 6 Structures of halogenated contaminants in possible admixture with chlorinated dibenzo-p-dixons and chlorinated dibenzofurans.

benzenes, polychlorinated naphthalenes, chlorophenols, polychlorinated diphenyl ethers, and polychlorinated-2-phenoxyphenols (predioxins), as illustrated in Figure 6. It is evident that a highly efficient cleanup procedure is a critical first step in the analysis of any environmental sample of chlorodioxins or chlorodibenzofurans. The second problem is the extreme difficulty of unequivocally assigning positions to isomers containing the same number of chlorine atoms, and third, the severe requirement in many cases of having an analytical sensitivity of at least 1 part per trillion (10^{-12} g). The latter aspect could perhaps best be illustrated by the following considerations. Baughman and Meselson [62,62] observed that no method existed which was sensitive enough to detect TCDD in animal tissues even after administration in some species of lethal doses. For example, in the guinea pig, one of most susceptible species of those that have been tested, the lethal single oral dose (LD_{50}) in males is 0.6 μg/kg of body weight. This means that if all the TCDD were retained, the level would be less than 1 ppb in the whole animal. The lowest reported limit of detection for TCDD in whole tissues in 1973 was 50 ppb [63]. Thus a guinea pig could be killed with TCDD and it would be impossible to establish this fact with the analytical procedures then in current use.

Because of its chemical stability and its lipophilic nature, the possibility has been suggested that TCDD released into the environment could accumulate in food chains. Earlier analytical techniques, such as gas chromatography per se, would be of minimal value in monitoring food chains for the buildup of TCDD. For example, the limit of detection of TCDD for the electron capture detector, the recognized keystone of most analytical procedures, is not much less than 1 ng (10^{-9} g).

The apparent need for more sensitive analytical procedures is even more apparent if, as Baughman and Meselson [62,63] state, one considers the possibility of sublethal toxic effects and allows a margin for a safety factor. For example, if a factor of about 100 is provided for nonlethal toxicity, and a further factor of 10 is allowed for a safety margin, in addition to allowing for the possible existence of species even more sensitive than the guinea pig, we would require a level of detection of $10^{-9} \times 10^{-2} = 10^{-12}$, or 1 part per trillion (1 part in 10^{-12}) for environmental monitoring. For a 1 g sample this would require a limit of detection of 1 pg (10^{-12} g).

In addition to high sensitivity, a requirement for any acceptable method is high specificity, because at very low levels, few confirmatory procedures could be employed to establish unambigously the identity of a particular compound.

Mass spectrometry in its various forms (e.g., high, medium, and low resolution, with or without interfacing to gas chromatographs) is the method that has been most widely employed for the analysis of chlorodibenzodioxins and chlorodibenzofurans in environmental samples and for the analysis of TCDD in environmental monitoring programs [64]. All the mass spectral methods that have been developed for the analyses of TCDD utilize the fact that the mass spectrum of TCDD is relatively simple and that the base peak is the molecular ion at m/e 320. As a result of the various possible combinations of the naturally occurring ^{35}Cl and ^{37}Cl isotopes in a tetrachloro compound, the signal for the molecular ion is a pentuplet with peaks at m/e 320, 322, 324, 326, and 328, with intensities in the ratio 77:100:49:10:1 [61,62,64]. In addition, the four chlorine atoms and the limited number of hydrogen atoms make the compound significantly mass deficient (e.g., the m/e 320 peak is actually 319.895), hence relatively easily resolvable from most other organic residues [61,62,64]. Figure 7 illustrates the mass spectrum of TCDD. The molecular ion (M^+) is at m/e 320; the ionizing voltage, 700 V; the source, 150°; and the asterisk denotes the impurity trichlorodibenzo-p-dioxin [61].

The original method of Baughman and Meselson [62] utilized a direct-probe high-resolution AEI MS-9 double-focusing mass spectrometer. The sensitivity was maximized by using the signal-averaging technique, wherein successive scans over a narrow mass range are added together to produce an integrated mass spectrum with a greatly improved signal-to-noise ratio for single-ion monitoring analysis. Typical instrumental conditions utilized by Baughman and Meselson were: source, 220°; resolution, 10,000; trap current, 1.0 mA; electron multiplier, about 3000 V; ionizing voltage, 70 eV; and time averaging, 4 scans/sec. Peak heights were measured at m/e 321.895 (corresponding to the isomer with one atom of ^{37}Cl and three atoms of ^{35}Cl). (The natural abundance of the chlorine isotopes are 75.53 and 24.47%, respectively.) The quantity of TCDD in picograms present in sample fractions to which TCDD had not been added was computed from the ratio of their mean peak heights to the mean peak heights found with added TCDD. [^{37}Cl]TCDD was added, and peak heights were measured at m/e 327.885 in order to compute the amount of [^{37}Cl]TCDD recovered. The recovery through the complete cleanup procedure was then calculated on the basis of the amount of [^{37}Cl] TCDD added to the sample at the beginning of the cleanup. The quantity of TCDD computed was corrected by the recovery factor obtained to give the final result [61,62,64].

Table 7 illustrates the original sample cleanup procedure of Baughman and Meselson for TCDD in human milk [61,62]. However, in the sample cleanup utilizing preparative GLC, the recovery was only 25%.

An improved cleanup procedure utilizing an alumina chromatography step eliminated interfering PCBs and DDE and was applied to the analysis of Vietnamese fish samples. Figure 8 depicts the mass spectra, showing reduction of DDE and PCB levels in fish residue by

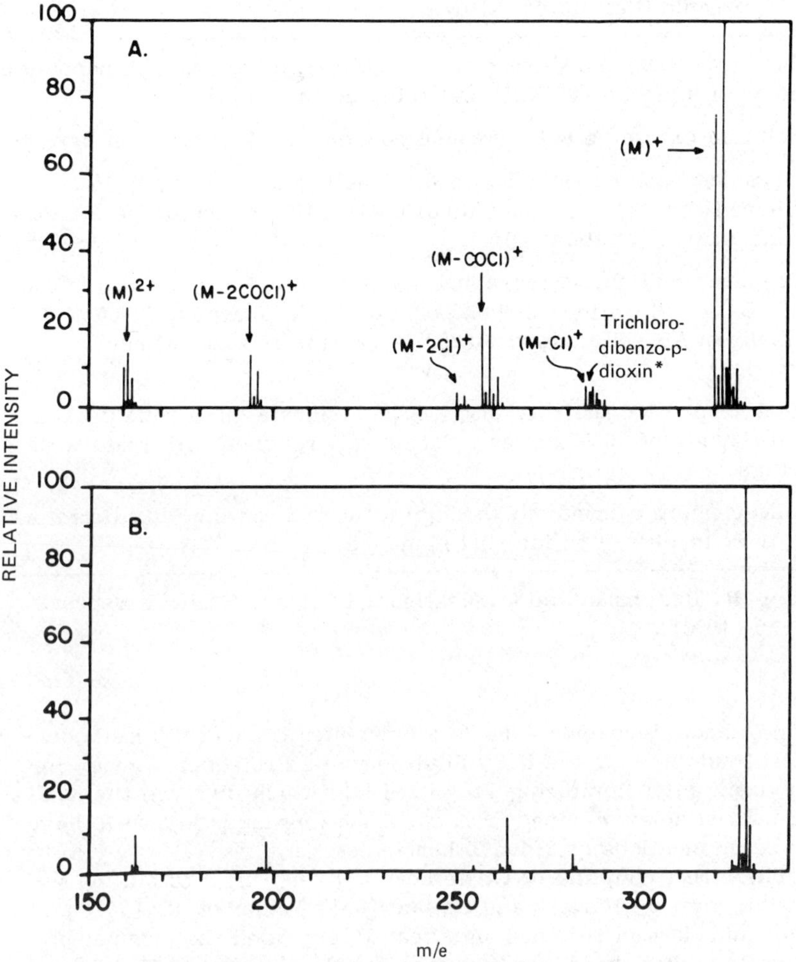

Figure 7 Mass spectra of (A) TCDD and (B) ^{37}Cl-labeled TCDD. The isotopic purity of the ^{37}Cl is 95.5%. The asterisk denotes an impurity. The multiplicity of lines associated with each major molecular species results from the presence of various isotopes of Cl and C. (From Ref. 62.)

means of alumina chromatography. The linearity of response for TCDD in the presence of beef liver residue is shown in Figure 9. The TCDD values are the amounts introduced into individual runs on the MS-9 mass spectrometer.

Less cumbersome procedures for directly measuring the recovery of TCDD in each sample by adding ^{37}Cl-labeled TCDD to the sample

Table 7 Sample Cleanup of TCDD in Human Milk

1. Ten gram sample of human milk combined with 10 ml of ethanol and 20 ml of aqueous 40% KOH and refluxed for 6 hr.
2. Solution extracted with 4 × 6 ml portions of 5% benzene in hexane.
3. Organic phase extracted with 4 × 8 ml portions of 85% H_2SO_4; filtered through a 10 mm i.d. column of 10 g of powdered Na_2CO_3, concentrated to about 10 μl.
4. Preparatively chromatographed by GLC on a 1 m × 1/4 in. column of 3% OV-101 methyl silicone polymer liquid phase on 50-60 mesh Anakrom AB solid support (200°C column; 30 ml/min helium carrier).
5. GLC trap: 150 mm × 1.5 mm i.d. borosilicate glass tube packed with 30 mm of 100-120 mesh glass beads retained with glass wool plugs.
6. GLC cleanup carried out through a thermal conductivity detector, with m-terphenyl as internal standard.

Source: R. Boughman and M. Meselson, Environ. Health Perspect. 5, 27-35 (1973).

have now been developed. Table 8 illustrates the cleanup methodology for TCDD adopted by the U.S. Environmental Protection Agency for its Environmental Monitoring Program [64], which involved the analysis of beef fat samples obtained from cows' grazing lands known to have received applications of 2,4,5-T herbicides.

The direct coupling of GC to both low- and high-resolution MS recently shown by Harless and Oswald [65], Taylor et al. [66], and Shadoff and Hammel [67] has significantly extended the original MS techniques of Baughman and Meselson for the analysis of TCDD. Direct coupling via separators to remove carrier gas offers several distinct advantages. It eliminates the trapping and subsequent handling steps that appear to be the cause of low recoveries [64], and there is no generation of high-ion-source pressures from vaporization of the sample. With increased pumping capacity at the source, the gas chromatographic effluent can be routed directly into the mass spectrometer, eliminating the separator and hopefully, minimizing sample loss [64].

McKinney [64] has stressed that with GC-MS, three different degrees of specificity must be obtained in order for a signal to be assigned to TCDD. These are: (1) the retention time of TCDD must

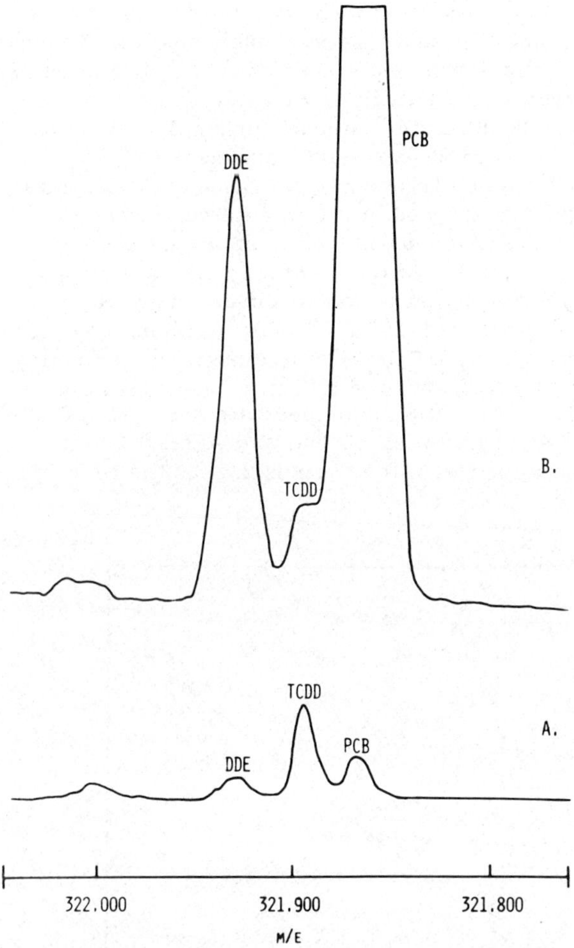

Figure 8 Mass spectra showing reduction of DDE and PCB levels in fish residue by means of alumina chromatography. Following the sulfuric acid cleanup step, the residue in hexane is added to a column of activated alumina: (A) trace from the material eluted by 20% CH_2Cl_2 in hexane after the column was first eluted with 20% CCl_4 in hexane; (B) trace obtained from a similar 20% CH_2Cl_2-in-hexane elution after the column was first eluted with 1% CH_2Cl_2 in hexane. Elution with 1% CH_2Cl_2 in hexane was reported to be effective in reducing the amount of PCB residues. Elution with 20% CCl_4 is clearly even more effective and was used routinely in obtaining the results reported here. (From Ref. 62.)

be correct, (2) response at both m/e 320 and m/e 322 must be correct, and (3) the observed isotope ratio must also be correct. Low-resolution GC-MS can be used as a screening method since once the samples are prepared, the actual running of the samples and interpretation of the data is straightforward and relatively low cost equipment is used. Then high-resolution GC-MS need only be used for confirmation, thus decreasing the load on this type of expensive equipment [64].

It is illustrative to further examine several cases of TCDD isolation and analysis. As part of a broad study to determine whether TCDD is accumulating in the environment due to approved uses of 2,4,5-T-based herbicides, samples of fish, water, mud, and human milk were collected from areas in Texas and Arkansas where these herbicides were used and were analyzed for TCDD by Shadoff et al. [67]. No TCDD was detected by a GC-MS procedure with a detection limit that averaged less than 10 parts per trillion. The instrumentation consisted of an LKB-9000 GC-MS, equipped with a 6 ft 3% OV-3 silicone column operated at a resolution of 400, and AEI-MS 30 interfaced to a Pye 104 GC equipped with the same column at the LKB-9000.

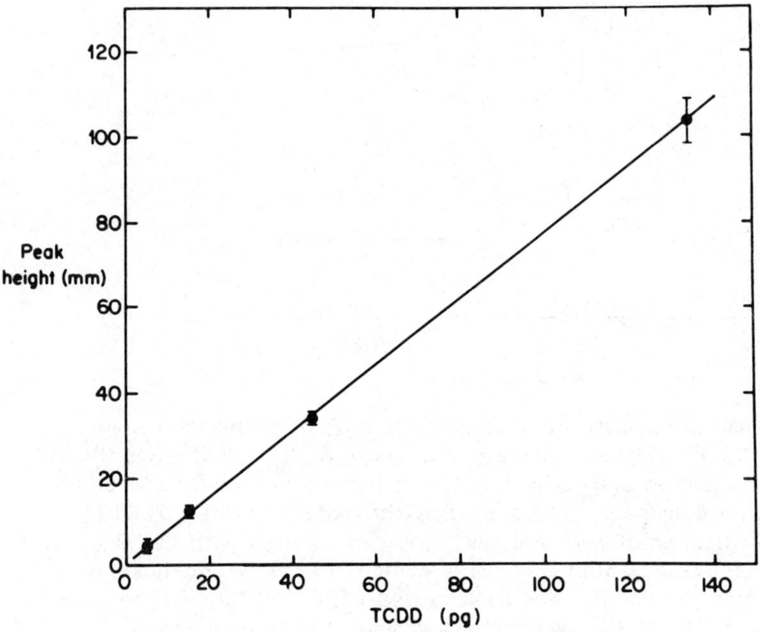

Figure 9 Linearity of response for TCDD in the presence of beef liver residue. The TCDD values are the amounts introduced into individual runs on the MS-9. (From Ref. 62.)

Table 8 Cleanup Methodology for TCDD Adopted by U.S. Environmental Protection Agency for Its Environmental Monitoring Program

1. Weigh a known quantity of homogenized sample into flask (optimal sample range 10 to 20 g).
2. Fortify sample with [^{37}Cl]TCDD (e.g., 2 ppb was added to 10 g.
3. Saponify with ethanol-40% KOH (heating under reflux for about 2 hr).
4. Extract saponified solution with four equal portions of hexane and combine hexane extracts.
5. Wash combined hexane extracts with one portion of 1 N KOH.
6. Wash hexane extracts with about four portions of concentrated H_2SO_4 until hexane layer appears colorless.
7. Wash hexane extract with one portion of aqueous Na_2CO_3.
8. Dry hexane by percolating it through a column of anhydrous Na_2CO_3.
9. Concentrate hexane and chromatograph on two separate columns (Woelm Neutral Alumina-Activity Grade 1).
10. For both columns: elute first with CCl_4 and discard; then with methylene chloride and collect the fraction (eluate contains TCDD).
11. Evaporate methylene chloride eluate. Replace with benzene and evaporate again to a final volume of about 60 μl. Seal in a glass melting-point capillary tube until analyzed.

Source: Data from Ref. 61.

The MS 30 was operated at a resolution of 3000 (medium) or a resolution of 9000 or 12,000 (high). The instrument was tuned to monitor the m/e 320 and 322 molecular ions of TCDD and the response calibrated with standard solutions of TCDD. The cleanup procedure for human milk and fish tissues for TCDD analysis is shown in Table 9.

A *neutral* procedure for the cleanup of TCDD in environmental tissues was reported by O'Keefe et al. [68] in 1976 (Table 10). This method avoids the use of acidic or basic conditions, which could, under certain conditions, conceivably lead to the formation of TCDD from precursor compounds.

McKinney [64] and others have suggested that direct saponification of tissue homogenates be avoided whenever possible. It has also been shown that ^{14}C-labeled TCDD can be extracted quantitatively from rat liver with chloroform-methanol by the procedure of Bligh and

Table 9 Cleanup Procedure for Human Milk and Fish Tissues for TCDD Analysis

1. Milk samples (20 g) or fish tissue (10 g) hydrolyzed with 10 ml of ethanol and 20 ml of 40% KOH by heating on a steam bath for 1 hr.
2. KOH solution extracted with a 4 × 10 ml portions of hexane. (Ethanol added to break emulsions if any formed.)
3. Combined hexane extracts washed with 10 ml of H_2O and then with 10 ml portions of concentrated H_2SO_4 until acid layer was nearly colorless (about 4 washes).
4. After a 10 ml H_2O wash, hexane evaporated under stream of air.
5. Residue from hexane extraction dissolved in 0.5 ml of hexane and added to a column of silica (4 × 50 mm) together with 2 × 0.5 ml hexane washes of container.
6. Effluent discarded and column eluted with 2 ml of 20% benzene in hexane (v/v). Effluent containing TCDD fraction evaporated to dryness; residue dissolved in hexane and added to alumina column (Fisher A540 activated at 140°C, 4 × 50 mm).
7. Column washed with 12 ml of 20% CCl_4 in hexane (v/v) followed by 1 ml of hexane. Washings discarded.
8. Column then eluted with 4 ml of 20% methylene chloride in hexane (v/v).
9. Effluent (containing TCDD) evaporated to 0.2 ml under air; residual solution transferred to vial using hexane solvent and evaporated; retained for analysis.

Source: Data from Ref. 67.

Dyer [69]. Hence it has been recommended that tissue extracts be used rather than tissue homogenates, since with the latter it is difficult to prevent the formation of emulsions that cause irreproducible losses [64,69,70].

Albro and Corbett [70] recently described procedures for the extraction and cleanup of animal tissues for subsequent determination of mixtures of chlorinated dibenzodioxins and dibenzofurans (Table 11). Utilizing this procedure, Albro and Corbett routinely obtained a 100 ± 2% recovery of a variety of chlorinated dibenzodioxins and dibenzofurans when total lipids were extracted. In contrast, extractions involving tissue digestion and saponification with KOH or NaOH, either at room temperature or under reflux [62], can cause extensive damage. For example, up to 60% of octachlorodibenzodioxin can be

Table 10 Neutral Procedure for the Cleanup of TCDD Residues in Environmental Tissues

1. Extraction of solids with either methylene chloride or an ether-hexane mixture, depending on the sample matrix.
2. TCDD is separated from lipid components and from chlorinated derivatives (DDE and PCBs) by liquid adsorption chromatography on columns of MgO, Celite, alumina, and Florisil.
3. Cleanup extracts are analyzed by mass spectrometry.
4. Recoveries of [^{37}Cl]TCDD (as internal standard) ranged from 71 to 87% in bovine milk samples to 77 to 108% in beef fat samples.
5. Advantage of neutral method: reduces the possibility of formation of TCDD from precursor compounds which is possible under certain acidic or basic conditions.

Source: Data from Ref. 68.

lost or destroyed at room temperature, and over 90% under reflux utilizing earlier procedures [62]. Only an 88 to 90% recovery of TCDD has been found if alkali is used, even at room temperature [62].

The sulfuric acid cleanup procedure described by Albro and Corbett [70] causes no detectable change in the *concentrations* of chlorinated dibenzodioxins or dibenzofurans in the CCl_4 layer, and only a 5% loss of nonchlorinated dibenzofuran (the worst case). It was found that sulfuric acid can easily handle up to 150 mg of triglyceride per ml of acid, but only about 50 mg of total liver lipid per ml of acid.

After correcting for recovery of the carbon tetrachloride phase in the preliminary cleanup the procedure described by Albro and Corbett [70] regularly accounts for 95% of 1 ng spikes of various di-, tetra-, hexa-, hepta-, and octachlorodibenzo-p-dioxins overall. Recoveries were also shown to be equal or greater for dibenzofurans than for dibenzo-p-dioxins in analogous cleanup procedures [70]. The final product from the procedure described by Albro and Corbett [70] has been found suitable for analysis at the parts per trillion level by GC-mass spectrometry both in electron impact (multiple-ion monitoring) and negative-ion chemical ionization modes [71].

The negative chemical ionization mass spectrometric procedure using oxygen as reagent gas appears to have considerable potential for chlorinated dioxin analysis [64,71,72]. It has recently been described by Hunt et al. [72] as a sensitive method (low-picogram range) for detecting and differentiating TCDD from PCBs, DDT, and DDE. About 80% of the ionization of TCDD under these conditions appears to result from the formation of one fragment ion at m/e 176, which may occur in

Table 11 Extraction and Cleanup Procedure for Animal Tissue for Determination of Mixtures of Chlorinated Dibenzodioxins and Dibenzofurans

1. Preliminary cleanup involves leaching of lipid residues [obtained from $CHCl_3$-CH_3OH (2:1) extractions of tissues] into CCl_4.
2. This fraction is partitioned against concentrated H_2SO_4, centrifuged at 200 rpm, the CCl_4 solution passed through a column of anhydrous Na_2CO_3, rinsed with fresh CCl_4, concentrated to dryness on a rotary evaporator at 40°C. Residue leached into n-hexane-methylene chloride (93:3, v/v).
3. Chromatographic cleanup involves adding this sample onto dry-packed column (0.5 to 0.7 cm diam) of 3 g of Fisher A-540 Alumina. Fraction I eluted with 28 ml of n-hexane-methylene chloride (93:3); fraction II eluted with 30 ml of n-hexane-methylene chloride (80:20).
4. Fraction II blown nearly dry under N_2 at room temperature for analysis.

Source: Data from Ref. 70.

a region relatively free of interfering signals. The negative chemical ionization mass spectra of 13 chlorinated dibenzodioxins have been obtained. Major peaks resulted from the exchange of oxygen for chlorine (M - 19) in isomers where chlorine is ortho to oxygen and from the formation of radical anions (m/e 142, 176, 210, 244) due to cleavage of ether linkages in the parent dioxin molecule. TCDD can be distinguished from all other tetrachlorodioxin isomers by its unique structure, which has no chlorine substituents ortho to oxygen [64].

There are additional recent separative techniques of note. Stalling [73] described laboratory investigations concerned with the isolation of TCDD residues from Agent Orange. Chromatography columns (12 × 1 cm i.d.) of Amoco Charcoal (PX-21) suspended on polyurethan foam absorbed almost 100% of the TCDD present in up to 10 ml of Agent Orange. Recovery of TCDD residue from these columns with 300 ml toluene washes averaged 99%. When necessary, additional cleanup of TCDD extracts was effected with an alumina adsorption column (Fisher A-450 activated at 130° overnight column, 1 cm i.d. × 10 cm) and elution with 20% methylene chloride in petroleum ether. It is noted, however, that GLC analysis of purified TCDD extracts from Agent Orange strongly suggested the presence of chlorinated naphthalenes as interfering contaminants. A 3% OV-1 (w/w) on Chromosorb WHP, 6 ft long column operated at 200° was satisfactory for the GLC separation of TCDD.

Stalling [74] earlier utilized columns of coconut charcoal to effect the separation of TCDD from Agent Orange, utilizing benzene as the eluting solvent.

Stalling et al. [75] also described the utility of an improved gel permeation chromatography (GPC) system which when combined with sequential adsorption or affinity chromatography could simplify residue analysis of environmental contaminants and minimize interferences. The GPC lipid cleanup system used Bio-Beads SX3 (styrene-divinyl benzene copolymers) and ethyl acetate or toluene-ethyl acetate as the solvent. Further, use of ethyl acetate in this system permitted the retention of chlorinated dibenzofurans, chlorinated dibenzo-p-dioxins, and chlorinated-naphthalenes on a Darco-charcoal column sequential to the GPC column. In general, the elution order for Darco-charcoal is analogous to reverse-phase chromatography. In addition, Darco has a high affinity for planar fused-ring aromatic compounds. This affinity is particularly advantageous in retaining the chlorinated dibenzodioxins, benzofurans, and naphthalenes. These derivatives were best recovered by benzene-reflux extraction of the small columns (2.5 cm i.d. × 30 cm; and 1.0 cm i.d. × 60 cm), allowing the hot benzene to percolate the Darco for 6 hr. Recovery of 0.06 μg TCDD and 0.5 μg/g octachlorobenzo-p-dioxins was 90% from the column and 75% for the combined gel permeation column-Darco charcoal system.

Some PCB constituents, chlorinated diphenylethers, and hexachlorobenzene were partially retained by the Darco-charcoal column. These compounds were eluted with toluene-petroleum ether (20:80).

Ramstad et al. [76] recently described the automated cleanup of herbicides by adsorption chromatography for the determination of TCDD. The automated system employs a low-cost silica column for the separation and collection of TCDD from the 1-isobutyloxy-2-propyl ester of 2,4,5-T in commercial herbicide preparations. The separation is accomplished on silica gel using a solution of 1:4 benzene-hexane. Under these conditions, the TCDD passes through the column essentially unretained, while the more polar ester is held up on the packing. To prepare the column for another sample, the adsorbed molecules must be removed from the silica surface and this is accomplished by eluting with a more polar solvent combination such as 15:85 (v/v) tetrahydrofuran (THF)-benzene. More than 400 runs have been achieved on a single 1 m × 5 mm "high-purity" silica gel column to date. The standard deviation for the same ester, analyzed 36 times, was 0.002 ppm at an average TCDD concentration of 0.026 ppm, with no measurable cross-contamination from sample to sample.

Following the Seveso accident in 1976, a large area south of the trichlorophenol-producing plant was polluted by a chemical mixture consisting primarily of trichlorophenol but also containing TCDD. In the emergency period, the analyses were carried out by a simple procedure consisting of extraction and mass fragmentography without prior cleanup. However, subsequently, more refined methods were needed to define the borders of the contaminated area, to monitor soil penetration of TCDD, and to check laboratory and field decontamination techniques further.

Soil samples were found by Camoni et al. [77] to be best extracted with methanol plus methylene chloride. The cleanup procedure consisted of a sulfuric acid treatment and chromatography on a multilayer column (Celite + H_2SO_4/silica gel) followed by alumina column chromatography. Sulfuric acid treatment and the use of a multilayer column were very effective in destroying most of the organic materials and removing more polar compounds. The clear, colorless solution thus obtained may contain common soil pollutants such as PCBs and DDE, which may interfere in the TCDD determination. Hence the utility of alumina column chromatography, which provides a useful means of separating TCDD from PCB's, DDE, and other interfering compounds which are eluted in the first fraction with light petroleum-methylene chloride (9:1). The second column fraction obtained with methylene chloride (containing the TCDD) has been found to be sufficiently clean for mass fragementographic analysis. Although the second fraction from the alumina column may contain other polychlorinated dibenzo-p-dioxins and polychlorinated dibenzofurans, no interference was found in the mass fragmentographic determination of TCDD, as was earlier shown by Buser and Bosshardt [78]. TCDD was identified by its chromatographic retention time and the simultaneous presence of the molecular ion at m/e 320 and the two isotopic ions at m/e 322 and 324 with the correct intensity ratios. Absolute amounts are calculated by comparing the intensity of the m/e 322 peak present in the sample with that obtained on injecting a comparable and known amount of TCDD standard.

As noted earlier (Table 2), several positional isomers exist for most individual polychlorinated dioxins and dibenzofurans. Often, isomers of both series have similar retention times and are difficult to separate. Although high-resolution gas chromatography using capillary columns would seem to be useful for such separations, suprisingly, very little has thus far been reported on its application for the analysis of PCDDs and PCDFs. This was suggested by Buser [79] to be due in part to the very low volatility of these compounds (eluting in the range up to n-C_{30} to n-C_{37}-alkanes) and hence requiring a high quality of the capillary columns used.

Buser [79] recently reported that high-resolution gas chromatography is applicable to the analysis of PCDDs and PCDFs. The high separation efficiencies of glass capillary columns could be maintained for the trace analysis of these very high boiling chlorinated derivatives using an isothermal splitless injection technique and an electron capture detector of low internal volume. Thin-film narrow-bone glass capillary columns (22 m × 0.3 mm i.d.) containing OV-101, OV-17,

Table 12A Observed Retention-Time Ranges of PCDDs and PCDFs on Glass Capillary Columns

Compound	Retention-time ranges relative to octa-CDD on:		
	OV-101[a]	OV-17[a]	SILAR 10C[a]
Tetra-CDDs	0.13-0.18	0.10-0.15	0.12-0.22
Penta-CDDs	0.20-0.27	0.16-0.24	0.18-0.30
Hexa-CDDs	0.32-0.41	0.28-0.38	0.31-0.43
Hepta-CDDs	0.56-0.63	0.52-0.63	0.54-0.62
Octa-CDD	1.000	1.000	1.000
Tetra-CDFs	(0.10-0.14)	(0.09-0.12)	0.11-0.19
Penta-CDFs	0.17-0.24	0.14-0.23	0.15-0.25
Hexa-CDFs	0.29-0.42	0.25-0.40	0.24-0.50
Hepta-CDFs	0.51-0.65	0.47-0.66	0.44-0.66
Octa-CDF	0.978	1.025	0.933

Source: Reprinted with permission from Ref. 79, H. R. Buser, High-resolution gas chromatography of polychlorinated dibenzo-p-dioxins and dibenzofurans, Anal. Chem. *48*, 1553-1557; © 1976 American Chemical Society.

Table 12B Dimensions, Operating Conditions, and Properties of Glass Capillary Columns[a]

	Column I, OV-101	Column II, OV-17	Column III, Silar 10C
Length (m)	22	22	22
i.d. (mm)	0.32	0.34	0.34
T (°C)	225	225	225
t_r (min)	33.4	31.8	26.9
I	3055	3420	3645
n	42500	43400	34000
HETP (mm)	0.52	0.51	0.65

[a] t_r, retention time; I, retention index; n, theoretical plate number; HETP, height equivalent to a theoretical plate of octa-CDD at operating temperature T.

Source: Reprinted with permission from Ref. 79, H. R. Buser, High-resolution gas chromatography of polychlorinated dibenzo-p-dioxins and dibenzofurans, Anal. Chem. *48*, 1553-1557; c 1976 American Chemical Society.

and Silar 10C allowed lower operating temperatures (205 to 225°) and sbowed greatly increased separation efficiencies compared to conventional packed columns. Table 12A and 12B lists the retention-time ranges for the individual compounds of both PCDDs and PCDFs (values reported relative to octa-CDD) and the dimensions, operating conditions, and properties of three glass capillary columns, respectively. As with the polychlorinated biphenyls, on OV-101 and OV-17 the retention times increase with increasing chlorine content, whereas on Silar 10C, some overlapping of retention ranges occur. Figure 10 illustrates chromatograms of sodium pentachlorophenate samples I and II on OV-101 glass capillary column at 225°, employing isothermal splitless injection and electron capture detection (tritiated scandium foil). The actual concentrations of individual PCDDs and PCDFs for both samples are listed in Table 13, as previously obtained using mass fragmentography and a packed column [79].

Although the *quantitative* aspects have not yet been fully investigated, it was suggested by Buser [79] that high-resolution GLC with capillary columns as described may offer an attractive alternative to conventional GLC with highly specific detection techniques (such as

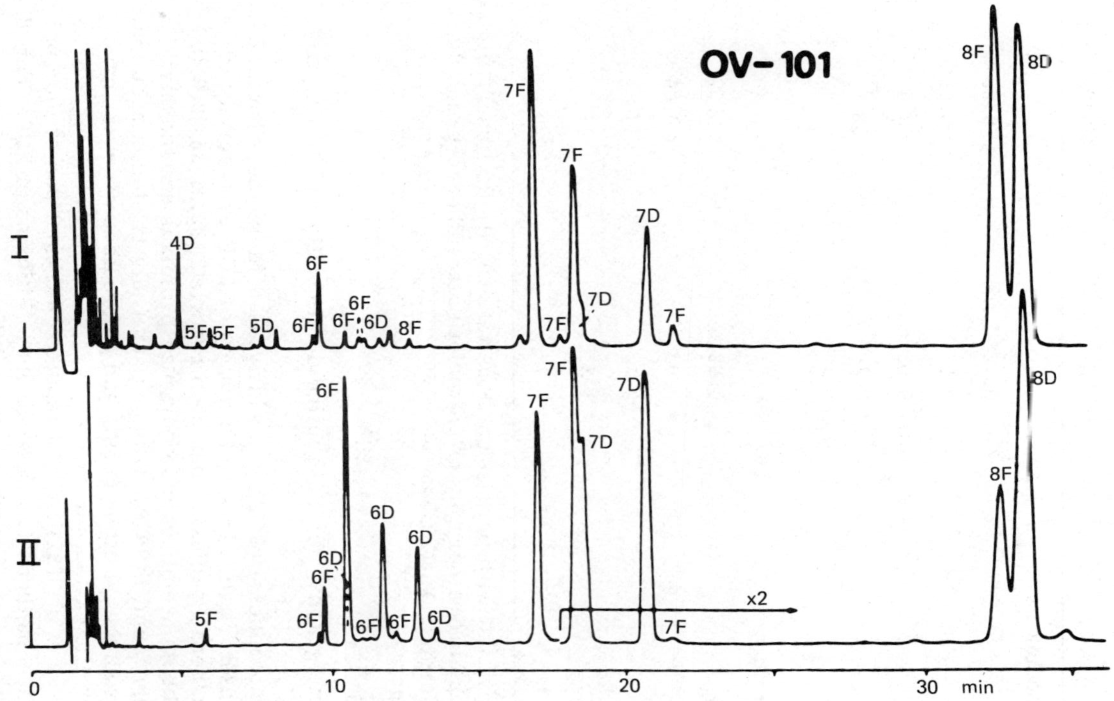

Figure 10 Chromatograms of PCP-Na samples I and II on OV-101 glass capillary column at 225°; ECD, isothermal splitless injection; other experimental conditions given in text. (From Ref. 79, reprinted with permission from H. R. Buser, High-resolution gas chromatography of polychlorinated dibenzo-p-dioxins and dibenzofurans, Anal. Chem. *48*, 1553-1557; © 1976 American Chemical Society.)

Table 13 Content of PCDDs and PCDFs in Two Commercial PCP-Na Samples as Determined by Mass Fragmentography

Compound	Content (ppm)	
	Sample I	Sample II
Chlorodibenzodioxins		
Tetra-	0.12	0.05
Penta-	0.03	< 0.03
Hexa-	< 0.03	3.4
Hepta-	0.3	38
Octa-	1.5	110
Chlorodibenzofurans		
Tetra-	< 0.02	< 0.02
Penta-	< 0.03	< 0.04
Hexa-	0.7	11
Hepta-	1.3	47
Octa-	2.1	26

Source: Reprinted with permission from Ref. 79, H. R. Buser, High-resolution gas chromatography of polychlorinated dibenzo-p-dioxins and dibenzofurans, Anal. Chem. *48*, 1553-1557; © 1976 American Chemical Society.

mass fragmentography) for the routine determination of PCDDs and PCDFs.

Pentachlorophenol (PCP) is a widely used fungicide, slimicide, and wood preservative. The contamination of PCP by a variety of chlorinated dibenzo-p-dioxins has been reported [32,33,35,80,81]. The hexa-, hepta-, and octachlorodibenzo-p-dioxins are the ones most commonly found in PCP. Other structurally related compounds, such as chlorodiphenyl ether (CDE) and chlorodibenzofurans, have been found in the extracts of PCP.

Villanueva et al. [82] in 1975 reported a comparison of four published analytical methods for chlorodibenzo-p-dioxins in PCP. For all methods, only one lot of technical grade PCP was analyzed, in order to keep the chlorinated dibenzo-p-dioxin level constant. Hence variation in results could be attributed to the analytical method employed. The methods used were: (1) Firestone [83] and Firestone et al. [33], (2) Jensen and Renberg [80], (3) Crummett [84] and Crummett and Stehl [85], and (4) Rappe and Nilsson [86]. The Firestone method involves the extraction of the nonacidic material in the PCP sample with petroleum ether, concentration of this extract, and then addition of the extract to an alumina column. The eluate from the column was shaken with concentrated sulfuric acid, passed through a column of sodium sulfate and sodium carbonate, and concentrated for analysis by electron capture-GLC. The Jensen method involved the extraction of the nonacidic material in the PCP sample with ether-hexane (1:1) concentration of the extract, treatment with diazomethane, and concentration for electron capture-GLC. With the Crummett method, the acidic components were removed by means of an ion exchange column, using ethanol-chloroform (1:3) as a solvent and eluent. The eluate was concentrated and analyzed by EC-GLC. In the Rappe method, PCP was treated with diazomethane and then analyzed by EC-GLC. In all the methods the chlorodibenzo-p-dioxins were estimated by EC-GLC using the peak height technique and available chlorinated dibenzo-p-dioxin standards. GLC-mass spectrometry was employed to confirm the presence of the chlorinated dibenzo-p-dioxins and to identify other contaminants in the PCP. A Varian 2100 gas chromatograph with a tritium detector was equipped with a 6 ft × 0.25 in. o.d. U-shaped glass column parched with 3% OV-1 on 80-100 mesh Supelcoport. The column temperature was 220°; detector, 200°, and injector, 235°. The nitrogen flow as 65 ml/min at 52 psi. Mass spectral analysis was accomplished on an LKB 9000 equipped with a mass marker (±0.3 mass unit) and interfaced to a 10 ft × 0.25 in. o.d. coiled Pyrex glass column parched with 3% SE-30 on 60 to Chromosorb GLDMCS treated and acid washed; the column temperature was 230°, and helium flow rate was 70 mg/min at 12 psi.

The levels of chlorinated dibenzodioxins in PCP obtained by the four methods of analysis, as determined by EC-GLC, are listed in Table 14 and illustrate the wide variations as a function of the analytical method. The gas chromatograms resulting from each of method are shown in Figure 11A-D. No correction was made for recovery. The Jensen and Crummett methods agree fairly well, while the Firestone method gave somewhat lower results, and the Rappe method, which has no cleanup step, gave extremely high results. The percent recovery of octachlorodibenzo-p-dioxin is shown in Table 15. The Crummett and Jensen methods gave the best recovery values. The sample of technical grade PCP was also found by electron capture GLC and GLC-MS to contain hydroxychlorodiphenyl ethers.

Table 14 Electron Capture-GLC Results of Pentachlorophenol Analysis

Method	Chlorinated dibenzo-p-dioxin (CDD) levels (ppm)		
	Hexa-CDD	Hepta-CDD[a]	Octa-CDD
Firestone	109	439	204
Jensen	551	903	1517
Crummett	429	962	1255
Rappe	-	3798	8042

[a]Based on OCTA-CDD standard.

Source: Reprinted with permission from Ref. 82, E. C. Villanueva, R. W. Jennings, V. W. Burse, and R. D. Kimbrough, A comparison of analytical methods for chlorodibenzo-p-dioxins in pentachlorophenol, J. Agric. Food Chem. *23*, 1089-1091; © 1975 American Chemical Society.

Table 15 Percent Recovery of OCTA-CDD

Method	Level of OCTA-CDD (ppm)		
	100	1000	10,000
Firestone	57	47	-
Jensen	96	65	-
Crummett	99	93	-
Rappe	77	80	105

Source: Reprinted with permission from Ref. 82, E. C. Villanueva, R. W. Jennings, V. W. Burse, and R. D. Kimbrough, A comparison of analytical methods for chlorodibenzo-p-dioxins in pentachlorophenol, J. Agric. Food Chem. *23*, 1089-1091; © 1975 American Chemical Society.

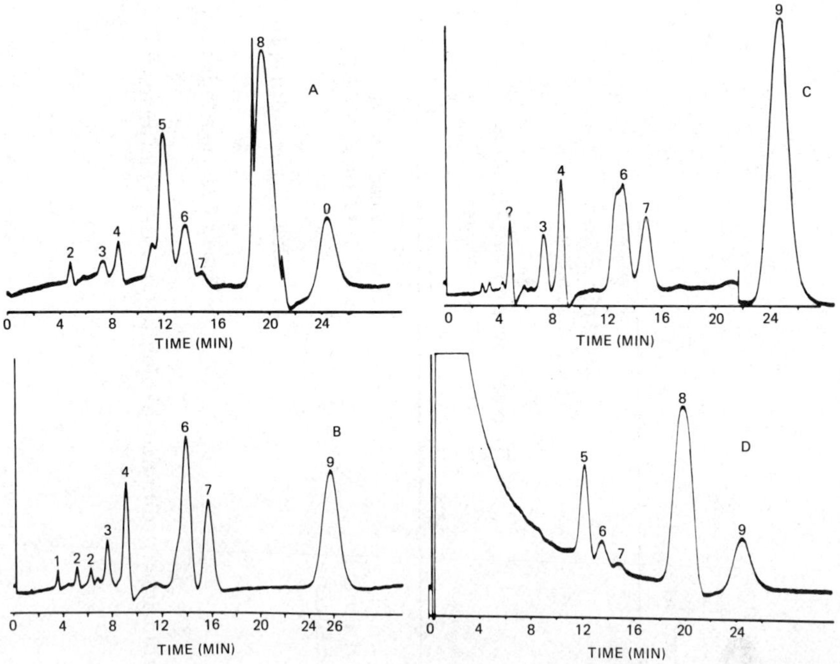

Figure 11 Gas chromatograms resulting from PCP analysis after treatment (A) by Jensen method, (B) by Firestone method, (C) by Crummett method, and (D) by Rappe method: 1, hexa-CDE; 2, hepta-CDE; 3, hexa-CDF and octa-CDE; 4, hexa-CDD and octa CDE; 5, methylated pre-hepta-CDD; 6, hepta-CDD and hepta-CDF; 7, hepta-CDD; 8, methylated pre-octa-CDD; 9, octa-CDD and octa-CDF. (From Ref. 82, reprinted with permission from E. C. Villanueva, R. W. Jennings, V. W. Burse, and R. D. Kimbrough, A comparison of analytical methods for chlorodibenzo-p-dioxins in pentachlorophenol. J. Agric. Food Chem. *23*, 1089-1091; © 1975 American Chemical Society.)

An additional scheme of analysis for the determination of chlorinated dioxins and dibenzofurans and their separation from PCBs, polychlorobenzenes, and polychlorodiphenylethers in commercial PCP is illustrated in Figure 12.

Levin and Nilsson [87] reported the results of numerous analyses of wood dust from several sawmills in Sweden and showed that 2,3,4,6-tetrachlorophenol, pentachlorophenol, chlorophenoxy phenols (Cl_5, Cl_6, Cl_7, Cl_8), chlorodibenzofurans (Cl_6, Cl_7), and chlorodibenzo-

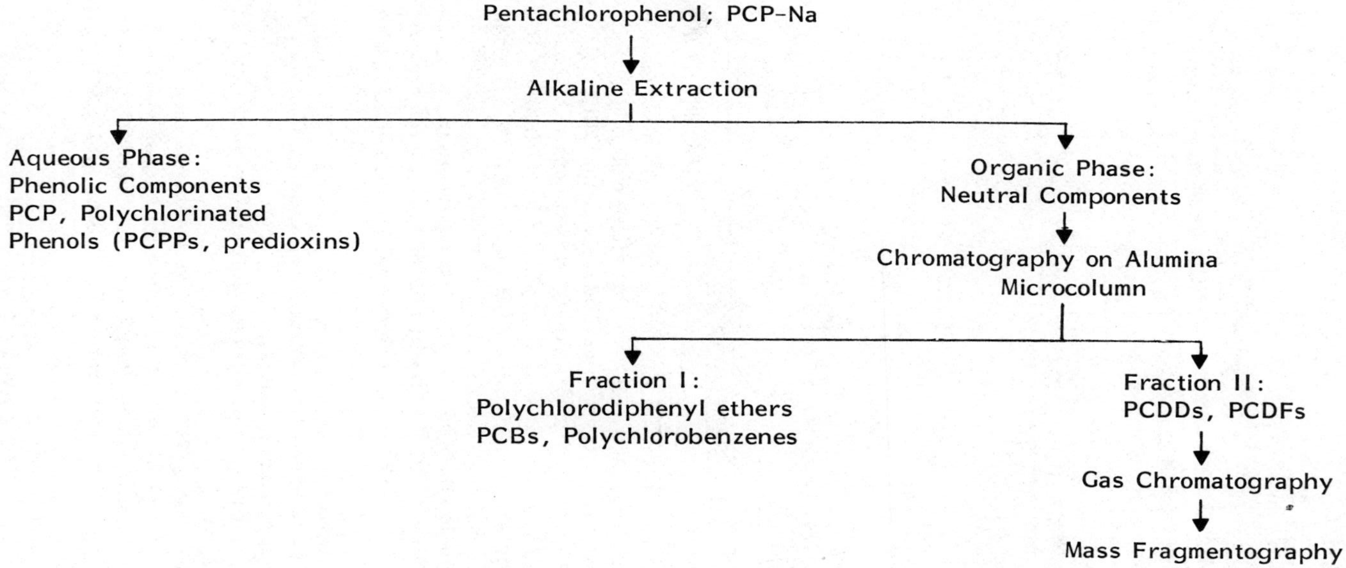

Figure 12 Scheme of analysis for determination of polychlorinated dibenzo-p-dioxins and dibenzofurans in commercial pentachlorophenols. (From Ref. 78.)

Table 16 Extraction-Adsorption Chromatography Procedure for Trace Contaminants in Pentachlorophenol

1. Dissolve sample in aqueous caustic. Extract with hexane.
2. Hexane extract passed through a disposable bed of silica gel which retains any chlorophenols, chlorophenoxy phenols, or other polar impurities extracted from the aqueous solution.
3. Hexane solution then passed through a disposable bed of basic alumina which retains chlorodioxins, chlorodibenzofurans, and chlorodiphenyl ethers while any chlorobenzenes or chlorobiphenyls present are eluted with benzene.
4. A 10 ml portion of 25% CCl_4 in hexane is then passed through the column to elute the chlorodiphenyl ethers selectively.
5. The chlorodibenzodioxin fraction is eluted by passing 5 ml of 50% methylene chloride in hexane through the column.
6. Effluent evaporated to dryness under nitrogen at room temperature. Residue is redissolved in $CHCl_3$ and analyzed by liquid chromatography.

Source: Reprinted with permission from Ref. 88, C. D. Pfeiffer, T. J. Nestrick, and C. W. Kocher, Determination of chlorinated dibenzo-p-dioxins in purified pentachlorophenol by liquid-chromatography, Anal. Chem. *50*, 800-804; © 1978 American Chemical Society.

dioxins tend to accumulate in the work environment. Analyses carried out on wood dust from sawmills using wood previously treated with pentachlorophenol show as much as 100 ppm octachlorodibenzodioxin in the wood dust.

Liquid chromatography is a potentially attractive alternative to GLC and GLC-mass spectrometry for analyzing samples on a routine basis because of the relatively low cost of the equipment and the rapid separations possible. Pfeiffer et al. [88] reported a rapid liquid chromatographic method for the determination of hexa-, hepta-, and octachlorodibenzo-p-dioxins in purified pentachlorophenol (PCP). Impurities that are present in commercial PCP, including chlorodiphenyl ethers, chlorinated dibenzodioxins, chlorophenoxyphenols, chlorodibenzofurans, polychlorinated benzene, and polychlorinated biphenyls, are quantitatively isolated from the matrix by an extraction column chromatography procedure as illustrated in Table 16. Figure 13 illustrates an example of the liquid chromatographic separation for a typical sample of purified pentachlorphenol. This chlorinated dibenzodioxin fraction concentrate was obtained from 2.5 g of pentachlorophenol with the residue dissolved in 1.0 ml of $CHCl_3$. The

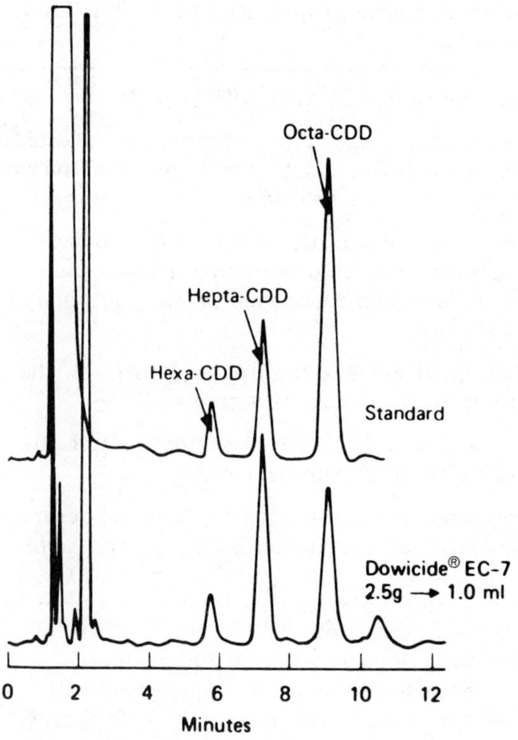

Figure 13 Determination of chlorinated dibenzo-p-dioxins in pentachlorophenol. Column, ODS Zorbax; conditions in the text. Standard concentrations: hexa-CDD 2.0 μg/ml; hepta-CDD 8.5 μg/ml; octa-CDD 25 μg/ml. (From Ref. 88, reprinted with permission from C. D. Pfeiffer, T. J. Nestrick, and C. W. Kocher, Determination of chlorinated, dibenzo-p-dioxins in purified pentachlorophenol by liquid-chromatography, Anal. Chem. *50*, 800-804; © 1978 American Cancer Society.)

sample contained 0.6 ppm hexa-, 5.2 ppm hepta-, and 5.2 ppm octachlorodibenzodioxins. Detection limits of 50 ppb for hexa-, and 100 ppb for hepta- and octachlorodibenzodioxins may be achieved by reducing the volume of $CHCl_3$ used to dissolve the chlorodibenzodioxins fraction to 250 μl. Further evidence of method validity was obtained by analyzing 10 samples by both LC and the GC-MS method of Blaser [88]. The results are summarized in Table 11. Generally, the two techniques compare favorably. The major advantages of the LC technique of Pfeiffer et al. [88] are that sample concentrates are analyzed in a 12 min separation with detection limits of 100 ppb and the entire analysis can be completed in 1 hr.

Table 17 Chlorinated Dibenzofuran Concentrations[a] in Polychlorinated Biphenyls

PCB	4-Cl	5-Cl	6-Cl	Total
Aroclor 1248 (1969)	0.5 (25)	1.2 (60)	0.3 (15)	2.0
Aroclor 1254 (1969)	0.1 (6)	0.2 (12)	1.4 (82)	1.7
Aroclor 1254 (1970)	0.2 (13)	0.4 (27)	0.9 (60)	1.5
Aroclor 1260 (1969)	0.1 (10)	0.4 (40)	0.5 (50)	1.0
Aroclor 1260 (lot AK3)	0.2 (25)	0.3 (38)	0.3 (38)	0.8
Aroclor 1016 (1972)	nd[b]	nd[b]	nd[b]	-
Clophen A-60	1.4 (17)	5.0 (59)	2.2 (26)	8.4
Phenoclor DP-6	0.7 (5)	10.0 (74)	2.9 (21)	13.6

[a]Expressed as μg/g PCB. Values in parentheses represent quantity as percentage of total dibenzofuran.
[b]nd, not detected (<0.001 μg/g).
Source: Ref. 103, reprinted from Nature (Lond.) *256*, 305-307; © 1975 Macmillan Journals Ltd.

Dolphin and Wilmott [89] have shown that chlorinated dibenzodioxins could be separated from PCBs and chlorinated naphthalenes, DDE, and DDT by HPLC on microparticulate alumina. This separation could form the basis of a rapid screening method for the determination of TCDD in environmental samples. Important advantages of HPLC are the reduced sample preparation compared to GLC and the elimination of sample volume reduction, with its inherent risk of volatile compounds. The separations were curved out on a Pye Unicam LC3 liquid chromatograph equipped with a variable-wavelength UV detector. For high-sensitivity work the instrument was coupled with an electron capture detector. Chlorinated dibenzofurans could interfere with the lower-substituted dioxins. Where the lower-substituted chlorinated dioxins and chlorodibenzofurans are to be quantified, HPLC must be followed by mass spectrometric analysis.

Dolphin and Willmott [89] suggested that HPLC can be used in the quantitative analysis of chlorodioxins in a number of ways. For example, at the higher concentrations found in a simple matrix such as commercial chlorophenols, analysis could be performed on a single column with either an ultraviolet (UV) or a LC/EC detector, depending on the sensitivity required. For more complex matrices (e.g., surface water, soil, and foodstuffs), a series combination of alumina and silica columns can be used to give improved selectivity and lower detection limits.

A number of chlorinated dibenzodioxins have been found in food grade oleic acids and emulsifiers prepared from the oleic acids and fleshing greases isolated from hides treated with pentachlorophenol. Contamination of cattle hides with PCP and dioxins is likely since PCP is used as a preservative during hide processing both in the United States and abroad [90,91].

Firestone [83] recently reported that 14 of 15 U.S. commercial gelatins examined contained hexa-, hepta-, and octachlorodioxins at levels from 0.1 to 28 ppb of total dioxins. Levels of individual dioxins as low as 0.01 ppb were detected. Three bulk gelatins of Mexican manufacture contained from 24 to 28 ppb of total dioxin. In addition, levels of up to 0.4 ppb of heptachlorofuran and 0.4 ppt octachlorofuran were found in 10 of the gelatins. No TCDD was found in any of the samples at a limit of detection of 0.2 to 0.4 ppb. It should be noted that two types of gelatin are produced domestically: type A by acid hydrolysis of pork skins and type B by alkaline hydrolysis of cattle bones and hides [92]. Both types are used in the food and pharmaceutical industries in the United States. Current annual consumption of gelatin in the United States is estimated at 57 million pounds of domestic production and 13 million pounds of imports.

The presence of chlorinated dibenzo-p-dioxins and furans (and PCP) in the consumer (market) samples is suspected to be due to blending of PCP-contaminated imported gelatin with domestic gelatin

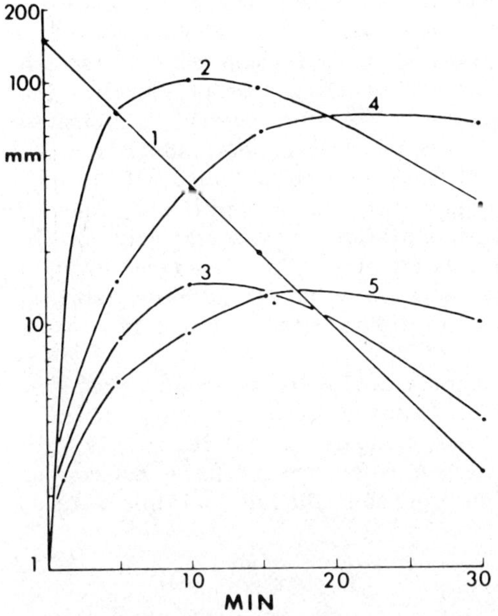

Figure 14 Photodechlorination of octachlorodibenzo-p-dioxin (OCDD); 200 ng/500 liters of hexane solution. GLC peak height (mm) versus irradiation time (min) at 253.7 nm. (1) OCDD; (2) 1,2,3,4,6,- 7,9-HpCDD; (3) 1,2,3,4,6,7,8-HpCDD; (4) 1,2,4,6,7,9-HCDD; and (5) 1,2,3,6,7,9-HCDD. EC-GLC column temperature, 210°. (From Ref. 83, reprinted with permission from D. Firestone, Determination of polychlorinated dibenzo-p-dioxins and polychlorodibenzofurans in commercial gelatins by gas-liquid chromatography, J. Agric. Food Chem. *25*, 1274-1280; © 1977 American Cancer Society.)

by the manufacturer [83]. The presence of hexa-, hepta-, and octachlorodioxins and penta-, hexa-, and heptachlorofuran in one of the Mexican samples was confirmed with GLC-mass spectrometry.

Photodechlorination was shown by Firestone [83] to be useful for confirmation of octachlorodioxins in the samples. Earlier work by Kim et al. [93] demonstrated that dioxins undergo photochemical dechlorination in methanol or hydrocarbon solvents under UV irradiation. First-order kinetic data are obtained. The mechanism of photo dechlorination involves breakage of the carbon-chlorine bond and hydrogen atom addition. The initial products formed are isomers (n - 1) of chlorodioxins, where n is the number of chlorine atoms on the dioxin ring prior to UV irradiation. The number and position of the chlorine atoms on the dioxins ring affect dechlorination in a predictable manner, so that the decomposition rate and composition of the dechlorination products can be used to identify the starting dioxins (Fig. 14).

Considerable efforts have been made to develop methods for controlling the purity of the chlorinated phenols per se as well as their agricultural and industrial products. The determination of chlorinated dibenzo-p-dioxins and dibenzofurans in the products listed above requires the use of standards and reference compounds. Of the large number of possible isomers of these trace contaminants, very few are commercially available and their preparation or synthesis may both be difficult or time consuming. Another factor to be considered is the high toxicity of some of these compounds, which thus necessitates extensive precautions to prevent ill effects if their synthesis is to be attempted [94].

The use of pure samples of individual chlorinated dibenzo-p-dioxins and dibenzofurans may be required for direct calibration of detector responses in a quantitative analysis. In addition, it is often desirable to have available *qualitative* reference mixtures that contain a variety of different chlorinated dibenzo-p-dioxins and dibenzofuran

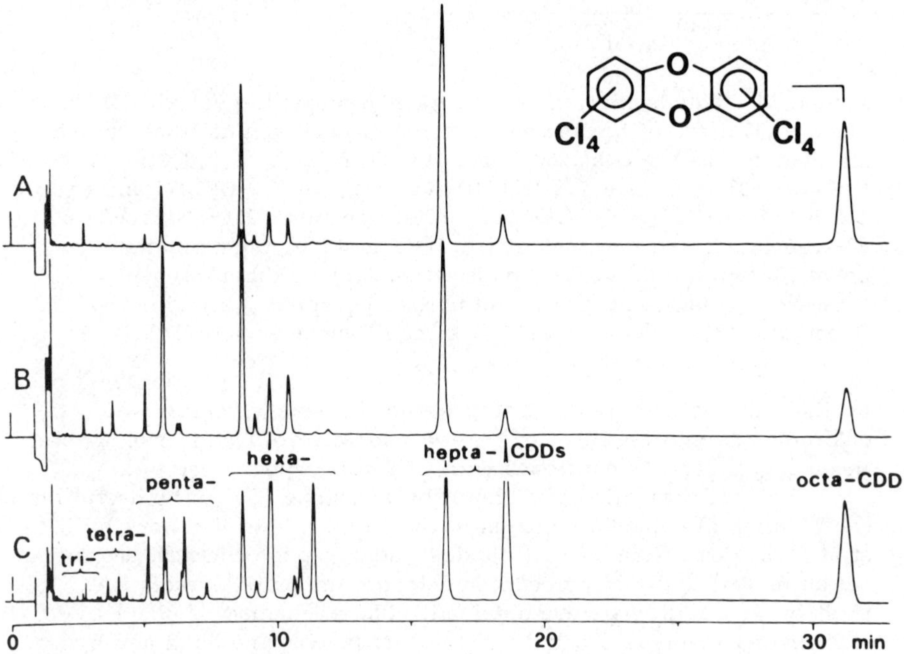

Figure 15 Chromatograms of UV- and gamma-irradiated octa-CDD. Conditions: OV-17 glass capillary column at 225° with ECD and isothermal splitless injection. (A) 4 hr UV, (B) 24 hr UV, and (C) 4 hr gamma-irradiation. Peak identifications as indicated. (From Ref. 94.)

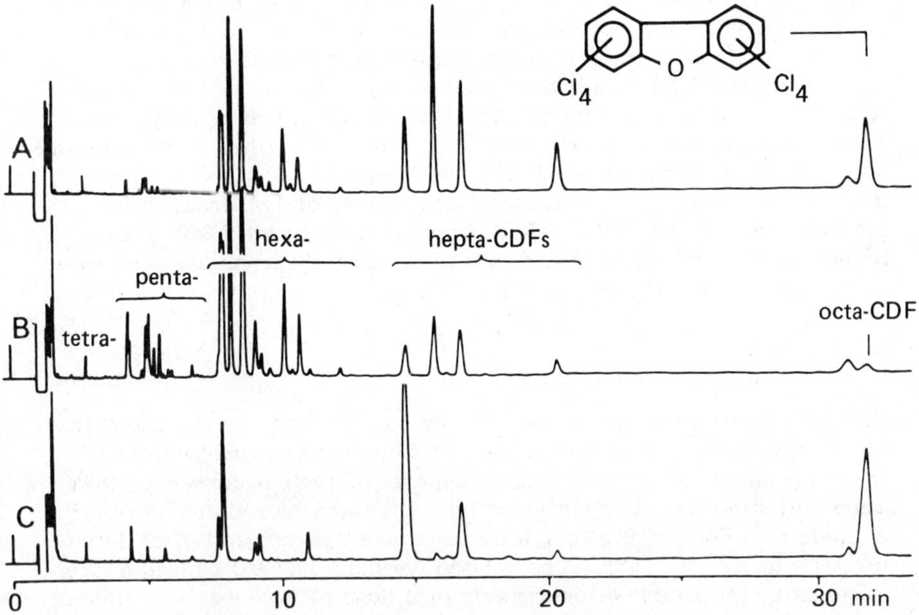

Figure 16 Chromatograms of UV- and gamma-irradiated octa-CDF. Conditions: OV-17 glass capillary column at 225° with ECD and isothermal splitless injection. (A) 4 hr UV, (B) 24 hr UV, and (C) 4 hr gamma-irradiation. Peak identifications as indicated. (From Ref. 94.)

components. Although the exact concentration of the individual components may not be known, these qualitative standard mixtures can be used to determine gas chromatographic, mass spectrometric, and other data on individual compounds for which pure samples are not available.

Buser [94] recently described the utility of reductive dechlorination by ultraviolet and gamma irradiation of the nontoxic, commercially available octachlorodibenzo-p-dioxin and dibenzofuran. This apparently easy and safe technique, requiring a minimum of sample handling, permitted the preparation of qualitative standard mixtures of some PCDDs and PCDFs. For example, the resulting mixtures of the penta-, hexa-, and heptachloro compounds were subsequently used for the development of methods for the determination of these compounds in commercial pentachlorophenol and other chlorinated phenols. Under the conditions investigated, dechlorination of octachlorodibenzo-p-dioxin and octachlorodibenzofuran to lower chlorinated dibenzo-p-dioxins and dibenzofurans appears to be a major reaction pathway. Reductive dechlorination has been previously shown to be the major reaction pathway in the photolysis of a number of PCDDs and PCDFs in organic solvents [95-98]. Nucleophilic displacement reactions may occur in polar (aqueous) solutions.

The ultraviolet irradiations were carried out on 4 ml of sample solution placed in 1 cm quartz cuvettes, placed approximately 8 cm from a mercury UV lamp and irradiated from 1 to 24 hr. Gamma irradiation was carried out on 10 ml of solution in PTFE-capped borosilicate glass vials, using a ^{60}Co source at dose levels of 1.4 Mrad/hr for periods ranging from 1 to 16 hr. Chromatograms of UV and gamma-irradiated octachlorodioxin and octachlorodibenzofurans are illustrated in Figures 15 and 16, respectively [94].

IV. CHLORODIBENZOFURANS

While the focus thus far in the chapter has been on the chlorodioxins (primarily TCDD), it is also important to stress the toxic nature of the chlorodibenzofurans as well as aspects of their occurrence, formation and analysis. For example, tri- and tetrachlorodibenzofuran in a single oral dose of 0.5 to 1.0 μg/kg caused severe and often lethal necrosis in rabbits [55]. The related compound TCDD caused a liver necrosis in the rabbit after a single oral dose of 0.05 mg/kg. Chicks fed 5 μg/kg per day of 2,3,7,8-tetrachlorodibenzofuran died within 8 to 15 days [99]. The toxicity to chicks is thus similar to that for 2,3,7,8-tetrachlorodibenzo-p-dioxin (TCDD) as reported by Schwetz et al. [100]. While the tetragenic potential of TCDD is well established, that of chlorinated dibenzofurans have not, thus far.

Vos et al. [101] calculated a maximum dose per egg of 0.2 μg of pentachlorodibenzofuran (obtained from the PCB-Clophen-A60) that caused 100% embryonic mortality when injected into the air cell of chicken eggs. The analogous effect was obtained with 0.05 μg of hexachlorodibenzo-p-dioxin.

In 1970, Vos et al. [101] identified polychlorinated dibenzofurans at the ppm level in several PCBs of German and French origin (e.g., Clophen A-60 and Phenoclor DP-6, respectively). The toxic effects of the PCBs were subsequently found to parallel the levels of chlorinated dibenzofurans. In 1975, several additional chlorinated dibenzofurans were found by Bowes et al. [102] in the PCB (Clophen A-60) originally examined by Vos et al. [101]. Further investigations by Bowes et al. [103] led to the detection by high-resolution mass spectrometry of the same type of chlorinated dibenzofurans (e.g., tetra-, penta-, and hexa-) in American samples of PCBs (e.g., Aroclors) (Table 17). Values reported in Table 17 represent a total of those compounds found in 400 ml Florisil column fractions from the original column chromatography of 1.0 to 2.0 g of PCBs in 400 ml hexane. A total of 10 to 12 isomers were identified in each PCB by GLC and mass spectrometry [103]. The most abundant chlorinated dibenzofurans had the same retention time as 2,3,7,8-tetra- and 2,3,4,7,8-pentachlorodibenzofurans.

Studies in 1974 by Roach and Pomerantz [104] indicated the presence of unidentified tri-, tetra-, and possibly pentachlorodibenzofurans in components of the Japanese PCB, Kanechlor 400. It should be noted that Kuratsune et al. [105] in 1972 identified Kanechlor 400 as the agent responsible for Yusho, a toxic syndrome in humans who had ingested contaminated rice oil.

Bowes et al. [106] in 1975 reported the presence of 2,3,7,8-tetra- and 2,3,4,7,8-pentachlorodibenzofurans at levels ranging from 0.08 to 0.83 μg/g of PCB in two additional Kanechlor samples (e.g., 200 and 500) as well as in Arochlors 1248 and 1254 (Table 18).

Although there is no evidence to date that chlorinated dibenzofurans are present in wildlife samples, these data allow one to estimate their potential concentrations. If the dibenzofurans were present in tissue in the same amounts relative to the PCB, the range of concentrations of the dibenzofurans isomers identified in the study of Bowes et al. [106] (Table 18) would be approximately 25 to 250 pg/gram of fresh weight in Great Lakes herring gull (*Larus Argentatus*) livers found to contain 300 ppm of PCB [103].

As large quantities of PCBs have entered the global environment [107-110] it can be assumed that the contaminant dibenzofurans also have been released in proportional amounts. Their persistence, effects, and significance remain to be determined.

Buser et al. [111,112] reported that under pyrolytic conditions (500 to 700°) commercial PCBs (e.g., Aroclors 1254 and 1260) yield PCDFs at the percent level. Up to 60 PCDFs were detected using high-resolution GLC and mass spectrometry. Among the major components found were the highly toxic 2,3,7,8-tetra- and 2,3,4,7,8-pentachlorodibenzofurans [111,112].

Buser et al. [111,112] recently reported that fly ash from an industrial heating facility and a municipal incinerator contained a pattern of PCDF isomers very similar to those found in the pyrolysis of commercial PCBs suggesting that PCBs were the precursors of the PCDFs found in fly ash.

We touched earlier on a specific PCB mixture, Kanechlor 400, as the agent responsible for Yusho, a toxic syndrome which in 1968 had effected more than 1200 persons in southwest Japan. They were intoxicated by consuming a commercial rice oil contaminated with 1000 ppm of the PCB Kanechlor KC400. This rice oil, known as Yusho oil, was found to contain 5 ppm of chlorinated dibenzofurans [113]. This level of chlorodibenzofuran in the PCB, which had contaminated the rice oil, was more than 250 times higher than in the ordinary Kanechlor KC400 samples.

Clinical aspects associated with Yusho include chloracne, blindness, and systemic gastrointestinal symptoms, with jaundice, edema,

Table 18 Concentration of Chlorinated Dibenzofuran Isomers in PCB (μg/g of PCB)

Structure of compound	PCB			
	Aroclor 1248	Aroclor 1254	Kanechlor 200	Kanechlor 500
2,3,7,8-Tetrachloro-	0.33	0.11	0.10	0.19
2,3,4,7,8-Pentachloro-	0.83	0.12	0.10	0.08

Source: Ref. 106.

and abdominal pain. Chloracne is very persistent, with some patients showing evidence of it after 3 years. The severity of the disease varied with age, being greatest from adolescence through 40 years of age. The disorder *generally* cleared when exposure to the offending agent was discontinued [114]. Newborn infants of poisoned mothers had skin coloration due to the presence of PCB via placental passage. Residues of PCB have been found in fetal tissue [115].

Exposure levels to the oil were calculated at approximately 15,000 mg/day. The lowest reported figures allow an estimate of a minimal positive effect level at 3 mg of PCB/day over several months. However, the average doses associated with significant disease in the Yusho incident were much higher and were in the range 30 mg/day. The latency period between the ingestion of the oil and the onset of clinical signs and symptoms was estimated at 5 to 6 months [116].

Rappe et al. [117], using GLC and high-resolution mass spectrometry, identified the 2,3,7,8-tetrachloroisomer as the major chlorinated dibenzofuran component in the Yusho oil.

A more definitive analysis of chlorinated dibenzofurans in Yusho oil as well as used Japanese samples [118] was reported by Buser et al. [119], who employed a simplified cleanup procedure and high-resolution GLC and mass spectrometry.

Table 19 illustrates the cleanup procedure employed for the analysis of Yusho oil [119]. A modified cleanup procedure was employed for the used PCB (Mitsubishi-Monsanto T 1248 sample). This PCB sample had been used in a heat exchanger for 2 years. In the cleanup procedure the silica column was replaced by an additional

Table 19 Cleanup Procedure for Yusho Oil Analysis

1. Yusho oil (100 mg) added to a silica (0.5 g) microcolumn (150 × 5 mm) using a disposable Pasteur pipet.
2. Chlorinated compounds (PCBs and PCDFs) eluted in 6 ml of n-hexane with almost complete retention of rice oil on the column.
3. After concentration, eluate is rechromatographed on basic alumina microcolumn (10 g of Woelin) in Pasteur pipet by elution with 10 ml each of 2% and 50% methylene chloride in n-hexane. Most of the PCBs eluted in first fraction. PCDFs and other chlorinated tricyclic aromatic compounds eluted in second fraction.
4. Last fraction concentrated to 50 μl and a 2 μl aliquot used for analysis by GLC and mass spectrometry.

Source: Ref. 119.

alumina column to remove the bulk of the PCBs. Although the final sample extract contained significant quantities of the lower PCBs, this did not affect the mass specific detection of PCDFs.

In addition to some other chlorinated compounds, the final extracts of the Yusho oil and the used PCB contained small quantities of polychlorinated naphthalenes (PCNS). Although PCNS can give response at the m/e values used for the PCDFs (hexa-CN: $M^+ + 6 = 338$; pentachlorodibenzofuran: $M^+ = 338$, with few exceptions), these compounds elute prior to the proper retention range of the PCDFs [112].

GLC-mass spectrometric analysis was accomplished using a Finnigan 4000 quadrupole instrument with EI source and a coupled 50 m × 0.37 mm i.d. OV-17 glass capillary column. The presence of the PCDFs could be confirmed for all major isomers from complete mass spectra through the presence of the molecular ions (M^+), the ion clustering being due to the chlorine isotopes and the major fragmentation (M^+ - COCl, etc).

The amount (μg/g) of PCDFs in Yusho oil and in used Japanese PCB were as follows:

	Tri-	Tetra-	Penta-	Hexa-
Yusho rice oil	0.15	1.4	2.5	1.6
Used Japanese PCB	4.2	4.5	5.5	1.4

The level of 2,3,7,8-tetrachlorodibenzofuran in these samples was 0.45 (Yusho) and 1.25 μg/g (PCB), respectively. The combined level of the PCDFs in the Yusho oil (5.6 μg/g) agrees well with the value of 5 ppm reported by Nagayama [113] (the Yusho oil contained 1 mg of PCB/g) [114]. Figure 17 illustrates mass fragmentograms of the elution of tri- to hexachlorodibenzofurans in purified sample extracts of Yusho rice oil. The pattern of the PCDFs in the Yusho oil was found to be very similar to that of the PCDFs formed from the pyrolysis of commercial PCBs [113]. Among the tetrachloro dibenzofurans, the major isomer present in both the Yusho oil and the used PCB is the toxic 2,3,7,8- isomer (peak 44, Fig. 17). This isomer was also one of the major isomers found from the pyrolysis of commercial PCBs. The toxic 2,3,4,7,8-pentachlorodibenzofuran (peak 68, Fig. 17) is a major constituent of the PCDFs in Yusho rice oil, Japanese used PCB, and in pyrolyzed commercial PCBs [112]. Other tetra-, penta-, and hexachlorodibenzofuran isomers found in Yusho oil and Japanese used PCB and identified by co-chromatography with authentic standards were: 1,3,7,9-tetra- (peak 27); 1,2,3,7,8-penta- (peak 60); 2,3,4,6,8-penta- (peak 61); 1,2,3,4,8-penta- (peak 62; and 2,3,4,6,7,8-hexachlorodibenzofuran (peak 85).

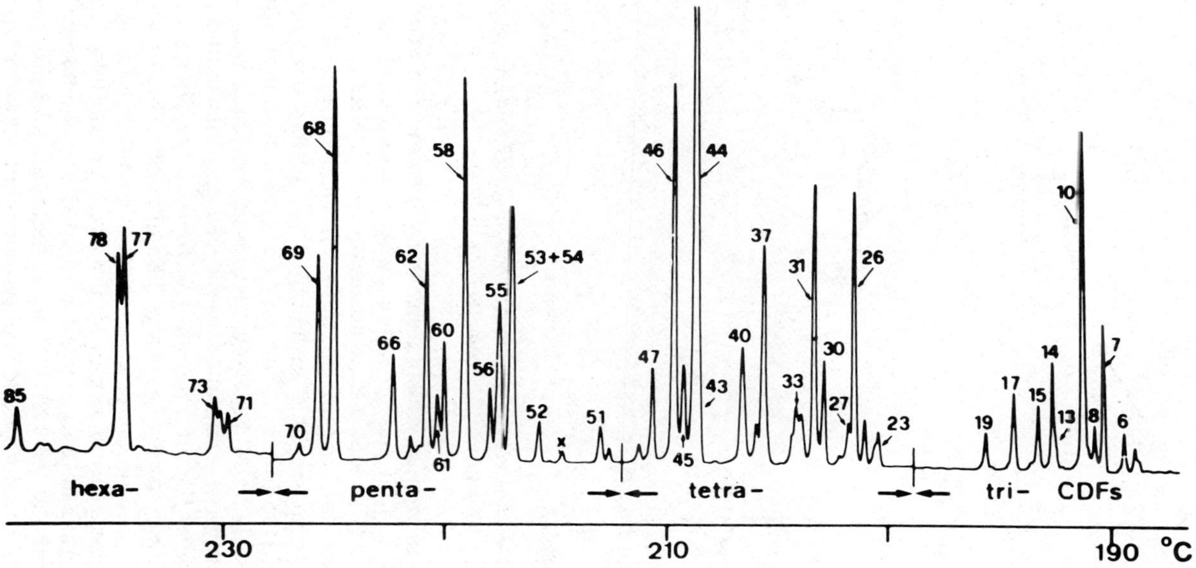

Figure 17 Mass fragmentograms (50 m OV-17 glass capillary column, m/e 270, 304, 338, and 372), showing elution of tri- to hexa-CDFs in Yusho oil. Peak identifications and column conditions: see the text. Sensitivities: 1 to 2 V f.s. (From Ref. 119.)

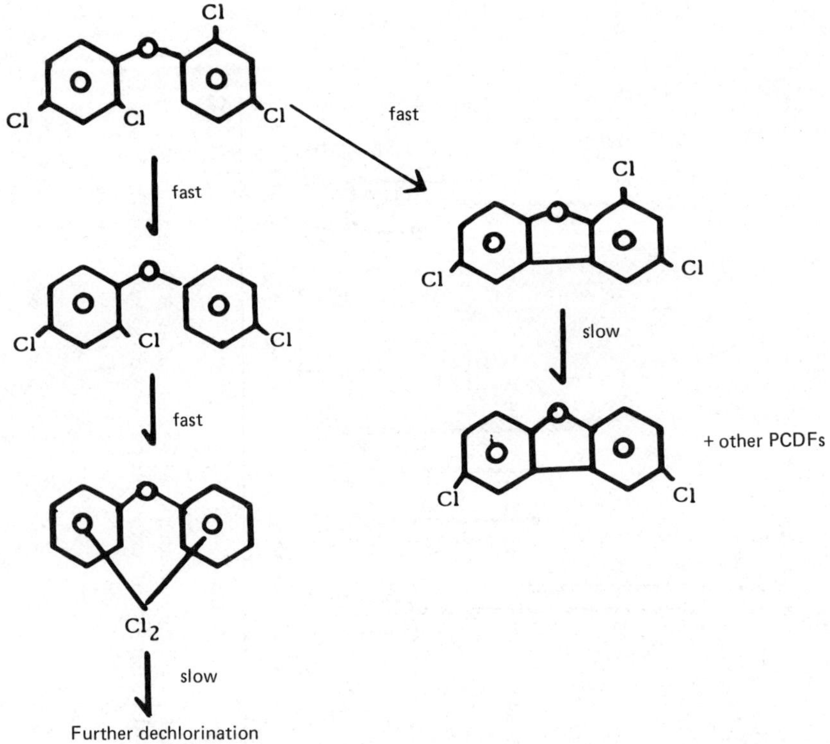

Figure 18 Possible pathways of photochemical degradation of polychlorinated diphenyl ethers. (From Ref. 120.)

Those results show a striking similarity between the PCDF isomers present in the Yusho oil and in the used Japanese PCB. The PCBs of these two samples (Kanechlor KC400 and Mitsubishi-Monsanto T 1248) have the same chlorine content and both were used in a heat-exchange system for long periods. This similarity in the PCDFs was suggested by Buser et al. [119] to add a new link between Yusho and PCBs.

Norstrom et al. [120] reported that irradiation of polychlorodiphenyl ethers, impurities found in commercial polychlorinated phenols, resulted in the formation of chlorodibenzofurans, and in one case this could be used as a synthetic method. The photochemical breakdown of the polychlorinated diphenyl ethers was suggested to follow two competitive pathways, as shown in Figure 18. For example, 2,4,4'-trichlorophenol ether on UV irradiation yielded 2,8-dichlorodibenzofuran. The irradiation of 2,2',4,4'-tetrachlorodiphenyl ether yielded 2,2',4-trichlorodibenzofuran and dichlorodiphenyl ether as the main photoproducts (Fig. 18). The authors suggested that since photochemical formation of the highly toxic chlorodibenzofurans from the much less toxic chlorodiphenyl ethers can be a reaction of environmental significance, the levels of chlorinated diphenyl ethers in commercial chlorophenols should be minimized [120].

There are two additional aspects of the chemical relationship between the PCBs and the chlorinated dibenzofurans that should be noted. Crosby and Moilanen [121] reported evidence for the photochemical conversion of certain PCBs to PCDFs in very low yields. In a limited study, the formation of chlorodibenzofurans was shown to occur under sunlight irradiation and in the laboratory using sunlight-simulating conditions. Two different orthochlorinated biphenyls (e.g., 2,5-dichloro- and 2,2',5,5'-tetrachloro-) were found to produce approximately 0.2% steady-state yields of a monochlorodibenzofuran.

Limited studies regarding the photochemical decomposition of the chlorodibenzofurans indicate that relatively rapid destruction of these derivatives may take place in the environment [121,122].

Since reductive dechlorination is a major route of chemical alteration of the PCDFs, the possibility exists that dechlorination of highly chlorinated debenzofurans to the more toxic congeners of lower chlorine content (e.g., tetrachlorodibenzofurans) can occur. The extent to which specific chlorinated biphenyls, found as *major* constituents of commercial PCB mixtures, or the mixtures per se can be photochemically converted to PCDFs is yet to be determined.

Two possible mechanisms for the formation of chlorinated dibenzofurans from PCBs in the environment are illustrated in Figure 19, both

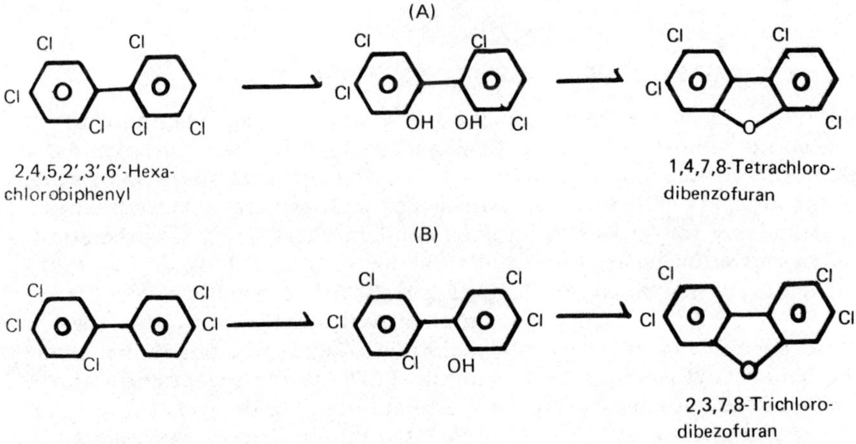

Figure 19 Possible mechanisms for the formation of chlorinated dibenzofurans from PCBs in the environment. (From Ref. 119.)

of which involve hydroxy derivatives as intermediates. Hydroxylation is a very likely route of metabolism of PCBs. (Ring-hydroxylated metabolites of PCBs have been reported as well as polar oxygenated compounds in photolytic products of PCBs.) It is of importance to note that transformation of only 0.002% of a major constituent of an Aroclor mixture to the corresponding chlorinated dibenzofuran would produce concentrations in the mixture corresponding to the values reported by Vos et al. [101,123] as being toxicologically significant.

Considering the chlorodibenzofurans as the toxicologically most significant class of chemical impurities found in PCB mixtures, the question may well be asked: What portion or to what extent can the observed effects noted in animals and humans from exposure to PCB mixtures be attributed to chlorodibenzofurans? At present, it is doubtful whether this question can be answered quantitatively. There are a number of severe analytical problems in the separation, identification, and quantification of the chlorinated dibenzofurans in various PCB mixtures, analogous to those considered previously for the chlorodibenzodioxins. Only a relatively small number of the 135 possible chlorinated dibenzofurans have been identified in PCB mixtures. The toxicity of these compounds can be expected (analogously to the chlorinated dibenzodioxins) to vary with both the number and the ring position of chlorine atoms in the molecule. Because of the very limited number of high-purity isomeric chlorinated dibenzofuran reference standards, toxicity data on these specific compounds are not readily available.

To date, chlorinated dibenzofurans have not been reported in foods. Analytical procedures to detect chlorinated dibenzofurans in the parts per trillion (10^{-12}) range, analogous to the chlorinated dibenzo-p-dioxins, would appear to be necessary.

V. NEW ASSAY APPROACHES

Although stress has been placed on GLC and GLC-MS techniques in the preceding review of the analytical methodology of the chlorodioxins and chlorodibenzofurans, it should be noted that several other approaches to the analysis of environmental samples of these trace contaminants (particularly for TCDD) have been considered [64]. These include radioassays, bioassays, and radioimmunoassays. Poland et al. [124] reported studies on the binding of [^{3}H]TCDD to hepatic cytosol from C57B1/6J mice. A small pool of high-affinity sites were found that stereospecifically and reversibly bind TCDD. It was suggested that the hepatic cytosol species that binds TCDD is the receptor for the induction of hepatic aryl hydroxylase activity [125]. Currently, the greatest limitation of use of this in vitro binding assay as a radioassay procedure is the poor stability of the TCDD binding species (e.g., even at 0° it is stable for only a few hours). TCDD is also a potent

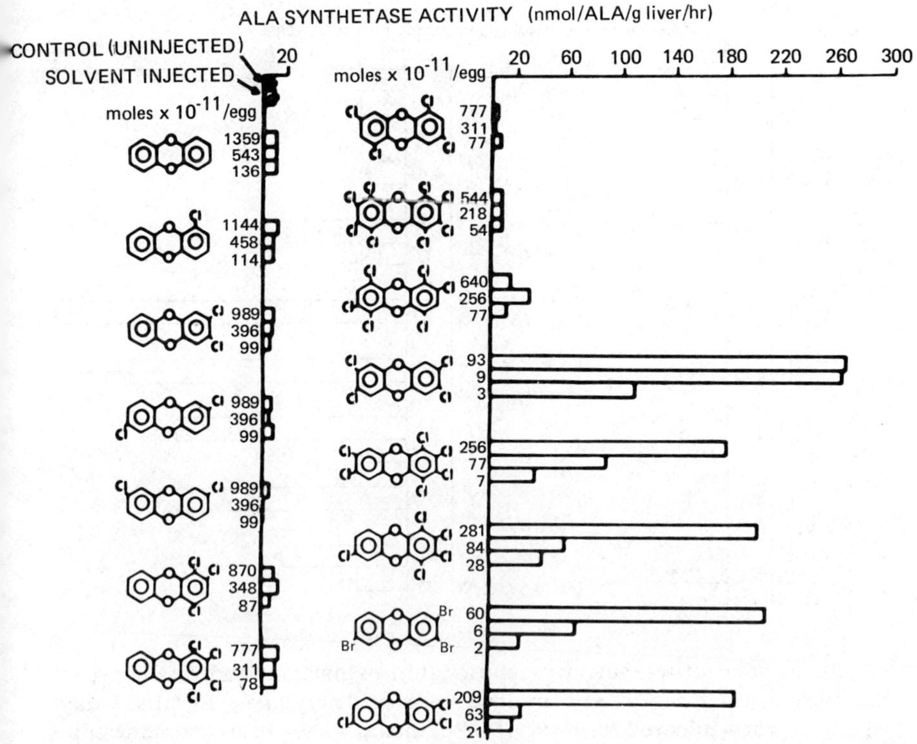

Figure 20 Structure-activity relationships of the halogenated dibenzo-p-dioxins: induction of ALA synthetase. Seventeen-day embryos were injected with the solvent (p-dioxane) or solvent containing the dioxin tested and enzyme activity was assayed 48 hr later. Uninjected control values (n = 9), do not differ appreciably from solvent injected controls (n = 12). Each bar for the test groups represents the value for a single group of three to five pooled livers. (From Ref. 125.)

inducer of ACA synthetase and aryl hydrocarbon hydroxylase in the chick embryo liver, as demonstrated by Poland and Glover [125] (Fig. 20 and 21, respectively). The sensitivity of induction of aryl hydroxylase by TCDD and other chlorodioxins suggests that this response might be a very valuable screening bioassay to detect the presence of the toxic dioxins in environmental samples or commercial pesticides. However, it should be stressed that the nonspecificity of the response rigidly requires that the samples tested be extracted to remove polycyclic hydrocarbons, and that the test is only collaborative, not definitive for TCDD and related dibenzo-p-dioxins [125].

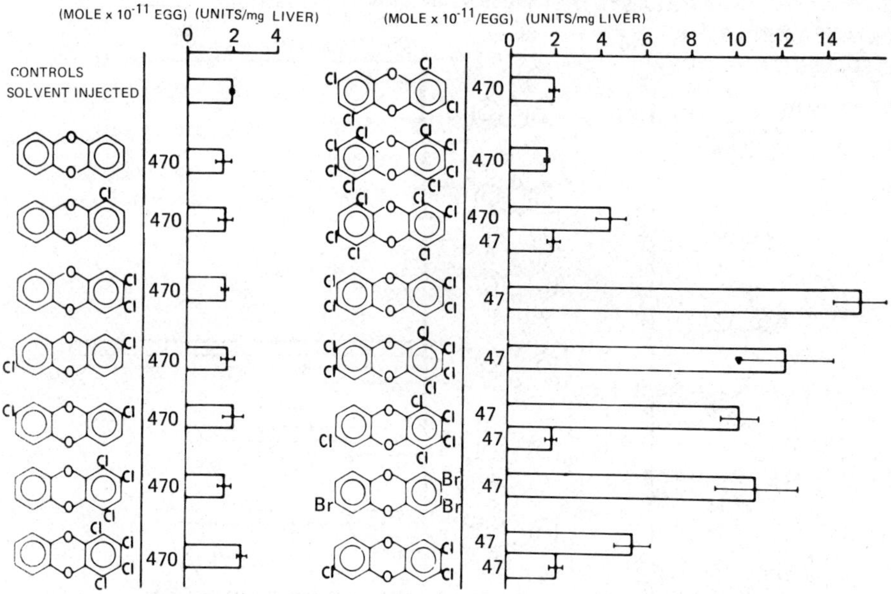

Figure 21 Structure-activity relationship of halogenated dibenzo-p-dioxins: inductions of aryl hydrocarbon hydroxylase. Eighteen-day embryos were injected with 25 μl of p-dioxane or p-dioxane containing the test dioxin, and enzyme activity was assayed 24 hr later. Each bar represents the mean ± standard error of four groups of pooled livers, except for the control and TCDD groups, where n = 12. (From Ref. 125.)

A somewhat similar bioassay reported by Bradlow et al. [126] is based on the dose levels that produce a 50% induction of maximal aryl hydrocarbon hydroxylase activity in a rat hepatoma cell culture system. This assay appears to be sensitive enough to allow detection of TCDD in the low-picogram range and has already been employed to a limited extent for the screening of several environmental samples for chlorodioxins in parallel with GLC identification. It was also noted that the LD_{50} doses in guinea pigs and dosages that produce 50% induction of maximal aryl hydrocarbon activity in the rat hepatoma cell culture system have certain similarities in magnitude and direction [64,126].

Difficulties in the development of a radioimmunoassay method for TCDD have been described by McKinney [64]. The focal point of difficulty to date has been to render the TCDD molecule antigenic. Although Chae et al. [127] have synthesized suitable haptens (e.g., 1-amino-3,7,8-trichlorodibenzo-p-dioxin and 1-amino-2,3,7,8-tetrachlorodibenzo-p-dioxin), much work remains to be done to determine antibody sensitivity, specificity, cross reactivity, and matrix effects. Although the method is not expected to be specific for TCDD alone, it may be specific for the general class of dioxins with two or more chlorines in the 2,8 and/or 3,7 positions [64].

VI. CONFIRMATORY TECHNIQUES

A confirmatory technique, which would be limited to the detection of low-nanogram levels, is the measurement of the differences in the visible and electron spin resonance spectra obtained when chlorodioxins are exposed to acidic oxidizing media/trifluoromethanesulfonic acid (TFMS acid) [128]. This technique of Pohland et al. [128] is based on the formation under these conditions of cation radicals from the various chlorinated dibenzo-p-dioxins:

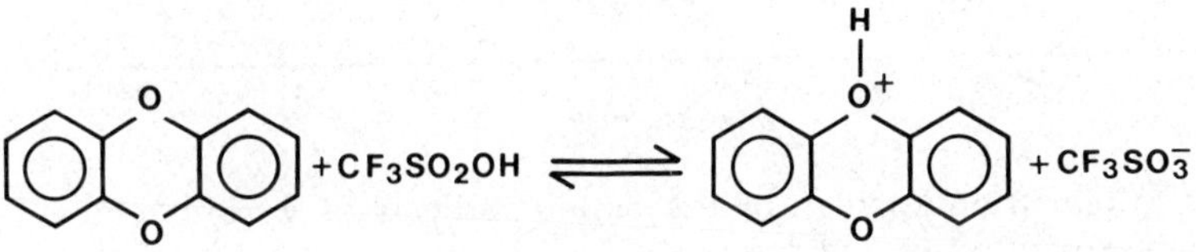

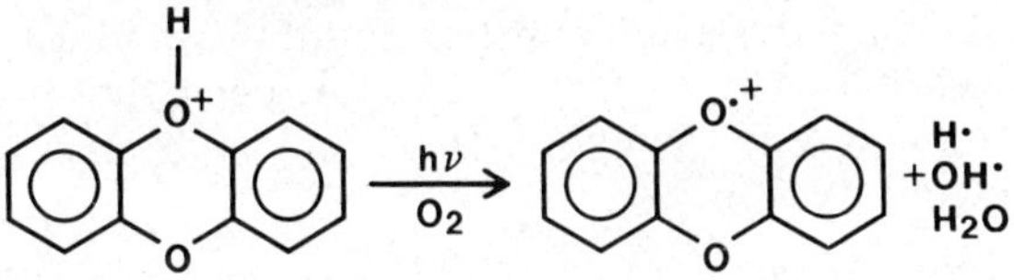

which can readily be differentiated on the basis of either their visible or their electron spin resonance spectra. The typical spectra of a series of cation radicals of various chlorinated dioxins presented in Figure 22 show the relative ease with which these materials can be recognized solely on the basis of the position of the absorption maxima. Figure 23 illustrates the ESR spectra of two isomeric tetrachlorodioxins. This type of hyperfine structure was obtained only on degassed samples and in these cases, UV irradiation was used to generate the free radicals.

Another confirmative technique is that of photolysis to distinguish qualitative and quantitative differences in the decomposition products of different isomers [64,129]. According to McKinney, this technique may be best suited for confirmation of octachlorodibenzodioxin. GC

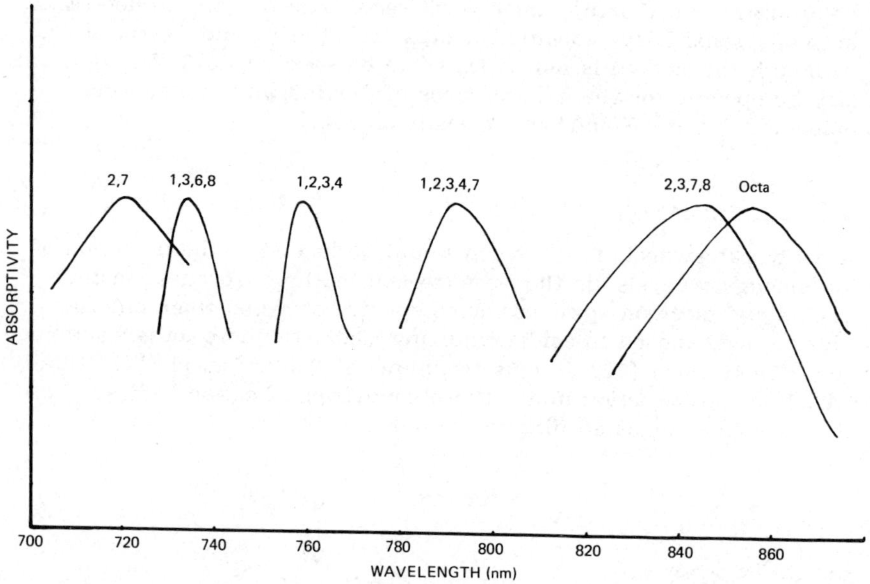

Figure 22 Absorption spectra of the cation radicals of various chlorinated dibenzo-p-dioxins. (From Ref. 128.)

with electron capture detection or GC-MS is used to establish the fingerprint patterns of the photolytic decomposition patterns. The technique is dependent on the availability of suitable standard materials. In addition, sample matrix effects have not been thoroughly investigated for the photolytic technique [64].

VII. DECONTAMINATION

In the foregoing overview, stress has been placed on the toxicity of various chlorodioxins (primarily TCDD) as well as on the lesser known chlorodibenzofurans. This of necessity has required the elaboration of requisite techniques for their safe handling and decontamination.

Although there is an expanding amount of work being done (primarily as a result of the Seveso, Italy, episode), only four different techniques of decontamination have been proposed: (1) incineration, (2) chlorinolysis, (3) soil biodegradation, and (4) solubilization and photodecomposition in aqueous solutions.

Although the first method is undoubtedly the safest as far as complete TCDD destruction is concerned, the use of very high temperatures (about 800 to 1000°) [11,130] is precluded for many laboratories and facilities lacking the requisite equipment and further, it

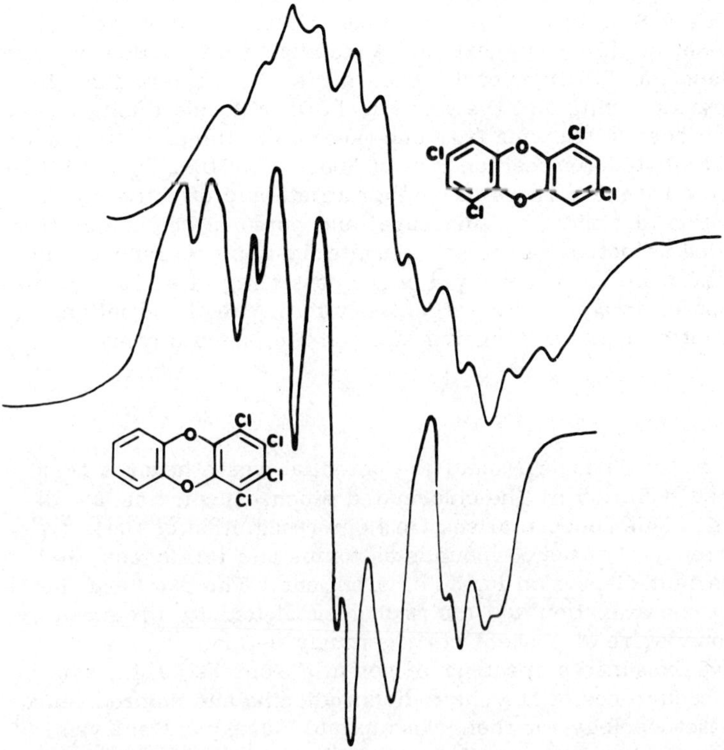

Figure 23 ESR spectra in TFMS acid with ultraviolet irradiation. (From Ref. 128.)

does not allow any recovery of contaminated materials, where required or feasible. Chlorinolysis is also a destructive procedure involving high chlorine pressures and temperatures for conversion of organic compounds to carbon tetrachloride [11].

Soil biodegradation of TCDD appears to be a promising technique [11]; however, it is now feasible only for cultivatable soils.

The technique of Botre et al. [131], involving TCDD solubilization and photodecomposition in aqueous solution, would allow the recovery of contaminated materials treated with aqueous solutions and the photodecomposition of both TCDD and the solubilizing agent. To date, photodecomposition is the most rapid method of TCDD degradation. This is achieved using a catamic surfactant, 1-hexadecylpyridinium chloride, which acts as an energy transfer agent in the photodecomposition process, thus increasing the TCDD decomposition rate in this micellar solution. In experimental studies, the time required for total TCDD decomposition when exposed to UV irradiation at 254 to 356 nm in a 0.02 M hexadecylpyridinium chloride solution was only 4 hr. Botre et al. [131] suggest that a stabilizing interaction between the surfactant and TCDD molecules occurs with π - π interactions between the pyridine ring and the aromatic TCDD molecule taking place, leading to an energy transfer from one molecule to the other which enhances the photodecomposition rate of "bound" TCDD. This method was suggested by the authors to be appropriate and effective for the decontamination of buildings, furniture, and personal belongings from TCDD, as well as potentially to soil decontamination. A particularly attractive feature of this technique is the possibility of a rapid photodecomposition of an aqueous detergent solution, with the simultaneous degradation of both the solubilizing and polluting agents [131].

VIII. SUMMARY

There is increasing concern about the potential health hazards from environmental pollution by the chlorinated dibenzo-p-dioxins and dibenzofurans. This concern arises from our recognition of the extraordinary potency of these compounds as toxins and teratogens, and their inadvertant dispersion in the environment. The extent of the environment contamination and the mechanism of toxicity produced by these compounds are at present not rigorously defined.

We have examined a spectrum of potential sources (e.g., synthetic) and occurrence of the chlorodibenzodioxins and chlorodibenzofurans and methodology for their cleanup and subsequent analysis. Stress has been placed on the difficulties of separation and identification of the many isomers in both classes per se as well as from co-contaminants such as the PCB, chlorinated benzenes, naphthalenes, diphenyl ethers, phenols, predioxins, DDT, and DDE.

Elaborate methods for the cleanup and analysis of environmental samples currently permit the monitoring of levels of chlorodioxins (primarily TCDD) and possibly chlorodibenzofurans in the parts per trillion (10^{-12}) range. Although special high-resolution mass spectral techniques have generally been used to achieve the desired high sensitivity and specificity, it is recognized that application of these methods to environmental samples has been complicated by cost, time, and additional factors, such as effects of sample matrix and size, that are involved in the analyses of the samples and interpreting the data.

New assay approaches, confirmatory techniques, and aspects of decontamination were also discussed.

REFERENCES

1. S. Ueo. 2,6-Dichlorobiphenylene oxide. Bull. Chem. Soc. Jap. *16*, 177 (1941).
2. W. Sanderman, H. Stockman, and R. Caston. Pyrolysis of pentachlorophenol. Chem. Ber. *90*, 1960 (1957).
3. K. D. Courtney, D. W. Gaylor, M. D. Hogan, H. L. Falk, R. R. Bates, and I. Mitchell. Teratogenic evaluation of 2,4,5-T. Science *168*, 864-866 (1970).
4. G. L. Sparschu, F. L. Dunn, and V. K. Rowe. Study of teratogenicity of 2,3,7,8-tetrachlorodibenzo-p-dioxin. Food Cosmet. Toxicol. *9*, 405 (1971).
5. Environmental Protection Agency. Pesticide Programs--Rebuttable Presumption Against Registration and Continued Registration of Pesticide Products Containing 2,4,5-T. Fed. Reg. *43*(78) 17116-17147 (1978).
6. J. Walsh. Seveso: The questions persist, where dioxin created a wasteland. Science *197*, 1064-1067 (1977).
7. IARC, Monographs on the Evaluation of the Carcinogenic Risk of Chemicals to Man, Vol. *15*: Some Fumigants, The Herbicides 2,4-D and 2,4,5-T, Chlorinated Dibenzodioxins and Miscellaneous Industrial Chemicals. International Agency for Research on Cancer, Lyon, France, 1977, pp. 41-102.
8. J. P. Van Miller, J. J. Lalich, and J. R. Allen. Increased incidence of neoplasms in rats exposed to low levels of 2,3,7,8-tetrachlorodibenzo-p-dioxin. Chemosphere *9*, 537-544 (1977).
9. E. E. McConnell, J. A. Moore, J. K. Haseman, and M. W. Harris. The comparative toxicity of chlorinated dibenzo-p-dioxins in mice and guinea pigs. Toxicol. Appl. Pharmacol. *5*, 259-266 (1973).
10. L. Fishbein. Trace organic contaminants in the environment: I. Chlorinated dioxins and dibenzofurans. Int. J. Ecol. Environ. Sci. *2*, 69-81 (1976).
11. P. C. Kearney, E. A. Woolson, A. R. Isensee, and C. S. Helling. Tetrachlorodibenzodioxin in the environment: sources, fate and decomposition. Environ. Health Perspect. *5*, 273-277 (1973).
12. S. Jensen and L. Renberg. Contaminants in pentachlorophenol: chlorinated dioxins and predioxins. Ambio *1*, 62-67 (1972).
13. M. J. Mercier. 2,3,7,8-Tetrachlorodibenzo-p-dioxin--An Overview. Report to European Economic Communities (EEC), May 1978.
14. C. A. Nilsson, A. Norstrom, K. Anderson, and C. Rappe. In Pentachlorophenol: Chemistry, Pharmacology and Environmental Toxicology, (K. Ranga Rao, ed.). Environmental Science Research Series, Vol. *12*. Plenum Press, New York, 1978.

15. U.S. Tariff Commission. Synthetic Organic Chemicals: Production and Sales, TC Publ. 479, Washington, D.C., 1970.
16. M. H. Milnes. Formation of 2,3,7,8-tetrachlorodibenzodioxin by thermal decomposition of sodium 2,4,5-trichlorophenate. Nature (Lond.) *232*, 395-396 (1971).
17. G. May. Chloroacne from the accidental production of tetrachlorodibenzodioxin. Br. J. Ind. Med. *30*, 276-283 (1973).
18. M. J. Mercier. 2,3,7,8-Tetrachlorodibenzo-p-dioxin: an overview. In Proceedings of the Expert Meeting on the Problems Raised by TCDD Pollution. (A. Berlin, A. Buratta, and M. T. Vandervenne, Eds.). Milan, 1976, in press (1977).
19. H. G. Langer, T. P. Brady, and P. R. Briggs. Formation of dibenzodioxins and other condensation products from chlorinated phenols and derivatives. Environ. Health Perspect. 5, 3-7 (1973).
20. L. Jirasek, J. Kalensky, and K. Kubeck. Acne chlorina and porphyria cutanea tarda during the manufacture of herbicides, II. Cesk. Dermatol. *49*, 145-157 (1974).
21. D. Firestone. The 2,3,7,8-tetrachlorodibenzo-p-dioxin problem: a review. Ecol. Bull. (Stockholm) *27*, 39-52 (1978).
22. C. Rappe. Chemical background of the phenoxy acids and dioxins. Ecol. Bull. (Stockholm) *27*, 28-30 (1978).
23. R. W. Storherr, R. R. Watts, A. M. Gardner, and T. Osgood. Steam distillation technique for the analysis of 2,3,7,8-tetrachlorodibenzo-p-dioxin in technical 2,4,5-T. J. Assoc. Off. Anal. Chem. *54*, 218-219 (1971).
24. C. S. Helling, A. R. Isensee, E. A. Woolson, P. D. J. Ensor, G. E. Jones, J. R. Plimmer, and P. C. Kearney. Chlorodioxins in pesticides, soils and plants. J. Environ. Qual. *2*, 171-178 (1973).
25. C. Rappe, H. R. Buser, and H. P. Bosshardt. Identification and quantification of polychlorinated dibenzo-p-dioxins (PCDDs) and dibenzofurans (PCDFs) in 2,4,5-T ester formulations and herbicide orange. Chemosphere 5, 431-438 (1978).
26. J. N. Huckins, D. L. Stalling, and W. A. Smith. Foam charcoal chromatography for analysis of polychlorinated dibenzodioxins in herbicide orange. J. Assoc. Off. Anal. Chem. *61*, 32 (1978).
27. B. Ahling, A. Lindskog, B. Jansson, and G. Sundstrom. Formation of polychlorinated dibenzo-p-dioxins and dibenzofurans during combustion of 2,4,5-T formulation. Chemosphere *8*, 461-468 (1977).
28. H. R. Buser and C. Rappe. Identification of substitution patterns in polychlorinated dibenzodioxins by mass spectrometry. Chemosphere 7, 199 (1978).

29. C. Rappe, S. Marklund, H. R. Buser, and H. P. Bosshardt. Formation of polychlorinated dibenzo-p-dioxins (PCDDs) and dibenzofurans (PCDFs) by burning or heating chlorophenates. Chemosphere *3*, 269-281 (1978).
30. W. Sandermann, H. Stockmann, and R. Casten. Pyrolysis of pentachlorophenol. Chem. Ber. *90*, 690-692 (1957).
31. M. Tomita, S. Ueda, and M. Narisada. Dibenzo-p-dioxin derivatives. XXVII. Synthesis of polyhalodibenzo-p-dioxin. J. Pharm. Soc. Jap. *79*, 186-189 (1959).
32. E. A. Woolson, R. F. Thomas, and P. D. J. Ensor. Survey of polychlorodibenzo-p-dioxin content in selected pesticides. J. Agric. Food Chem. *20*, 351-358 (1972).
33. D. Firestone, J. Ress, N. L. Brown, R. P. Barron, and J. N. Damico. Determination of polychlorodibenzo-p-dioxins and related compounds in commercial chlorophenols. J. Assoc. Off. Anal. Chem. *55*, 85-92 (1972).
34. H. R. Buser. Analysis of polychlorinated dibenzo-p-dioxins and dibenzofurans in chlorinated phenols by mass fragmentography. J. Chromatogr. *107*, 295-310 (1975).
35. E. C. Villaneuva, V. W. Burse, and R. W. Jennings. Chlorodibenzo-p-dioxin contamination of two commercially available pentachlorophenols. J. Agric. Food Chem. *21*, 739-740 (1973).
36. N. P. Buu-Hoi, G. Saint-ruf, P. Bigon, and M. Mungane. Preparation proprietes et identification de las "dioxine" (tetrachloro-2,3,7,8-dibenzo-p-dioxine) dans les pyrolysats de defoliants a base d'acide trichloro-2,4,5-phenoxy acetique et des esters et des vegetaux contamines. C. R. Acad. Sci. Ser. D. *273*, 708-711 (1971).
37. R. H. Stehl and L. L. Lamparski. Combustion of several 2,4,5-trichlorophenoxy compounds: formation of 2,3,7,8-tetrachlorodibenzo-p-dioxin. Science *197*, 1008-1009 (1977).
38. A. L. Young. Ecological Studies on a Herbicide-Equipment Test Area. Report AFATL-TR-74-12. Air Force Armament Laboratory, Eglin Air Force Base, Fla. 1974.
39. R. H. Stehl, R. R. Papenfuss, R. A. Bredeweg, and R. W. Roberts. Degradation of 2,4,5-T. Presented at the 162nd National Meeting of American Chemical Society, Washington, D.C., Sept. 1971.
40. K. Anderson, H. P. Bosshardt, H. R. Buser, S. Marklund, and C. Rappe. In Chlorinated Phenoxy Acids and Their Dioxins (C. Ramel, Ed.). Ecol. Bull. (Stockholm) *27*, 26 (1978).
41. T. R. Plumb, L. A. Norris, and M. L. Montgomery. Persistence of 2,4-D and 2,4,5-T in chaparral soil and in vegetation. Bull. Environ. Contam. Toxicol. *17* (1977).
42. E. E. McConnell, J. A. Moore, J. K. Haseman, and M. W. Harris. The comparative toxicology of chlorinated deibenzo-p-dioxins isomers in mice and guinea pigs. Toxicol. Appl. Pharmacol. *37*, 146 (1976).

43. A. Poland, E. Glover, and A. S. Kende. Stereospecific, high affinity binding of 2,3,7,8-tetrachlorodibenzo-p-dioxin by hepatic cytosol. J. Biol. Chem. *251*, 4936 (1976).
44. H. R. Buser. Polychlorinated dibenzo-p-dioxins; separation and identification of isomers by gas chromatography and mass spectrometry. J. Chromatogr. *114*, 95 (1975).
45. H. R. Buser, H. P. Bosshardt, and C. Rappe. Identification of polychlorinated dibenzo-p-dioxin isomers found in fly ash. Chemosphere. *2*, 165-172 (1978).
46. A. P. Gray, S. P. Cepa, and J. S. Cantrell. Intervention of the Smiles rearrangement in synthesis of dibenzo-p-dioxins: 1,2,3,6,7,8- and 1,2,3,7,8,9-hexachlorodibenzo-p-dioxin (HCDD). Tetrahedron Lett., 2873 (1975).
47. A. S. Kende and M. R. Decamp. Smiles rearrangements in the synthesis of hexachlorodibenzo-p-dioxins. Tetrahedron Lett., 2877 (1975).
48. K. Olie, P. L. Vermeulen, and O. Hutzinger. Chlorodibenzo-p-dioxins and chlorodibenzofurans and trace components of fly ash and flue gas of some municipal incinerators in The Netherlands. Chemosphere *8*, 455-459 (1977).
49. H. R. Buser and H. P. Bosshardt. Polychlorierte Dibenzo-p-dioxine, Dibenzofurane und Benzole in der asche kommunaler und industrieller Verbrennungsanlagen. Mitt. Geb. Lebensmittelunters. Hyg. *69*, 191-199 (1978).
50. L. M. Dalderup. Safety measures for taking down buildings contaminated with toxic material, II. T. Soc. Geneesk. *52*, 616-623 (1974).
51. A. Hay. Toxic cloud over Seveso. Nature (Lond.) *262*, 636-638 (1976).
52. S. Zedda. La lezione della chloroacne. In Kmesa, una rapina di saluti, di lavoro, e di teritorio. (G. Ceruti et al., Eds.). Mazzotta, Milan, 1977, pp. 17-43.
53. P. I. A. Gruppo, B. Mazza, and V. Scatturin. Kmesa: come e perche. Sapere *796*, 10-36 (1976).
54. R. L. Rawls and D. A. O'Sullivan. Italy seeks answers following toxic release. Ghem. Eng. News, (27-35, Aug. 23, 1976).
55. P. J. Goldman. Schwetste akute Chlorakne durch Trichlorophenolzersetzungsprodukte. Arbeitsmed. Sozialmed. Arbeitshyg. *7*, 12-18 (1972).
56. H. Bauer, K. H. Schulz, and U. Spiegelberg. Berufliche Vergiftungen bei der Herstellung von Chlorophenol-Verbindungen. Arch. Gewerbepathol. Gewerbehyg. *18*, 538-555 (1961).
57. A. P. Poland, D. Smith, G. Metter, and P. Possick. A health survey of workers in a 2,4-D and 2,4,5-T plant with special attention to chloracne, porphyria cutanea tarda and psychologic parameters. Arch. Environ. Health *22*, 316-327 (1971).

58. P. Dugois, P. Amplard, M. Aimard, and G. Deshors. Acne chlorique collective et accidentelle d' un type nouveau. Bull. Soc. Fr. Dermatol. Syphiligr. *75*, 260-261 (1968).
59. L. Jirasek, J. Kalensky, and K. Kubeck. Acne chlorina and porphyria cutanea tarda during the manufacture of herbicides. C.S. Dermatol. *48*, 306-317 (1973).
60. D. G. Crosby, A. S. Wong, J. R. Plimmer, and E. A. Woolson. Photo-decomposition of chlorinated dibenzo-p-dioxins. Science *173*, 748-751 (1971).
61. R. Baughman and M. Meselson. An improved analysis for tetrachlorodibenzo-p-dioxins. In Chlorodioxins--Origin and Fate, Am. Chem. Soc. Monogr. No. 120. American Chemical Society, Washington, D.C., 1973, pp. 92-104.
62. R. Baughman and M. Meselson. An analytical method for detecting TCDD (dioxin): levels of TCDD in samples from Vietnam. Environ. Health Perspect. *5*, 27-35 (1973).
63. E. A. Woolson, D. J. Ensor, W. L. Reichel, and A. L. Young. Dioxin residues in lakeland sand and Bald Eagle samples. In Chlorodioxins--Origin and Fate, Am. Chem. Soc. Monogr. No. 120. American Chemical Society, Washington, D.C., 1973, pp. 112-118.
64. J. D. McKinney. Analysis of 2,3,7,8-tetrachlorodibenzo-para-dioxin in environmental samples. Ecol. Bull. (Stockholm) *27*, 53-66 (1978).
65. R. L. Harless and E. O. Oswald. Low and high resolution gas chromatography/mass spectrometry (GC-MS) method of analysis for the presence of 2,3,7,8-tetrachlorodibenzo-p-dioxin (TCDD) in environmental samples. Presented at the 24th American Society for Mass Spectrometry Meeting, San Diego, Calif. May 1976.
66. M. L. Taylor, R. L. C. Wu, C. D. Miller, and T. O. Tiernan. Levels of TCDD in environmental and biological samples as determined by gas chromatography-high resolution mass spectrometry. Presented at the 24th American Society for Mass Spectrometry Meeting, San Diego, Calif., May 1976.
67. L. A. Shadoff, R. A. Hummel, L. Laparski, and J. H. Davidson. A search for 2,3,7,8-tetrachlorodibenzo-p-dioxin (TCDD) in an environment exposed annually to 2,4,5-T herbicides. Bull. Environ. Contam. Toxicol. *18*, 478-484 (1977).
68. P. W. O'Keefe, M. Meselson, and R. W. Baughman. A neutral clean up procedure for TCDD residues in environmental samples. Presented at the 90th Annual Meeting of the Association of Official Analytical Chemists, Washington, D.C., Oct. 18-21, 1976.
69. E. C. Bligh and W. J. Dyer. A rapid method for total lipid extraction and purification. Can. J. Biochem. Physiol. *37*, 911-917 (1959).

70. P. W. Albro and B. J. Corbett. Extraction and cleanup of animal tissues for subsequent determination of chlorinated dibenzo-p-dioxins and dibenzofurans. Chemosphere 7, 381-385 (1977).
71. J. R. Hass, M. Friesen, and M. K. Hoffman. Manuscript in preparation, cited in Refs. 63 and 69.
72. D. F. Hunt, T. M. Harvey, and J. W. Russell. Oxygen as a reagent gas for the analysis of 3,3,7,8-tetrachlorodibenzo-dioxin by negative ion chemical ionization mass spectrometry. J. Chem. Soc. Chem. Commun. 5, 151-152 (1975).
73. D. L. Stalling. Laboratory Investigations Concerned with Charcoal Sorption of TCDD in Herbicide Orange. Fish-Pesticide Research Laboratory. 3rd Quarterly Report, June 17, 1976.
74. D. L. Stalling. Laboratory Investigations Concerned with Charcoal Sorption of TCDD in Herbicide Orange. Fish-Pesticide Research Laboratory, Sept. 26, 1975.
75. D. L. Stalling, J. Johnson, and J. N. Huckins. Automated gel-permeation, carbon chromatographic cleanup of dioxins, PCBs, pesticides and industrial chemicals. Environ. Qual. Safety, Suppl. *3*, 12-18 (1975).
76. T. Ramstad, N. H. Mahle, and R. Matalon. Automated cleanup of herbicides by adsorption chromatography for the determination of 2,3,7,8-tetrachlorodibenzo-p-dioxin. Anal. Chem. *49*, 386-390 (1977).
77. I. Camoni. A. DiMuccio, D. Pontecorvo, and L. Vergori. Cleanup procedure for extraction of soil samples in the determination of 2,3,7,8-tetrachlorodibenzo-p-dioxin. J. Chromatogr. *153*, 233-238 (1978).
78. H. R. Buser and H. P. Bosshardt. The determination of polychlorinated dibenzo-p-dioxins and dibenzofurans in commercial pentachlorophenols by combined gas chromatography-mass spectrometry. J. Assoc. Off. Anal. Chem. *59*, 562-569 (1976).
79. H. R. Buser. High-resolution gas chromatography of polychlorinated dibenzo-p-dioxins and dibenzofurans. Anal. Chem. *48*, 1553-1557 (1976).
80. S. Jensen and L. Renberg. Contaminants in pentachlorophenol chlorinated hydroxydiphenyl ethers. Ambio *1*, 62-65 (1972).
81. J. Plimmer, J. Ruth, and E. Woolson. Mass spectrometric identification of the hepta- and octa-chlorinated dibenzo-p-dioxins and dibenzofurans in technical pentachlorophenol. J. Agric. Food Chem. *21*, 90-93 (1973).
82. E. C. Villanueva, R. W. Jennings, V. W. Burse, and R. D. Kimbrough. A comparison of analytical methods for chlorodibenzo-p-dioxins in pentachlorophenol. J. Agric. Food Chem. *23*, 1089-1091 (1975).

83. D. Firestone. Determination of polychlorinated dibenzo-p-dioxins and polychlorodibenzofurans in commercial gelatins by gas-liquid chromatography. J. Agric. Food Chem. *25*, 1274-1280 (1977).
84. W. Crummett. Personal communication, Apr. 2, 1973, cited in Ref. 81.
85. W. B. Crummett and R. H. Stehl. Determination of chlorinated dibenzo-p-dioxins and dibenzofurans in various materials. Environ. Health Perspect. *5*, 15-25 (1973).
86. C. Rappe and C. Nilsson. An artifact in the gas chromatographic determination of impurities in pentachlorophenol. J. Chromatogr. *67*, 247-253 (1972).
87. J. O. Levin and C. A. Nilsson. Chromatographic determination of polychlorinated phenols, phenoxyphenols, dibenzofurans and dibenzodioxins in wood-dust from worker environments. Chemosphere *7*, 443-448 (1977).
88. C. D. Pfeiffer, T. J. Nestrick, and C. W. Kocher. Determination of chlorinated dibenzo-p-dioxins in purified pentachlorophenol by liquid-chromatography. Anal. Chem. *50*, 800-804 (1978).
89. R. J. Dolphin and F. W. Wilmott. Separation of chlorinated dibenzo-p-dioxins from chlorinated congeners. J. Chromatogr. *149*, 161-168 (1978).
90. D. Firestone. Etiology of chick edema disease. Environ. Health Perspect. *5*, 59-66 (1973).
91. P. F. Lewis. Personal communication, cited in Ref. 87.
92. Gelatin Manufacturers of America, Inc. Gelatin. GMA, New York, 1973.
93. P. Kim, G. G. Yang, D. Firestone, and A. E. Pohland. Photochemical dichlorination of chlorinated dibenzo-p-dioxins. Presented at the First Chemical Congress of the North American Continent, Mexico City, Nov. 1975.
94. H. R. Buser. Preparation of qualitative standard mixtures of polychlorinated dibenzo-p-dioxins and dibenzofurans by ultraviolet and Γ-irradiation of the octachloro compounds. J. Chromatogr. *129*, 303-307 (1976).
95. J. R. Plimmer, U. I. Klingebiel, D. G. Crosby, and A. S. Wong. In Chlorodioxins--Origin and Fate, Adv. Chem. Ser. 120. American Chemical Society, Washington, D.C. 1973.
96. D. G. Crosby, A. S. Wong, J. R. Plimmer, and E. A. Woolson. Photodecomposition of chlorinated dibenzo-p-dioxins. Science *173*, 748-749 (1971).
97. O. Hutzinger. S. Safe, B. R. Wentzell, and V. Zitko. Photochemical degradation of di- and octachlorodibenzofuran. Environ. Health Perspect. *5*, 267 (1973).

98. R. H. Stehl, R. R. Papenfuss, R. A. Bredeweg, and R. W. Roberts. The stability of pentachlorophenol and chlorinated dioxins to sunlight, heat and combustion. In chlorodioxins--Origin and Fate, Adv. Chem. Ser. No. 120. American Chemical Society, Washington, D.C., 1973, pp. 119-125.
99. J. A. Goldstein, J. D. McKinney, G. W. Lucier, J. A. Moore, P. Hickman, and H. Bergman. Effects of hexachlorobiphenyl isomers and 2,3,7,8-tetrachlorodibenzofuran (TCDF) on hepatic drug metabolism and porphyrin accumulation. Pharmacologist. *16*, 239 (1974).
100. B. A. Schwetz, J. M. Norris, G. L. Sparschu, V. K. Rowe, P. J. Gehring, J. L. Emerson, and C. G. Gerbig. Toxicology of chlorinated dibenzo-p-dioxins. Environ. Health Perspect. *5*, 87-98 (1973).
101. J. G. Vos, J. L. Koeman, H. L. Van Der Maas, M. C. ten Noever de Brauw, and R. H. Vos. Identification and toxicoological evaluation of chlorinated dibenzofurans and chlorinated naphthalenes in two commercial polychlorinated biphenyls. Food Cosmet. Toxicol. *8*, 625 (1970).
102. G. W. Bowes, B. R. Simoneit, A. L. Burlingame, B. W. De Lappe, and G. W. Risebrough. The search for chlorinated dibenzofurans and chlorinated dibenzodioxins in wildlife populations showing elevated levels of embryonic death. Environ. Health Perspect. 5, 191-198 (1973).
103. G. W. Bowes, M. J. Mulvihill, B. R. Simoneit, A. L. Burlingame, and R. W. Risebrough. Identification of chlorinated dibenzofuran in American polychlorinated biphenyls. Nature (Lond.) *256*, 305-307 (1975).
104. J. A. G. Roach and I. H. Pomerantz. The findings of chlorinated dibenzofurans in a Japanese polychlorinated biphenyl sample. Bull. Environ. Contam. Toxicol. *12*, 338-342 (1974).
105. M. Kuratsune, T. Yoshimura, J. Matsuzaka, and A. Yamaguchi. Epidemiologic study on Yusho, a poisoning caused by ingestion of rice oil contaminated with a commercial brand of polychlorinated biphenyls. Environ. Health Perspect. *1*, 119-128 (1972).
106. G. W. Bowes, M. J. Mulvihill, M. R. DeCamp, and A. S. Kende. Gas chromatographic characteristics of authentic chlorinated dibenzofurans, identification of two isomers in American and Japanese polychlorinated biphenyls. J. Agric. Food Chem. *23*, 1222-1223 (1975).
107. I. C. T. Nisbet and A. F. Sarofim. Rates and routes of transport of PCBs (polychlorinated biphenyls) in the environment. Environ. Health Perspect. *1*, 21-38 (1972).
108. S. Jensen, A. G. Johnels, M. Olsson, and G. Otterlind. DDT and PCB in marine animals from Swedish waters. Nature (Lond.) *224*, 247-250 (1969).

109. R. W. Risebrough, P. Reiche, D. B. Peakall, S. G. Herman, and M. N. Kirven. Polychlorinated biphenyls in the global ecosystem. Nature (Lond.) *220*, 1098-1102 (1968).
110. J. H. Koeman, M. C. ten Noever de Brauw, and R. H. deVos. Chlorinated biphenyls in fish, mussels, and birds from the River Rhine and The Netherlands coastal area. Nature (Lond.) *221*, 1126-1128 (1969).
111. H. R. Buser, H. P. Bosshardt, and C. Rappe. Formation of polychlorinated dibenzofurans (PCDFs) from the pyrolysis of PCBs. Chemosphere 7, 109-119 (1978).
112. H. R. Buser, H. P. Bosshardt, C. Rappe, and R. Lindahl. Identification of polychlorinated dibenzofurans in fly ash and PCB pyrolyses. Chemosphere 7, 419-429 (1978).
113. J. Nagayama, M. Kuratsune, and Y. Nasuda. Determination of chlorinated dibenzofurans in Kanechlors and "Yusho oil." Bull. Environ. Contam. Toxicol. *15*, 9-13 (1976).
114. M. Goto and K. Higuchi. The symptomology of Yusho (chlorobiphenyl poisoning) in dermatology. Fukuoka Acta Med. *60*, 409-443 (1969).
115. T. Kojima, H. Fukumoto, and J. Makisumi. Chlorobiphenyl poisoning-gas chromatographic detection of chlorobiphenyl in rice oil and biological materials. Jap. J. Legal. Med. *23*, 415 (1969).
116. DHEW Final Report of Subcommittee on the Health Effects of Polychlorinated Biphenyls and Polybrominated Biphenyls. Washington, D.C. 1977.
117. C. Rappe, A. Gara, H. R. Buser, and H. P. Bosshardt. Analysis of polychlorinated dibenzofurans in Yusho oil using high resolution gas chromatography-mass spectrometry. Chemosphere *6*, 231-236 (1977).
118. M. Morita, J. Nakagawa, K. Akiyama, S. Mimura, and N. Isono. Detailed examination of polychlorinated dibenzofurans in PCB preparations and Kanemi Yusho oil. Bull. Environ. Contam. Toxicol. *18*, 67-73 (1977).
119. H. R. Buser, C. Rappe, and A. Gara. Polychlorinated dibenzofurans (PCDFs) found in Yusho oil and in used Japanese PCB. Chemosphere 5, 439-449 (1978).
120. A. Norstrom, K. Andersson, and C. Rappe. Formation of chlorodibenzofurans by irradiation of chlorinated diphenyl ethers. Chemosphere *1*, 21-24 (1976).
121. D. G. Crosby and K. W. Moilanen. Photodecomposition of chlorinated biphenyls and dibenzofurans. Bull Environ. Contam. Toxicol. *10*, 372-377 (1973).
122. O. Hutzinger, S. Safe, P. R. Wentzell, and V. Zitko. Photochemical degradation of di- and octachlorodibenzofuran. Environ. Health Perspect. 5, 267-271 (1973).

123. J. G. Vos and J. H. Koeman. Comparative toxicology study with polychlorinated biphenyls in chickens with special reference to porphyria, edema formation, liver necrosis and tissue residues. Toxicol. Appl. Pharmacol. *17*, 656-668 (1970).
124. A. Poland, E. Glover, and A. S. Kende. Sterospecific high affinity binding of 2,3,7,8-tetrachlorodibenzo-p-dioxin by hepatic cytosol. J. Biol. Chem. *251*, 4936-4946 (1976).
125. A. Poland and E. Glover. Studies on the mechanism of toxicity of the chlorinated dibenzo-p-dioxins. Environ. Health Perspect. *5*, 245-251 (1973).
126. J. A. Bradlow, D. Sims, and D. Firestone. Cell culture-enzyme induction bioassay for detection of toxic dibenzo-p-dioxin components in fish and animal products. Presented at the 90th Annual Meeting of Association of Official Analytical Chemists, Washington, D.C., Oct. 18-21, 1976.
127. K. Chae, L. Cho, and J. D. McKinney. Synthesis of 1-amino-3,7,8-trichlorodibenzo-p-dioxin and 1-amino-2,3,7,8-tetrachlorodibenzo-p-dioxin as haptenic compounds. J. Agric. Food Chem. *25*, 1207-1209 (1977).
128. A. E. Pohland, G. D. Yang, and N. Brown. Analytical and confirmative techniques for dibenzo-p-dioxins based on their cation radicals. Environ. Health Perspect. *5*, 9-14 (1973).
129. D. Firestone. Personal communication, cited in Ref. 63.
130. H. G. Langer, T. P. Brady, L. A. Dalton, T. W. Shannon, and P. R. Briggs. Thermal chemistry of chlorinated phenols. Paper presented at the 162nd Meeting of American Chemical Society, Washington, D.C., 1971, Abstr. Pest. Sect. No. 83.
131. C. Botre, A. Memoli, and F. Alhaique. TCDD solubilization and photodecomposition in aqueous solutions. Environ. Sci. Technol. *12*, 335-336 (1978).

Index